PERCEPTION

PERCEPTION

THIRD EDITION

Robert Sekuler

BRANDEIS UNIVERSITY

Randolph Blake

VANDERBILT UNIVERSITY

McGRAW-HILL, INC.

New York   St. Louis   San Francisco   Auckland   Bogotá   Caracas
Lisbon   London   Madrid   Mexico City   Milan   Montreal   New Delhi
San Juan   Singapore   Sydney   Tokyo   Toronto

PERCEPTION, 3rd edition
International Editions 1994

Exclusive rights by McGraw-Hill Book Co. - Singapore for manufacture and export. This book cannot be re-exported from the country to which it is consigned by McGraw-Hill.

Credits and Acknowledgments appear on pages 555-556, and on this page by reference.

    7 8 9 0 **SLP FC** 2 0 9

This book was set in Bembo by Ruttle, Shaw & Wetherill, Inc.
The editors were Jane Vaicunas and Jean Akers;
the production supervisor was Leroy A. Young.
The cover was designed by Circa '86.
The photo editor was Kathy Bendo.

Library of Congress Cataloging-in-Publication Data

Sekuler, Robert.
    Perception / Robert Sekuler, Randolph Blake. - 3rd ed.
        p.   cm.
    Includes bibliographical references and index.
    ISBN 0-07-056085-4 (alk. paper)
    1. Perception.   I. Blake, Randolph.   II. Title.
BF311.S434   1994
152.1-dc20   93-1128

When ordering this title, use ISBN 0-07-113683-5

Printed in Singapore

ROBERT SEKULER is the Louis and Frances Salvage Professor of Psychology at Brandeis University and Research Professor of Biomedical Engineering at Boston University. At Brandeis, where he served as the university's chief academic officer, he is also a member of its National Center for Complex Systems. Sekuler earned his Ph.D. at Brown University in 1964 and then held a postdoctoral fellowship at the Massachusetts Institute of Technology. Subsequently, he was on the faculty at Northwestern University for twenty-four years, where he was John Evans Professor of Neuroscience, and had the rank of professor in the departments of psychology, ophthalmology, and neurobiology. He chaired Northwestern's department of psychology and served as Associate Dean in the College of Arts and Sciences. A leader in the fields of motion perception and perceptual changes in aging, Sekuler has published more than 130 scientific papers and has contributed chapters to various books including *The Handbook of Perception, The Handbook of Sensory Physiology,* and the *Oxford Textbook of Geriatric Medicine.* A former Chair of the Committee on Vision of the National Academy of Sciences, Sekuler directed the Academy's studies of "Aging Workers and Visual Impairment" and its study of "Vision and Aging" and co-edited the book *Aging and visual function.* Sekuler has served on the board of the Hugh Knowles Center on Hearing and its Preservation and on the Sensory Physiology Advisory Panel of the National Science Foundation. He is a fellow of the American Psychological Society, the Optical Society of America, and the American Association for the Advancement of Science; he is a member of the Society for Neuroscience, the International Neural Network Society, the Psychonomic Society, the Association for Research in Vision and Ophthalmology, and the Bessie Buxton Branch of the American Begonia Society.

RANDOLPH BLAKE is currently professor and chairman of the Department of Psychology at Vanderbilt University, Nashville, Tennessee. Prior to this appointment he was on the faculty of Northwestern University for fourteen years. He received his Ph.D. from Vanderbilt in 1972 and then spent two years as a postdoctoral fellow in the Sensory Sciences Center at the University of Texas Graduate School of Biomedical Sciences. Blake has published extensively in major psychology and neuroscience journals and has contributed chapters to edited books including *Models of the Visual Cortex, Frontiers of Visual Science,* and *Development of Perception.* His research, supported by grants from the National Science Foundation and the National Institutes of Health, focuses on visual perception with particular emphasis on binocular vision, motion perception and the neural bases of pattern perception. In recognition of his research contributions, Blake received a Career Development Award from the National Institutes of Health and the American Psychological Association's Early Career Award for Distinguished Scientific Contribution. In 1987 Blake was elected as a Fellow of the American Association for the Advancement of Science and in 1991 a Fellow of the American Psychological Society. He is a past member of the Committee on Vision of the National Academy of Sciences/National Research Council and the Sensory Sciences Advisory Panel of the National Science Foundation. During 1992 he was a Fellow of the Japan Society for the Promotion of Science; during that time he delivered talks on his work at major universities throughout Japan. His hobbies include bicycling, music, and collecting textiles.

CONTENTS

Human beings have always wondered about how they perceived the world in which they lived. In modern times, this age-old wonder has inspired behavioral and biological scientists to take up a systematic study of perception. Building on the cumulative efforts of all these people, this book explains seeing, hearing, touching, smelling, and tasting to students of perception.

ORGANIZATION AND COVERAGE. The introductory chapter summarizes the motivations that inspire people to study perception as well as the various approaches that such study can take. It also outlines the framework on which the entire text is constructed. Chapters 2 through 7 discuss seeing—the biological bases of vision and the perception of pattern, color, and depth. The treatment of seeing concludes in Chapter 8 with an essay on the perception of visual events. The most detailed chapters in the book are Chapters 9 and 10 on hearing, Chapter 11 on touch, and Chapter 12 on smelling and tasting. Chapter 13 concludes the text with a consideration of the important interactions between knowledge and perception.

SPECIAL FEATURES. Our book has several noteworthy features. Central topics are presented in historical context, underscoring that the contemporary study of perception is part of an unfolding intellectual process. At the same time, our source materials are strongly biased toward items only recently published. Because we want students to appreciate developments at the frontiers of perception, we give thorough coverage to "hot," rapidly developing topics. For example, one chapter provides a comprehensive treatment of recent discoveries concerning visual agnosias; another highlights the amazing plasticity of sensory systems; and a third chapter details the latest thinking on signal transduction in hearing. This special stress on the most recent work demonstrates that perception is a living and growing field.

The extensive program of more than 300 illustrations, nearly all either new or redrawn for this edition, is another of this book's most important features. Our combined forty years of teaching have taught us that students don't always see in a diagram exactly what was intended. In fact the ability to "read" a graphic is a skill that, like any other skill, requires practice. So instead of merely directing student readers to look at the figure, we have crafted and coordinated the text, figures, and figure captions to ensure proper interpretation of the illustrative material. In addition, we have given extra care to the graphic presentation of complex ideas. Such ideas are often conveyed in this book by a short series of illustrations, with each illustration in a series introducing additional concepts. This approach enables every reader to get the point—even those who are novices at interpreting graphs and diagrams. Finally, illustrations that depict previously published experimental results have been adapted and redrawn to maximize clarity and consistency of presentation.

VOCABULARY AND METHODS OF PERCEPTUAL RESEARCH (GLOSSARY AND APPENDIX). Because the study of perception draws on many different disciplines—physics, chemistry, anatomy, psychology, and several branches of medicine, among others—its technical vocabulary incorporates the terminology of those disciplines. Beginning students of perception are often bewildered by the flood of new terms that they must master. Recognizing this problem, we have introduced only those terms that are absolutely necessary to the discussion. Where it's likely to aid memory or understanding, we explain the term's origin. Also, each term is carefully defined when it is first used, and all these terms appear in a Glossary at the back of the book.

We have kept detailed, abstract descriptions of research methods to a minimum. Where appropriate, we explain particular methods in enough detail that the student reader can appreciate the methods and whatever constraints they impose on results and conclusions. Various methods for studying perception are discussed within the context of the specific problems that they were designed to solve. By integrating methods and results, we hope to facilitate the reader's genuine appreciation of both. An Appendix provides much additional information about conventional behavioral methods for studying perception. The Appendix also describes contemporary variants of those methods: forced-choice procedures, sensory decision theory, and adaptive psychophysical methods. The Appendix grounds these methods in their historical context, enabling the student to understand not only the methods but also the reasons for their development.

LINKS TO EVERYDAY LIFE. In *Talks to Teachers* (1892), William James advised teachers how best to adapt psychology's principles to the classroom. In one chapter, James urged teachers to recognize and exploit the natural interests that students bring to any topic. He suggested that abstract facts and new ideas are most readily assimilated when they have been linked to matters that students find inherently interesting, particularly matters that relate to their own lives. In our own classrooms and while writing this book we have kept James's good advice in mind. Perception is not just an abstract, scientific discipline, but an integral and fascinating part of everyday life. Recognizing this fact, our book consistently relates scientific research on perception to the reader's own perceptual experiences. To underscore the relationship between science and everyday experience, we present many simple, interesting demonstrations that readers can perform on their own with little or no equipment. Also, in order to anchor the discussion in the reader's own experience, the text emphasizes the everyday behavioral needs that seeing, hearing, smelling, tasting, and touching are designed to satisfy—the functions of perception. This functional approach to perception is highlighted by the many discussions, throughout the text, of clinical disorders and their intriguing perceptual consequences. Some students will be interested in learning about these disorders for personal reasons; all students should find that the study of perceptual disorders provides insight into the nature of normal perception.

INTEGRATION. William James advised also that teachers take care to connect new ideas and facts with what students have already learned. "Associate the new with the old in some natural and telling way, so that the interest, being shed along from point to point, finally suffuses the entire system of objects of thought." In his own textbook, *The Principles of Psychology,* James followed this counsel, to great success. Our textbook, too, tries to follow James's advice. We have attempted to make our treatment of perception an integrated one, in part by linking ideas across chapters. These linkages reflect the fact that different areas in perception often utilize similar techniques and related theoretical ideas. Our text is integrated in another way, blending anatomy, physiology, and psychophysics. The information and ideas from each of these three approaches have been carefully selected to ensure a coherent, complete presentation. Structure and function become more comprehensible and memorable when they are integrated. We would like to think that James would approve.

KEY CHANGES FOR THIS EDITION. Instructors who have used an earlier edition of this book will be pleased that the new edition adheres to the same general thematic approach and organization. There are, however, a number of notable changes that provide a fresher, more lively portrayal of the field of perception. You will find, for example, that no fewer than four different chapters communicate important findings from studies that exploit the rapidly evolving techniques of brain imaging.

In Chapter 1 the main change is a new discussion of computational approaches to various areas of perception. Our aim in reworking Chapter 1 was to establish the principle that, whatever their diversity, all areas of perception draw on shared principles and face common challenges. In this spirit, some of the philosophical material in Chapter 1 has been revised in order to give a stronger and clearer treatment of these important foundational issues. Chapters 2 and 3 contain important new references and figures. In its expanded treatment of multiple visual representations, or maps, within the brain, Chapter 4 gives new emphasis to the advantages and difficulties created by distributed representations. Chapter 5 now includes an expanded treatment of ideas derived from the Gestalt movement. Chapter 6, on color vision, is enhanced by new ideas on the genetics and evolution of color vision. Chapter 7 goes into more detail on some of the so-called monocular depth cues, particularly those cues that are of great interest to researchers probing machine vision. This chapter also now includes discussion of the perception of visual direction. The chapter on motion perception, Chapter 8, now includes coverage of the latest work on the cortical regions that play special roles in the analysis of global motion. The treatment of eye movements has been sharpened, and discussions of reafference and of structure from motion added. Chapter 9, the first of two chapters on hearing, boasts a strengthened treatment of masking and critical bands and coverage of new discoveries on the biophysics of signal transduction in the cochlea. Chapter 10 takes new notice of an important idea in recent research into hearing: the idea of auditory organization. In particular, we have strengthened the discussion of how the auditory system picks out, from the entire acoustic environment, those acoustic features that arise from a single event; additional material on speech perception now appears in this chapter. The chapter on taste and smell integrates new findings on the basis of olfactory transduction and the behavioral conse-

quences of taste disorders. New material on brain processes in smell and taste are added. The chapter on touch perception, which made its debut in the second edition, attracted much favorable comment from readers. For the current edition, we expanded this chapter by adding important new material on haptics, the coordinated interaction between touch and active exploration of the near-environment. Also, the treatment of plasticity in the somatosensory system has been expanded. Chapter 13, which focuses on knowledge and perception, has been broadened and reorganized around a new taxonomy of the four main modes of interaction between knowledge and perception. The treatment of several topics, including imagery, memory, perceptual agnosias, and unconscious perception, has been expanded to reflect significant new findings. The Appendix, on behavioral methods, now notes the utility of theoretical, "ideal" observers that can provide benchmarks for real, human performance. The special-topics boxes are considerably reduced in number, with some of their material now integrated into the text itself.

We have mentioned just some of the additions and revisions in this third edition. Users of earlier editions will also notice the book's attractive new layout and the fact that virtually every drawing has been redone for this edition. Scrutiny of the reference list reveals that close to 250 references are new to this edition, with most of these new references representing contributions that were published in the last three years.

ROBERT SEKULER
RANDOLPH BLAKE

ACKNOWLEDGMENTS

In preparing various editions of the book, we benefitted greatly from a great many people's comments and suggestions. Special credit, though, should be given to those individuals who reviewed various chapters and sections. These include:

Martin S. Banks, University of California at Berkeley
William P. Banks, Pomona College
Linda M. Bartoshuk, Pierce Foundation, Yale University
Patrick J. Bennett, University of Toronto
Ira H. Bernstein, University of Texas at Arlington
Irving Biederman, University of Southern California
Richard Bowen, Loyola University of Chicago
Edward Carterette, College of William and Mary
Carol Christensen, Vassar College
James E. Cutting, Cornell University
Peter Dallos, Northwestern University
David S. Emmerich, State University of New York, Stony Brook
Trygg Engen, Brown University
Lewis O. Harvey, Jr., University of Colorado at Boulder
Mary Hayhoe, University of Rochester
Morton Heller, Winston-Salem State University
Leo Hurvich, University of Pennsylvania
Jon H. Kaas, Vanderbilt University
Eileen Kowler, Rutgers University
Susan J. Lederman, Queen's University
Herschel W. Leibowitz, Pennsylvania State University
Robert M. Levy, Indiana State University
Jack Loomis, University of California at Santa Barbara
Dennis McFadden, University of Texas at Austin
Walter Makous, University of Rochester

Michael Merzenich, University of California at San Francisco
Ennio Mingolla, Boston University
John Mollon, Oxford University
Kenneth Nakayama, Harvard University
William Newsome, Stanford University
Matthew Olson, Hamline University
Robert O'Shea, Otago University
Robert Pachella, University of Michigan
Robert Patterson, Washington State University
Nancy Perrin, Portland State University
Steve Poltrok, University of Denver
James R. Pomerantz, Rice University
Tim Pons, National Institutes of Health
Keith Rayner, University of Massachusetts at Amherst
Allison Sekuler, University of Toronto
Justine Sergent, Montreal Neurological Institute
Margaret Shiffrar, Rutgers University
James Todd, The Ohio State University
Joseph Verillo, Syracuse University
Benjamin Wallace, Cleveland State University
Brian Wandell, Stanford University
William H. Warren, Jr., Brown University
Gerald S. Wasserman, Purdue University
Scott N. J. Watamaniuk, Smith-Kettlewell Institute
John S. Werner, University of Colorado
David H. Westendorf, University of Arkansas
Frances Wilkinson, McGill University
David R. Williams, University of Rochester
William A. Yost, Loyola University of Chicago
James L. Zacks, Michigan State University

While we were writing the first two editions of this book we were fortunate to occupy adjoining offices and laboratories. Our physical proximity made it easy for us to share materials, ideas, comments, and suggestions. It also enabled us to do much of the writing while we both sat at one personal computer that had been outfitted with twin keyboards. Because we now find ourselves separated by about 1,000 miles (1,600 km), for the third edition we had to find other means to support our close, highly interactive collaboration. One solution was a series of intense home-and-home visits—Blake to Concord, Massachusetts, and Sekuler to Nashville, Tennessee. For our more usual interaction, though, we depended on the Internet, that wonderful electronic network spanning the United States and the world. Almost daily, our Macintosh computers and their modems sent ideas, draft text, diagrams and illustrations back and forth. The Internet helped us, also, to send ideas and draft sections to colleagues around the world, for their input and suggestions. Finally, we adopted common word-processing software that suited our style of joint authorship; this software made it easy to highlight proposed changes, deletions, and additions.

Our electronic closeness allows both of us to take full responsibility for every word in the book. Of course, files, comments and drawings shared over an electronic network are not the same thing as sitting side by side, but they proved to be an acceptable substitute. Both of us have strong feelings and fond memories of weekend sessions when we carried on prolonged, high-speed elec-

tronic dialogues over some matter or other. For two months toward the end of the project, the Internet kept us in touch despite the fact that Blake was working in Japan and despite our separation by fourteen time zones. Researchers are adapting computer technology in order to create what is known as virtual reality, computer-mediated experiences that substitute for—and sometimes improve on—the real thing. In this spirit, we were delighted that the speed and ease of our largely electronic collaboration made us into what we can call virtual colleagues.

Thanks are owed to our students and colleagues, and a special note of gratitude to our wives, Susan and Elaine, and our children, Stacia, Allison, Erica, and Geoff for their tolerance and good humor during our preoccupation with this project. Finally, we thank the excellent editorial and production staff at McGraw-Hill, in particular Jane Vaicunas, psychology editor; Beth Kaufman, assistant editor; and Jean Akers, senior editing supervisor. Finally we are pleased to acknowledge the contribution of Alice Jaggard for a careful and thoughtful job of copy editing.

ROBERT SEKULER
RANDOLPH BLAKE

PERCEPTION

Introduction to Perception

The world is filled with objects and events that combine to create a kaleidoscope of potential information. Though much of that information is irrelevant for people's daily needs, some of it is absolutely essential. So that they can use this information effectively, human beings are equipped with specialized machinery for capturing this information and for translating it into the language of the nervous system. In translated form, the selected information is digested by the brain, culminating in an awareness of the objects and events in the environment. The awareness then guides people's actions in the world around them.

As we've just described it, **perception** entails a sequence of interrelated events. To understand perception completely requires knowing all the components of that sequence and the ways the components interact. To begin, we must specify the nature of the environment in which we live, for this environment determines what there is to perceive. Aspects of the environment are specified using terms derived from physics, because stimulation comes in various forms of physical energy: thermal, mechanical, acoustic, and electromagnetic. The physical energy that initiates the chain of events is called a **stimulus** (plural, "stimuli").

Next, it is necessary to understand how the nervous system converts the patterns of physical energy into neural events. Known as **sensory transduction,** this conversion process requires an understanding of the specialized sensory receptors such as those contained in the eye and the ear. Once this transduction has been achieved, objects and events are represented solely as patterns of neural impulses within the various sensory nerve fibers. From this point on, all further elaboration and editing of the sensory information must be performed using this neural representation.

A complete understanding of perception must include a thorough description of the appearances of objects and events: we have to be able to describe systematically the sights, sounds, smells, and tastes that populate our conscious experiences. In addition to describing how things appear to us, we must also specify how our abilities to detect, discriminate, and recognize objects are governed by the information available to our senses. And, in a similar vein, we must understand the behavioral consequences of sensory stimulation. Together, these represent formidable challenges. Not surprisingly, diverse techniques have been developed for systematically cataloging the performance of our perceptual systems and relating that information to patterns of physical stimulation. The enterprise of relating physical stimulation to perceptual events is known as **psychophysics.** By specifying the relation between physical and perceptual events, psychophysics provides important clues to unraveling the intervening events.

According to the view spelled out above, perception consists of a sequence, stretching from events in the physical world external to the perceiver, through the translation of those events into patterns of activity within the perceiver's nervous system, culminating in the perceiver's experiential and behavioral reactions to those events. This sequence is schematized in Figure 1.1. Let's now

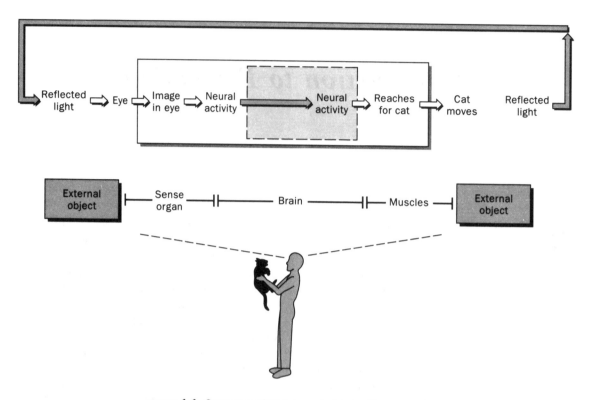

FIGURE 1.1 Sequence of major events involved in perception.

consider several important implications of this way of thinking about perception.

PERCEPTION IS A BIOLOGICAL PROCESS

In this book, we approach perception as a *biological* process. For events in the world to be perceived, any information about those events must be registered by the sensory nervous system. The noted neuroscientist Vernon Mountcastle has described this constraint very vividly:

Each of us lives within . . . the prison of his own brain. Projecting from it are millions of fragile sensory nerve fibers, in groups uniquely adapted to sample the energetic states of the world around us: heat, light, force, and chemical composition. That is all we ever know of it directly; all else is logical inference. (1975, p. 131)

Mountcastle is pointing out that sensory nerve fibers are the only link to the external world; they alone provide the communication channels to reality. If environmental events fall outside the range of sensitivity of the sensory channels, those events will not be experienced directly. It may be possible to detect some of these events indirectly, however, using specialized instruments. Such instruments work in one of two ways. Some amplify physical energy, making weak signals strong enough to stimulate the senses. For example, a microscope can magnify objects otherwise too small to be seen by the naked eye. Other instruments convert energy that is *outside* the normal bounds of the senses into a form that is within those bounds. For instance, Geiger counters can warn about the presence of radioactivity, a form of energy that cannot be sensed directly. In either case, though, such instruments are being used to extend the reach of the sensory system.

It may be difficult to accept that your rich perceptual world encompasses only a small, restricted portion of the entire universe. Because one's conception of reality is so intimately determined by subjective experience, it seems unnatural to distinguish between one's "perception of the world" and the "world itself." Yet to understand perception fully, you have to make this distinction. Perhaps a few examples will enable you to appreciate what we mean by the limited scope of your perceptual world.

Consider, for instance, how various species of animals probably experience the world. It is well documented that not all animals have the same sensory systems. Consequently, various species have access to different universes of physical events. Dogs can hear sounds in regions of the frequency spectrum where humans are deaf; bees are able to navigate using a quality of light, polarization, that is outside the realm of human visual experience. And there are chemical substances that evoke no experience of odor for humans and yet elicit strong olfactory responses in certain animals. In general, there is no single "environment" that all animals live in. Members of different species interact with their physical and biological worlds in ways that reflect their own unique requirements and capabilities. As Box 1.1 shows, although all animals inhabit the same *physical* world, their *perceptual* worlds may differ radically.

In fact, not all humans have equivalent sensory systems. For instance, some people have defects of the eye that prevent them from experiencing the full range of colors that other people see. There are also certain people who cannot taste one of the bitter substances in coffee because of an abnormality in their taste system. These and similar examples that we shall bring up throughout this book underscore the dependence of perception on the sensory nervous system.

Recognition of perception as a biological process underscores another important point: perception is a symbolic activity (Frisby, 1980). A "symbol" is something that stands for something other than itself. Your name is a symbol for you; you are much more than just your name, but in many circumstances your name represents you. A road map is also a symbol, representing the highways and terrain over which you may wish to travel. Running your finger along some highway on a map is much different from traveling the actual road, but one symbolizes the other.

Each of your percepts is associated with some characteristic activity in your brain (hence we say that perceptual states are produced by brain states). This fact gives perception the status of a symbolic process. Suppose you listen to some sound. Your experience, the percept, is certainly not the same as the sound itself; however, the percept does represent that sound. In this case, the symbols are not the sort that we usually think of—a screech of brakes, the trill of a cardinal, the crescendo of an orchestra. Instead, the symbols are the various brain states that stand for these sounds. Just like those of other kinds of symbols, however, the properties of these symbols are not the same as the properties of the things being symbolized: in your brain, the representation of a loud explosion is neither loud nor explosive.

Evidently, the brain has a constant need for input from the external world. When that input is reduced or eliminated, the sensory systems lapse into a kind of disorderly conduct that yields hallucinations, sometimes quite bizarre. Input to the brain can be shut off by placing a person in an environment that drastically reduces all sensory stimulation (Bexton, Heron, and Scott, 1954; Siegel, 1984) or as a result of diminished function in a particular sensory channel. For example, in about 10 to 15 percent of people with eye disease, impaired vision evokes realistic and complex visual hallucinations (Schultz and Melzack, 1991). Similarly, following amputation of a body part, many people experience "phantom limbs," compelling and very painful hallucinations that the missing body part is still present (Melzack, 1992). Both the visual hallucinations and the phantom limbs are generated by activity within the brain.

Normal perception seems to occur immediately and without much effort. Nonetheless, we should not lose sight of the fact that even the simplest perceptual experiences result from a complex series of neural events involving exten-

Box 1.1 *Seeing the Invisible*

It's hard even to imagine what it must be like to sense forms of energy that humans ordinarily cannot sense (Nagel, 1982). But one can get an inkling of this experience. Normally, humans cannot see electromagnetic radiation in the portion of the spectrum called infrared. This form of radiation is usually associated with heat, including the body heat of living creatures. If infrared is sensed at all, it is experienced as warmth on the skin. Although some animals, notably certain snakes, have specialized sense organs that allow them to detect and respond to objects on the basis of the infrared energy radiated by those objects, humans are fairly insensitive to infrared.

To give you some idea of what it might be like to see infrared radiation, we have prepared the two accompanying photographs. The photograph on the left shows a scene taken with ordinary black and white film; this film is about as *in*sensitive to infrared as the human eye is. That is why pictures taken with such film look "normal." The photograph on the right shows the same scene taken with film that is sensitive to infrared; it reveals things (areas of heat and cold) in the scene that humans ordinarily would not see. Thus, for instance, the water in the right-hand photo appears dark because it is cold.

Although the differences between these pictures are interesting, we can't really claim that the photographs provide much insight into the experiences of those infrared-sensitive snakes. In some cases, their infrared-sensitive organs are not even part of their eyes, so they probably wouldn't be *seeing* the infrared. The photographs do remind us, though, that the human perceptual world is not the only one possible.

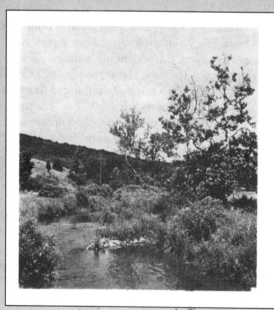
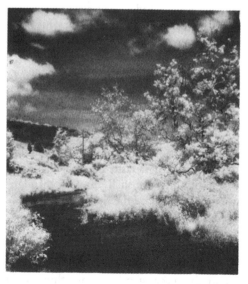

sive interactions among numerous brain cells. These interactions, which bear a formal resemblance to the interactions in an electronic circuit, can be thought of as computations. The computations that shape the symbolic representations in the brain work on environmental information picked up by the eyes, ears, and other sensory organs. Using this information, the brain computes the properties of objects and events (such as their size or their distance from the point of observation).

The philosophy that guides contemporary work in perception is termed **materialism**—it asserts that perceptual experience depends on the operation of the nervous system, with no requirement for the involvement of some noncorporeal force. The materialistic viewpoint has been well expressed by the late Roger Sperry, the Nobel Prize-winning brain scientist from the California Institute of Technology. According to Sperry, perceptual experience is a "functional property of brain processing, constituted of neuronal and physicochemical activity, and embodied in, and inseparable from the active brain" (1980, p. 204).

Although materialism holds that perception is based on neural events in the brain, it does not imply that one could dissect a brain and thereby locate those experiences. Again, Sperry put it quite well:

Once generated from neural events, the higher order mental patterns and programs have their own subjective qualities and progress, operate and interact by their own causal laws and principles which are different from and cannot be reduced to those of neurophysiology. (1980, p. 201)

To illustrate further what he had in mind, Sperry offered the example of a wheel rolling downhill. The wheel

carries its atoms and molecules through a course in time and space and to a fate determined by the overall system properties of the wheel as a whole and regardless of the inclination of individual atoms and molecules. The atoms and molecules are caught up and overpowered by the higher properties of the whole. One can compare the rolling wheel to an ongoing brain process or a progressing train of thought in which the overall organizational properties of the brain process, as a coherent organizational entity, determine the timing and spacing of the firing patterns within its neuronal infrastructure. (1980, p. 201)

In other words, though one's experiences have a physical basis, they cannot be entirely reduced to a set of physical components; equally important are the spatial organization of those components, how they interact with one another, and how both spatial organization and communication change with time. If another analogy would help, consider what would happen if you took a television set completely apart and examined all its components in an effort to understand how it worked. The proper function of the television set demands a particular spatial arrangement of parts as well as a certain sequence of signals in time. The "secret" of the set's operation would have completely eluded you and could not be found in the pile of parts left after the set had been dismantled. And certainly from the parts alone, it would be impossible to deduce the function of a television set.

Not everybody agrees with the materialistic perspective. Some prominent scientists, including John Eccles (1979), another Nobel Prize winner, subscribe to an alternative view. This alternative, **dualism,** is often associated with the seventeenth-century French philosopher René Descartes. Dualism holds that perceiving (like any other "mental" function) is not solely a phenomenon of the physical brain. Instead, it also entails some special, nonphysical substance—the mind or the soul—that interacts with the brain. Many people find dualism persuasive because they are puzzled over how perception, a personal, subjective experience, can be caused by brain processes, which are certainly not experiences. They object to materialism's basic claim: a quantity of one sort—neural activity—can cause a quantity of so different a sort—perception.

According to John Searle, though, no logical barrier prevents cause-and-effect relationships between entities of radically different sorts. In fact, denying that such relationships are possible betrays a misunderstanding of cause and effect itself (1987, p. 223). To drive his point home, Searle draws on the discipline of physics. Physicists commonly distinguish between large-scale macro phenomena and smaller-scale micro elements, postulating causal relationships between the two, even though macro and micro entities are quite different from one another. Take some examples offered by Searle. Heat and lightning are macro-level phenomena; molecular movements and electrical discharges are elements on the micro level. Physics teaches us that a macro phenomenon can be *caused* by the behavior of micro elements: we say that heat is caused by molecule movements or that lightning is caused by electrical discharge. Moreover, either macro phenomenon can be equated to the behavior of its micro elements. Therefore, we can say that heat is the mean kinetic energy of molecule movements or that lightning is an electrical discharge.

Paul Churchland (1986) has elaborated the main arguments against dualism. Here we'll mention two of them. Against the claim that perception is independent of what happens in the brain, Churchland cites numerous instances where the condition of the brain dramatically alters perception; throughout the following chapters, we give many examples of perception disordered by brain damage. Against the claim that perception is far too complicated to be the product of things as simple as nerve cells, research on neural networks shows that one can create extraordinarily complex, sophisticated systems out of very simple components, undercutting the need to postulate other, more intelligent agents (Nadel, Culicover, Cooper, and Harnish, 1989; Bechtel and Abrahamsen, 1991). As a result, one can account for complex, intelligent aspects of perception without recourse to elements that are themselves complex or intelligent.

John Searle elegantly expressed the view adopted by most investigators in the field of perception:

Mental phenomena, whether conscious or unconscious, whether visual or auditory, pains, tickles, itches, thoughts, and all the rest of our mental life, are caused by processes going on in the brain. Mental phenomena are as much a result of electrochemical processes in the brain as digestion is the result of chemical processes going on in the stomach and the rest of the digestive tract. (1987, p. 220)

As you will learn, perception is a major area of advance in understanding the relation between brain and mind; adoption of the materialist position has facilitated those advances greatly.

PERCEPTION INVOLVES ACTION

Perceiving usually requires some action on the part of the perceiver. Often, one must look in order to see, searching the visual environment until the desired object of regard is located. Likewise, to make a faint sound audible, one must sometimes turn an ear in its direction. When one touches an object, it is more easily identified if explored with the fingers. All these examples are a reminder that perception is an *active* process, an idea especially championed by James J. Gibson (1966). This active process works to guide behavior, thereby stimulating even more activity. Once an object has been perceived, one decides whether to approach or avoid it. Hearing a noise, one might reply vocally or one might find it wiser to remain very quiet. Having identified an object by touch, one may discard it or try to keep it. In each case behavior depends on *what* is perceived.

Perception's action orientation raises an interesting distinction among the various senses that has to do with the proximity of the perceiver to the object of perception. Touch and taste require direct contact between the perceiver and the source of stimulation. Because of this restriction, taste and touch can be considered **near senses.** The sense of smell is also effectively a near sense. Volatile chemicals from an odorous substance are diluted with distance, so smell works more effectively for substances in the general vicinity of the nose. Seeing and hearing, in contrast, can be thought of as **far senses,** or **distance senses.** The eyes and ears can pick up information originating from remote sources; in this respect, they function like a ship's radar. They allow one to make perceptual contact with objects located too far away for immediate grasp; they extend one perceptually out into the world beyond the fingertips and nose. These two senses serve as able substitutes for actual locomotor exploration of the environment, enabling one to explore the surroundings vicariously. They provide advance warning of approaching danger, and they guide the search for friends and desired objects. In general, hearing and seeing open up to you the large world that lies outside your reach. Imagine how vulnerable you would feel if you were denied access to all information picked up by your far senses; your whole world would shrink to the area within arm's reach. You would be able to sense objects only when you touched them or when they touched you. It is not surprising, therefore, that blindness and deafness, loss of the far senses, are considered so devastating.

Incidentally, this distinction between the near and far senses has an important behavioral consequence. Any crucial reaction called for by taste or touch must be executed swiftly. There is no time to decide whether a bitter substance is toxic—you spit it out reflexively. Nor do you first try to judge what is causing a burning sensation before you remove your hand from a hot object. In these cases, you act first and then consciously think about what it was that triggered your reflex action. However, in the case of the far senses—seeing and hearing—one is usually dealing with objects located some distance away. This distance permits the luxury of evaluating the potential consequences of one's actions.

WHY STUDY PERCEPTION?

Over the years, people have studied perception for a variety of reasons. Some of these reasons, as you will see, stem from practical considerations, such as the need to solve a particular problem. Other reasons do not reflect practical concerns but instead arise simply from intellectual curiosity about ourselves and the world we live in.

PRACTICAL REASONS FOR STUDYING PERCEPTION

The human senses evolved in an environment that was different in many ways from the one we live in now. Many of the challenges confronting the human senses today didn't exist in the more primitive environments for which these senses were designed. It's very important to know just what kind of perceptual demands can reasonably be placed on the human senses without compromising safety and sanity (Russell and Ward, 1982). As already mentioned, there is an optimum range of sensory stimulation within which the majority of people work and play most effectively. Intense stimulation—such as excessive noise, glaring light, and harsh smells—can impair immediate performance as well as damage the sensory nervous system. Through the study of perception, one can identify and correct potentially hazardous environmental conditions that threaten the senses and impair the ability to make decisions.

In a related vein, studying perception enables one to design devices that ensure optimal perceptual performance. Just think how often each day you come in contact with devices designed to communicate some message to you. Traffic lights, alarm clocks, telephones, and video displays are just a few of the myriad inventions that people rely on during work, play, study, even sleep. To be effective, these devices should be tailored to human sensory systems. It would be unwise, for example, to use a high-pitched tone as a fire alarm in a hotel, because elderly people have difficulty hearing such tones. Similarly, a traffic sign with blue lettering on a green background would be inefficient, since blue and green are more difficult to distinguish than other pairs of colors. In general, one wants the signs and signals in the environment to be easy to see and hear, which requires an understanding of human perceptual capacities and limitations.

Studying perception also makes it possible to design aids for individuals with impaired sensory function. Take hearing aids as an example. Most hearing aids amplify not only the sounds that the user wants to hear—such as a person's voice—but also other, unwanted sounds—such as traffic noises. Recognizing this problem, Richard L. Gregory developed a procedure that selectively amplifies just speech sounds (Gregory and Drysdale, 1976). This invention, which is now in wide use, grew out of earlier work on the ear's ability to respond selectively to particular sounds. Just over the horizon are even more sophisticated hearing aids that directly stimulate the auditory nerve, using implants driven by small microchip speech processors (Wilson et al., 1991). Designing aids for sensory-impaired people requires a solid understanding of the mechanisms of normal perception.

Let us turn to another practical reason. People in consumer marketing are very interested in human perception. For instance, companies in the food and beverage industry carefully test the perceptual appeal—the taste, smell, and appearance—of their products before marketing them. Advertising, too, capitalizes on perception research to package and market products in ways that will bring those products to the attention of consumers. There are even claims that subliminal sensory messages—pictures or words presented too briefly or too faintly to be consciously seen or heard—can improve one's memory or enhance self-esteem, although these claims are questionable (Greenwald, Spangenberg, Pratkanis, and Eskenazi, 1991).

So far, our practical reasons have focused on human perception. But as the following examples show, there are solid reasons for studying animal perception too. For one thing, animals can be trained to perform jobs that are beyond the sensory limits of humans. Dogs, because of their keen sense of smell, are adept at detecting odors that are too faint for the human nose. This is why dogs are frequently employed to sniff out illegal drugs or to trace the path of a suspect. In other instances, knowledge of an animal's sensory apparatus allows one to control that animal's behavior. For instance, agriculture scientists are now controlling cotton bollworms—moth larvae that damage crops—by spraying crop fields with a chemical that fools adult males into mating with moths of a different species. The chemical works by overwhelming the smell cues that normally guide the moths. As a result, the moths engage in promiscuous and ineffective mating behavior. As a final example, scientists study animals whose sensory capacity is impaired as a consequence either of congenital disorders or of some experimental manipulation such as sensory deprivation (Blake, 1978). These studies, in turn, are leading to new ideas concerning the bases and treatment of comparable sensory disorders in humans.

PERCEPTION AND PLEASURE

Probably in more primitive life styles (such as those of our primate ancestors) the lion's share of perceptual processing was devoted to survival—being on the alert to distinguish friends from foes and trying to locate the next meal. As civilization developed, these pressing demands have relaxed. As a result, civilized people enjoy the freedom to develop pastimes—the visual arts, music, cuisine—that engage their perceptual machinery in more amusing and creative ways. All these pastimes involve stimulation of the senses. Besides their immediate aesthetic and sensual qualities, these kinds of sensory experiences play an important role in the cultural heritage of societies. Through various forms of art, people are able to share the joys and pains experienced by others and to savor vicariously the thrill of discovery that originally inspired an artist. In brief, art embodies much of a culture's wisdom; relaxed demands on our perceptual machinery allow us the luxury to create and enjoy that embodment.

PERCEPTION AND INTELLECTUAL CURIOSITY

Practical and pleasurable concerns aside, learning about perception satisfies an intellectual curiosity about ourselves and the world we live in. Perception can be thought of as each individual's personal theory of reality, a kind of knowledge-gathering process that defines our view of the world. Because this perceptual outlook guides our activities, both mental and behavioral, we naturally find it fascinating to inquire about the bases of perception.

Natural curiosity leads to a variety of conjectures about perception. When looking at a newborn child, for instance, one cannot help speculating about what that infant sees and hears. Likewise, one is curious to know whether blind people really can hear sounds that escape the ears of sighted people. You may have wondered why colors seem to change depending on the time of day. As dusk approaches, greens take on a deeper richness, while yellows and reds lose some of their brilliance. And why does everyone effectively become color-blind under dim light conditions? One would like to know what sensory cues enable a displaced pet to journey hundreds of miles, eventually returning to its old home. And one grudgingly marvels at how adept mosquitoes are at locating one's bare skin in total darkness.

People are intrigued by their everyday experiences and curious about the bases of those experiences. This curiosity was long ago formalized in philosophy. For centuries, philosophers have argued about how human beings can know the external world. Their arguments reflected a concern about the validity of sense experiences. Though our concept of the world derives from the information of our senses, can those senses be relied on to tell the truth? Might we not be deceived about the world? Perhaps, as Plato suggested in Book VII of *The Republic*, we are like prisoners in a cave, cut off from the world so that we can see only a shadow of the world outside.

In fact, from earliest times, people knew that their senses were fallible. Realizing that sensory information was not totally dependable, philosophers became increasingly skeptical about anyone's ability to know the world as it really is. This skepticism reached full bloom during the late seventeenth and early eighteenth centuries. During that time, the British philosopher John Locke (1690/1924) made a crucial observation: water in a basin can feel either warm or cool to the touch, depending on where your hand has just been. If your hand has been in cold water, the basin's water would feel warm; if your hand has previously been in hot water, the water in the basin would feel cool. The apparent warmth or coolness of the water does not reside in the water itself; it is a quality that depends on the perceiver's own state. Since, to him, some perceived qualities of the external world seemed more subjective than others, Locke distinguished between primary qualities (real qualities, actually present in the object) and secondary qualities (resulting from an object's power to produce various sensations in us). Primary qualities included the bulk, number, motion, and shape of objects; Locke's secondary qualities included objects' color, sound, taste, and smell. Accordingly, we can rely on primary qualities to reflect accurately the nature of objects in the real world, but we must be cautious, or skeptical, about relying on secondary qualities in the same way.

This skepticism about the information of the senses was carried to greater extremes by David Hume in *A Treatise of Human Nature* (1739/1963). Hume rejected the distinction between primary and secondary qualities, banishing all sense experiences to the realm of the subjective and unreliable. Hume's pessimism about the possibility of ever understanding perception is represented quite well by the following comment from his *Treatise:*

As to those impressions which arise from the senses, their ultimate cause is, in my opinion, perfectly inexplicable by human reason, and it will always be impossible to decide with certainty whether they arise immediately from the object, or are produced by the creative power of the mind, or are derived from the author of our being. (Book I, Part III, Section V, p. 75)

There is good reason, though, to question this Humean skepticism (Schlagel, 1984). As knowledge of our senses has deepened, we have come to understand that lawful processes are responsible for what previously seemed to be mysterious sensory caprice. We know that holding one's hand in a basin of hot water initiates a process called adaptation, an alteration in the skin's temperature receptors. This process produces the thermal paradox that perplexed Locke. If we understand adaptation—how it grows with time, how long it lasts, and so on—Locke's paradox becomes less of a reason for skepticism. Suppose you put on some colored sunglasses. If they're strongly tinted, they'll change the way the world looks. But that's no reason to dismiss vision as inherently undependable. If you understand how the sunglasses alter the light that reaches your eye, and if you understand enough about vision itself, you should be able to explain the change in the way that the world looks. In fact, the senses are actually quite dependable—as long as you know enough about how they operate. For instance, you'd be able to take any arbitrary pair of sunglasses and predict quite accurately how the world will look through those glasses, or you'd be able to take any person's hand and a basin of water and predict exactly how warm that water will feel. Perception research, according to this view, can overcome the doubts of skepticism.

Since we are discussing attitudes about the relation between perception and reality, this is a good time to introduce a view that we'll mention from time to time in this book. This view, **naive realism,** is common among laypersons and beginning students of perception. "Naive realism is the view that what we know about the world is both unadulterated and unexpurgated with respect to even its most subtle details" (Shaw and Bransford, 1977, p. 18). In other words, the world *is* always exactly as it appears.

A simple test can determine whether someone is a naive realist; when asked, "Why does the world look to you the way it does?" the naive realist will answer, "Because it *is* that way." In other words, the properties of experience can always be completely and easily explained by the properties of the world itself. But this simple view of perception is wrong. For one thing, it cannot explain why different people experience the same environmental event differently. And this does happen, as you'll discover throughout this book. It is known that infants cannot see small objects that adults can see; it is known that young adults can hear some sounds that older adults cannot; and it is known that certain people are completely

oblivious to odors that others have no trouble smelling. Such facts challenge naive realism. We all live in the same *physical* world. If naive realism were a valid viewpoint, wouldn't our *perceptual* worlds be identical?

There's another reason for rejecting naive realism: a single, unchanging physical stimulus can change in appearance from one moment to the next. You can see examples of this in Figure 1.2. Note how the rhomboid at the left seems to fluctuate in appearance. At one moment line segment AB appears closest to you, whereas at another moment segment CD appears closest. The appearance of the figure at the right undergoes similar fluctuations. Now if perception were determined solely by the physical properties of the figures, their appearance should be stable. Such examples clearly demonstrate that one's perceptions have qualities not present in the physical attributes of the stimulus.

At the other extreme from naive realism is **subjective idealism,** the view that the physical world is entirely the product of the mind, a compelling mental fiction. This philosophical position is usually associated with the Irish philosopher George Berkeley, who capsulized the idea in the phrase "to be is to perceive." Carried to its extreme, this position leads to **solipsism,** the notion that only your mind exists and that all other worldly objects are perceptions of your mind.

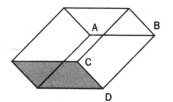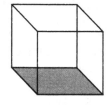

FIGURE 1.2 Transparent figures whose perspectives appear to fluctuate. The darkened surface in each figure seems sometimes to be an inner surface and sometimes an outer surface. The fluctuations of the rhomboid (left) were first noticed by L. A. Necker about 150 years ago while he was examining some crystals. Today these figures are known as Necker's rhomboid and Necker's cube.

This position can be entertaining to discuss among friends but is scientifically sterile. If there were no real world in which we exist, there would be no reason to study the relation between perceiving and that imaginary world.

Having rejected naive realism and solipsism, what do we propose about the relations between human perceptions and the real world? As we stressed earlier, we acknowledge the existence of the real world and assert that its existence does not depend on a perceiver. At the same time, we recognize the perceiver's own contribution to the process of perception. The perceiver's view of the world is necessarily inaccurate, because the perceiver's sensory system both *limits* the information that is available and *augments* the information that is available.

To show you more exactly what we mean by the perceiver's contribution, consider a familiar question: "Does a tree falling in the forest make a sound if there is no one around to hear it?" According to a solipsist, no tree, no forest, and no sound would exist in the absence of a perceiver. But according to our view, not only would the falling tree still exist even though no perceiver happened to be around, its fall would create acoustic energy in the form of air pressure waves. But would this constitute sound? If the term "sound" means a perceptual experience, then clearly the falling tree would not produce a sound. For the tree to produce a sound would require the presence of some organism with a sensory system capable of registering the available acoustic energy. But even this does not guarantee that the resulting experience would be what is normally called sound. It's conceivable that the organism that is present might not be able to hear, because it has no ears, but instead could *feel* the energy produced by the falling tree (in the same way that you can feel the wind blowing against your skin). To qualify as sound, the energy must strike the ears of a human—or some other creature with a nervous system like that of a human. What this boils down to is that the quality of one's sensory experience depends on events within the nervous system, as is underscored in Box 1.2.

To sum up: In order to understand perception as fully as possible, one must study not only the properties of the physical world but also those of the perceiver.

PSYCHOLOGICAL, BIOLOGICAL, AND THEORETICAL APPROACHES TO PERCEPTION

At the outset of this chapter we stated that perception entails a sequence of interrelated events. Furthermore, we said that to understand perception requires knowing something about each component of the sequence. Understanding these components requires the combined knowledge from several different scientific disciplines, ranging from biophysics to psychology. These disciplines use different levels of analysis, from the microscopic (studying the behavior of molecules) to the macroscopic (studying the behavior of whole organisms). For a complete picture, then, one needs to analyze perception at several different levels, each offering a unique and invaluable perspective. For a metaphorical illustration of what we mean by levels of analysis, look at Figure 1.3 (p. 14). It shows an aerial photograph taken over the Peruvian desert from a very great height. From this altitude, one can see a mammoth sand carving thought to be a thousand years old. The carving, made by people lost to history, is a figure nearly 1,600 meters long. It is so huge that it can be recognized only from a great height; standing on the ground, you would be unable to take in the entire carving. Thus, to appreciate the carving requires a particular level of analysis, namely, one a great distance above the carving. Suppose, though, that you wished to examine the details of the carving and what it was made of. Such examination would require quite a different level of analysis, one much closer to the ground.

This beautiful and mysterious desert carving dramatizes a point about perception: one must adopt different levels of analysis in order to answer all the significant questions about a subject. Consequently, we'll be adopting various levels of anal-

---

Box 1.2 *Hearing Lightning and Seeing Thunder*

Seeing and hearing are qualitatively different perceptual experiences; this is shown by the fact that people never confuse sight and sound. The same has been said for touch, taste, and smell. In fact, these qualitative differences form the basis for the classic five-part division of the senses—touch, taste, smell, hearing, and seeing. Our assumption in this book is that these subjectively different experiences are—each one—products of neural events within the brain. And yet those events, it is known, all boil down to patterns of nerve impulses within the brain. Since different experiences are represented by the same sort of events, how does the brain manage to distinguish one type of experience from another—sight from sound, and taste from smell? Let's consider this question as it applies to sight and sound.

It is tempting to answer by pointing out that sound waves, the stimulus for hearing, are fundamentally different from light energy, the stimulus for seeing. However, this argument is not adequate because the brain does not directly *receive* either sound waves or light

energy—it receives only tiny electrical signals called neural impulses. In other words, from the brain's perspective, all incoming signals are equivalent. But, you might point out, although they resemble one another, those neural impulses *arise* from different sources, namely, the eyes and the ears. And, you might continue, those sources *are* fundamentally different—they are specially designed to respond only to particular kinds of physical stimulation. Because of their specialized receptors, the eyes respond to light but not to sound, while the opposite is true for the ears. So, you might well conclude, the distinctiveness of seeing and hearing depends on the difference between the eyes and the ears.

This explanation is not adequate, though. Sensations of light and sound can be produced without the participation of eyes and ears. One can bypass them and stimulate the brain directly. During the course of brain surgery on awake, alert humans, neurologists sometimes need to stimulate the brain's surface electrically to determine exactly where they are working. Depending on the area of

---

ysis in our examination of perception. The three main levels of analysis that we'll explore are the *psychological, biological,* and *theoretical.*

Distinguishing among the psychological, biological, and theoretical approaches will help organize the discussion that follows. We repeat, though, that these approaches are not mutually exclusive, but are complementary; one simply cannot learn all one wants to know about perception from just one approach.

PSYCHOLOGICAL APPROACHES

First, there is no single psychological approach to perception; instead, there are many, each differing

from the others in various ways. Although they all use some behavioral reaction to stimuli as a way of studying perception, they differ in terms of *what* behavioral reaction is used. For instance, one might attempt to train a bird to fly to a red perch but not to a green perch. If the bird succeeds in learning this task, one might infer that the bird can tell red from green. (However, as indicated in Chapter 6, to justify this conclusion requires some additional tests.)

Similarly, a human being can be instructed to push one button whenever a red object is presented and to push another button whenever a green object is presented. For birds and humans, behavior is used to infer something about percep-

the brain stimulated, patients report very vivid sensations that seem quite real (Penfield and Perrot, 1963). For instance, stimulation at a point in the back of the brain can elicit sensations of light flashes, whereas stimulation at the proper spot on the side of the brain can cause the patient to hear tones. Here, then, are examples of qualitatively distinct sensations that arise from exactly the same sort of stimulation—a mild electric current. Note, though, that the patients did not *feel* the electric current—they "heard" it or "saw" it, depending on the brain region stimulated.

These observations force a surprising conclusion: that the critical difference between hearing and seeing depends not so much on differences between the eyes and the ears but on *where* in the brain the eyes and ears send their messages. This is actually a very old idea, dating back to Johannes Müller, a nineteenth-century German physiologist. Müller's theory, called the doctrine of **specific nerve energies,** states that the nature of a sensation depends on the particular set of nerve fibers stimulated. According to this doctrine, activity in the nerve from the eye will invariably produce visual sensations, regardless of how that activity was instigated. Nowadays, it is

recognized that sensory nerves travel to specific brain areas: the nerve from the eye travels to one place, the nerve from the ear to another. Thus the emphasis has shifted from the nerves themselves to their projection sites in the brain. It is now widely believed that the distinctiveness of sight and sound is related to the unique properties of the neural connections within different regions of the brain. At present, detailed information about these unique properties is lacking, although the issue has sparked lively debate (Puccetti and Dykes, 1978; Sur, Garraghty, and Roe, 1988).

The contemporary version of Müller's doctrine suggests a provocative thought experiment. Suppose you were able to reroute the nerve from your eye, sending it to the part of your brain that normally receives input from your ear. Suppose that while you were at it, you also rerouted the nerve from your ear, sending it to that part of your brain that normally gets visual information. Now imagine that with this revised nervous system, you are caught in a thunderstorm. You should *hear* a flash of lightning and then *see* a clap of thunder. Think about it.

tion. There are actually many specific techniques for studying perception, and we'll describe some of those techniques as the need arises. Now, though, let's not focus on the details of particular behavioral techniques; instead, let's analyze the methods along more general lines, grouping them according to their degree of *formality.* By "formality" we mean the extent to which stimuli and reactions to them are structured or controlled.

The least formal is the phenomenal/nauralistic method. "Phenomenal" means that the evidence used by the approach consists of one's conscious experiences. "Naturalistic" means that the evidence concerns responses to whatever stimuli occur naturally within the environment; there is no

attempt to modify these stimuli or create artificial ones.

Phenomenal/Naturalistic Approach. There are certain advantages to this least formal approach to perception. For one thing, it relies on the most readily obtainable data—experiences evoked by naturally occurring events. Such experiences might include the appearance of a sunset, the sound of a police siren, the taste of an artichoke. Everyone has untold numbers of such experiences throughout the waking hours. To study perception, then, you could collect and organize these experiences. Going one step further, you could discuss your perceptual experiences with other

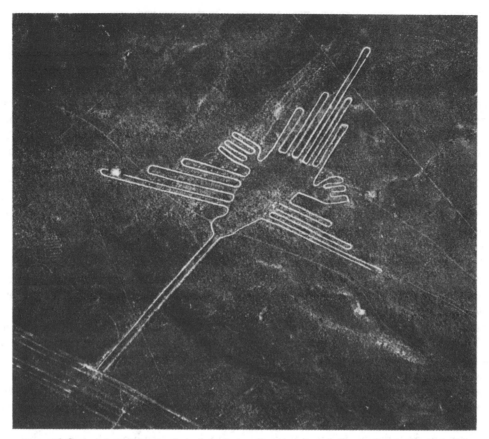

FIGURE 1.3   Aerial photograph of sand carving on Peruvian desert. (Georg Gerster/Comstock.)

people, for purposes of comparison. But what pitfalls would you encounter by following this program?

First, by restricting yourself to phenomenal descriptions, you would not be able to study perception in animals and preverbal infants, a serious limitation. Second, even working with humans who *can* verbalize their experiences, you would need to be wary. Verbal reports can be fallible and misleading. For one thing, not all people use words in the same way. Many people who are color-blind, for example, have learned to label colors much as color-normal people do, even though their experiences are surely very different.

Because verbal reports are usually made with such confidence, one may be misled into believing that they are a direct pipeline to experience. In fact, that assumption underlies the use of verbal reports as a way to examine perceptual experience. But the assumption is probably unwarranted, for there is reason to doubt that individuals *can* accurately describe their experiences, motives, or thought processes (Nisbett and Wilson, 1977); these often cannot be accessed at a conscious level. In some instances, moreover, people are motivated to avoid telling what they consider to be the truth about their experiences. Here's one instance. A malingerer is someone who pretends to have an illness or disability to get some special gain or avoid some responsibility. Feigned deafness is one form of malingering. Ask such a malingerer if he can hear, and you'll get no answer unless the question is communicated in writing, lip reading, or sign language. Then, the malingerer will assure you that he can't hear (a misleading verbal report). But there is a very clever, foolproof way to catch the malingerer: delayed auditory feedback. While the person is reading aloud, record his speech and, following a very short delay, play it back into his ears. If he is genuinely deaf, and not a malingerer, delayed auditory feedback will have no influence on his reading. But if he *can* hear, the delayed feedback of his own voice will invariably disrupt his speech.*

The word "feigns" implies that someone is purposely lying or pretending. But there are instances where a person's erroneous verbal reports don't really consitute lying. One such instance is **Anton's syndrome.** This syndrome, as rare as it is bizarre, involves complete blindness coupled with denial (the blind person denies that he or she is blind). The condition supposedly arises because two different areas of the brain have been damaged—the one needed for seeing and the one

---

* This example raises an interesting issue. What if the person insists that he cannot hear, even though the auditory feedback disrupts his speech? Should one automatically label the person a "malingerer"? Should one put more faith in the delayed feedback's interference than in his verbal report? It's conceivable that delayed feedback impairs speech at a preconscious level—in which case the person might be unaware of any disruption of his speech.

needed for knowing that you're seeing (Symonds and MacKenzie, 1957). This damage to the brain occurs quite suddenly—usually as the result of a stroke—and the victim of Anton's syndrome may walk around for quite some time bumping into things and having other mishaps until he or she becomes convinced that something is wrong. But immediately following damage to the brain, victims of Anton's syndrome confidently insist they can see. Asked to describe what is seen, the victim provides a very detailed answer but one that is a complete fabrication, as evidenced by its lack of correspondence to reality.

Anton's syndrome, besides underscoring the potential unreliability of verbal reports about perception, also points up a more general fact: perceptual experiences and knowledge of those experiences are two quite separate things. Many forces that people are not aware of can influence what they perceive. These unconscious influences include expectations, prior experience, and motivations (see Figure 1.4). Although such forces are distinct from the links that form the perceptual chain, the phenomenal approach would foreclose separating these two kinds of influences on perception. As you'll see in Box 1.3 (pp. 18–19), other, more formal approaches *do* allow one to separate the two.

Despite its limitations, the phenomenal/naturalistic approach to perception does have an important role to play. For more than a hundred

FIGURE 1.4 Look at this drawing for a while. If you cannot discern an animal, look at Figure 1.5 on page 16.

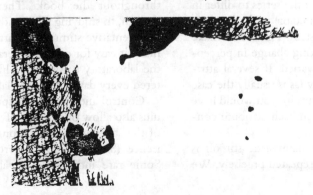

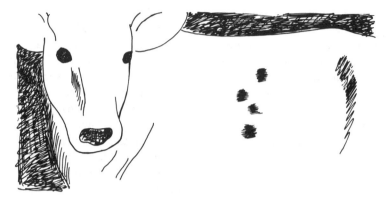

FIGURE 1.5 Outline drawing of the same animal depicted in Figure 1.4. Note how seeing this figure helps you interpret Figure 1.4. Surprisingly, this effect lasts for months.

years, careful and thoughtful observers have used this informal approach as a basis on which to build a more formal study of perception. This book will emphasize these more formal approaches; but it should not be forgotten that many of the ideas for formal study derive from this less formal method.

Experimental Approach. The phenomenal/naturalistic approach takes stimuli as they come in nature without controlling them. The approach is simple but not entirely satisfactory. For one thing, to study a particular aspect of perception usually requires access to a particular stimulus, which may not be available naturally. Moreover, you often need to use a whole series of stimuli—comparing the effect of each to the effects produced by its fellows. And the series you wanted might never occur naturally. For example, you might want the members of the series to differ in only one attribute (such as color) with all others (such as intensity) held constant. This would make it easy to ascribe any resulting change in perception to the attribute that varied. If several attributes varied simultaneously (as is usually the case with naturally occurring stimuli), you would have trouble knowing how much each attribute contributed to perception.

Another problem with naturalistic stimuli is that often they cannot be repeated precisely. We

mentioned earlier that the study of perception should be general: it should involve the perceptions of more than one person, and it should involve perceptions at more than just one moment. To satisfy the need to generalize requires repeated measures of perceptual responses. The same stimuli need to be presented again and again, under controlled conditions.

To understand perception fully, one must be able to control and manipulate stimuli. One must often use stimuli that never occur in nature. Such stimuli are sometimes criticized as being "nonecological," because they are not the stimuli for which perceptual systems evolved (Gibson, 1966). We feel, however, that their use can be valid since simple, artificial (nonecological) stimuli can often clarify the effects of more complex, naturally occurring stimuli. This point is well documented throughout the book. There is some merit, though, to studying perception using ecologically representative stimuli. In particular, such stimuli make it easy for one to generalize from studies in the laboratory to situations likely to be encountered every day outside the laboratory.

Control and careful manipulation of the stimulus also allow one to identify exactly *what* aspect of the stimulus underlies some perceptual experience (Stevens, 1951). Here's one illustration: Some rare individuals are able to discriminate among thousands of different wines by taste alone. To determine the basis of this remarkable ability, you could create a series of specially constituted wines that varied in their composition, and using this set of controlled stimuli, you could isolate the cues enabling such individuals to distinguish what most people cannot.

One also needs control over the stimuli in order to conduct two kinds of experiments that are the foundation of the scientific study of perception: matching and detection experiments. Matching experiments ask people to adjust one stimulus until it appears identical to another. This obviously requires stimuli that can be manipulated precisely. Detection experiments measure the weakest stimulus that a person can detect. Again, such experiments require stimuli whose intensities can be controlled.

* * *

As we've indicated, the psychological approach to perception uses a variety of methods, ranging from the simple and naturalistic to the highly structured and controlled. Each of these methods makes its own unique contribution. The Appendix describes some of the formal, structured methods. In addition, you'll encounter descriptions of various methods throughout the book, in the context of the research problems for which they were designed.

Although the psychological approach is useful in the study of perception, it leaves unanswered important questions about underlying neural processes. We turn now to a complementary approach that addresses those questions.

BIOLOGICAL APPROACHES

Recognizing the linkage between brain events and perception, some investigators seek to relate perceptual and biological results. Though such investigations can be challenging to carry out, their outcome often yields information that is fundamental to understanding perception. Here we'll sketch out some of the strategies used to relate physiology to behavior, without going into the details or the outcomes. In subsequent chapters,

you'll learn how these strategies are applied to answer specific questions about perception.

Lesion Technique. The oldest method for relating brain events to perception entails destroying some portion of the nervous system and then measuring associated changes in perceptual function. Called a **lesion,** this delimited area of brain damage can be created by application of strong electrical current to the targeted area, by injection of a chemical that kills nerve cells, or by surgical removal of brain tissue. Interpreted with proper caution, these studies can help specify the anatomical locus of neurons crucially involved in a given perceptual ability.

There are limitations, however, to the conclusions that can be drawn from lesion studies (Gregory, 1961), especially since lesions disrupt more than just the neural operations associated with the lesioned brain region. Destroying the Golden Gate Bridge would seriously interfere with the economic activity throughout the San Francisco bay area, but we wouldn't want to conclude that economic activity is localized on the Golden Gate Bridge. Likewise, lesioning a particular brain area may destroy an animal's ability to recognize certain stimuli, but it would be misleading to state that this brain region was solely responsible for analyzing those stimuli. By the same token, an animal may recover function following the destruction of brain tissue, but this doesn't mean that the lesioned area does not participate in that function normally—other brain areas may have taken over for the destroyed area. So, in summary, results from lesion studies can be strongly suggestive but seldom definitive.

It is worth noting that this strategy of creating a lesion and then determining its perceptual consequences is merely a systematic, experimental version of what happens when disease or trauma damages parts of the nervous system involved in perception. Naturally occurring lesions offer insights about the neural basis of human perception and have done so for centuries (Boring, 1942). However, since disease or trauma usually creates lesions that affect diverse areas of the brain, such

---

Box 1.3 *Should You Answer the Phone?*

Everyone has had the following maddening experience. While taking a shower, you faintly hear what sounds like the telephone ringing. Because of the shower's steady noise, though, you're not sure it *is* the phone. So do you decide yes and run, dripping wet, to answer it? Or do you conclude that it's only your imagination?

Your behavior in this situation depends on factors other than the loudness of the ringing sound. For instance, if you are expecting an important call, you will in all likelihood scurry out of the shower to see whether the phone is indeed ringing. If, in contrast, you're not expecting a call, you're more likely to attribute the ringing sound to the shower's own noises. Your decision about the reality of the sound, then, is influenced by your expectations. This example illustrates a significant principle, namely, that one's interpretation of sensory data depends significantly on nonsensory factors.

This dependence colors the way in which results from perceptual studies are interpreted. Imagine testing a person's hearing by presenting faint sounds and having the person say whether or not she could hear the sound. Performance on such a test can vary from one person to the next, and not just because some people have better hearing than others. Some people are simply more willing to take a gamble, asserting that they heard something even if they're not 100 percent certain (these people might also want to impress the tester with their keen hearing, say, if the hearing test is part of a job application). There are also more conservative people, who are not gamblers; in the hearing test, such people might require a much louder sound before they are willing to say that they heard it. Suppose that two people took a hearing test, one a conservative type, the other a gambler. On the basis of their performance on the hearing test, the tester might mistakenly conclude that the conservative had inferior hearing.

---

natural lesions may offer limited help in pinpointing the neural basis of some perceptual function.

Evoked Potential Technique. Another widely used procedure relates perceptual judgments made in response to a given stimulus with the electrical brain activity evoked by that same stimulus. Measured through small electrodes attached to a person's scalp, this brain activity is termed an **evoked potential (EP).** A popular strategy involves measuring the amplitude of the EP (a measure of level of brain activity) to stimuli that are barely detectable: does the magnitude of the EP mirror the ease with which a stimulus is detected? Here's one example of this strategy: A person viewing a very low-contrast visual pattern might press a button whenever that pattern faded into invisibility (which it will do from time to time). At the same time, brain activity evoked by that pattern could be measured, to see whether the level of evoked activity varied in synchrony with the appearance and disappearance of the pattern (Campbell and Kulikowski, 1972). To implement this procedure requires sensitive electronic amplifiers that boost the electrical signals measured from the scalp and skull. Because these signals are being recorded on the surface of the scalp, they are said to be massed responses, reflecting the waxing and waning of activity among several thousand individual brain

People *do* differ in the sensitivity of their sensory systems; some individuals, for instance, have a keener sense of smell than do others. But people *also* differ in their motivations, expectations, and willingness to gamble. As an aggregate, these latter differences can be labeled "motivational differences." In studies of perceptual abilities, it is important to distinguish between an individual's sensitivity and motivation. Toward this end, psychologists have developed several strategies for separating the two.

To tell whether a person can *really* hear an extremely faint sound, one needs more to go on than the fact that she is constantly saying that she hears a sound. Logically, one must also ensure that she does not make exactly the same claim when no sound whatever has been presented (Goldman, 1976). Many experiments on hearing, then, randomly intermix two types of test trials. On one type of trial, a weak sound is presented; on the other, no sound is presented. After each trial, the person says whether or not she heard a sound. Someone really interested in impressing the tester might say "Yes, I hear it" after every single trial. Of course, she'd be right every trial on which a sound actually occurred, but she'd be wrong every trial on which no sound occurred. From this result, the tester should realize that this person could not discriminate the presence of sound from the absence of sound. Omitting the sound and noting the subject's failure to recognize that omission allows the tester to separate the person's sensitivity to sound from other possible factors—such as the motivation to impress.

This general strategy is not limited to the study of hearing; similar methods are used with the other senses as well. To implement the strategy, psychologists have developed a set of sophisticated statistical techniques collectively known as signal detection theory. The Appendix provides additional details of signal detection theory. For a more thorough treatment of this topic, you may consult MacMillan and Creelman (1991), McNicol (1972), or Swets, Tanner, and Birdsall (1961). Meanwhile, before showering the next time, take the phone off the hook.

cells located near the electrode. Additional information can be derived from simultaneous recordings of brain activity from many electrodes covering much of the skull. Sampling over larger areas permits the researcher to compare the electrical activity a stimulus evokes in different regions of the brain.

The EP technique is also useful for studying individuals—such as human infants or animals—who are unable to report verbally on their perceptions. Being able to measure EPs from such individuals indicates that the evoking stimulus generates activity within the brain. Although this does not necessarily mean the individual perceives the stimulus, it confirms that a necessary condition for perception is satisfied. Using EPs, researchers have learned important facts about the visual world of infants (see Norcia and Tyler, 1985) and of animals (see Berkley and Watkins, 1971).

This technique, too, has its drawbacks. For one, the *failure* to record an EP doesn't necessarily mean the brain fails to register the evoking stimulus—the neural signals may just be too weak to be picked up or the recording electrodes may be misplaced on the scalp. For another, it is very difficult to pinpoint in exactly what region of the brain EP activity is arising. So, it is important to realize that the evoked potential provides a rather diffuse measure of brain activity picked up from tiny signals generated by large numbers of brain cells; the evoked potential only reflects omnibus brain activity.

Brain-Scan Techniques. In just the past decade, perception research has profited substantially from noninvasive techniques that create detailed pictures of the human brain. Under the right conditions, such pictures can reveal which regions of the human brain contribute to a given perceptual ability. Brain-scanning techniques, all of which produce detailed pictures or maps of the human brain, are based on differing technologies. The best-known technique, the **CAT scan** (CAT is an acronym for computer-assisted tomography), uses computer software to analyze the passage of x-rays through the head, exploiting the fact that different kinds of brain tissue differentially impede the passage of x-rays. For perception research, though, the most significant kind of brain scan is clearly the **PET scan** (PET is an acronym for positron emission tomography). Although CAT scans yield detailed information about brain structure, PET scans reveal the differential metabolic activity across the brain. So CAT is an anatomical tool; PET is a physiological one.

The PET scan capitalizes on the fact that active regions of the brain require additional amounts of energy. If a chemical required by this increased metabolism is made radioactive, one can visualize the accumulation of this ingredient in particular brain regions. In one procedure, a person first inhales a mixture of air and radioactively labeled carbon dioxide. From the person's lungs, the radioactive material, in trace amounts, enters the bloodstream and then dissipates rapidly. If, immediately after the inhalation, some local region of the brain were to increase in activity, its heightened metabolic rate would attract a stronger local flow of blood, bringing along with it additional radioactive material. Radioactive sensors are then able to register the location of this increased blood flow, allowing the construction of a picture of the distribution of radioactivity within the brain. The procedure can be taken one step further. The person can now be engaged in a particular perceptual task (for example, detect changes in the color of a geometric form) while the PET scan is being performed. It thus becomes possible to relate neural activity in specific brain regions with the execution of particular perceptual tasks (Corbetta et al., 1991). Despite its promise, PET scan suffers from a couple of limitations. First, it is impossible to pick up regional variations in activity in nearby brain areas; the PET tends to blur together variations in activity over small spatial regions. Second, the person must remain very still during the PET scan procedure, which precludes tasks involving head or body movements.

Single Cell Techniques. The techniques discussed so far all operate on a fairly coarse scale, one whose grain comprises thousands or more neurons. Techniques that provide finer-grain analysis are excellent supplements to what we have characterized as coarser techniques. In one fine-grain approach, the physiological responses of individual neurons are recorded while an alert, behaving animal, usually a monkey, engages in some perceptual task. While varying the difficulty of the task, the researcher tries to identify single neurons whose responses are strongly correlated with the animal's performance. Correlated activity suggests that those neurons form part of the neural machinery involved in the perceptual task. This approach, to be successful, must draw upon prior evidence about the locus of neurons thought to register information utilized in the task; otherwise, the research would degenerate into an unguided search for a needle in a haystack.

Once an investigator has identified a set of neurons that is believed to undergird a particular perceptual judgment, that hypothesis can be tested more directly. One can artificially stimulate the neurons by passing weak electrical current into them. If activity in those neurons is crucial, this boost in activity should alter an animal's performance on an associated perceptual task (Newsome, Britten, and Movshon, 1989). Note, however, that electrical stimulation activates not only those neurons in contact with the electrode but also other neurons connected to them. So it would be a mistake to assume that activity in those neurons *alone* is affecting the animal's behavior.

THEORETICAL APPROACHES

The previous two sections outlined strategies by which perception and its underlying neural events can be studied and ultimately related to one another. Borrowing some terms from computer science, one might say that these sections dealt with the *input* for perception, the *hardware* of the perceptual process, and its *output*. This metaphor ignores a crucial element, the *program*. Here, "program" refers to the set of instructions or rules that transforms input into output.

Sometimes people tend to confuse the program with the hardware on which the program runs. This confusion obscures an important distinction between the two. To reinforce the distinction between hardware and program, consider philosopher Daniel Dennett's discussion of an abacus:

Its computational task is to do arithmetic: to yield a correct output for any arithmetic problem given to it as input. At this level, then, an abacus and a hand-held calculator are alike; they are designed to perform the same "information-processing task." The algorithmic description of the abacus is what you learn when you learn how to manipulate it—the recipe for moving the beads in the course of adding, subtracting, multiplying, and dividing. Its physical description depends on what it is made of: it might be wooden beads strung on wires in a frame, or it might be poker chips lined up along the cracks in the floor, or something accomplished with a pencil and good eraser on a sheet of lined paper. (1991, p. 276)

In his influential book *Vision*, David Marr (1982) argued the value of studying perception on three complementary levels of abstraction. From most to least abstract, the levels are as follows: one can analyze perception as an information-processing problem; one can examine the set of rules (the program) used to solve the information-processing problem; finally, one can study the neural

machinery of perception and how that machinery executes the program. Marr insisted that some effort on the most abstract level ought to precede work on the other two levels.

If, like Marr, one describes perception as a solution to a problem, one needs to appreciate exactly what the problem is. An analogy may help. Suppose a friend tells you that she is thinking of a number between 1 and 20. Your job is to identify that number. You get one clue: the number is odd. Obviously, the clue does not give enough information to identify the number with certainty; it *underspecifies* the solution (as opposed to being told, for instance, that the number is the largest prime in the set). Generally speaking, the information provided to our sense organs underspecifies the true nature of objects in the world. Somehow, though, despite significant underspecification, the perceptual process manages to yield high-quality, useful representations of those objects.

Any computation, whether carried out by an electronic device or by a biological device, is only as good as its data and its processing rules. The brain's perceptual computations may be accurate or they may be in error, depending on the quality of information supplied by the senses and on the brain's predisposition to process that information in certain ways. However, if certain processing rules can lead to errors, why would the brain be predisposed to use those rules?

The information picked up by the senses is not just one random input after another; that information conforms well to particular, predictable patterns (Snyder and Barlow, 1988). These patterns arise from the very nature of the physical world itself, the world our senses have evolved in. For instance, in our world, objects tend to be compact. The various parts of any object tend to be near one another, not scattered at random all over the landscape. In our world, the surface color or texture of most natural objects tends to change gradually from one point to another rather than abruptly (Kersten, 1987). In our world, light tends to come from above rather than from below (Gregory, 1978). In our world, the hardness of a surface determines how sound energy is reflected from that surface (Handel, 1989).

If the brain's processing rules embodied these regularities, or constraints, that characterize the natural world, the brain's perceptual operation could be more efficient and rapid. Just as processing rules can be embodied within the microchips of an electronic device, rules that assume these regularities of the natural world could be embodied in the hardware of our brains (Ramachandran, 1988). We'll illustrate this with a detailed example.

Look at Figure 1.6, one of many interesting stimuli devised by Gaetano Kanizsa of the University of Trieste (1976). The figure conveys a strong impression of a white square resting atop four black circles. However, in creating the figure, we had only to make the four sectored disks; your perceptual system did the rest by creating the white square. It is widely believed that subjective contours, like the ones seen in Figure 1.6, occur because the visual system makes the quite reasonable assumption that nearer objects tend to occlude objects located farther away (see Figure 1.7 for examples). Designed to deal with naturally

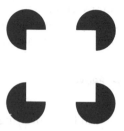

FIGURE 1.6 Subjective, or illusory, square. (Adapted from Kanizsa, 1976.)

occurring objects, the visual system treats Kanizsa's unnatural stimulus as though it were one object (a white square) occluding other objects (four black disks).

Several lines of evidence support the view that **subjective contours** reflect normal, built-in assumptions of the visual system. First, creatures other than humans do see subjective contours (Bravo, Blake, and Morrison, 1988), which is understandable since the visual systems of those creatures evolved in the same environment as ours; second, brain damage can selectively eliminate the

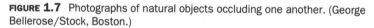

FIGURE 1.7 Photographs of natural objects occluding one another. (George Bellerose/Stock, Boston.)

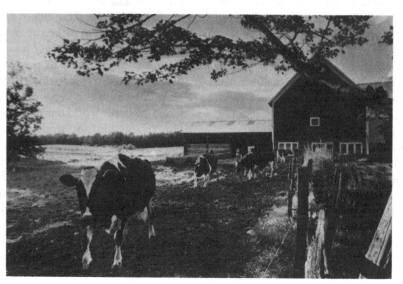

ability to see subjective contours (Stevens, 1983); finally, single neurons in the brains of monkeys respond to illusory contours, a point we'll revisit later in the book (von der Heydt, Peterhans, and Baumgartner, 1984). Fabrication or restoration of missing sensory evidence is not limited to vision; hearing performs a similar feat, when the situation warrants (Dannenbring, 1976; see Chapter 13).

In the last several paragraphs, we have been focusing on perception from an information-processing approach, one aimed at specifying the computational problems facing perception. This represents one form of theorizing within the field of perception. In general, the development of theories of perception, whether computational or not, sharpens our thinking, often translating qualitative observations into quantitative statements. These kinds of quantitatively explicit theories then serve to guide the design and implementation of experiments in perception; good theories tell us what to look for and, often, where to look.

SPECIAL CASES

Traditionally, the study of perception has focused on the "typical" perceiver—the normal adult human being. Because the majority of people fall within this category, that focus is understandable and sensible. This book follows that tradition. But additional important information about perception can be discovered by studying atypical perceivers—individuals who fall outside the category of normal adult human being. Such studies might involve perceivers who are infants, or nonhuman, or physiologically abnormal. Let's consider each of these special cases in turn.

To begin, we can examine perception *developmentally*—studying newborns, infants, children, and at the life span's other end, elderly people. Systematic changes in perception with age accompany developmental changes in the sense organs and central nervous system. Developmental work on perception thus offers one way to study the relation between sensory systems and perceptual experience.

Animals from nonhuman species represent another type of atypical perceiver. Although special sophisticated techniques are required to study animal perception, such work often repays the effort many times over. In this book, some of what you will learn about human perception comes from studying animals. A good deal is known about the anatomy and physiology of the sensory systems of several nonhuman species. This knowledge takes on added significance when it can be related to studies of perception in the same species.

Yet another approach to the study of perception exploits the consequences of certain disorders or diseases. Just as studying pathology illuminates the processes of health, studying the abnormal or deviant perceiver illuminates the normal processes of perception. If the physiological changes produced by some disease are known, as well as how perception is altered by that disease, it becomes possible to relate the physiological changes to the perceptual changes, thereby identifying the physiological basis for that aspect of perception. For example, current understanding of color vision's neural bases has benefited greatly from the study of people whose color vision is deficient. And even when the basis for some disorder is not fully understood, one can still capitalize on its perceptual effects, especially when those effects are rather specific. In particular, one may determine which aspects of perception are affected by the disorder and which are not. This, by inference, indicates which perceptual abilities depend on shared neural structures. For example, a person with misaligned (crossed) eyes can have diminished depth perception but still be able to see objects and judge whether those objects are moving or stationary. This implies that the disorder of eye alignment has selectively affected portions of the nervous system that are concerned with the analysis of depth information. In general, this kind of selective perceptual loss indicates that the affected perceptual abilities depend on parts of the nervous system different from those mediating the unaffected perceptual abilities (Hebb, 1949; Brindley, 1970).

The previous paragraphs described various categories of atypical perceivers. But atypical perception can also be produced in typical perceivers,

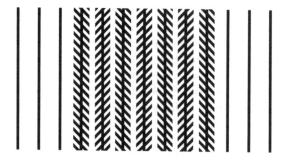

FIGURE 1.8 Zöllner's illusion of orientation.

by using unusual, provocative stimuli. Such stimuli provoke errors that highlight perception in ways that normal, error-free operation does not. This approach resembles the use of provocative tests in medicine, such as the stress electrocardiogram. In the case of perception, the easiest, most common provocative tests are stimuli that produce errors of perception called **illusions.** These errors can assume many forms, one of which was shown in Figure 1.6. To see another illusion, look at Figure 1.8. The long vertical lines are actually parallel, but the central ones appear tilted with respect to one another. This figure was devised by Franz Zöllner in 1860, and it is an example of an orientation illusion. At several places in this book you'll see that illusions are more than just fascinating novelties. It may seem odd, but the special, provocative stimuli that evoke illusions can reveal much about how humans process the ordinary, mundane perceptual information encountered every day; illusions highlight the processing rules inherent in perception.

UBIQUITOUS PROBLEMS: RECOGNITION AND PERCEPTUAL ORGANIZATION

Throughout the book, a couple of related issues will come up again and again, and for this reason deserve special mention. One is the recognition of objects and events, and the other concerns the organizational principles underlying perception. Let's briefly consider the two.

The English word "recognize" comes from the Latin prefix *re*, meaning "again," and the verb *cognoscere,* meaning "to know." So **recognition** signifies knowing again, and it is one of perception's essential functions. Recognition enables us to respond in a consistent fashion when the same object is seen, heard, tasted, smelled, or felt on different occasions and under very different conditions. Because you recognize your friends by sight, you can address them by name; because you recognize the voice of a loved one on the telephone, you can say things not meant for a stranger; because you recognize its distinctive hardness and texture, you can spit out an unwanted bone from a mouthful of fish. The rapidity and effortlessness with which all our senses recognize objects belie the difficulties that must be overcome.

Early in the process of recognition, the perceptual system must segregate an object or event from its background. When you are listening to someone over the phone, the sounds of that person's voice must be differentiated from background sounds such as music or children crying. This process of differentiation is called **segregation.** For segregation to occur, the various component sounds of that person's voice must be perceptually grouped, allowing them to cohere into a single perceptual object differentiated from background sounds. **Grouping** related elements into a larger coherent unit and segregating that larger unit from others are both important parts of recognition. When segregation fails, perceptual mistakes can result. Imagine encountering a man carrying in his arms a two-headed baby. You shudder at the horrible sight! Upon closer examination, you see that this strange "object" is, in fact, twins—their identical clothing and close proximity promoting perceptual grouping of the two into a single hideous object. The true state of affairs became apparent when you saw the toddlers' bodies moving in different directions.

We have given just a cursory overview of recognition and perceptual organization, but we'll return to both topics throughout the remainder of this book.

S U M M A R Y   A N D   P R E V I E W

This chapter lays out the framework for our analysis of perception, including the philosophical assumptions we'll be making. We have mentioned some of the practical and theoretical reasons for wanting to know more about perception. And we have outlined three distinct though complementary ways of understanding perception: the psychological, biological, and theoretical approaches. Now that this general framework is in place, the next chapter will begin to fill in the pieces, starting with some fundamentals about the organ we use for seeing. Although the book also covers hearing, taste, smell, and touch, it devotes somewhat more coverage to seeing. More is known about vision than about the other senses, and we believe vision represents the richest source of environmental information. This preeminence of vision is mirrored in the proportion of the human brain that is devoted to vision.

K E Y   T E R M S

Anton's syndrome
CAT scan
distance senses
dualism
evoked potential (EP)
far senses
grouping
illusions

lesion
materialism
naive realism
near senses
perception
PET scan
psychophysics
recognition

segregation
sensory transduction
solipsism
specific nerve energies
stimulus
subjective contours
subjective idealism

The Human Eye

T he visual system of any vertebrate con- sists of three major sections: *eyes,* which capture light and generate messages about that light; *visual pathways,* which transmit those messages from the eye; and *visual centers of the brain,* which interpret the messages in various ways. Because they all contribute to seeing, each component's function must be understood in or- der to understand how an organism sees. This chapter and the next one concentrate on the first of these components, the human eye; they discuss its anatomy (structure) and physiology (how it works). These chapters emphasize how the eye captures light and how the eye turns that light into neural messages that the brain can interpret. Chapter 4 will discuss the remaining two major sections of the mammalian visual system, the vi- sual pathways and the brain's visual centers.

All these chapters have features that require special comment. First, we don't spend time talk- ing about anatomy simply because we are fasci- nated with structure per se. We think structure is important because it influences how and what one can see. Second, although mainly interested in the *human* eye, we also consider the eyes of other animals, particularly animals whose environments and life styles differ from those of humans. Un- derstanding the uniqueness of human vision will heighten your appreciation of the processes in- volved in seeing. Finally, when we discuss struc- ture, we also consider how structural defects im- pair vision. We have included material on dysfunction because it, too, illuminates the inti- mate connection between structure and function.

In writing these chapters we were very much influenced by Gordon Walls's book *The Vertebrate Eye and Its Adaptive Radiations* (1942). He wrote eloquently about the eye, as the following statement demonstrates:

"Everything in the vertebrate eye means something." Except for the brain, there is no other organ in the body of which that can be said. It does not matter in the least whether a liver has three lobes or four, or whether a hand has five fingers or six, or whether a kidney is long and narrow or short and wide. But if we should make comparable changes in the makeup of a vertebrate eye, we should quite destroy its usefulness. Man can make optical instruments only from such materials as brass and glass. Nature has succeeded with only such things as leather and water and jelly; but the resulting instrument is so delicately balanced that it will tolerate no tamper- ing. (pp. iii–iv)

This brief extract argues convincingly that to understand vision, one *must* understand the eye's structure. We'll begin our actual discussion of the eye with a series of general questions about the nature of vision—*why* vision took the form that it did.

DESIGNING THE ORGAN OF VISION

WHY HAVE EYES THAT USE LIGHT?

The preceding chapter distinguished between the near and the distance senses, putting vision among the distance senses. By definition, a distance sense enables one to detect objects without having to come in immediate proximity to those objects. Hearing and seeing both endow one with this capacity. But vision enjoys a major advantage over hearing: it enables one to detect objects that make no sound. (Hearing offers many advantages of its own, including the ability to detect things that cannot be seen—but we'll get to that in Chapters 9 and 10.) Vision also provides important information about objects that hearing cannot give—for example, about an object's color, size, and shape. Such information is conveyed by light, the messenger that bridges the distance between oneself and the objects one sees.

Light is just one form of **electromagnetic radiation;** other familiar varieties include radio waves, infrared and ultraviolet radiation, microwaves, and x-rays. All these forms of energy are produced by the oscillation of electrically charged material. Since virtually all matter consists of oscillating (that is, wavelike) electrical charges, electromagnetic energy exists in abundance. An animal that can sense electromagnetic radiation benefits in several important ways.

First, electromagnetic radiation travels very rapidly (in empty space, at 186,000 miles, or ap-proximately 300,000 kilometers, per second). Any creature that is able to detect such radiation can pick up information from distant sources with minimal delay. Thus one sees events practically as soon as they occur. A second advantage of being able to sense electromagnetic radiation comes from its tendency to travel in straight lines. As a result of this tendency, images created by this radiation retain important geometrical characteristics of the object or objects that reflected the radiation toward the eyes. We'll come back to this point in a moment.

The frequency of electromagnetic radiation depends on the emitting material's mode of oscillation. In fact, electromagnetic radiation can be scaled or arranged along a spectrum according to the frequency of oscillation, with light occupying only a very small portion of that spectrum (see Figure 2.1). The frequency, or rate of oscillation, of light energy can be converted into units termed wavelengths. **Wavelength** is defined by how far the radiation travels between oscillations. High rates of oscillation mean that radiation will not travel very far between oscillations—hence a short wavelength. Figure 2.1 underscores an important point: light, the form of radiation on which we

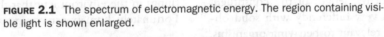

FIGURE 2.1 The spectrum of electromagnetic energy. The region containing visible light is shown enlarged.

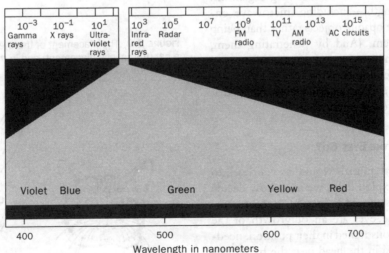

depend for sight, occupies only a very small portion of the electromagnetic spectrum. Actually, radiation from other portions of this spectrum *could* have been used to bridge the distance between the perceiver and objects of visual perception. So why do the eyes depend solely on this one, very narrow portion of the entire electromagnetic spectrum, the part known as light?

One reason for using light as a medium is that there is a lot of it in the world. Light's abundance ensures that creatures will have ample opportunity to use their light-sensing apparatus. It wouldn't have made much sense for early vertebrate "eyes" to depend on wavelengths in the ultraviolet range, for example, because most (but not all) of the energy in this short wavelength region of the spectrum is absorbed by molecules in the earth's atmosphere (mainly nitrogen and oxygen) and, consequently, never reaches the objects in our environment. Second, light is useful as a medium of information about the world because light interacts with the surface molecules of many objects. These interactions, in the form of reflection and absorption, allow light to convey information not only about the presence and absence of objects but also about the structure of those objects and their surfaces (Gibson, 1966). Energy from outside the "light" portion of the electromagnetic spectrum—because of the length of the constituent waves—interacts very differently with solid objects of the sizes relevant to behaving organisms. Longer wavelengths—including microwave energy—penetrate opaque objects rather than being reflected by them. (And by penetrating them, microwaves can more evenly heat objects and therefore are useful in cooking.)

In summary, eyes are a good idea, and eyes that use light are an even better idea.

WHERE SHOULD THE EYES GO?

Recognizing that animals would do very well to have eyes that exploit light, we must now decide *where* those eyes should be placed. Because embryologically the eyes are an outgrowth of the brain, they are constrained in their position, needing to be located in the head near the brain. But where exactly in the head should the eyes go? Nature has devised several different ways to position the eyes. In vertebrates, there are two popular designs for outfitting the head with a pair of eyes: they can be located in a *frontal* position, as are those of a human being or a cat; or they can be located in a *lateral* position, as are those of a rabbit (see Figure 2.2). Each strategy carries its own advantages: frontal eyes improve depth perception (as discussed in Chapter 7), whereas lateral eyes make it possible to take in more of the visual world at one time. As a rule, predatory animals—those who hunt and eat other animals—have frontally placed eyes, and those who are prey—animals taken as food—have laterally placed eyes. In other words, those needing excellent depth perception to stalk and capture have considerable binocular overlap of the two visual fields; those needing a more panoramic view of the environment in order to watch for predators have little binocular overlap.

WHY SHOULD THE EYES BE ABLE TO MOVE?

Because we lack panoramic vision, what humans can see at any one moment is rather limited (see Figure 2.3). And there is no guarantee that the eyes of humans will always be directed toward the things in the environment that they need to see. Fortunately, humans can compensate for their rel-

FIGURE 2.2 The placement of the eyes in the head of a cat (frontal eye placement) and in the head of a rabbit (lateral eye placement).

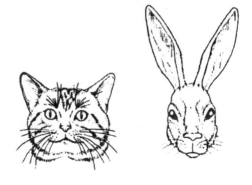

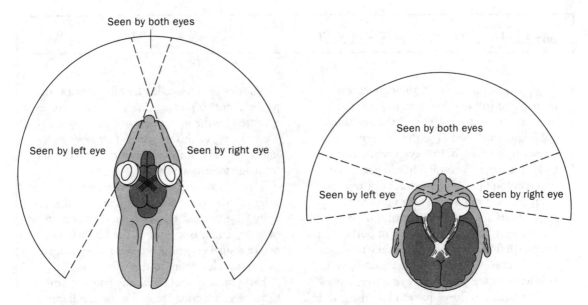

FIGURE 2.3 The extent of visual field of view for a rabbit and for a human. Note that the rabbit has almost completely panoramic vision, whereas the human's field of view encompasses only about 180 degrees.

atively narrow field of vision by being able to adjust where the eyes are directed (Gibson, 1966, p. 175). This is what you do when you look both ways before crossing a street. You also move your eyes because they are not uniformly sensitive; some parts of the eyes provide much better detail vision than do other parts. Think for a moment what you do when you notice something out of the corner of your eye. If you wish to see particular details of it, your eyes must move so that you're looking directly at those details.

Animals use various strategies for changing their field of view: they can move their bodies, turn their heads, or move their eyes. Some animals—owls for one—have very limited ability to move their eyes (Steinbach and Money, 1973). This comes about because their eyes are large and fit tightly into their sockets (Walls, 1942, p. 212). Rather than depending on eye movements, the owl relies on a relatively slower method for redirecting its gaze: it moves its entire head. But not all birds are our inferiors when it comes to eye movements. The European starling, now so numerous as to be a nuisance in most North

American or European cities, owes some of its success to its eye movements. Most birds, as they forage on the ground, need to look sideways in order to see what they're about to peck at. But starlings, whose skulls are quite narrow and whose eyes are extremely mobile, can turn their eyes far enough forward so that they can actually see between their opened jaws. Just as important—and amazing—is the starling's ability to instantly swing its eyes up and back to scan the skies behind its head for possible predators (Martin, 1987). Because it can watch for predators without having to turn its head, the starling remains relatively unobtrusive, another element of protection. With eye movements so well designed for both fruitful foraging and self-protection, it's no wonder that in just 90 years starlings have increased their numbers in North America from just 100 European imports to more than 200 million birds.

We typically think about eye movements as being intentional and, indeed, they are in most cases. However, even when trying to hold the eyes perfectly steady, we are not completely successful, which is fortunate. Box 2.1 explains why.

Box 2.1 *Eyes That Never Stand Still*

As we explain in the text, the extraocular muscles control the direction of gaze. Contractions of these muscles pull the eyeballs, guiding their direction so that objects of interest can be fixated. But even when you try to keep your eyes absolutely still, small random contractions of the extraocular muscles keep the eyes moving. These involuntary eye movements are usually too small for you to be aware of them, but they are important for seeing. Before explaining why they're important, though, we can describe a simple trick that lets you see your own eye movements.

The trick requires a pattern like the grid in the accompanying figure (Verheijen, 1963). First carefully fixate the black dot in the center of the pattern about 30 seconds, keeping your eyes as still as possible. Then quickly move your eyes to the white dot. Again, keep your eyes as still as possible. You'll see

an illusory pattern, called an **afterimage,** that jiggles slightly. The jiggling of the afterimage is caused by the movements of your eyes. You can prove this to yourself by now making large, intentional eye movements; the afterimage follows your eyes.

Here's how the demonstration works. The original 30-second period of fixation differentially fatigues the neurons over various parts of your retina. But because the black squares evoke a smaller retinal response, they fatigue your retina less than do the white squares. When you stop looking at the pattern, portions of your retina are in a state of differential, patterned adaptation. This differential adaptation produces an afterimage, such that areas that were white in the original now appear dark, whereas areas that were dark now appear light. Of course, the fatigued neurons are fixed in place in the eye's retina; it is as if

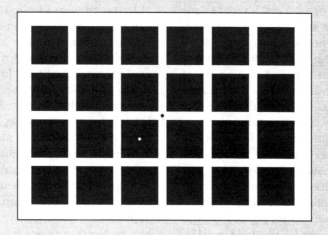

a negative image of the grid is temporarily imprinted on the back of the eye. Thus whenever you see the afterimage move, it must indicate that your eyes have moved—whether you intended them to or not. In the slight jiggling of the afterimage you are seeing the consequences of your own involuntary eye movements.

These small random eye movements are actually very important for vision; when they are eliminated, vision changes dramatically. For example, special optical systems have been developed that move whatever you're looking at in step with the movements of your eyes. This scheme produces a motionless, stabilized image on your retina. Here's one way to produce a stabilized retinal image. A small photographic transparency of some object is mounted on a special high-power contact lens that focuses the image on the retina. Since the contact lens moves along with the eye, the image of the transparency attached to this lens is stabilized on the retina. And the perceptual result is remarkable—within a few seconds, the object begins to fade from view, as if the brightness on a television screen were being reduced. Eventually the object disappears entirely, leaving nothing but a homogeneous gray field. So when the effects of normal involuntary eye movements are eliminated, vision is eliminated too (Pritchard, Heron, and Hebb, 1960; Riggs, Ratliff, Cornsweet, and Cornsweet, 1953).

The fact that stabilized retinal images fade and disappear is actually quite fortunate. If they didn't, you would be constantly annoyed by the images produced in your eyes

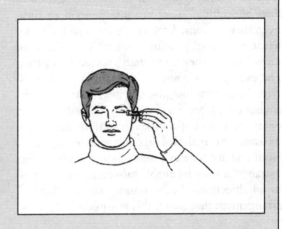

by blood vessels. Because they are in the path of light, these blood vessels cast shadows on your retina. Since the branches move along with your eye, their shadows are stabilized retinal images and, consequently, are invisible to you. However, you can "destabilize" them by moving a beam of light back and forth across the vessels. This causes their shadow to move back and forth slightly, enough to make them visible. The simplest way to produce this effect is with a small flashlight (a penlight). Looking straight ahead with eyes closed, place the penlight against the corner of your eye—the corner away from your nose, as is shown in the illustration. Gently rock the penlight back and forth. After a second or two you should begin seeing what look like the branches of a tree. These are the shadows of blood vessels in your eye. Once you get them into view, stop moving the flashlight and the branches will disappear within a few seconds, as the image returns to its normal, stabilized condition.

Humans can shift the position of their eyes with enormous speed. For instance, it takes less than one-fifth of a second for the eyes to turn from their extreme leftward position to their extreme rightward position. Not only do the eyes move rapidly, they move with great accuracy too. For example, as you read these lines, your eyes skip along from one place of interest to another, alighting with great precision on the desired letter or space. The cooperative interaction among the **extraocular muscles** (six for each eye) makes rapid and accurate eye movements possible. The extraocular muscles enable movement of the eyes in all directions. Let's consider the mechanical arrangement that makes this possible.

How the Eyes Move. Every muscle works by contracting and thereby pulling on the structure or structures to which the muscle is attached. In the case of the extraoculars, each muscle is connected at one end to an immovable structure, the eye socket of the skull, and at the other end to an object that is free to move, the eyeball. So when the extraocular muscle contracts, it pulls on the eyeball and moves it. The *amount* of movement depends on the strength of the muscle's contrac-

tion and on the action of the other muscles. The *direction* of movement depends on the place at which the contracting muscle is attached to the eyeball and skull, and on what the other muscles are doing. Because each extraocular muscle is attached to the eyeball at a different position, contraction of any particular muscle turns the eyeball in a characteristic direction. The following is a brief and simplified description of what the extraoculars do.

Each eye's muscles can be divided into two groups, one with four muscles and one with two. The larger group, the **rectus muscles,** run straight back from the eyeball. Muscles in the other, smaller group run obliquely back from the eyeball. One can understand the general principles of the eye's movements by looking just at muscles in the larger group.

Each rectus muscle is attached to the eyeball at a different location, in each case toward the front of the eyeball (see Figure 2.4). The other end of each rectus muscle is attached to the rear of the bony cavity holding the eyeball; this is the immovable end of the muscle. Whenever a rectus muscle contracts, it pulls the eyeball toward the place at which that muscle connects to the eyeball;

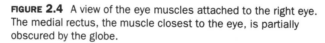

FIGURE 2.4 A view of the eye muscles attached to the right eye. The medial rectus, the muscle closest to the eye, is partially obscured by the globe.

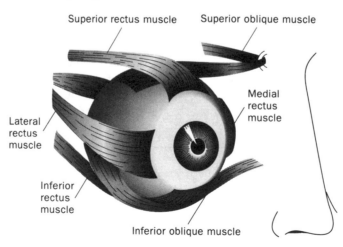

Superior rectus muscle

Superior oblique muscle

Medial rectus muscle

Lateral rectus muscle

Inferior rectus muscle

Inferior oblique muscle

when a rectus muscle relaxes, the eye turns back toward its original position.

One muscle, the *medial* rectus, attaches to the side of the eyeball closest to the nose. Thus when it contracts, the medial rectus rotates the eye toward the nose. Another muscle, the *lateral* rectus, has exactly the opposite effect. It is connected to the side of the eyeball farthest from the nose, so its contraction turns the eyeball laterally, away from the nose. The *superior* rectus muscle connects to the top of the eyeball, and its contraction elevates the eyeball, causing you to look upward. Its opposite number, the *inferior* rectus, is attached to the lower portion of the eyeball, and its contraction lowers the eye, causing you to look down.

Now let's consider how these muscles cooperate to move the eyes. Imagine that while looking straight ahead, you decide to glance leftward. Both eyes must move to the same degree and in the same direction. In order for you to look to the left, both the medial rectus of the right eye and the lateral rectus of the left eye must contract, while both the lateral rectus of the right eye and the medial rectus of the left eye must relax. You should be able to figure out for yourself what will happen if you now decide to glance rightward.

For the eye movements just described, both eyes have moved in the same direction—upward, leftward, and so on. Eye movements of this type are called **conjunctive** eye movements. But the eyes are capable of other types of movements as well, ones in which the eyes move in opposite directions—both may turn inward or both may turn outward. These are called **vergence** eye movements. For example, the left eye can turn rightward while the right eye turns leftward. As a result, both eyes turn inward, toward the nose. This movement aims the two eyes at a very close object straight ahead of you. This particular type of movement is called a convergent eye movement. To accomplish it, the medial rectus muscles of both eyes contract, while the lateral rectus muscles of both eyes relax. If you are looking at an object at arm's length and then bring it closer to you, your eyes converge, tracking the object. When the object moves away from you, your eye

muscles will engage in the opposite behavior, resulting in a divergent eye movement. We postpone further discussion of eye movements until Chapter 8.

HOW SHOULD THE EYES BE PROTECTED?

Vertebrate eyes are extremely complicated devices, occupying a very exposed position in the head. Various protective measures have evolved to compensate for their vulnerability. An outline of these protective mechanisms will provide a good introduction to the overall structure of the eye.

The eye is partially protected by virtue of its location within the **orbit,** a bony depression in the skull. Within the orbit, the eye is cushioned by heavy deposits of fat surrounding each eyeball. Without this orbital fat, blows to the head would be transmitted directly to the eye. But by absorbing such shocks, orbital fat cushions the eye against all but the most severe jolts.

The eyelids, movable folds of tissue, also protect the eye. The position of the upper lid relative to the lower one determines the opening through which the front of the eye is visible. The lids move relative to each other in various modes. For instance, they can open and close rapidly, in a small fraction of a second. Such closures of the lids, blinks, occur voluntarily as well as involuntarily. Blinks clean and moisten the front of the eye to keep it from drying out; they also protect the eye from objects that seem to be on a collision course with it, and they reduce light when so desired (as for sleep).

Under normal circumstances a blink occurs about once every 4 seconds (Records, 1979a, p. 19). The exact frequency varies from person to person, with emotional state, and with environmental conditions. When the air is very dry, the blink rate goes up, ensuring that the delicate front surface of the eye doesn't dry out. At the beginning of a casual conversation with someone, your blink rate may double; anger may further increase blink rate. You can see this for yourself by observing your friends under various conditions. Just be sure they don't know you're making these observations. Otherwise, they may attempt to alter their blink rate voluntarily (Doane, 1980).

From the instant the lids begin to close until they reopen, a blink takes roughly one-third of a second. For about half this time, the lids are completely closed, reducing the light by over 90 percent (Riggs, Volkmann, and Moore, 1980). If the room lights were momentarily dimmed by this amount, the blackout would be very noticeable. Why is it, then, that one never notices the same blackout when it is caused by a blink?

Volkmann, Riggs, and Moore (1980) tried to explain this puzzle. They believed that the part of the brain that signals the lids to close also produces a neural signal that suppresses, or temporarily shuts off, vision for the duration of the blink. Suppression would keep you from noticing that a blink had occurred. This hypothesis, although intriguing, is hard to test. The appropriate test would be to measure vision during a blink without having those measurements affected by the lids' closing. Volkmann and colleagues developed the following ingenious way to stimulate the eye so that the light reaching the retina would not be affected by lid closure.

The eyes lie directly above the roof of the mouth. Thus, a strong light focused on the roof of the mouth under one eye can stimulate the retina, causing the light to be seen whether or not the lids are closed. If the room lights were off and the only light reaching your eye came through the roof of your mouth, blinking would not affect the light reaching your eye. This arrangement makes it possible to measure the ability to see a dimming of the light at various times relative to a blink.

Volkmann and colleagues used a bundle of transparent plastic fibers to carry light to the roof of a person's mouth. By abruptly dimming the light, they determined the smallest reduction in light intensity visible to the person. Remember: All the light that could be seen came through the person's mouth, bypassing the lids. At the same time, Volkmann and colleagues used skin electrodes to measure when a blink occurred. Since a blink is produced by muscle contraction, it is easy to measure the electrical activity of the lid muscles and know from that activity when a blink begins and ends. These investigators found that dimming was much harder to see *during* a blink than *between* blinks. To be detected during a blink, the light had to be dimmed by an amount 5 times greater than it did between blinks.

This result proves that the nervous system suppresses vision just before and during each blink—keeping you from noticing visual blackouts. Without this suppression, 10 to 15 times per minute, you would be bothered by profound blackouts (Riggs, Volkmann, and Moore, 1981, p. 1079). Your visual system uses a temporary, well-timed suppression to protect you from the annoying but necessary behavior of your eyelids.

The lids of the eye can also change position in situations other than blinking. In conversation, the size of the opening between the lids provides a reliable clue as to how interested your listener is. Watch a friend's eyes closely; the opening between lids will average 8 millimeters (about $\frac{1}{3}$ inch). You'll probably notice a change in that opening as your friend's attention varies. When interest is high, the opening between lids increases to about 10 millimeters. Drowsiness or boredom reduces the size of the opening (Records, 1979a, pp. 15–17).

Tears, too, protect the eyes. Although usually associated either with emotional states or with slicing raw onions, tears are intended to protect the eyes in several ways. Tears are secreted from a gland situated in the upper, front portion of each orbit (under the upper lid). From there, they pass down over the cornea, moistening it, and then drain out of the eye through small openings in the lower nasal portion of each orbit. Finally, the tears drain onto the mucous membrane lining the nose's inner surface. This nasal membrane acts as an evaporator for the tears, which explains why you have to blow your nose when you have been crying. Tears contain an antimicrobial agent that helps protect the eye from certain bacteria present in the environment. In addition, the regular flow of tears flushes away debris, such as dust. Tears also lubricate the surface of the eyes so that blinking won't abrade the lids or scratch the front of the eyeball. The constant, very thin film of tears over the front of the eye minimizes the wear and tear produced by constant lid movement.

Having covered its ancillary features, we are now ready to discuss the structure of the eye itself.

THE STRUCTURE OF THE HUMAN EYE

To understand the human eye requires dealing with the details of ocular structure and function; but as an introduction, let's start with the major features. We can omit details until the second stage of our discussion, by which time you'll have a good idea where those details fit into the eye's grand scheme. In portraying these details, incidentally, texts often draw an analogy between the eye and a camera. Certainly, both are optical devices designed to record visual images on light-sensitive material (film, in the case of the camera; photoreceptors, in the case of the eye). And the two do have components in common (mechanical, in the case of the camera; biological, in the case of the eye). So where appropriate, we will point out these analogies. But don't be misled—the analogy is limited. For instance, eyes work best when they are moving (recall Box 2.1),

whereas a camera is designed to be held still. In this and the next few chapters, we'll point out other instances where the analogy fails.

The human eye is very nearly spherical, with a diameter of approximately 24 millimeters (nearly 1 inch), or slightly smaller than a Ping-Pong ball. It consists of three concentric layers, each with its own characteristic appearance, structure, and primary function. From outermost to innermost, the three layers are the **fibrous tunic,** which protects the eyeball; the **vascular tunic,** which nourishes the eyeball; and the **retina,** which detects light and initiates neural messages bound for the brain. Figure 2.5 illustrates this three-layered arrangement. Note also from this figure that the eye is partitioned into two chambers, a small anterior chamber and a larger vitreous chamber. Thus the basic layout is three concentric layers and two chambers, plus the iris, pupil, and lens.

THE OUTERMOST, FIBROUS TUNIC

When looking directly at someone's eye, you see only about one-sixth of its outer surface; the rest lies hidden behind the lids and other protective structures. The "white" of the eye is part of the outermost, fibrous coat. Since this white part is

FIGURE 2.5 Cross section of human eye, showing major layers and structures. View is from above the left eye.

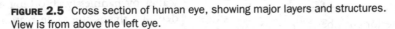
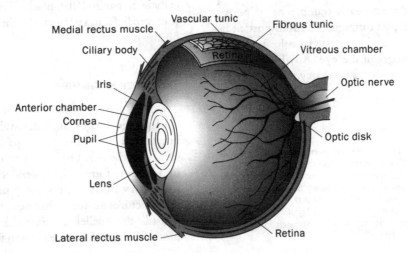

made of tough, dense material, it is called the **sclera,** from a Greek root meaning "hard."*

The sclera averages about 1 millimeter in thickness, and microscopic inspection reveals that it's made of tightly packed, interwoven fibers running parallel to the sclera's surface. These densely packed fibers give the sclera its toughness. Actually, the sclera has to be tough because pressure inside the eyeball is double that of the atmosphere. If the sclera were more elastic, that pressure could cause the eyeball to become deformed. Among other consequences, deformation would ruin the quality of one's sight. We'll return to the importance of the eyeball's shape later, when we discuss the eye as an optical instrument.

At the very front of the eye, this outer coat loses its white coloring and becomes so transparent that it's difficult to see it in the mirror. However, if you look at someone else's eye from the side, you will notice a small bulge on the front of the eye. This bulge is called the **cornea,** a term from the word for "hornlike," meaning that the cornea is composed of material similar to that in an animal's horn. So why is the cornea transparent? The major reason is that the fibers of the cornea are arranged in a neater, more orderly fashion. In addition, greater transparency is made possible by the fact that the cornea has no internal blood supply of its own. Since blood and the requisite vessels would reduce the passage of light, the cornea draws its nourishment from the clear fluid in the anterior chamber.

Because the cornea is transparent, it permits more light to pass through. This is important because the cornea plays a crucial role in the formation of images in the eye. Anything that disturbs the cornea's transparency, therefore, will reduce the quality of these images and, hence, the quality of vision. For self-protection, the cornea has extremely high sensitivity to touch. Foreign bodies contacting the cornea trigger a sequence of protective responses, including lid closure and tear production.

THE MIDDLE, VASCULAR TUNIC

For most of its course, the vascular tunic hugs the wall of the eyeball, and only toward the front of the eyeball does it pull away from the wall. We'll begin by considering the rear two-thirds of this middle layer, the part that fits snugly against the wall of the eyeball.

Most of the middle layer consists of a dark, heavily pigmented, spongy structure called the **choroid.** The choroid averages about 0.2 millimeters in thickness and contains a network of blood vessels, including capillaries. Blood from these capillaries nourishes many cells in the retina, the innermost of the eye's three layers. Without that nourishment—oxygen and nutrients—those cells, which are vital for vision, would die.

The choroid's heavy pigmentation also reduces light scatter, the tendency for light to bounce around randomly within the eyeball, which would reduce the sharpness of images formed inside the eye. The choroid's pigmentation reduces scatter by harmlessly absorbing extra light. Incidentally, this is the same reason the inside of a camera is painted flat black. The paint absorbs scattered light and protects the sharpness of images on the film.

THE ANTERIOR CHAMBER

Toward the front of the eye, this middle, choroidal layer no longer hugs the wall of the eyeball but instead runs more or less parallel to the front surface of the eye. Over this part of its course, the middle layer forms a long slender structure called the **ciliary body.** This spongy network of tissue manufactures **aqueous humor,** the watery fluid that fills the smaller, anterior chamber of the eye located behind the cornea and in front of the lens.

---

* Most parts of the eye have names related to their character or appearance. Knowing the origin of some of these names can help you appreciate the structure of the eye. Our explanations come from a book, *On Naming the Parts of the Human Body,* written in the second century A.D. by Rufos of Euphesus, a city located in what is today Turkey. We have drawn on an excellent translation by Stephen Polyak (1941, p. 96).

The aqueous humor serves a number of major maintenance functions: it transports oxygen and nutrients to several of the structures it bathes, and it carries away their waste products. Elsewhere in the body, blood performs these functions, but inside the eye, blood would interfere with light transmission and make seeing difficult or impossible. Therefore, in place of blood, the crucial optical components of the eye—the cornea and lens—rely on aqueous as their source of nourishment.

The aqueous serves another function as well. Filling the anterior chamber, this fluid maintains the shape of the eyeball. If there were too little fluid in the anterior chamber, the eye would become deformed, like an underinflated basketball. It doesn't though, because cells in the ciliary body are constantly producing new aqueous to keep the supply of nutrients from becoming exhausted. The creation of new fluid also prevents the buildup of high concentrations of waste products.

There is a limit, however, to how much aqueous the anterior chamber can hold. So a balance must be achieved between the rate of creation of the fluid and the rate at which it is drained from the eye. Sometimes the balance is not maintained and too much aqueous accumulates in the eye. Excess aqueous accumulates either because of overproduction or because of improper drainage out of the anterior chamber. Drainage can be blocked or slowed down if the outlets for aqueous (which lie at the junction of ciliary body and cornea; see Figure 2.6) become squeezed shut or clogged. Pressure builds up within the eye, and if the pressure remains high for too long, vision can be impaired permanently. This is the most common cause of blinding eye disease in North America—**glaucoma.**

THE IRIS, PUPIL, AND LENS

The Iris. As it folds inward, away from the wall of the eye, the ciliary body gives rise to the **iris,** a circular patch of tissue that gives your eye its characteristic color: brown, blue, green, gray, and at least in the case of one famous actress, violet

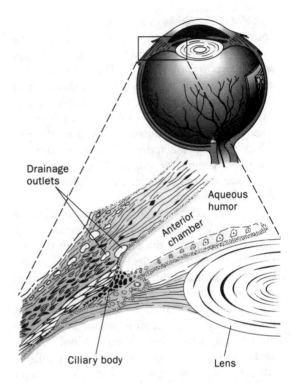

FIGURE 2.6 Enlarged view of anterior chamber, showing the eye's drainage system. The small box in the inset shows the region of the eye represented in the enlarged drawing.

(Howard, 1983). This variety of colors makes the name "iris" very appropriate, for it comes from the Greek word for "rainbow."

The iris actually consists of two layers, an outer layer containing pigment, and an inner layer containing blood vessels. If the outer layer is heavily pigmented, the iris will appear brown. But if this outer layer is lightly pigmented, someone looking at the iris can actually see the back layer through the front one. In this case, the iris will look blue or some other light color. The color results from a combination of the pigmentation of the front layer and the color of the blood vessels in the back layer. If the iris's front layer had no pigment, the rear layer would become very noticeable, giving the eye a pinkish hue. This occurs in albino humans, who, because of a genetic defect, have greatly reduced pigmentation (see page 61).

The Pupil. Looking in a mirror at the center of your own iris, you'll see a round black region, the **pupil.** The pupil is actually an opening, or gap, within two sets of muscles. The inner set runs circularly around the pupil. When this circular band of muscles contracts, the pupil gets smaller. Another set of muscles runs radially out from the edge of the circular muscles, away from the pupillary opening. When the radial muscles contract, the pupil widens, or dilates. These changes in pupil size control the amount of light reaching the back of the eye.

The size of the pupil at any given moment depends on several factors. First, it depends on the light level to which the eye is exposed: the size of the pupil decreases as the level of light increases. In young adults, the pupil diameter varies from about 8 to 9 millimeters down to 1.5 to 2 millimeters, a fourfold variation. The amount of light passing through the pupil is proportional to the pupil's *area,* which is itself proportional to the square of pupil diameter. Thus, as the pupil diameter varies over a range of 4 to 1, the amount of light the pupil admits to the eye varies over a range of 16 to 1. In older adults, the pupil responds to light by changing size, but its largest opening is less than half that of the average 20-year-old. As a result, less light gets into the eyes of very old people.

Besides light level, the size of the pupil depends on other events that influence the autonomic nervous system. In particular, excitement, fear, or sexual interest can change the size of the pupil. Some people, such as professional gamblers and jewel merchants, are quite adept at sensing emotional state on the basis of a person's pupil size (Hess, 1965). This has been appreciated for some time, and countermeasures have been developed—including dark glasses to hide the pupils.

Although large pupils allow more light into the eye, smaller pupils can sometimes offer an advantage (Cornsweet, 1970). Suppose you are looking at an object about 2 or 3 meters away. While you're looking at that object, other objects—those much closer or much farther away—will tend to appear somewhat blurred. The range of distances over which objects will appear sharp varies with the size of the pupil. This range is sometimes called the **depth of field.** The easiest way to demonstrate the depth of field is to substitute a camera for your eye. In taking the photographs shown in Figure 2.7, the photographer varied the size of the camera's aperture to simulate the effects of changing pupil size. The photograph on the left was taken with a large aperture; the one on the right, with a small aperture. Note that on the left, very few objects appear sharp. With a large aperture, the objects that were not precisely at the distance for which the camera was focused appear blurred. The other photograph was taken without changing the focus but with a smaller aperture. Now, more objects appear well focused—the range of distances over which objects can be situated and still be adequately focused has increased.

The Lens. One very important optical element of the eye, the **crystalline lens,** lies right behind the iris. The lens takes its name from its resemblance to a lentil, or bean. In adults, the lens is shaped like a very large aspirin tablet, about 9 millimeters in diameter and 4 millimeters in thickness. The lens consists of three distinct parts: an elastic covering, or *capsule;* an *epithelial layer* just inside the capsule; and the *lens* itself. As you might expect, each of these parts has its own job to do.

In fact, the thin, elastic capsule around the lens has two jobs. First, it moderates the flow of aqueous humor into the lens, helping the lens retain its transparency to light. Second, the elastic capsule molds the shape of the lens—varying its flatness and, thereby, the lens's optical power. This variation in optical power is called **accommodation.**

The lens never stops growing. Throughout the life span, the outer, epithelial layer of the lens continues to produce protein fibers that are added to the surface of the lens. Consequently, those protein fibers nearest the center of the lens are the oldest (some were present at birth), whereas the fibers on the outside are the youngest. Between birth and age 90 years, the lens quadruples in thickness and attains a weight of 250 milligrams

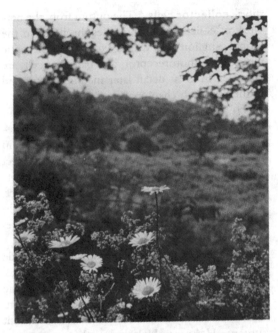 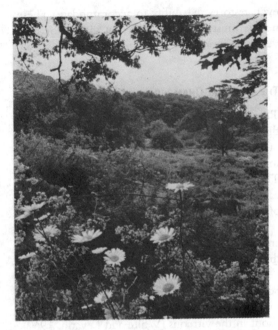

FIGURE 2.7 The degree of blur in a picture depends on the size of the aperture of the camera. The sharp photo on the right was taken through a smaller aperture than was used in taking the photo on the left, thus increasing the depth of field in the right-hand photograph. (Glyn Cloyd.)

(Paterson, 1979). In the center of the lens the old fibers become more densely packed, producing **sclerosis,** or hardening, of the lens. We'll describe the importance of sclerosis later in this chapter.

To provide for good vision, the lens must be transparent—light must be able to pass through it easily and with little loss. This transparency depends on the material out of which the lens is made. Of all the body's parts, the lens has the highest percentage of protein, and its protein fibers are lined up parallel to one another, maximizing the lens's transparency to light. Anything that disturbs this alignment—such as excess fluid inside the lens—reduces transparency.

An opacity (or reduced transparency) of the lens is called a **cataract.** While some cataracts are minor—barely reducing the transmission of light—others cause blindness. Cataracts are common in elderly people, but they can also occur in the young. In fact, certain populations (Arabs and

Sephardic Jews, for instance) have a very high incidence of congenital cataracts—lens opacities at birth. These opacities severely degrade the stimulation received by the eye, and this can be serious. At birth, the visual nervous system is immature and its proper development depends on normal stimulation of the eye. Deprived of that proper stimulation, the immature visual nervous system develops abnormally (Hubel, Wiesel, and LeVay, 1977). Realizing this fact, many physicians now remove congenital cataracts as early in life as possible.

Surgical removal of a cataractous lens has become more or less routine today. Since the lens contributes to the total optical power of the eye, removal of the lens must be accompanied by some form of optical compensation. Powerful spectacles or contact lenses can be worn, or alternatively, a plastic lens can be surgically inserted inside the eye, replacing the missing biological lens (Applegate et al., 1987). None of these alternatives, however, restores the ability to accommodate. These people must, then, use different glasses for near versus far vision.

THE VITREOUS CHAMBER

The vitreous chamber accounts for nearly two-thirds of the total volume of the eye. This larger of the eye's two chambers is bounded by the lens in front and the retina on the sides and in the rear. This chamber is filled with a transparent fluid called **vitreous,** a substance with the consistency of egg white.

Encased in a thin membrane, the vitreous is anchored to the inner wall of the eyeball. Unlike the aqueous, the vitreous is not continuously renewed, which means that debris can accumulate. Sometimes you become aware of this debris, in the form of **floaters,** small opacities that float about in the vitreous (White and Levatin, 1962). If you are looking at a bright, uniform surface, the floaters cast shadows on the back of the eye, producing little dark spots that dart about immediately in front of you. Although floaters are usually harmless, dense or persistent floaters may be a symptom of a more serious, vision-threatening condition that requires treatment.

THE RETINA

The innermost of the eye's three layers, the retina resembles a very thin, fragile meshwork, which explains its name—*rete* is Latin for "fisherman's net." Although no thicker than a postage stamp, this delicate structure has a complex, layered organization. Figure 2.8 shows how a section of the retina would look if viewed from the side. The arrows represent the direction taken by incoming light. Notice that in this view, the retina lies just below the vitreous, with the choroid underneath the retina. The incoming light must pass through a complex of neural elements before reaching the **photoreceptors** which are actually responsible for converting light energy into neural signals. Those neural signals, in turn, pass through a network of diverse cells we lump together under the

rubric **collector cells.*** The output from the network of collector cells provides the input to the retinal ganglion cells whose axons form the optic nerve. The photoreceptors and ganglion cells are discussed in great detail later in this chapter and in the next two chapters.

To a large degree, the retina's complexity reflects its origins. Embryologically, the retina derives from the same tissue out of which the brain itself develops. So the retina is actually a direct extension of the central nervous system. This affinity with the brain has one unfortunate aspect, though: damaged retinal cells, like damaged brain cells, are not replaced. The visual consequences are permanent.

The eye, besides being a window to the outside world, also provides a window through which someone else can look into the body. In fact, the eye is the only place where the nervous system and blood supply can be viewed directly, without surgery. Hermann Helmholtz, the nineteenth-century physicist, physician, mathematician, and philosopher, is credited with the invention of the **ophthalmoscope,**† a simple device for seeing the internal structures of the living human eye, including its retina. Today, variants of Helmholtz's instrument are widely used to examine the inside of the eye and to monitor the health of the central nervous system and blood supply. Millions of examinations are made with this instrument every year, usually using a hand-held, battery-powered model with which you may be familiar.

Retinal Landmarks and Blood Supply. Figure 2.9 (p. 42) shows what is seen when one looks

---

* These so-called collector cells consist of three major classes of neurons: bipolar cells, amacrine cells, and horizontal cells. Together these gather and modify information registered by the receptors. A detailed description of these three classes of cells can be found in Dowling (1987).

† Actually, Charles Babbage, who developed a mechanical digital computer in the middle of the eighteenth century, made a working model of an ophthalmoscope some years before Helmholtz but didn't pursue the project (Rucker, 1971).

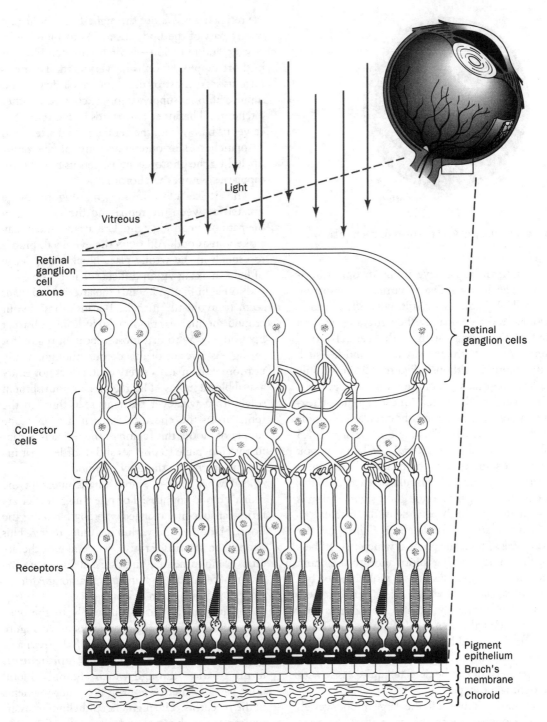

Light

Vitreous

Retinal ganglion cell axons

Retinal ganglion cells

Collector cells

Receptors

Pigment epithelium

Bruch's membrane

Choroid

FIGURE 2.8 Cross section of the retina. The small box in the inset shows the region of the eye represented in the enlarged drawing.

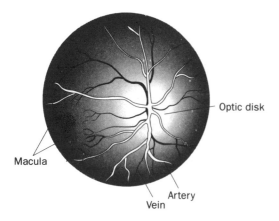

Optic disk

Macula

Artery

Vein

FIGURE 2.9 The inside of the back of the human eye.

into a normal human eye using an ophthalmoscope. The living retina is virtually transparent (Records, 1979b). As a result, what the ophthalmoscope reveals is mainly the structures lying in front of the retina—such as the central retinal artery—and the structures lying behind it—such as the choroid. Although Figure 2.9 shows only the rearmost one-sixth of the retina, it does highlight several of the retina's most significant features. Look first at the nearly circular area indicated by the arrows. This region, measuring 1.5 millimeters, is called the **macula.** When you look directly at some object, the image of that object is centered within the macula of each eye; this part of the retina is vital for good sight. Vision is most acute right in the middle of the macula.

Consider another landmark in Figure 2.9, the **optic disk.** This is the point at which nerve fibers exit the retina, carrying information to the brain. Generally, the optic disk has a pinkish color because of small blood vessels on its surface; these nourish part of the optic nerve. Loss of this pink color signifies the presence of some circulatory problem that could eventually starve the optic nerve and impair vision. Fortunately, such changes in color can be detected quite easily with the ophthalmoscope.

Notice in Figure 2.9 the large blood vessels that run outward from the optic disk; these are labeled "artery" and "vein." The arterial branches supply blood to a large part of the retina. Since the retina has just about the highest metabolic rate of any part of the body, its access to blood—for oxygen and nutrition—is vital. So when blood is in short supply, vision is hit very hard. To minimize its risk, most of the retina has a dual blood supply; if one supply is obstructed, the other pitches in. The inner two-thirds of the retina receives its blood from the central retinal artery and its branches. The outer one-third of the retina (including the photoreceptors) gets its blood from capillaries within the choroid.

The arteries and veins shown in Figure 2.9 are situated between the retina and the vitreous, in the path of incoming light. This arrangement may strike you as odd. Although the eye needs blood, too much in the wrong place blocks the passage of light, making vision difficult or impossible.

Notice in Figure 2.9 that the arteries and veins seem to avoid the macula. Because they detour around the macula, blood vessels do not obstruct light on its way to that most important region for seeing. As a result of this detour, though, a tiny portion of the macula's very center does not enjoy a dual blood supply. This region gets nourishment solely from whatever nutrients seep through the retina from the choroid. Since it has only one supply of blood, this region of the retina is particularly vulnerable to diseases and disorders that interrupt or impede the flow of blood.

But what sorts of things might interrupt the retina's blood supplies? For one thing, feeder arteries can become clogged, thereby blocking the flow of blood to and within the inner retina. This happens in arteriosclerosis ("hardening of the arteries") and sometimes in sickle cell disease, a condition of relatively high incidence among Africans and people of African descent.

Impairment of the blood supply to the *outer* retina also has disastrous consequences. As Figure 2.8 shows, the outermost layer of the retina, a single layer of cells, the **pigment epithelium,** forms a barrier through which choroidal blood must pass in order to nourish the outer segments of the receptors. The pigment epithelium transfers oxygen, nourishment, and vitamin A from the choroidal circulation to the rods. A steady supply of vitamin A is required for the synthesis of the receptors' light-sensitive pigment, as will be discussed in more detail later in this chapter.

The pigment epithelium has one other role: waste disposal. Material that has been shed by the receptors is taken up and recycled within the pigment epithelium; if the debris accumulates, it can eventually impede the transfer of nutrients. So anything that keeps pigment epithelium cells from performing their tasks will cause photoreceptor starvation and, eventually, death.

Among the forces that may harm the pigment epithelium is aging. Age-related macular degeneration, a condition that causes a progressive loss of vision, accounts for about one-half of the cases of blindness among the elderly. Currently, the minority of cases of age-related macular degeneration can be arrested, but not reversed, if treated early by means of laser surgery.

Diabetes is another common disease that can affect the retina's blood supply. This disease is marked by disordered insulin metabolism that causes too much sugar to accumulate in the diabetic's blood. By means not completely understood, the excess sugar promotes the development of a cataract in the eye's crystalline lens. The cataract then reduces vision. But diabetes has another serious consequence for vision. In some diabetics, the retina's blood supply is severely reduced. Sensing that it is being starved for oxygen (carried in the blood), the retina generates a chemical to stimulate the growth of new, large blood vessels. Growing new blood vessels may sound like an excellent solution to the problem, but it brings devastation of its own. The thick new vessels grow out of control, blocking light and causing eventual blindness. In the last decade, lasers have been used very successfully to stop the growth of these new vessels.

THE EYE AS AN OPTICAL INSTRUMENT

Vision requires that light entering the eye be captured and then converted, or transduced, into electrical activity that can be processed by neural elements in the eye and in the brain. In order for you to see the world around you, the pattern of light reaching the retina should mirror the distribution of light in the scene being viewed. This light distribution, or **retinal image** as it's called, is the raw material on which the retina works. The fidelity of the retinal image depends on a host of factors, including the way various ocular structures interact with the incoming light. Obviously then, to appreciate the workings of the retina first requires understanding something about the image it receives.

Light brings the eyes information about objects in the environment. But how does light acquire that information in the first place? Initially, light originates from a source such as the sun or a light bulb. This is called emitted light. However, for purposes of seeing, the more important form of light is that which is reflected off objects and surfaces. It is this reflected light that picks up and carries information about perceptually relevant objects and events (Gibson, 1966). How is this accomplished?

Surfaces absorb some, but not all, of the light shining on them; the portion of light not absorbed is reflected by the surface. Objects with high reflectance usually appear "light," whereas objects with low reflectance appear "dark." For example, this page has a reflectance of about 80 percent, whereas the print on this page has a reflectance of about 10 percent. Abrupt changes in reflectance usually signal discontinuities in a surface, such as those demarcating edges, corners, or the like (see the top drawing in Figure 2.10). More gradual changes in reflectance usually correspond to curved surfaces (see the middle drawing in Figure 2.10).

There are other kinds of differences in the ways in which surfaces reflect light. For example, some surfaces reflect light evenly in many different directions. Lacking highlights—areas of particularly strong reflection—such surfaces appear dull or matte. Other surfaces reflect light in only one or in very few directions, giving the surface highlights and making it appear glossy (Greenberg, 1989). These differences can be seen in the bottom drawing in Figure 2.10. In other words, reflected light conveys information about the texture of surfaces.

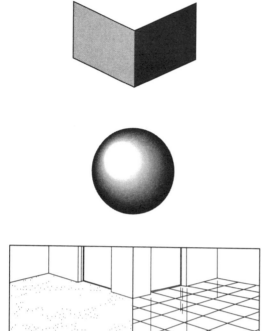

FIGURE 2.10 The top drawing illustrates how abrupt changes in reflectance signal the presence of an edge. The middle drawing illustrates how gradual changes in reflectance signal the presence of a smooth surface. The bottom drawing shows how reflected light specifies the texture of a surface.

These are just some of the ways in which objects in the environment "sculpt" light and provide potential information. But before that potential can be realized, three prerequisites must be satisfied. First, the light must be sufficiently intense to penetrate the eye, reaching the photosensitive material in the retina. In fact, about 50 percent of the light striking the cornea is reflected or absorbed before reaching the retina (Cornsweet, 1970, p. 24). This can have practical consequences under conditions of very dim illumination (Hess, Sharpe, and Nordby, 1990).

Second, the distribution of light—the retinal image—must be properly focused. Think of an object as a set of very small points. To produce a sharp image of that object, light from any of its points should form a small, compact pattern on the retina. A blurred image would be created if each small point in space was imaged as a large, spread-out distribution on the retina. In this case, distributions from neighboring points on the retina would overlap, blurring one another's boundaries and making it difficult to see separate, individual points. Among other consequences, blur would make reading impossible, because the individual letters would be indistinguishable. Some effects of blur are illustrated in Figure 2.11.

Finally, the pattern of light falling on the retina must preserve the spatial structure of the object from which it is reflected. If that spatial structure is preserved, light arising from two adjacent points in space—from neighboring parts of an object, for instance—will fall on adjacent points of the retina. A distribution of light that preserves the spatial ordering of points in space is called an **image.** If the light distribution on the retina were scrambled or spatially random, it would be useless as a source of information about the structure and layout of objects.

IMAGE FORMATION IN THE HUMAN EYE

The sharpness of images formed on the retina depends mainly on two factors. The first is the optical power of the cornea and crystalline lens (where "optical power" means ability to bend, or refract, light). The other factor controlling image sharpness is the size of the eyeball, particularly the eyeball's length from front to back. In a camera, a good picture requires that the film be just the right distance from the lens. In the eye, the same thing holds: the retina must be the right distance from the crystalline lens. Some eyes are too short, others are too long; either condition impairs vision.

The optical power of the eye is not constant, though. By changing its shape somewhat, the crystalline lens automatically changes its optical power. This automatic change, called accommodation, helps one see objects clearly, regardless of their distance from the eye. To appreciate how these components of the eye contribute to vision, we'll have to consider the behavior of light and its interaction with these components. To simplify

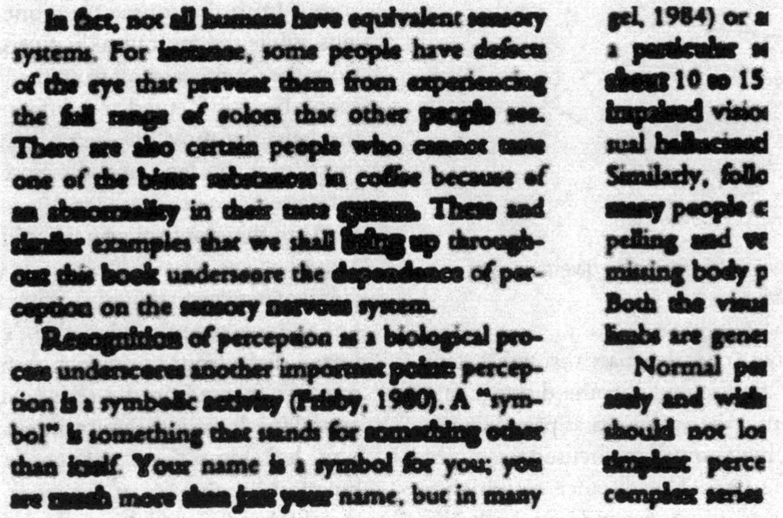

In fact, not all humans have equivalent sensory systems. For instance, some people have defects of the eye that prevent them from experiencing the full range of colors that other people see. There are also certain people who cannot taste one of the bitter substances in coffee because of an abnormality in their taste system. These and similar examples that we shall bring up throughout this book underscore the dependence of perception on the sensory nervous system.

Recognition of perception as a biological process underscores another important point: perception is a symbolic activity (Frisby, 1980). A "symbol" is something that stands for something other than itself. Your name is a symbol for you; you are much more than just your name, but in many

gel, 1984) or a particular s about 10 to 15 impaired vision sual hallucinat Similarly, follo many people c pelling and ve missing body p Both the visua limbs are gene Normal pe sorely and with should not los simplest perce complex series

FIGURE 2.11 Effect of blur on the legibility of text. (For a legible version, you can find these paragraphs on page 3.)

our analysis of image formation, we'll begin with a very small object: a single point in space that emits light. The same analysis works for other, more complex visual objects, since we can think of them as consisting of a large set of points. But dealing with just one point will simplify our explanation of the rudiments of image formation.

In the eighteenth century, Thomas Young showed that light could be treated as though it consisted of waves. Upon dropping a pebble into a pond, you'll see wavefronts spreading out from the place where the stone hit the water. The stone corresponds to our point of light, and radiating out from the point is a set of spherical wavefronts (see Figure 2.12). Light that spreads out in this way is said to be **divergent.** Divergent light cannot form a well-focused image—a point—unless something is done to reverse its divergence. Let's examine how the eye accomplishes this feat. Certain optical devices can counteract light's tendency to diverge. One such device is a convex lens, which gets its name from its shape. Once a diverging wavefront passes through a strong convex lens, the paths of neighboring points on the wavefront get progressively closer together and eventually converge to a single point. After pass-

ing through this point, light diverges once again. Figure 2.13 illustrates this effect of a convex lens.

Lenses differ in their ability, or power, to converge light. A highly convex lens converges light more strongly than does a mildly convex lens. As

FIGURE 2.12 Light waves radiate out from a source of light in a way that resembles the ripples produced when a pebble is dropped into a pond.

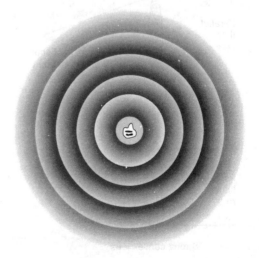

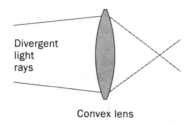

FIGURE 2.13 A convex lens focuses diverging light.

Figure 2.14 shows, rays that pass through a lens of lower power are focused at some distance farther from the lens, whereas rays that pass through a convex lens of high power are focused to a point very close to the lens. The distance at which a lens brings light to focus depends on both the power of the lens itself and the degree of divergence of the light striking the lens. To converge the light, a convex lens must overcome, or null, the light's divergence. This is demonstrated in Figure 2.15: a lens of constant power is shown converging light of three different degrees of divergence. The most strongly divergent light

FIGURE 2.14 Convex lenses of different power bring light to focus at different distances. If the light rays striking the lens are parallel, the spot at which the light converges to a point is called the *focal point*.

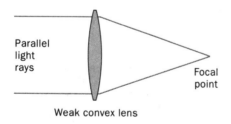

Weak convex lens

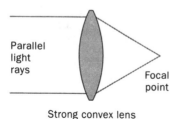

Strong convex lens

comes from the source positioned closest to the lens, while the most weakly divergent light comes from the source farthest from the lens. In addition, each object is focused at a different distance from the lens: the most divergent light is focused farthest from the lens, and the least divergent light is focused closest to the lens.

With these optical principles in mind, consider a human eye that is looking at an object sufficiently far away that light coming from that object has essentially zero divergence. To form a useful image, light from the object, as from any object, must be focused on the retina. Since cornea and crystalline lens both contribute to image formation, let's lump them together, calling the combination "the optics of the eye." How powerful should those optics be in order to produce a sharp retinal image of that distant object? For the retinal image to be sharply focused, the optics' power must match the length of the eyeball—specifically, the distance from the lens to the retina.

This idea is shown in Figure 2.16 (p. 47). The top eyeball is just the right length, given the power of its optics. As a result, the distant object is brought to focus exactly on the retina. Such an eye is described as **emmetropic** (meaning "in the right measure or size").

The middle panel shows an eye that is too long, given the strength of its optics. Although an image *is* formed, that image is formed in front of the retina, rather than on it. In fact, the rays have begun to diverge again by the time they reach the retina, so the image on the retina is blurred. Such an eye is described as **myopic,** or nearsighted, because near objects will be in best focus.

The bottom panel in Figure 2.16 shows an eye that is too short for its optics; an image is formed on the retina, but it, too, is not well focused and hence the image is blurred. Actually, for this eye the best-focused image would lie behind the retina—if light were able to pass through the retina. Such an eye is described as **hyperopic,** or farsighted, because far objects will be in best focus.

What are the perceptual consequences of a mismatch between an eye's length and its optics? You've seen that in myopic or hyperopic eyes, light does reach the retina, but that it is not sharply

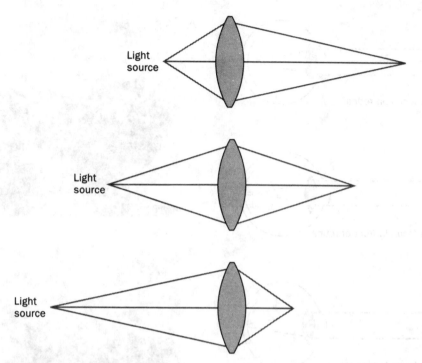

FIGURE 2.15 The spot at which a convex lens brings light to a point depends on the degree of divergence of the light arriving at the lens.

focused. When an eye of the wrong size looks at a distant point, the resulting image on the retina will be a circular patch, not a point. Thus the point in space will appear blurred, or indistinct.

The degree of blur depends on the extent to which the eye is too short, or too long: the greater the mismatch between the eye's optics and its length, the worse the blur. The photographs in Figure 2.17 illustrate how the world might appear to a properly focused eye (panel A), to an eye that is only one-third of a millimeter too long (panel B), and to an eye that is 2 millimeters too long (panel C). Remember that when we describe an eye as "too long" or "too short," we mean this in relative terms. "Too long" and "too short" are defined relative to the power of the eye's optics.

The blur in panels B and C is so striking that it is hard to imagine that many people actually suffer for years unwittingly with that much blur or more. They go through their entire childhood and adolescence never realizing that their vision

is defective. For reasons that are explained below, if their vision is blurred from myopia, they may have trouble seeing the chalkboard clearly; if the blur comes from hyperopia, they may have trouble reading for prolonged periods. Unfortunately, the difficulties they experience in school may be mistakenly attributed to poor learning abilities rather than to poor vision.

Since much of the human race is afflicted with these problems, it's worth some time to consider various errors of image formation in the eye and what steps can be taken to correct those errors.

Hyperopia. Imagine an eye whose length and optical power are properly matched. For that eye, a distant object would be in proper focus on the retina. Recall that proper focus demands an object just far enough from the eye so that wavefronts from the object, when they strike the eye, will be diverging at the right rate. If that same eye were shortened—making it hyperopic—by even a frac-

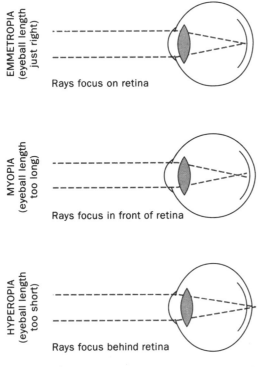

FIGURE 2.16 Image formation in emmetropic, myopic, and hyperopic eyes.

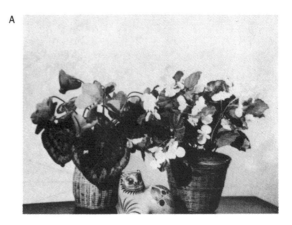

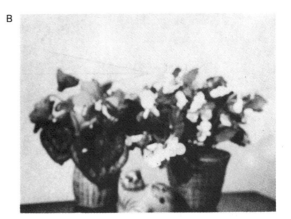

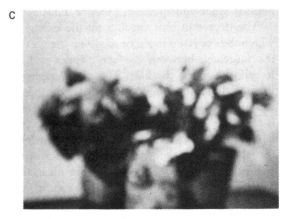

FIGURE 2.17 Focus influences the quality of the image. Panel A simulates the image formed by an emmetropic eye; panel B, by a mildly myopic eye; and panel C, by a more severely myopic eye. (Glyn Cloyd.)

tion of a millimeter, the distant object would no longer be focused as well on the retina. The plane in which the image would be focused best would lie behind the retina, not right on it (see top panel of Figure 2.18). In its shortened state, this eye's optics would be too weak even for light coming from an object so distant that it is not diverging at all. If it has to deal with light from closer objects (even more strongly diverging), the eye will misfocus the light by even more.

A person with hyperopia—a hyperope—can alleviate this problem by accommodating, increasing the eye's optical power. This enables the hyperope to produce focused images of objects, provided the eye is not too hyperopic and provided the objects are not too close. Accommodation makes the lens more convex, thereby increasing its power and allowing well-focused images to be formed on the retina. The middle panel of Figure

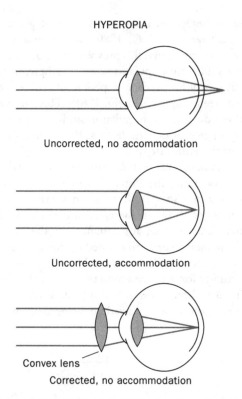

HYPEROPIA

Uncorrected, no accommodation

Uncorrected, accommodation

Convex lens

Corrected, no accommodation

FIGURE 2.18 Mild hyperopia can be overcome either by accommodation or by placing a convex lens in front of the eye.

2.18 shows how accommodation helps the hyperope bring an object into better focus on the retina.

But the hyperope pays a price for constant accommodation. First, there are limits to the amount of accommodation that the human eye can produce. As a result, if the eye is much too short and the resulting hyperopia substantial, the hyperope may be unable to accommodate enough for close work, such as reading. Second, even if the hyperope could accommodate enough to read, accommodation requires maintained muscular effort. The very strong, prolonged accommodation, as might be required in order to read, triggers eyestrain, headaches, and nausea (Daum, 1983).

Fortunately, there is an alternative. Since the hyperopic eye cannot make incoming light converge rapidly enough, the light is not focused on the plane of the retina. The problem can be corrected by placing a convex lens in front of the cornea. With such a lens, the total optical power of the eye will be approximately the sum of the eye's own inherent optical power plus the power of the supplementary lens. This increased total optical power allows distant objects to be focused on the retina with little or no accommodation. As a result, the hyperope will need less accommodation when doing close work and will suffer less accommodative strain. The bottom panel of Figure 2.18 illustrates how this added convex lens helps the hyperope see near objects without accommodation.

Myopia. Start again with an eye whose length and optical power are well matched. If that eye were lengthened, making it myopic, a distant object would be focused best not right on the retina, but somewhere in front of it (top panel, Figure 2.19). This situation could be rectified if we moved the object closer to the myopic person, or conversely, if we moved the myopic person closer to the object. Sometimes, of course, neither of these approaches is practical. Nor is it possible for the blur to be corrected by accommodation. In

FIGURE 2.19 A concave lens in front of the eye can correct myopia.

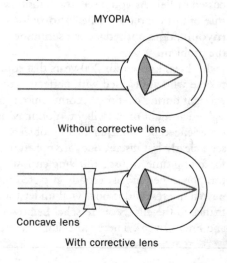

MYOPIA

Without corrective lens

Concave lens

With corrective lens

fact, increasing the power of the crystalline lens increases the overall optical power of the eye, worsening the blur. Fortunately, there is an effective solution to myopia: alter the effective optical power of the eye by placing the proper spectacle lens in front of, or the proper contact lens on, the eye.

What sort of corrective lens would the myopic eye need? We could correct the myopic eye by adding a concave lens (which causes light to *diverge*, combating the myopic eye's tendency to make light *converge* too much). The bottom panel in Figure 2.19 shows how such a lens helps focus an otherwise misfocused target on a myope's retina.

In many countries, myopia is so common that it poses a costly public health problem. For example, in the United States about 20 percent of the adult population is myopic and cannot see distant objects in sharp focus without glasses or contact lenses (NRC, 1989). It is important to note, however, that this prevalence is not uniform across different populations. For example, in Hawaii nearly 80 percent of people of Chinese descent are myopic (Baldwin, 1981). This study and other comparative population studies suggest the importance of genetic factors. But genetics is far from the entire story.

Prevalence varies also with environmental factors, including the visual demands of a person's occupation. So, people who do a great deal of near work show an increased incidence of myopia. This is true, for instance, in the case of submariners. They are cooped up for months on end in very small quarters, with little or no opportunity for distance vision (Kinney et al., 1980). Closer to home, a number of studies have documented the slow but steady development of my-

---

Box 2.2 *Myopia as a Sometime Thing*

Some conditions have the power to diminish even the best vision, converting emmetropes into myopes, though only temporarily. Because this error in the eye's optical power is temporary, it differs from myopia that we discussed earlier. As you'll see, the transitory nature of this condition, called **anomalous myopia,** does not reduce the seriousness of the problem.

It's been known for 200 years that some people who are blessed with perfectly good eyesight during daytime become quite nearsighted at night or at twilight. You may have experienced this yourself: nearby objects are seen clearly but distant ones are not. Ignored for a long time as just a puzzling curiosity, this phenomenon has recently attracted renewed interest and is now well understood, thanks to the efforts of Herschel Leibowitz and Fred Owens. There exist dramatic individual differences in the severity of anomalous myopia (Owens, 1984): some people show virtually no myopia at low light levels, whereas others become extremely nearsighted.

Low light is not the only condition that elicits a temporary myopia. Even in daylight, many individuals become myopic in featureless environments, such as a large open field, or when viewing a clear, cloudless sky. The amount of nearsightedness an individual experiences in such a featureless environment is strongly related to the nearsightedness experienced at twilight (Leibowitz and Owens, 1975). One suspects then that both "open field myopia" and twilight myopia arise from a common cause. And both are subsumed under the general rubric, anomalous myopia.

What causes this condition? At low light levels or in open fields, there is no powerful

opia among college students (NRC, 1989). The importance of environmental factors is clinched by a study in which monkeys spent their waking time on the equivalent of near work. In order to simulate near work, newborn monkeys were reared so that there was nothing for them to see more than 50 centimeters from their eyes. Over a 3-year period, these rearing conditions led to severe, permanent myopia (Young, 1981). And as Box 2.2 describes, certain conditions produce a temporary, reversible form of myopia.

Presbyopia. Myopia and hyperopia affect many individuals. But the eye's focus can be disturbed in yet another way that *everyone* will sooner or later experience.

As people get older, their ability to accommodate decreases. As Figure 2.20 shows, the trend begins very early in life and continues until about age 70 (Carter, 1982). For the average 20- or 30-year-old, this loss has no practical consequence; people that age still have sufficient ability to accommodate. But upon reaching the mid-forties, the average person can no longer accommodate sufficiently to bring very close objects into focus. Reduced accommodation arises from various sources, including sclerosis of the lens and reduced elasticity of the lens's capsule (Koretz and Handelman, 1988). Severely diminished ability to accommodate is called **presbyopia,** meaning "old sight." In addition, an old lens is very sluggish in executing even the small shape changes of which it is still capable. This lengthens the time required to change gaze from near to distant objects, and vice versa, causing potential problems in driving and similar tasks.

You have probably seen signs of presbyopia in people who are beyond 40 years of age but have

stimulus to control the amount of accommodation. Freed from stimulus control, accommodation returns to a preferred neutral, or resting, level. The eye becomes myopic because that resting level is more suited to seeing near objects than very distant ones. In other words, the resting state of accommodation, in many people, does not produce a perfectly relaxed lens with minimal optical power. Instead, the resting state of accommodation leaves the lens focused for relatively nearby distances. Using laser-based instrumentation, Leibowitz and Owens (1975) confirmed that in the dark, most people's eyes tended to focus at some intermediate distance, not optical infinity. The actual distance varied widely among people, with an average value of about 0.67 meters.

The existence of anomalous myopia poses a potentially serious safety threat (Owens, 1984). Imagine you are the pilot of an airplane flying through the nighttime sky or the driver of a car speeding over a dark country road. In both conditions, accommodation will revert to its resting level. This will tend to blur and diminish the visibility of any object that appears within the field of view at a distance other than that associated with the resting level. If you are a pilot, the blurred object might be another aircraft; if you are driving a car, it could be a pedestrian.

Like other refractive errors, anomalous myopia can be remedied optically. Leibowitz and Owens (1976) measured the resting level of accommodation for various individuals and then fitted them with concave corrective lenses of the appropriate power. These glasses, although inappropriate for daylight, nonmyopic conditions, produced impressive improvements in drivers' nighttime vision. Perhaps, sometime in the future, drivers and pilots will be routinely outfitted with in dividually prescribed glasses for nighttime use. The benefits, in lives saved, could be substantial.

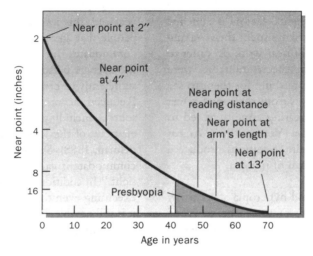

FIGURE 2.20 The *near point*—the closest distance at which an object can be seen without blur—increases with age.

yet to wear glasses or contact lenses. To see clearly, they have to hold reading material at arm's length or even beyond. They may comment that they wished their arms were a bit longer. But a more realistic solution is not too hard. A convex lens in front of the eye substitutes for the crystalline lens's own diminished ability to become sufficiently convex.

Benjamin Franklin, the American statesman and inventor, was about 47 years old when he found that he could no longer read without spectacles. However, his reading glasses made distant objects too blurred. Constantly having to switch from one pair of glasses to another annoyed him, so Franklin invented bifocals—glasses having two separate lenses in front of each eye, with the more strongly convex lens filling the bottom of the frame. Looking down at reading material, Franklin could take advantage of the extra help given by that lens. Looking slightly upward, he could see the world through a less powerful convex lens, allowing him clear vision of distant objects.

Astigmatism. So far, our discussion of image formation in the eye has emphasized the role of the crystalline lens. The cornea, though, contributes more than the lens toward the formation of

a sharply defined retinal image. More precisely, the cornea contributes about two-thirds of the eye's total optical power, with the crystalline lens contributing the rest (see Box 2.3, p. 54). As in the case of the lens, the cornea's shape determines its power—the more spherical the cornea, the more strongly will it converge incoming light. When the cornea is misshapen, the retinal image will be distorted. The most common distortion of shape produces a visual problem called **astigmatism.**

You can test yourself for astigmatism by using the spoke pattern in Figure 2.21. Look at the center of the spoke pattern. Without shifting your

FIGURE 2.21 Chart for testing astigmatism.

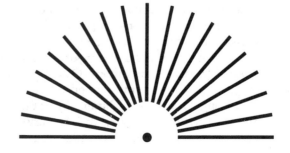

gaze, note whether some lines look lighter or less black than others. If they do, you may have astigmatism. This condition causes lines of one orientation to be well focused on the retina while lines of another orientation (different by 90 degrees) are poorly focused. If you wear glasses that correct an astigmatism, you may want to take this test twice, once with your correction and again without it. You can easily determine whether your glasses correct an astigmatism. While looking through one lens, slowly rotate the glasses through a 90-degree angle and note whether the lines in the chart change in appearance. If they do, your glasses contain a correction for astigmatism.

Almost all eyes have some degree of astigmatism, because the cornea is almost never perfectly shaped. But for some people the astigmatism may be severe enough to interfere with perception. Figure 2.22 illustrates how severe astigmatism can distort the appearance of a common, everyday scene. Astigmatism can be corrected by providing a lens that compensates for the cornea's distortion by an equal and opposite distortion of its own.

* * *

The previous section detailed the optical components responsible for forming images on the back of the eye. Now we're ready to resume looking at this back portion of the eye—the retina—which serves as the screen on which the image is cast. You may be surprised to learn that this screen is actually located *behind* a complex network of nerve cells; the carefully formed image must pass through this network before the image can be registered by the photoreceptors. This would be like projecting a motion picture film in a theater in which there are clumps of bushes located in front of the screen. Let's take a look at this odd but apparently successful arrangement.

A SIDEWAYS LOOK AT THE RETINA

Figure 2.23 (p. 56) shows a thin slice of the retina viewed from its side. This slice was created by carefully removing the retina from the eye,

FIGURE 2.22 The photograph at the right was taken using a lens that simulates astigmatism. (Glyn Cloyd.)

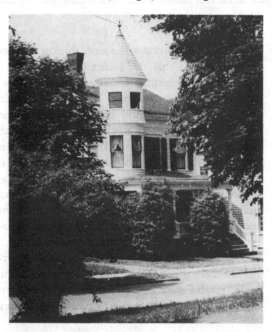 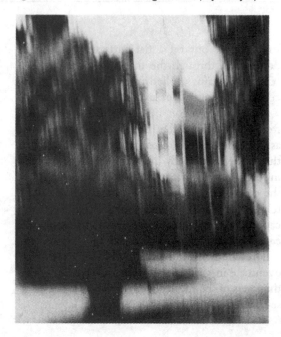

Box 2.3 *Seeing Under Water*

The next time you go swimming, try this experiment. Hold your hand under water and, with your head out of the water, look at your hand. Now, keeping your hand where it was, put your face into the water with eyes open. Looking at your hand, you'll notice it doesn't look as sharp and clear as it did when your eyes were out of the water. The reason is that the cornea has effectively been eliminated as part of the eyes' optical system.

When light moves from air into the cornea, the path it travels is altered. This alteration, or bending, of light is called **refraction.** The amount of refraction depends on the difference between air and the material out of which the cornea is made. Under water, light enters the eye not from air but from the water itself. Because of the strong similarity between water and the material out of which the cornea is constructed—a large percentage of the cornea is water—light from the water

is bent very little as it enters the cornea. Thus when under water, the eye has effectively no cornea. Putting your face under water has reduced the optical power of your eye by about two-thirds, so it's no wonder you can't see so well. Of the eye's usual optical system, only the crystalline lens remains functional. But steps can be taken to restore the effectiveness of your cornea under water. A transparent diving mask keeps water away from direct contact with your corneas, allowing them to work just as they did with your face out of water.

Other creatures also need to use their eyes under water but don't have access to face masks. How do they do it? If an animal spends all its time under water, there's no problem; its eye is designed so that the cornea contributes little optical power anyway. The lens is strong enough to do all the necessary light bending. Most fish eyes have ex-

stretching it out on a flat surface, and cutting downward, through the thickness of the retina. (Chemical stains applied in the laboratory make certain types of cells or layers visually prominent.)

The cross section in Figure 2.23 was taken from the center of the retina, the region known as the macula. This cross section is arranged so that if it were actually in an animal's eye, incoming light would first pass through the *top* part of the cross section. Notice the location of the photoreceptors, those specialized neurons that actually capture the light. They are situated toward the *bottom* of the drawing. This means that before light can reach them and initiate the responses that eventuate in vision, light must traverse the entire thickness of the retina. Let's think about the consequences of this seemingly backward layout.

Not all the retina is of the same thickness. Note in Figure 2.23 that the retina thins out in the center of the macula, forming a pit called the **fovea** (in Latin, *fovea* means "pit"). The retina in the foveal neighborhood is thin because some overlying structures have been peeled away. This thinness is crucial for sharp vision. The reason is that as light goes through the retina, some of it is absorbed or scattered before it can reach the photoreceptors. The thinness of the retina's fovea minimizes these problems. In fact, this thinness may be an absolute necessity. Most regions of the retina contain not only photoreceptors but also an entire array of other neurons that gather information from the receptors and pass it along to the brain (recall Figure 2.8). Normally, these neurons lie directly above the receptors with which they

tremely powerful convex crystalline lenses—a perfect adaptation to their aquatic world.

But what about animals who spend some time above water and some below? They face the same problem that humans do. We'll consider two particularly interesting creatures who solve this challenge in different ways. Think about the problem that a diving bird faces. Flying along, it looks for fish swimming near the surface of the water below. When it spots a fish, the bird dives into the water and tries to snatch the fish. But as soon as it enters the water, the bird's cornea will lose its optical power, handicapping the bird visually. Some diving birds avoid this effect by using the equivalent of an adjustable face mask. The cormorant, for instance, has a thick but partially transparent eyelid that closes when the bird enters the water. Keeping water from coming into contact with the bird's cornea, the lid preserves much of the cornea's optical power.

But some animals face a situation that is even more demanding optically. Instead of going into and out of the water, these creatures are simultaneously both in and out of the water. The most famous of these creatures is *Anableps anableps,* a freshwater fish found in South and Central America. Because some of its food supply consists of insects above the water, anableps swims along the surface of the river, its eyes half under water and half above water. Anableps has a rather interesting adaptation to this peculiar environmental niche. The upper portion of anableps's eye (the part that is exposed to air) is distinct from the lower portion (the part that is exposed to water). Anableps has two pupils in each eye (one below and the other above the water). In addition, the lower half of its lens is more powerful than the upper half. Anableps is commonly referred to as *cuatro ojos* (Spanish for "four eyes"), but having four eyes rather than two suits anableps's life style very well indeed.

communicate. In the fovea, though, their cell bodies are displaced, producing a circular mound that surrounds the foveal pit. This displacement reduces the obstacles to the passage of incoming light to this particularly important region of the retina (Hughes, 1977).

With this overview of image formation and the retina firmly in mind, let's now consider how the photoreceptor cells in the retina sense the presence of light and initiate the process of seeing.

THE PHOTORECEPTORS

The human eye contains two major classes of photoreceptors: **rods** and **cones.** In humans, each eye contains about 120 million rods and approx-imately 8 million cones. Typical examples of the two types of photoreceptors are shown in Figure 2.24. The two types derive their names from their appearance. The tip of a cone is tapered, resembling a spruce tree or an empty ice cream cone. In contrast, the tip of a rod has straighter sides and a blunt end—it is rodlike. But their differences go well beyond shape. In fact, functional differences between the two types of photoreceptors determine the life style of their owners. Creatures who have a preponderance of rods in their retinas, such as the owl, are active at night. Creatures who have a preponderance of cones, such as the squirrel, tend to be active only during daylight hours. Because human beings have duplex retinas, containing both types of photoreceptors, their activity is not limited to a fixed part of the day-night cycle.

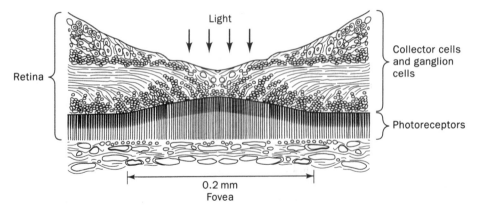

FIGURE 2.23 A sideways view of the central portion of the human retina. (Redrawn from Polyak, 1941.)

Think back to the analogy between the eye and a camera: the eyes' photoreceptors would be analogous to the camera's film. Because human eyes contain two types of photoreceptors, they

FIGURE 2.24 A single rod photoreceptor and a single cone photoreceptor, magnified approximately 1,500 times.

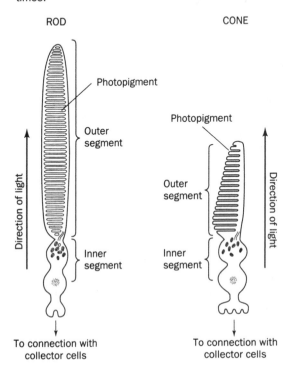

resemble a camera that holds two different kinds of film at once. The type of film in a camera—color versus black and white—determines what kind of pictures are produced. The eye has two different kinds of "film" (rods and cones) at once. And this duplex nature of the retina produces some interesting idiosyncrasies in the way humans see.

Because the kinds of photoreceptors that creatures have determine the properties of their vision—including what they can see, when they can see it, and how it looks to them—those photoreceptors deserve detailed consideration.

THE GEOGRAPHY OF RODS AND CONES

Rods and cones differ not only in their shapes and numbers but also in their geographical distributions. Looking within a very small portion of retina at the center of the macula discloses only cones, no rods. Looking far from the macula, you will find predominantly rods, with only a scattering of cones. Our two types of "film," then, are distributed across the eye in very different ways.

Figure 2.25 shows the density of rods and cones in samples taken from various parts of the retina. A sample from the very center of the macula is represented over the center of the horizontal axis; samples taken at various distances, leftward and rightward, from the macula are represented above other points on the horizontal axis. Cones are

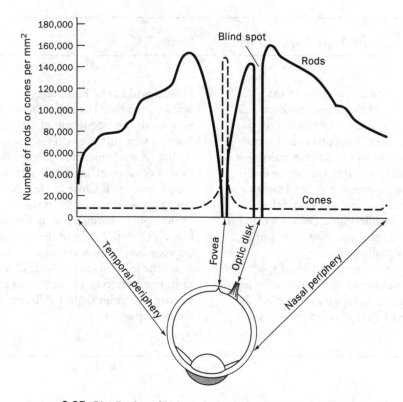

FIGURE 2.25 Distribution of rods and cones over the extent of the retina of the right eye, as seen from above. In the left eye, the nasal and temporal areas of the retina would appear reversed, but the relative distributions of rods and cones would be the same. Note the complete absence of rods within the fovea, where cones abound.

packed densely in the very center of the human macula; about 150,000 cones occupy an area 1 millimeter square (about the size of this letter: o). Note the systematic decrease in the number and proportion of cones as you move away from the center of the macula, and a corresponding increase in the number of rods. In fact, about 7 millimeters away from the fovea—along the retina in a direction toward the nose—rods reach a density approximately the same as that found for cones in the center of the macula. Various parts of the retina make their own characteristic contributions to vision because the prevalence of rods and cones differs from one retinal region to another.

Notice the interruption in the plots shown in Figure 2.25. This gap reflects the complete ab-

sence of photoreceptors at the optic disk. Because you cannot see without photoreceptors, you are actually "blind" within that area of retina where there are no receptors. We referred earlier to an analogy between the retina and photographic film. In this analogy, the optic disk resembles a defective area of the film, on which the factory neglected to put any light-sensitive chemical. If that defective film were used in a camera and developed, the resulting picture would have a noticeable blank region. Surprisingly though, people almost never notice the large gap that the optic disks create in their retinas. Box 2.4 will help you see what you've been missing all these years.

The array of more than 100 million photoreceptors in each eye converts the retinal image into

Box 2.4 *A Gap in Your Visual Field*

"Optic disk" is the name given to the place where the axons of the retinal ganglion cells come together to form the optic nerve. Because this region of the retina contains no photoreceptors, it cannot support vision—it is literally a blind spot. Note that we're distinguishing between a region defined anatomically, the optic disk, and a region defined perceptually, the blind spot. Before we go on about the blind spot, you may want some proof that it actually exists.

Of course you cannot *see* a blind spot (though you can see an optic disk, using an ophthalmoscope). What you can see are the consequences of your blind spot—an object imaged within this blind region of your retina will be invisible. The figure below will help you see the consequences of this blind spot. Making sure that the book is propped up at right angles to the tabletop, view the figure from a distance of about 60 centimeters (about two feet). Close the left eye and, using your right eye only, stare at the fixation cross in the figure. At this viewing distance, the black disk to the right of the cross should fall on your optic disk and therefore disappear. Since the location of the optic disk varies from one person to the next, you may have to stare at a point slightly different from the fixation cross.

X

Fixation cross

a neural image that will be transmitted to the brain. The quality of information contained in the neural image is set, in large part, by the way the photoreceptors are distributed over the retina. If each square millimeter of retina contains too few receptors, part of the spatial detail present in the retinal image will not be captured in the neural image, and consequently, some spatial detail will not be perceived.

To capture the detail in the retinal image, the photoreceptors take simultaneous samples of the light intensities at various retinal sites. If there are too few photoreceptors to create a sufficient number of different samples, some spatial detail will be lost. Imagine, for example, looking at a pattern of alternating dark and light bars. If your eyes are focused properly, the image on your retina will contain variations in light intensity that correspond to the pattern's bars. In order for you to perceive the details of the pattern, though, your photoreceptors' responses must capture those details.

To see how this might work, consider Figure 2.26. In each panel of that figure, the alternating dark and light bars constitute a pattern that is imaged on the retina; as you can see, the pattern in panel B is relatively coarse compared with the one in panel A, whereas the patterns in panels C and D are relatively fine. In each panel, striped cylinders represent a series of photoreceptors that are evenly spaced across some region of the retina. Finally, each photoreceptor's response to the light falling on it is shown by the height of the black bar immediately below the photoreceptor. Note

The demonstration of the existence of a blind spot represented a milestone in understanding the eye. Edmé Mariotte, the French scientist who discovered the blind spot in 1668, did not simply stumble upon it by accident (Mariotte, 1668/1948). Instead, his dissection of human eyes suggested to him that vision might be impaired in the region of the optic disk. This was the first time that anyone had predicted a previously unknown perceptual phenomenon simply from an anatomical observation. From the geometry of the eyeball, including the location of the optic disk, Mariotte correctly predicted where stimuli would have to be placed relative to a fixation point in order for the image to fall on the optic disk. Mariotte also confirmed that there were individual variations in the precise location of the blind spot, corresponding to individual variations in the optic disk itself.

It's been claimed that England's "merry monarch," Charles II, exploited the retina's blind spot to "behead" symbolically members of his court who were in disfavor (Rushton, 1979). After placing them at the right distance from his throne, Charles would adjust his gaze so that the head of his "victim" was imaged on the king's optic disk. Although this is an intriguing story, the more so because Charles II's father had in fact been beheaded, Adam Reeves (1982) describes the story as "a baseless canard" against Charles II. Frankly, we're not sure who's correct.

While you were looking for your own blind spot, you may have noticed something strange. When the black disk disappeared, you didn't see even a shadow or other residue of the disk; the background appeared uniformly white. This is a common phenomenon called *completion*, or "filling in." The blind spot has been cleverly exploited by Ramachandran (1992) to study the filling-in phenomenon in some detail. His article, which contains some delightful demonstrations, concludes that completion of vision across the blindspot is just one instance of a more general process called interpolation; this aspect of perception we shall take up in Chapter 7.

that a receptor stimulated by a bright bar responds more strongly than does a receptor stimulated by a dark bar.

In panel A, the pattern's bars match the spacing of the receptors, and therefore, the distribution in response magnitude from receptor to receptor accurately mirrors the variation of light in the retinal image (and, hence, in the pattern actually being looked at). In other words, each dark stripe and light stripe in the stimulus has a counterpart in the response of a receptor; all the stimulus information is captured by the receptor array. Panel B demonstrates that the same array would also give a faithful representation of a pattern that is coarser than the spacing of the photoreceptors.

But there is an upper limit to the information that any receptor array can capture. When a pattern gets too fine for that array, the receptors can no longer produce a faithful representation. For the array shown, the pattern in panel C exceeds the limit imposed by the receptor spacing. Although the pattern consists of eight dark and eight light stripes, the photoreceptor responses indicate (erroneously) the presence of just three, quite broad, dark and light bars.

If one knows how the photoreceptors are packed, it's possible to calculate the finest pattern that any particular array of receptors could reproduce (Yellott, 1982). In the foveas of most young adults, the photoreceptors are packed very densely, in an orderly arrangement that produces a near-constant distance between neighbors. As one progresses away from the center of the retina, the distances increase between neighboring receptors and the orderliness of the packing diminishes (Hirsch and Miller, 1987). When the photoreceptors are photographed end-on, they suggest a carefully laid mosaic, such as one would make out of small, hexagonal tiles. In the center of the retina, this remarkably orderly and tightly packed mosaic allows the photoreceptor array to reproduce the finest details that the eye's optics can transmit to the retina.

Panel C showed that when a pattern's details

are too fine, relative to the arrangement of receptors, information is lost. There is one way to prevent this: simply pack the receptors more tightly together. This is illustrated in panel D. Note that a tighter packing produces a receptor array that manages to capture the variation in this relatively fine pattern. Of course, even this densely packed array could be fooled if one made the fine pattern even finer.

In panel C of Figure 2.26, not only do the receptors fail to capture the relatively finely detailed pattern; their responses actually create a different, illusory, coarse pattern. The creation of illusory, coarse patterns from real, finer ones is called **aliasing.** This process comes about when a photoreceptor mosaic is relatively coarse compared to the fine detail in the pattern imaged on the mosaic.

In the human eye, the photoreceptor mosaic is well matched to the spatial detail in the image, so aliasing normally isn't experienced. But it can be. When two weak laser beams are imaged in the eye's pupil, the two beams interact (add and subtract from one another) to set up very finely detailed patterns on the retina, far finer than could be produced with normal light. These laser-generated patterns are so fine, relative to the receptor

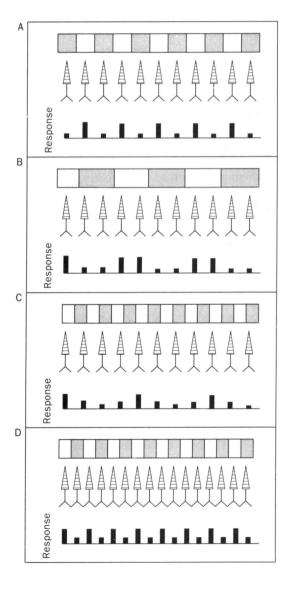

FIGURE 2.26 In each panel, A through D, the top row of alternating dark and light rectangles represents the distribution of stimulus light across some section of the retina; the middle row of cone-shaped objects represents the distribution of photoreceptors across that same section of retina. In the bottom row, labeled "Response," the height of each dark bar represents the magnitude of response generated by the corresponding photoreceptor. Note the variation in the stimulus among the panels: individual dark/light regions are of intermediate size in panel A, are widest in panel B, and narrowest in panels C and D. Note also the variation in spacing between photoreceptors: the spacing is constant from panel A through panel C, but is reduced in panel D. As the text indicates, the responses of the photoreceptors in panels A, B, and D accurately reproduce the spatial distribution of stimulus light on the retina. But in panel C the narrow dark/light regions would give rise to the illusory appearance of broad dark/light regions. See the text for details.

packing, that they do produce aliasing in the eye. The character of these illusory patterns reveals how densely packed the human photoreceptors are and how orderly the packing is (Williams, 1988). Incidentally, aliasing effects can be produced outside the eye as well. You may have noticed some aliasing on television, when someone's suit has a fine pinstriped pattern. Television's coarse sampling of the pinstripes creates wavy, coarse stripes.

We've commented admiringly on the exquisite packing of photoreceptors in the central retina of the human adult and on the contribution of that packing to the excellence of vision. The situation is quite different, though, for young infants. It takes about 4 years for an infant's retina to reach its final, adult state. During that time, photoreceptors migrate toward the center of the retina from the periphery, a migration that creates the pit known as the fovea. Even as late as 15 months of age, the distance between neighboring photoreceptors of the central retina is twice the comparable value in the adult eye (Yuodelis and Hendrickson, 1986). Although some of infants' poor visual acuity arises from the immature state of their brains, the lion's share results from immaturity at the retinal level (Banks and Bennett, 1988; Teller and Movshon, 1986).

An analogous, though far less dramatic, change occurs at the other end of the life span. In old age, the packing of receptors in the central retina changes because of cell death and other factors (Weale, 1986). Undoubtedly, this contributes to the drop in acuity that accompanies aging (Owsley, Sekuler, and Siemsen, 1983).

Although retinal anatomy and retinal function follow parallel courses, in some humans, retinal anatomy and retinal function are permanently arrested at the infant stage. These humans, whose skin, hair, and eyes lack pigmentation, have a genetic disorder known as albinism (Abadi and Pascal, 1989). Melanin, the pigment that can give color to skin, hair, and eyes, is particularly abundant in the macular region of the normal retina. The melanin promotes the inward migration of photoreceptors and the formation of the foveal pit. The albino eye, lacking melanin, does not have much receptor migration and never develops a foveal pit. As a result, the number of photoreceptors per unit area in the central retina of the albino eye is far below that of pigmented adults. Hugh Wilson and colleagues have studied the vision of human albinos and liken their central retinal anatomy and function to that of a normal 10-month-old (Wilson, Mets, Nagy, and Kressel, 1988). All these unusual cases—infants, the aged, and albinos—reinforce the idea that the retina's photoreceptor mosaic sets important limits on the information that can be extracted from the retinal image.

THE FIRST STEP TOWARD SEEING

Light registers its presence on the retina by interacting with special light-sensitive molecules contained within the photoreceptors. Each of these molecules, called **photopigments,** consists of two components: a very large protein, *opsin,* and another component, *retinal,* derived from vitamin A. The retinal is the same for all human photopigments, but the molecular structure of the opsin varies, giving different photopigments their characteristic properties.

Normally, the two components are tightly connected, producing a stable molecule that won't break up spontaneously. But when light strikes a molecule, the molecule changes shape, or *isomerizes,* thereby releasing energy. Once this shape change occurs, the photopigment molecule is no longer stable and its two components undergo a series of changes, eventually splitting apart. This change in shape alters the flow of electric current in and around the photoreceptor. The entire chain of events—from absorption to isomerization to current flow—occurs in less than a thousandth of a second. To appreciate how this chain of events leads to seeing, let's look more closely at the absorption of light by the photoreceptor.

Exposing a photoreceptor to light from various regions of the wavelength spectrum makes it possible to measure how much of that light is actually absorbed and, therefore, stimulates the photoreceptor. When this is done, one finds that for any given receptor there is one wavelength of light that most strongly stimulates the receptor—that is, there is one wavelength to which the receptor is most sensitive. Rods give their biggest response when stimulated with approximately 500 nanometers (the wavelength of light is measured in **nanometers,** billionths of a meter); shorter or longer wavelengths give a diminished response. This response is illustrated in Figure 2.27. In order to appreciate the stimulus to which rods are most sensitive, you should know that under daylight conditions, light of 500 nanometers looks bluish-green.

The corresponding story for cones is somewhat more complicated, since the wavelength at which sensitivity is optimum depends on *which* type of cone is being studied. There are three distinct classes of cones. One is maximally responsive to light of about 440 nanometers, a second class responds best to light of 530 nanometers, and a third class has its peak response at 560 nanometers. The responses of these three classes of cones are shown in Figure 2.28 as functions of the wavelength of stimulating light. Again, to help you understand these stimuli, consider that under daylight conditions, light of 440 nanometers looks violet, light of 530 nanometers looks green, and light of 560 nanometers looks yellow.

FIGURE 2.27 This graph shows how the amount of light absorbed by rod photoreceptors varies with the wavelength of the light.

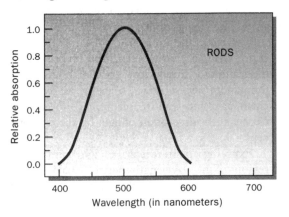

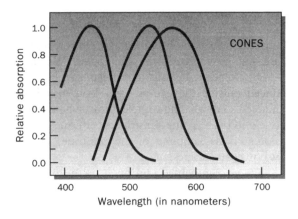

FIGURE 2.28 This graph shows how the amount of light absorbed by each of three types of cone photoreceptors varies with wavelength.

The curves shown in Figures 2.27 and 2.28 underscore an important feature of human vision. The curves separate electromagnetic radiation that one *can* see ("light") from electromagnetic radiation that one *cannot* see. For example, one cannot see infrared radiation (wavelengths longer than 700 nanometers) because human photopigments do not respond to wavelengths that long.

The following story dramatizes how photopigments determine what one can see. During World War II, the United States Navy wanted its sailors to be able to see infrared signal lights that would be invisible to the enemy. Normally, it is impossible to see infrared radiation because, as pointed out earlier, the wavelengths are too long for human photopigments. In order for humans to see infrared, the spectral sensitivity of some human photopigment would have to be changed. Vision scientists knew that retinal, the derivative of vitamin A, was part of every photopigment molecule and that various forms of vitamin A existed. If the retina could be encouraged to use some alternative form of vitamin A in its manufacture of photopigments, the spectral sensitivity of those photopigments would be abnormal, perhaps extending into infrared radiation. Human volunteers were fed diets rich in an alternative form of vitamin A but deficient in the usual form. Over sev-

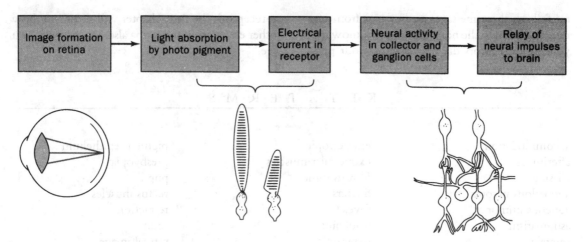

FIGURE 2.29 The three boxes at the left of the figure summarize the events discussed in this chapter; the remaining boxes represent the topics of the next two chapters.

eral months, the volunteers' vision changed, giving them greater sensitivity to light of longer wavelengths. Though the experiment seemed to be working, it was aborted. The development of the "snooperscope," an electronic device for seeing infrared radiation, made continuation of the experiment unnecessary (Rubin and Walls, 1969). Still, the experiment demonstrates that photopigments select what one can see; changing those photopigments would change one's vision.

To actually see, though, requires more than just a change in the photoreceptors' own electrical state. Messages about the presence of light must be transmitted from the receptors to their collector cells, retinal ganglion cells, and finally to the brain. Neuronal cells in the retina communicate with one another by means of chemicals called **transmitter substances.** These transmitter substances bridge the very small gap, or **synapse,** that separates cells. Light-induced variations in the electrical state of a photoreceptor cause changes in the amount of transmitter substance that the photoreceptor secretes. Because changes in amount of transmitter substance are related to the number of isomerizations, the concentration of this chemical communicates to a collector cell how much light is falling on the photoreceptor. The leftmost three boxes in Figure 2.29 summarize the events that we've been describing; the remaining boxes represent the concerns of the next two chapters.

S U M M A R Y A N D P R E V I E W

This chapter has laid out the basic design of the human eyeball, emphasizing the good fit between its structure and the job it must do. Because vision depends on an interaction between light and the eye, we also considered how light itself manages to capture information about the environment, information that is conveyed by light. This led us to a discussion of the eyeball's optical characteristics and various common imperfections in those characteristics. The chapter ended with the capture of light by photopigment molecules and the first step toward seeing—photoreceptor responses that are communicated to other neurons in the retina and eventually to the brain. The next chapter follows these messages as they pass from one retinal neuron to the next. You already know that your vision mirrors the properties of your pho-toreceptors; the next chapter will show you how other elements in the retina also control what you see.

K E Y   T E R M S

accommodation
afterimage
aliasing
anomalous myopia
aqueous humor
astigmatism
cataract
choroid
ciliary body
collector cells
cones
conjunctive
cornea
crystalline lens
depth of field
divergent
electromagnetic radiation

emmetropic
extraocular muscles
fibrous tunic
floaters
fovea
glaucoma
hyperopic
image
iris
macula
myopic
nanometers
ophthalmoscope
optic disk
orbit
photopigments
photoreceptors

pigment epithelium
presbyopia
pupil
rectus muscles
refraction
retina
retinal image
rods
sclera
sclerosis
synapse
transmitter substances
vascular tunic
vergence
vitreous
wavelength

The Eye and Seeing

A s detailed in the previous chapter, light is absorbed by pigment in the photoreceptors, which triggers the flow of electric current in the photoreceptors, culminating in the release of a chemical transmitter substance. These events were characterized as "the first step toward vision." In this chapter, we examine further steps in this sequence of events.

Each photoreceptor performs one simple job: it gauges the amount of light it is receiving. This results in about 130 million separate messages, each one specifying the light level falling on the tiny region of the eye occupied by a photoreceptor. This array of messages is then passed on to other cells in the retina, collector cells, as we termed them. These collector cells have a more complicated assignment: to reorganize those millions of raw messages into a more manageable, useful form. After all, our eyes are used to see *objects* and *events,* not points of light. The collector cells begin this reorganizational process by translating the raw messages they receive into descriptions of visually important information about edges, textures, and thus, objects.

The extraction of biologically relevant information about objects is a crucial function for the retina. However, before one can gauge how well the system performs this function, it is necessary to define *what* is meant by "information about objects." From the standpoint of vision, what defines an object? And what must the retina do in order to reorganize the photoreceptors' raw messages into information about objects?

Think back to our discussion of image for-

mation in the preceding chapter. There we noted that by reflecting and absorbing light, objects "sculpt" the light that eventually falls on the retina. Consequently, when it reaches the retina, the amount of light reflected from some object usually differs from the amount of light reflected from the object's surroundings. The key word is "differs." If there were some way of registering when neighboring retinal regions were being illuminated by *different* amounts of light, one would be on the way to identifying an object's edges or borders—places where the amount of reflected light changes. If one is interested in objects and edges, one is *not* interested in regions of the retina over which the light level remains constant. Homogeneous, or uniformly illuminated, regions of the retina probably do not represent the image of an edge. To identify an edge, the retina needs to note where there are *differences* between the light levels at adjacent locations. As you'll see, many retinal cells are designed to do precisely that: respond to differences between adjacent levels of light.

Our immediate goal, then, is to understand how the retina condenses and reorganizes the multitude of messages supplied by the photoreceptors. Then we shall want to consider how the condensation and reorganization actually affect the appearance of objects and their surfaces. There are various approaches that we could take to the retina's reorganization of information. Since the network of collector cells plays a major role in this reorganization, we could work through the details of how one stage after another of collector cells alters the message it has received. However, our primary interest is in the messages sent to the brain by the retina. Therefore, let's take a more direct approach. For the moment, let's skip to the **retinal ganglion cells,** the neurons responsible for the last stage of processing within the eye itself.

During our discussion, keep in mind that the ganglion cells, although they do respond to visual stimulation, do not themselves absorb light; they are *not* photoreceptors. Ganglion cells process neural information that other cells have received directly from the photoreceptors. Without input from these other collector cells, the ganglion cells would be blind to everything happening in the visual world.

Moreover, you must realize that ganglion cells can signal the outcome of their processing only by generating **action potentials,** brief electrical discharges carried by the nerve fibers of the ganglion cells to more central visual stages within the brain. So whatever a ganglion cell has to "say" about a visual stimulus must be expressed using this one-"word" vocabulary. This restriction actually applies to *all* further stages of visual processing—neurons talk to one another in a language composed entirely of action potentials, or neural impulses, as they are sometimes called. Particular neurons speak up with a burst of impulses only upon the appearance of particular types of visual stimuli. By virtue of their early position in this chain of visual processing, retinal ganglion cells set this neural dialogue in motion. Let's examine now what the ganglion cells have to say.

THE RETINAL GANGLION CELLS

The human eye contains roughly 1 million retinal ganglion cells. Comparing this figure to the 130 million receptors in the eye, you know from the outset that ganglion cells must be condensing the raw messages from the receptors. Imagine you are handed a 1,000-word essay and told to reduce it to 8 words—without losing the essentials of its message. To meet this editing challenge, you must identify the essay's major points and then rephrase them, condensing so as to retain the essence of

the original. The retinal ganglion cells face the same kind of problem: they must collate messages from the more numerous photoreceptors and summarize those messages in a biologically relevant way. How do the ganglion cells accomplish this job?

The most direct way to tackle this question is to determine what kinds of visual stimuli are best able to activate these cells. Figure 3.1 illustrates the experimental procedure for determining a visual cell's preferred stimulus. An experimental animal, a monkey in this case, is shown facing a screen. A tiny, fine-tipped wire called a **microelectrode** is surgically placed into the part of the visual system under study, in this case, the optic nerve (which comprises the axons of the ganglion cells). The probe can be positioned close enough to an individual ganglion cell axon so that the electrode picks up the action potentials (neural impulses) arising from just that cell. One can then monitor the number of action potentials generated by this single cell, and try to influence the cell's activity level by presenting various sorts of visual stimuli on the screen. This technique, called **single cell recording,** has been successfully employed to determine what kinds of visual stimuli it takes to activate cells at different stages within the visual system. Here we are interested in the retina. In effect, we wish to ask the ganglion cells, "What sort of visual stimulus do you respond most strongly to?"

Before presenting *anything* on the screen, you discover that the ganglion cell is already active; the electrode is picking up an irregular but persistent chatter of action potentials from the cell. This spontaneous activity continues even when the monkey is in complete darkness. To provide a pictorial representation of this neural activity, you can plot the occurrence of individual action potentials over time; this is done in Figure 3.2. In each of the three panels, the small vertical lines are meant to represent single action potentials from one retinal ganglion cell; time is traced out along the horizontal axis. Looking at panel A, you see the impulses occurring in the absence of visual stimulation—this is the spontaneous activity of the cell.

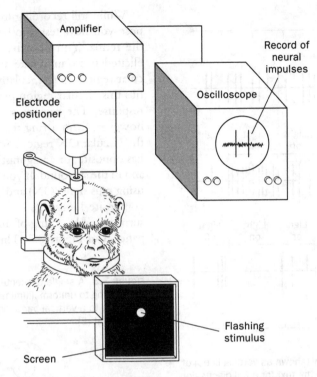

FIGURE 3.1 Laboratory setup for recording action potentials from single neurons. The placement of the recording electrode governs which stage of the visual nervous system will be examined. In the case shown, the electrode would pick up action potentials generated in the axons of the retinal ganglion cells.

Since it is spontaneously active when no light is present, the cell must signal the presence of light (a change from no light) by a change in its level of activity. Suppose your job is to discover what it takes to produce that *change* from spontaneous activity. Knowing that photoreceptors (from which the ganglion cells receive input via collector cells) are small, you start by moving a small spot of light around over the screen. By doing this, you are moving the spot of light around over the monkey's retina, stimulating photoreceptors wherever you move the spot. So, in effect, your job is to search for an area of the retina where the image of the spot of light will influence the ganglion cell's level of activity.

As we proceed with our example, it is very important to keep the following in mind: different regions on the screen in front of the monkey correspond to different areas on the retina of the monkey. To maintain this correspondence, it is necessary for the monkey's eye to remain perfectly still. If the monkey moved its eye around during the experiment, you could never be certain where your spot of light would fall on its retina. By immobilizing the eye, you can specify the retinal position of your spot of light in terms of its location on the screen. You might know, for instance, that positioning the spot in the center of the screen places the image of the spot on the center of the monkey's eye, in the macula. With this in mind, let's start our experiment.

By exploring with the spot of light on the screen, you discover a region of the retina where the spot causes an increase in the activity of the

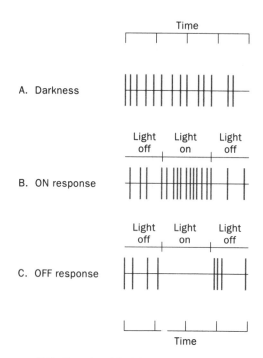

FIGURE 3.2 Neural activity (shown as vertical lines) of retinal ganglion cells. See the text for a full discussion.

While still recording from this same cell, suppose you now test at other, nearby locations on the retina. You find that ON responses can be elicited from anywhere within a restricted, circular region; in fact, enlarging your spot so it just fills this circular region produces a very vigorous response. The regions giving an OFF response, however, form a ring that completely surrounds the circular ON region. So the same spot of light has opposite, or antagonistic, effects in the center and in the surround. If you label these two regions using plus signs (ON) and minus signs (OFF), the composite looks like a small circle of plus signs surrounded by a ring of minus signs, as shown in panel A of Figure 3.3. This spatial layout of ON

FIGURE 3.3 A single ON-center retinal ganglion cell (A) responding to uniform illumination (B), to a dark/light edge (C), to a vertical bar of light (D), and to an oblique bar of light (E).

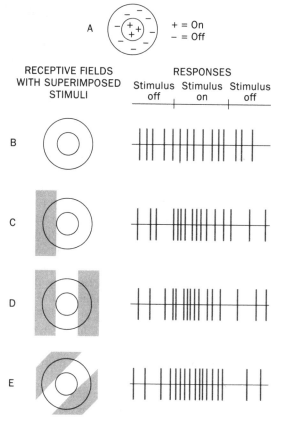

cell from which you're recording. Concentrating on this region, you discover that the cell gives a burst of impulses when you turn the light on within this area; when you turn the light off, the cell's activity quickly settles back to the background (spontaneous) level. This outcome is shown in panel B of Figure 3.2. Next, you test a neighboring area of the retina in the same way. Now you find just the opposite result—turning the light on causes the activity level to drop *below* the background level. But when you turn the light off, the cell emits a short, vigorous burst of impulses. This second outcome is illustrated in panel C. So, this cell responds in two antagonistic ways, depending on where you place the light spot on the screen and, hence, on the retina. In one region it responds to an *increase* in light, whereas in the other it responds to a *decrease* in light. To distinguish these two kinds of responses, let's call the first an "ON response" and the second an "OFF response."

and OFF regions actually arises from interconnections among the precursor collector cells and their inputs onto the ganglion cell. Look back at Figure 2.8 to see a schematic of those connections—notice how some of the collector cells form laterally extensive contacts with the ganglion cells. These lateral connections provide the underlying circuitry for the composite ON and OFF regions.

Light placed anywhere *outside* this donut-shaped composite has no influence whatsoever on this cell's activity. In other words, only light falling within this restricted, concentrically shaped area of the retina is registered by this ganglion cell. This area constitutes that cell's **receptive field**—the patch of retina within which a cell's activity may be influenced. (The term "receptive field" was coined by H. K. Hartline [1938] in his classic work on retinal ganglion cells in the frog.) The concept of a receptive field is extremely important for understanding visual processing. As you will come to appreciate in this chapter and the next one, the receptive field serves as a kind of template with which a cell gauges the pattern of light falling within a restricted area of the retina. In effect, a visual stimulus must fit into the receptive field in order to activate a cell.

To illustrate what we mean, let's consider the receptive field mapped out in panel A of Figure 3.3. Can you picture an optimal visual stimulus for this cell, one that would produce the most vigorous increase in neural activity? First, imagine illuminating the entire retina, in effect, filling the cell's receptive field with light. As shown in panel B of Figure 3.3, the cell gives only a weak response to uniform illumination. This is because such a stimulus produces opposite effects in the center and surround; the two antagonistic regions compete with one another, resulting in a near stand-off. This interaction between antagonistic regions is often called **lateral inhibition.**

Now imagine what happens when an edge is positioned in the manner shown in panel C. The ON-center portion of the receptive field receives an increase in light, its preferred stimulus, while a good portion of the surround receives a reduced level of light, its preferred stimulus. The net result

is a vigorous response from the cell. As panels D and E show, the cell would also respond well to bars of light positioned appropriately within the receptive field. Incidentally, because these center/surround areas are nearly always concentrically arranged, ganglion cells will respond well regardless of whether the edge is oriented vertically, horizontally, or diagonally. The orientation of an edge or bar is irrelevant so long as the edge or bar is positioned appropriately within the receptive field.

This antagonistic arrangement of center and surround within the receptive field enables the retinal ganglion cell to perform a major editing job. Lateral inhibition has enabled the cell to condense the messages from a patch of photoreceptors into a single statement: "I detect a light/dark boundary." By accenting the *difference* in light levels on adjacent areas of the retina, the cell has begun the process of extracting perceptually relevant information.

Although the cell just described does signal differences in light level, it monitors a very limited region of the retina. To learn more about the editing process initiated by retinal ganglion cells in general, other cells must be studied. You do this by moving the microelectrode to record action potentials from another cell, and repeating the steps outlined above. We can now summarize what has been discovered from studying cell after cell in this fashion.

RECEPTIVE FIELD LAYOUT

Nearly all ganglion cells have concentrically arranged receptive fields, composed of a center and a surround that respond in an antagonistic fashion. Some of those cells have ON centers and OFF surrounds, like the receptive field illustrated in Figure 3.3. (Box 3.1 discusses one interesting perceptual phenomenon thought to result from these cells.) Other cells have just the opposite layout, with an OFF center and an ON surround. An example of this latter type of cell is shown in Figure 3.4 (p. 71). There are about as many ON-center cells as there are OFF-center cells; both types respond best to light/dark boundaries. The

Box 3.1 *Blacker Than Black*

Because of its spontaneous activity, an ON-center cell sends the brain a stronger message when no light falls in its receptive field than it does when its surround alone is illuminated. This curious state of affairs suggests the possibility that some light may actually appear darker than no light at all. In fact, surrounding a dim area with a sufficiently intense light does make that dim area appear darker than an area that contains no light whatever. Probably the intense surround derives the activity of ON-center ganglion cells *below* their spontaneous levels, signaling the brain that something blacker than black is present (Brown and Mueller, 1965).

Spontaneous activity shows up in everyday life, too. Think about what it's like to wake up in the middle of the night in an absolutely dark room. Usually the room doesn't appear totally black. In fact, many people experience dim, illusory, swirling lights, the result of spontaneous activity in the visual system (Hurvich and Jameson, 1966).

Some artists exaggerate discontinuities in intensity in order to highlight the outline of figures in their work. If an artist wants to create the deepest possible black region in some painting, he or she must do more than simply use black paint. Even if that black paint reflected no light at all (which isn't really pos-

sible with paint), receptive fields in which the black paint was imaged would still be sending spontaneous messages to the brain. To reduce those messages to a minimum, the artist surrounds the black paint with an area of white or other light-colored paint. The contrast between the two areas intensifies the blackness produced by the black paint. Floyd Ratliff (1972) gives a good introduction to the uses of lightness illusions in art.

Mature artists are not the only people who take advantage of lightness illusions; parents and children do, too. Many children have a hard time falling asleep unless conditions are just right. Not only must it be past their appointed bedtime but also conditions outside must confirm that it is bedtime—it must *look* sufficiently dark outside. Some wise parents take advantage of a lightness illusion to hasten bedtime—as some children realize. The Finnish-American poet Anselm Hollo captured this idea by putting the following words into the mouth of a 4-year-old:

> *switch on the light*
> *so it gets dark outside*
> *and we can go*
> *to bed.*
>
> *(1977, p. 30)*

receptive fields on the ON-center cells and OFF-center cells overlap to make up a mosaic covering the entire retina. As a result, whenever light falls on a limited patch of the retina, that light is bound to affect a number of retinal ganglion cells of both types, producing opposite effects in the two. Don't imagine, though, that these opposite effects cancel one another; at higher stages of the visual system, information from ON-center and OFF-

center cells remains segregated, allowing information from both types to be used (Wässle, Peichl, and Boycott, 1981). Moreover, behavioral studies of animals in which activity within the ON cells has been disrupted reveal that the ON and OFF cells support different aspects of vision (Schiller, Sandell, and Maunsell, 1986). With the ON cells inactivated, animals have difficulty detecting increments in light, whereas light decre-

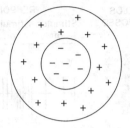

FIGURE 3.4 A receptive field of an OFF-center retinal ganglion cell.

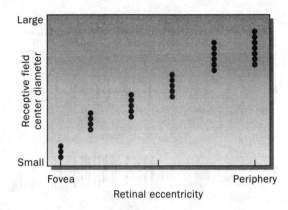

FIGURE 3.5 Graph showing how the sizes of receptive field centers increase with distance from the fovea. The size of the entire receptive field is larger than just the center diameter, since the entire receptive field consists of a center *and* a surround.

ments are readily perceived. Low-contrast objects are also more difficult to see without a functioning ON system. In general, the existence of ON and OFF systems seems to expand the range of visual events to which we are sensitive.

RECEPTIVE FIELD SIZE

The sizes of receptive fields vary systematically with retinal location (Wiesel and Hubel, 1960; de Monasterio and Gouras, 1975). Receptive fields in the center of the retina, within the macula, are quite small, with some on the order of 0.01 millimeters. Cells with these centrally placed receptive fields monitor tiny areas of the visual world wherever the monkey is looking. As you move away from the macula into the periphery of the retina, you find that the receptive fields grow increasingly larger; in fact, 10 millimeters away from the fovea, receptive field centers may be as large as 0.5 millimeters, 50 times larger than their foveal counterparts. Cells with these peripherally placed receptive fields collect information from larger areas of the retina. Figure 3.5 graphs the relation between receptive field size and retinal location. The horizontal axis represents the retinal location around which the receptive field was centered; "fovea" stands for the center of the macula. The vertical axis is the diameter of the center portion of the receptive field. Note that with increasing **eccentricity**—deviation from the center of the retina—the size of receptive fields tends to increase.

The graph in Figure 3.5 reveals another im-

portant fact. At each of the various eccentricities, we have data for more than just a single receptive field. Comparing data collected at the same eccentricity, we see that not all receptive fields at that eccentricity have exactly the same size. Because these size differences occur at a single locality on the retina, the phenomenon is known as *local variation.* So the sizes of receptive fields differ in two ways: first, they vary with retinal eccentricity; second, they vary locally.

Think what this variation in receptive field size means for the sort of stimulus that would be best suited to activate a particular cell. As shown in Figure 3.6, there is one bar width size (panel B) that elicits the best response from that cell; bars smaller (panel A) or larger (panel C) than this produce a less than optimum response. As you can see in Figure 3.7, cells with small receptive fields will respond best to small objects, while those with large receptive fields will prefer larger objects. This principle suggests that analysis of object size may be inaugurated in the retina.

TWO TYPES OF RETINAL GANGLION CELLS

So far we've distinguished retinal ganglion cells on the basis of receptive field size as well as on the basis of center type (ON versus OFF). But

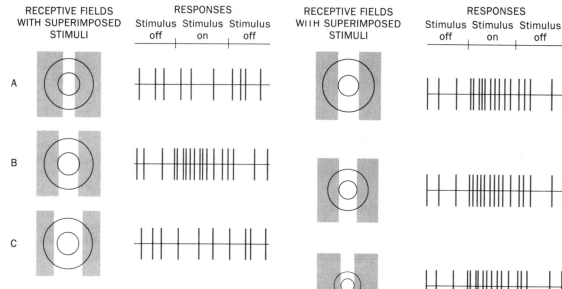

FIGURE 3.6 A single ON-center receptive field responding to bars of light of varying width.

FIGURE 3.7 Three ON-center receptive fields with different-sized receptive fields responding to bars of light of matching width.

retinal ganglion cells differ in other ways, some of which are particularly relevant for understanding vision. These differences form the bases for classifying ganglion cells into one of two groups, the **M cells** and the **P cells** (Shapley and Perry, 1986), with M standing for "magnocellular" and P for "parvocellular"; these two terms refer to the two classes of brain cells to which the M and P cells relay their neural impulses. Let's survey some of the major differences between these two cell types.

First, seen under a microscope, M cells are larger than P cells, and the portion of the cell carrying information out of the retina, the **axon,** is thicker in M cells. This means that neural impulses travel more rapidly to the brain over M-cell axons, since the conduction velocity of neural impulses increases with axon thickness. Second, these two types of cells differ greatly in number, with approximately 80 percent of all primate ganglion cells belonging to the P class. Third, at any given retinal eccentricity, the receptive fields of P cells are several times smaller than the receptive fields of M cells; this difference is responsible for much of the vertical scatter in receptive field size

seen in Figure 3.5. This difference in field size between P and M cells means that P cells will respond better to small objects than will M cells (recall Figure 3.7). Fourth, M cells respond well to very small differences in light levels in center and surround; P cells require larger light differences before they will respond strongly (Kaplan, Shapley, and Purpura, 1988). This distinction between cell types suggests that M cells may be especially important for the perception of objects of low contrast, such as dark gray letters on a medium gray background; P cells may be more important for seeing high-contrast objects, such as black letters on a white background. Fifth, M cells respond well even when a visual stimulus is turned on and off very quickly, whereas P cells respond poorly if at all to such a temporally modulated stimulus. This difference in temporal sensitivity means that M cells are better able to register transient visual events, such as the presence of a rapidly moving object.

The sixth difference between M and P cells is especially intriguing, for it probably relates to color vision (Lennie, 1984). For P cells, an excitatory response is evoked only when the receptive field is stimulated with light of a particular color (for example, red); P cells are inhibited by the presence of another, quite different color (for example, green). For M cells, in comparison, color makes no difference—they respond to light regardless of color. To understand this important difference between P and M cells, imagine looking for a ripe, red apple lying on a lawn of green grass. If the apple and grass reflect the same amount of light (that is, if they are equal in lightness), the M ganglion cells would fail to signal the presence of the apple—everywhere you looked, the responses of the M cells would be the same. The P cells, however, would solve the problem: as your gaze roams over the grass, a P cell sensitive to red would be silent until your gaze brought the image of the apple into the P cell's receptive field, thus evoking a robust response.

Although P and M cells constitute the lion's share of neurons in the retina (roughly 90 percent of the total), there are other, less well-studied cell types. These other cell types send their axons to phylogenetically older regions of the brain that are probably involved in the control of eye and head movements; these other cell types are also thought to provide the visual information that drives circadian rhythms. The P and M cells, in contrast, project to higher brain centers mediating visual perception. As you will learn, nature has gone to some lengths to keep separate the information carried to these higher centers by the P cells and the M cells. In the next chapter, we shall learn more about the separate pathways formed by the P cells and M cells in the retina and shall discuss further their possible roles in visual perception.

* * *

This completes, then, our abbreviated survey of the ganglion cells of the retina. By examining the workings of the retinal ganglion cells, you have learned several important things about the processing of visual information within the eye. You now know that this processing begins with the photoreceptors—they act like an array of tiny photocells, each specifying the level of light falling within the purview of the photoreceptor. These 130 million messages about light intensity are then passed on to a complex network of collector cells that integrate information from groups of neighboring photoreceptors. The results of this integration are conveyed to the retinal ganglion cells. Because of the center/surround organization of their receptive fields, the vast majority of ganglion cells are designed to detect differences in light level, or *contrast*, as it is called; these cells are much less concerned with the overall level of light.

And in some of these cells this center/surround organization is designed to extract information about color contrast. This kind of local receptive field analysis is performed over the entire retina by the 1 million or so ganglion cells in the eye. Hence everything you see must have registered its presence within this retinal machinery. The particulars of this machinery necessarily influence the *way* you see. There is no other route to visual perception but through the retinal ganglion cells.

The remainder of this chapter relates certain properties of vision to events occurring in the retina. A few of these events transpire in the photoreceptors, while most others occur at the level of the retinal ganglion cells. It's important that you understand what we mean when we claim that some property of vision is caused by the idiosyncrasies of some retinal cell. We are *not* saying that conscious visual perception occurs in the retina. Most visual scientists think that the process called "vision" actually takes place somewhere in the brain, not in the eye.

Instead, we're saying that events in the retina *shape* vision by emphasizing some information (such as differences in light level) and by de-emphasizing other information (such as uniformities). For example, retinal ganglion cells respond very strongly to discontinuities in illumination, and this operating principle reveals itself, sometimes vividly, in visual experience. Potentially important information, in other words, gets accentuated. In contrast, retinal cells fail to respond to images composed of wavelengths longer than 700 nanometers, meaning that the brain receives no information about such images. So some information gets ignored. Thus even though sight occurs in the brain, the retina preordains much of what we can and cannot see. Brindley (1970) and Teller (1989) discuss the logical bases for attributing some perceptual event to the behavior of some particular physiological process.

PERCEPTUAL CONSEQUENCES OF CENTER/SURROUND ANTAGONISM

The preceding section emphasized the antagonism between the center and the surround of a retinal ganglion cell's receptive field. The net response of such a cell is the sum of these two opposed influences. This antagonistic arrangement, which serves to reorganize the receptors' raw information, can explain some intriguing perceptual illusions, two of which are considered in the following sections.

MACH BANDS

Ernst Mach was an Austrian physicist and philosopher who made important contributions to a number of scientific disciplines during the last part of the nineteenth century and the early part of the twentieth. (The speed of sound is given as Mach numbers.) We're concerned here with just one small part of his work. The interested student will find an excellent, highly readable account of Mach's life and work in Ratliff (1965).

Mach became interested in the connection between light's intensity and the resulting sensation. His basic approach was to create various patterns out of paper and then to note how the perception of lightness varied from one part of the pattern to another. Many of the patterns that Mach developed caused him to see things that could not easily be explained by the corresponding distribution of light reflected from those patches of paper. Mach had the great insight that these idiosyncrasies of perception were caused by antagonistic influences within the retina. Because we have much more information about retinal physiology and anatomy than was available to Mach, we are able to infer

that these idiosyncrasies are caused by the center/surround antagonism evidenced in the receptive fields of retinal ganglion cells.

The upper portion of Figure 3.8 shows one of the kinds of patterns Mach developed. The graph below the pattern specifies the actual distribution of light intensity in the pattern. The horizontal axis of the graph represents position in the pattern; the vertical axis shows how much light the pattern reflects at that position. From left to right, the graph shows the level of intensity in the pattern increasing in a stepwise fashion. Thus the pattern really consists of a number of bars, each of uniform intensity and each giving way abruptly to another level.

When you look at the pattern itself, though, you'll notice some things that seem not to correspond with the graph. In particular, the lightness of each bar does not appear uniform. Take, for example, one of the bars in the middle. One

FIGURE 3.8 The lightness of each stripe in the pattern (upper portion of the figure) varies even though the intensity of each stripe is constant (lower portion of the figure).

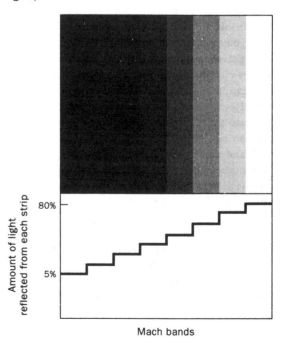

Mach bands

edge—near the bar's left-hand, darker neighbor—seems extra light, whereas the other edge—near the bar's right-hand, lighter neighbor—seems extra dark. In other words, the *lightness* varies even though the *intensity* does not. Most people describe the edges of each bar as having bands, extra dark and extra light regions. These bands—**Mach bands**—are named for the first person to study them systematically.

These bands, no matter how vivid they may seem, are illusory; they don't exist on the paper, only in your head. To understand where they come from, consider how the retinal ganglion cells respond to such a pattern of bars. When one looks at the pattern in the upper part of Figure 3.8, a distribution of light is produced on the retina, similar to the distribution shown by the graph in the lower part of Figure 3.8. This distribution of light is broad enough so that it extends across the receptive fields of many retinal ganglion cells. To simplify the discussion, let's consider only three adjacent bars from the pattern (see Figure 3.9). Suppose that the image of the three bars falls on some small number, say five, of ON-center receptive fields (though this assumption is not crucial to our point). These ganglion cells are each responsible for signaling the brain about the

intensity of light falling within their individual receptive fields. What sorts of messages would the brain get if these cells were stimulated by the pattern shown in the upper part of Figure 3.8?

To see what response any cell would give, we must weigh how much light falls in each of its two regions. (Remember the convention: "plus" indicates an ON region, "minus" indicates an OFF region.) Let's take the three easiest ones first. Receptive field A (leftmost ganglion cell in Figure 3.9) receives the least light, field E the most, and field C an intermediate amount of light. The responses produced by each cell will be proportional to the amount of light falling within their receptive fields. So the bar "seen" by A will seem the dimmest, that seen by E the brightest, with the bar seen by C appearing intermediate to the two. That leaves fields B and D as the interesting cases.

Receptive field B's center is stimulated by the same level of light as A's. Their respective surrounds, however, are *differentially* stimulated. All of A's surround is dimly illuminated, thereby producing little antagonism to combat the response produced by the center. Although the left part of B's surround is similarly illuminated, the right part is stimulated by the higher light level of the middle bar. As a result, the surround of B generates *more* antagonism than does the surround of A, *diminishing* the overall response of B to a level below that of A. Consequently, the region seen by B appears darker than that seen by A; B creates a dark Mach band.

Now consider fields D and E. The net response from D will be larger than that from E because D's surround is partially stimulated by the reduced light from the center bar, rather than by the higher level from the right-hand bar. As a result, D's surround generates *less* antagonism to its center's response, yielding a net response that is *greater* than that from E. So the region seen by D will appear lighter than that seen by E; D creates a light Mach band.

This treatment of Mach bands just barely scratches the surface. The scientific literature on this fascinating topic is quite large and, as Mach himself anticipated, it has taught us much about the human retina. One important lesson taught

FIGURE 3.9 Possible neural explanation of Mach bands.

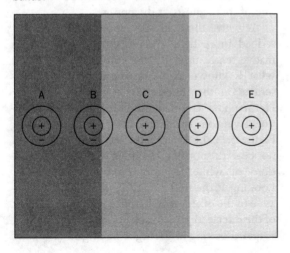

by Mach bands is the distinction between intensity on one hand, and lightness, on the other. **Intensity** is a physical variable, something that a light meter can measure; **lightness** is a psychological, or perceptual, variable, whose measurement requires a visual system.* Often, the two—intensity and lightness—covary, with surfaces reflecting more intense light appearing lighter. But Mach bands show that the correlation is not perfect. Although intensity changes in a stepwise fashion, lightness does not. Of course, this discrepancy arises from the processing of contour information through a system that has center/surround antagonism. And there is an advantage to such a system. By intensifying the contours demarcating objects, the process that produces Mach bands makes objects more conspicuous.

Mach bands are not the only way the retina's center/surround antagonism manifests itself. Let's consider another interesting manifestation.

THE HERMANN GRID

About a decade ago, one of America's well-known private universities published what turned out to be a beguiling cover on the catalog of its course offerings (Figure 3.10). When the catalog was distributed, it generated a stir: viewers experienced what seemed to be spots that disappeared whenever they tried to look directly at them. By inspecting Figure 3.10, you can experience these

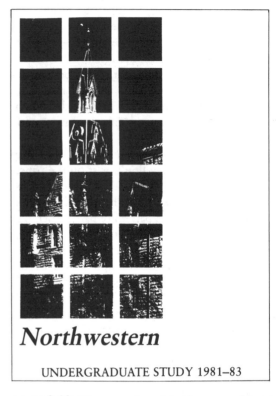

Northwestern

UNDERGRADUATE STUDY 1981–83

FIGURE 3.10 The cover of a catalog from one of America's outstanding institutions of higher education.

---

* The terms "brightness" and "lightness" are sometimes used interchangeably, but they should be differentiated. Among experts, the term "brightness" refers to the amount of light that appears to be arising from a given spatial location; for instance, we may speak of the brightness of the light reflected from, say, a piece of white paper. Brightness also refers to the perceived level of illumination produced by an emitting source; for instance, we may speak of the brightness of a room light. "Lightness" is a property of surfaces of objects illuminated by light; it depends on the amount of light reflected from the surface (which itself depends on both the amount of light illuminating the object and the amount of that illumination reflected by the surface). Lightness ranges from black, through shades of gray to white. A sheet of white paper is always lighter than a sheet of gray paper, but the gray sheet may look brighter when it is in direct sunlight as compared with when it is in the shade. To reiterate, brightness refers to light, lightness to surfaces.

illusory spots in most of the intersections between a horizontal and a vertical white stripe. Note, too, that when you move your eyes to look *directly* at one of these ghosts, it disappears.

Actually, these illusory spots were first described more than a century ago. The pattern inadvertently used by the university resembled what is known as a **Hermann grid,** first described in the nineteenth century by Ludimar Hermann, a German physiologist. More traditional versions of Hermann's grid are shown in Figure 3.11. Looking at the left-hand grid, you'll notice dark spots located in most of the intersections of white horizontal and vertical stripes. Looking at the middle grid (a photographic negative of the other), you'll notice light spots in most of the intersections of black horizontal and vertical stripes. Looking at the right-hand grid (a smaller

On surround, of antres.
Intersection = most light, so surrounds ↑ firing

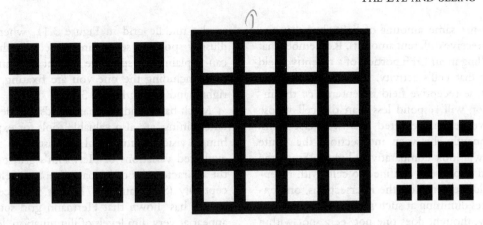

FIGURE 3.11 Three conventional versions of Hermann grids.

version of the one on the left), you'll see dark spots at *all* the intersections. Although they are vivid, every one of these spots is illusory. Where, then, do they come from, and why do they appear where they do? It is generally accepted that these illusory spots are the product of center/surround antagonism within receptive fields of retinal ganglion cells.

We'll make use of ON-center receptive fields to explain why spots are seen in the left-hand grid. Two questions must be answered. First, why are the spots that you see located only at intersections between horizontal and vertical stripes, not elsewhere? Second, why do you *not* see a spot located

within the intersection you look directly at? To answer the first question, we've drawn receptive fields on Hermann's grid (Figure 3.12). This allows you to compare how the retinal image of the grid would affect the two receptive fields shown, one being stimulated by an intersection and the other being stimulated by part of a white stripe that is not at an intersection.

To determine the response of either retinal ganglion cell, we must analyze how each of its components—center and surround—would be affected by the grid pattern. Assume that a viewer gazes steadily on the spot labeled "fixation point." Now, note that the centers of both receptive fields

FIGURE 3.12 A possible neural explanation of Hermann grids.

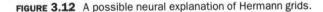

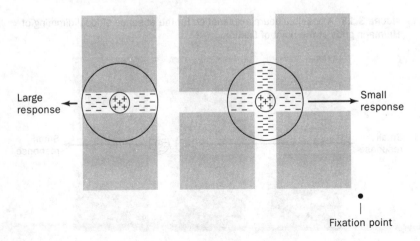

Large response

Small response

Fixation point

receive the same amount of light, but the surrounds receive different amounts. Remember that light falling in an OFF portion of a receptive field reduces that cell's activity. This means that the cell whose receptive field is centered *on* the intersection will respond less than the cell whose receptive field is centered *between* intersections. Consequently, between intersections the white stripes will look comparatively lighter. Since the reduced response is confined to cells with receptive fields centered on the intersections, one experiences dimming at such locales—gray spots.

Why, though, does one not see a spot within the intersection one is looking directly at? Recall that receptive fields vary in size according to their eccentricity, the smallest receptive fields coinciding with the fovea. When you look directly at an intersection, you are using receptive fields whose centers and surrounds are so small that *both* fit completely within the width of a stripe. We've illustrated this in Figure 3.13. Assume that a person fixates the right-hand intersection of the grid. As you can see, these small receptive fields all receive the same amount of stimulation within their centers and surrounds. Consequently, all the cells around the region of fixation will give the same response—whether on the intersection or not. As a result, there will not be any local dimming at the intersection.

To test your understanding of these ideas, see whether you can apply this same line of reasoning to the middle grid in Figure 3.11, where light illusory spots are seen. Finally, see whether you can explain why spots are seen at *every* intersection, including the one you are fixating, in the right-hand grid in Figure 3.11.

Mach bands and Hermann grids, besides being entertaining, are also valuable tools for exploring human vision. Some visual scientists have cleverly exploited variations of Hermann's grid to study the characteristics of human receptive fields perceptually (Spillmann, 1971). For instance, Wist (1976) has shown that Hermann grid spots disappear at very dim levels of illumination, levels at which the influence of the donut-shaped surround portion of a ganglion cell receptive field drops out, leaving only a center response.

Work by Jeremy Wolfe (1984) suggests that the ganglion cell account of Hermann's grid is oversimplified. First, Wolfe demonstrated that as the number of intersections in a Hermann's grid grows, so too does the strength of the illusory spots seen at the intersections. In a second experiment, Wolfe showed that the regular spacing of the intersections plays an important role as well. Although the explanation offered here is probably basically correct, Wolfe's results suggest the operation of an additional perceptual process that responds to global influences (over large regions of the field) as well as to influences that are spatially localized.

One routinely encounters objects in the envi-

FIGURE 3.13 A possible neural explanation for the absence of local dimming of Hermann grids at the point of fixation.

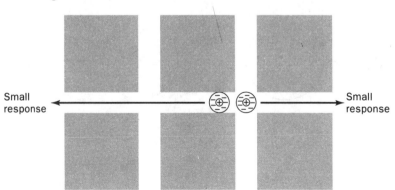

Small response ← → Small response

ronment that have the same effect on the visual system as do Mach bands and Hermann grids (Ratliff, 1984). The borders of these objects appear similarly exaggerated, though usually not as blatantly as the ones illustrated in Figures 3.8 and 3.11. You should realize that borders set objects apart from one another, which is precisely why retinal processing concentrates on signaling information about borders. Mach bands and Hermann grids simply highlight the presence of processing machinery that one relies on all the time. This reliance is further underscored by other important visual consequences of antagonism between center and surround. To see what these are, let's perform two more experiments with retinal ganglion cells.

TWO MORE CENTER/SURROUND EXPERIMENTS

In the first experiment, let's compare how a retinal ganglion cell responds when its center is stimulated by light of different intensities while its surround is subjected, in turn, to no illumination, some illumination, and finally, intense illumination. Suppose that we are recording from a retinal ganglion cell of the ON-center variety. Finding the cell's receptive field center, we focus a small spot of light within just that area, avoiding the surround altogether. The test spot is turned on for a second and the resulting number of impulses is recorded. After repeating this procedure with test spots of varying intensities, we plot the results as the curve labeled A in Figure 3.14. The graph's vertical axis represents the number of impulses; the horizontal axis represents the light intensity that evoked each response.

At the extreme left of the horizontal axis is plotted the spontaneous activity of the cell—the activity when no light is present at all. The graph reveals that several different very weak intensities of light fail to change the cell's spontaneous activity. Notice the arrow extending from curve A to the horizontal axis of the figure. It indicates the weakest intensity of light that will evoke a response appreciably different from that occurring with no light at all. In a sense, this is the minimum

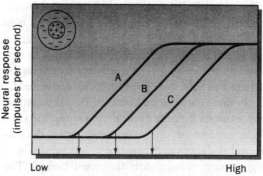

FIGURE 3.14 Graph showing the response of an ON-center ganglion cell to light of varying intensity falling on the center of the cell's receptive field. The three curves represent the effect of different intensities of surrounding stimulation.

amount of light the cell can "distinguish" from complete darkness.

As the spot's intensity grows, the cell's response grows larger. This steadily increasing response is important if the response of such a cell is to carry information about the intensity level of light in some scene. Finally, at some high intensity, the response of the cell *saturates*: further increases in intensity fail to produce corresponding increases in response. As far as this cell is concerned, all spots more intense than the point of saturation are indistinguishable from one another; from the cell's viewpoint, all such spots are equally light.

Now suppose this experiment is repeated with one modification. The small spot again falls in the receptive field center, but now the surround is illuminated, too. The cell's response under this arrangement is shown by curve B in Figure 3.14. Again, we vary the intensity of the spot in the receptive field center and note the number of impulses evoked by each. What are the differences between curves A and B? For both, arrows extending to the horizontal axis indicate the dimmest intensities that will produce an appreciable change in the cell's spontaneous response rate. As you can see, when the surround is illuminated, the center must be more strongly stimulated in order to change the cell's response. More generally, adding light in the surround reduces the response produced by any given intensity of light in the center. This is another demonstration of antagonistic forces at work; light has opposite effects on the ganglion cell's activity, depending on where the light shines within its receptive field.

Before considering how these antagonistic forces might influence vision, let's repeat the same basic experiment one more time. Again, the surround is illuminated constantly, but now with a light more intense than that used before. The results—the cell's response to various intensities of light in the center—are shown by curve C in Figure 3.14. With this strongest light in its surround, the cell requires an even more intense light in its *center* before its response can increase noticeably.

Lightness Contrast and Constancy

Now let's consider how vision is affected by ganglion cells that behave in the way shown in Figure 3.14. Assume that as its response grows, the ganglion cell is signaling the brain that light intensity is increasing.* With this assumption in mind, consider Figure 3.15. The two graphs in this figure add several features to what you saw in Figure 3.14. The left-hand graph indicates the three different intensities of light that produce the same response—a *constant response*—from the ganglion cell with various surrounds. This line of constant response is represented by a broken line parallel to the horizontal axis. The vertical arrows extending from each of the three curves to the horizontal axis point up the three different spot intensities that produce the same response from the ganglion cell.

The right-hand graph of Figure 3.15 analyzes the cell's response in a different way. Now we are interested in the magnitude of response produced by a central spot of *fixed intensity*. This line of fixed intensity is represented by a broken line

parallel to the vertical axis. The horizontal arrows extending from each of the three curves to the vertical axis point up the cell's response to this intensity with various surrounds.

In the left graph, the line of constant response indicates that with various lights in the receptive field's surround, different intensities of *center* stimulation are required to produce the same response. Alternatively, in the right graph, the line of fixed intensity indicates that with various lights in the surround, the same intensity of center stimulation will produce different responses. Both graphs highlight the same idea: the cell's response to a stimulus falling in its receptive field center is affected by the level of stimulation in the receptive field surround. Thus the messages that the brain will get about exactly the same stimulus will vary depending on how much light is falling in the receptive field surround.

From the behavior illustrated in these two graphs, one might conclude that ganglion cell responses provide unreliable information about lightness. Does this seeming unreliability disqualify ganglion cells as carriers of lightness information? The answer is no. Although the cell's behavior (as represented in Figure 3.15) would certainly produce errors of perception, the errors would have two sorts of consequences, one good and one not so good. Let's consider the not so good one first.

The right-hand graph of Figure 3.15 showed that a retinal ganglion cell could send the brain rather different messages about a spot of fixed intensity, depending on what other light happened to fall in the cell's surround. Translating this into perceptual terms, objects identical in intensity could appear different in lightness. In fact, such an outcome is experienced; Figure 3.16 demonstrates this effect, called **lightness contrast.** The two center spots are equal in *physical* intensity, but they appear different in lightness. To verify that both center spots are identical in intensity, you must eliminate the influence of their surrounds. Cut a hole just slightly smaller than either spot in a piece of paper. Position the hole over each spot in turn, occluding the surround in each case. By looking only at the spots,

---

* The following analysis holds for ON-center cells. A corresponding, separate analysis could be made for OFF-center cells whose increased activity signals increasing darkness.

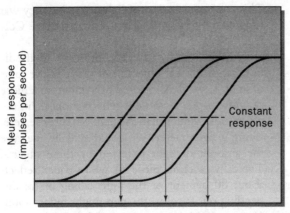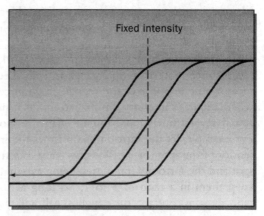

Intensity of light falling on receptive field's center

FIGURE 3.15 Two graphs showing the response of an ON-center ganglion cell to light of varying intensity falling on the center of the cell's receptive field. The left graph shows that a single, constant response (broken horizontal line) can be produced by several different intensities, depending on the amount of light falling on the cell's surround. The right graph shows that a fixed intensity of light (broken vertical line) can produce several different levels of neural response.

without contamination by their surrounds, you will see that both are identical in lightness. This proves that the different surrounds are responsible for the differences in perceived lightness. This perceptual outcome means that one's judgments of lightness can be in error by a substantial amount—seemingly a disadvantageous consequence.

Lightness contrast represents a case where the *same* physical intensity can yield differences in perceived lightness. The converse also occurs—*different* physical intensities can yield the *same* lightness. This routinely happens when you view an

object under different levels of light. Under such conditions, your perception of lightness tends to remain constant despite variations in the amount of light falling on the retina. This phenomenon is called **lightness constancy.** You can demonstrate lightness constancy for yourself. Hold an object, such as an aspirin tablet, under strong light, and notice how light the object looks. Then dim the lights. As the amount of light falling on the object drops, so too does the amount of light reflected from the object to your eye. Nonetheless, its lightness remains unchanged over a fairly wide range of light levels. This constancy of perceived lightness is the good perceptual error alluded to above.

Why do we characterize constancy as "good"? You might argue that lightness constancy means the human visual system is flawed—perception of light intensity fails to keep pace with the actual changes in light reflected from the aspirin tablet. But in fact, it's lucky that perception fails in this manner, for it allows recognition of an object even when the level of illumination changes drastically. Because of this "flaw," the surface appearance of an object remains constant despite changes in the level of illumination of that surface. After

FIGURE 3.16 Demonstration of simultaneous lightness contrast. Both central disks are physically the same.

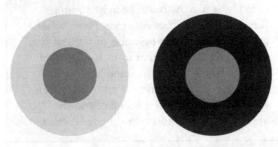

all, one is more concerned with seeing objects than with judging the level of illumination of those objects.

To understand how lightness constancy works, return once more to retinal ganglion cells. Let's measure the response of the retinal ganglion cell when a light of intensity x is flashed inside a surround several times more intense than the spot. For example, let the surround be 3 times the intensity of the spot, or $3x$. We now vary *both* the spot and the surround intensities, being careful to keep them in a ratio of 3 to 1. So long as this ratio remains constant, the ganglion cell will give the same neural response when the spot appears within the center. Assuming the retinal ganglion cell's response signals lightness, this invariant response means that lightness of the spot will remain constant even though the actual light from the spot is changing. The same result holds for most other ratios between the spot and its surround.

This ratio explanation of lightness constancy was suggested by Hans Wallach of Swarthmore College (1963).

Now let's apply this ratio principle to the illumination of real objects, not just circular spots of light. Lay a dark-colored pen down on a piece of white paper. Because it reflects more light, the paper looks lighter than the pen. No surprise here. Using a light meter, we could actually measure the amount of light reflected by these objects. Typically, a clean piece of white paper reflects about 80 percent of the light falling on it; depending on its color, the pen might reflect about 10 percent, giving us a ratio of 8 to 1.

Now take a strong desk lamp and shine its light on both pen and paper. More light is falling on the pen than before you turned the lamp on. Consequently, more light is being reflected from the pen into your eyes. But the pen looks no lighter than before (lightness constancy). The rea-

---

Box 3.2 *When Lightness Constancy Fails*

Usually lightness constancy works and keeps you from erroneous interpretations of what you are seeing. But when constancy fails, it fails dramatically, as the following incident suggests. One of us (R.S.) woke up, looked at his wife, and was shocked. Overnight, a large patch of her hair had turned silvery white (it had been brown the night before). He could not imagine what terrible nightmare could possibly have made her hair go white in just a few hours.

Reaching over to touch the strange patch, he discovered the silvery appearance was illusory. In fact, when he touched her hair, his hand also turned silvery. Despite this temporary disfigurement of his hand, he was relieved that he wouldn't have to break the news about her hair to his wife.

But why did this illusion occur? The partially open shutters passed a narrow beam of light into the room, illuminating part of his sleeping wife's hair though not illuminating anything else in the room. The psychologist Adhemar Gelb showed in 1929 that this sort of arrangement—illumination confined to one object with no illumination of its surround—tends to defeat constancy. Perhaps you've had a more common version of this experience while walking in a forest. Suddenly, you chance upon a large, shiny coin on the ground. Bending down to pick it up, you discover it is a leaf that had been illuminated by a narrow beam of light coming through the branches of a tree. Here, again, constancy failed; the lightness of the leaf was so much inflated relative to its background that the leaf appeared to shine like silver.

Some researchers have tried to relate this breakdown of lightness constancy to the viewer's lack of knowledge, a cognitive exson is that with the lamp on, more light is also being reflected from the paper. Since the ratio (8:1) of light from the paper to light from the pen is unchanged, with more light coming from *both,* perceived lightness is unchanged. Recent research shows just how robust the ratio explanation can be. Under the proper conditions, observers show lightness constancy even though the overall level of illumination varies by more than 1 million to 1 (Jacobsen and Gilchrist, 1988). Of course, if you did something to alter that ratio (such as illuminating *just* the pen), lightness constancy would fail: the lightness of the pen would change as you varied the amount of light falling on it alone. And, as Box 3.2 shows, under certain conditions, lightness constancy does indeed fail.

* * *

We've just seen how the properties of retinal ganglion cell receptive fields can account for the way

vision accentuates differences between adjacent levels of illumination. Because ganglion cells collect their information from the photoreceptors, the cells' behavior reflects the preferences and peculiarities of those photoreceptors. Bearing in mind that the relation between retinal ganglion cells and the photoreceptors is particularly important for vision, we'll now turn to that relation.

SENSITIVITY VERSUS RESOLUTION

ASPECTS OF CONVERGENCE

Earlier we noted that over the entire retina, information from 130 million photoreceptors converges onto about 1 million retinal ganglion cells. This suggests an average convergence, over the entire retina, of about 130 to 1. But this statistic is actually a little misleading.

planation. Usually, these researchers follow the line taken by Hermann Helmholtz (1909/1962), namely that lightness constancy depends on an "unconscious inference" about the true conditions of stimulation. In this view, constancy breaks down when the viewer is confused about the actual level of illumination. According to this theory, lightness judgments should be corrected if the confusion is corrected. Yet incorrect unconscious inferences cannot account for the failure of lightness constancy. For instance, even after R.S. recognized its illusory nature, the silvery appearance of his wife's hair persisted. Knowledge of the correct stimulus conditions did not override the illusory perception of lightness (see also Hurvich and Jameson, 1966).

These failures of lightness constancy, and the inability of mental effort to remedy them, reinforce the idea that lightness constancy depends on lateral interactions within the visual system, interactions that are initiated by the

registration of different amounts of light from adjacent areas of the field.

Although the ratio between the amounts of light reflected from two adjacent retinal areas does seem to explain many aspects of lightness constancy (and its failures), these ratios don't tell the whole story. Alan Gilchrist (1977) studied the lightness of a gray piece of paper seen against various backgrounds. When the piece of paper appeared in front of or behind the background, the paper's perceived lightness changed. These changes occurred even though the amount of light reflected from the paper and from the background were unchanged.

Here, then, lightness perception varied despite the fact that adjacent retinal areas received fixed amounts of light. Similar results have been reported by others, too (for example, Gogel and Mershon, 1969). In another paper, Gilchrist (1988) described how lightness constancy and lightness contrast are influenced by yet other factors.

Suppose we examine the number of receptors and the corresponding number of ganglion cells locally in different small patches throughout the retina, ranging from the macula into the periphery. For each patch of retina we can calculate the degree of convergence by taking the ratio of number of receptors to number of retinal ganglion cells. This calculation reveals two important facts. First, the convergence ratio varies widely and systematically from one part of the retina to another; second, near the center of the macula, the convergence ratio is close to unity—about one ganglion cell per receptor—whereas in the periphery of the retina, the ratio is several hundred to one. In other words, there is a strong connection between retinal eccentricity and amount of conver-

gence. The connection is so strong that it suggests the operation of some grand plan. What might that plan be? To answer this question, we need to explain what is gained and what is lost by this neural convergence. And as we proceed, keep in mind that the extent of convergence of receptors onto ganglion cells is directly related to the sizes of the receptive fields of those ganglion cells: the greater the number of receptors innervating a given ganglion cell, the larger that cell's receptive field. This principle is illustrated schematically in Figure 3.17. At the top are shown schematically two ganglion cell receptive fields, one small (left) and one large (right). Note that the number of photoreceptors contributing input, via the collector cells, to the small receptive field is fewer than

FIGURE 3.17 A ganglion cell receiving input from just a few receptors (left-hand example) has a smaller receptive field and, thus, responds best to small stimuli. A cell receiving input from more receptors (right-hand example) has a larger receptive field and responds poorly to small stimuli.

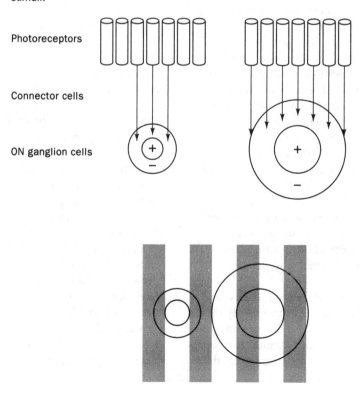

Photoreceptors

Connector cells

ON ganglion cells

the number contributing input to the larger receptive field. We'll get to the bottom part of the drawing in a moment.

To picture the consequences of convergence, consider an extreme form of convergence. Suppose your eye had only a single retinal ganglion cell—a convergence ratio of 130 million to 1. In effect, your entire retina would be the receptive field for this solitary cell. How would your vision differ from its present form? It's certain that your vision would be changed in two ways, one for the good, one for the bad.

We'll start with the bad. With only one retinal ganglion cell to tell your brain what the eye saw, you would not be able to read or watch television. In fact, you would be able to do very few of the things for which you now use your eyes. Imagine the problem faced by the brain whose only link to the visual world was this one retinal ganglion cell. The brain would have difficulty distinguishing different distributions of light. Many distributions would have the same effect on the cell. You would confuse letters of the alphabet and be unable to recognize your friends by sight. In brief, your resolution would be awful—not a good situation.

The term **"resolution"** refers to the ability to distinguish differences in the spatial distribution of light in the image. The best-known measure of resolution is **visual acuity,** which we shall discuss in a moment. With only one retinal ganglion cell to "describe" the image on the retina, your resolution would be nil. So long as the total light falling on the retina remained constant, you wouldn't be able to distinguish one letter of the alphabet from another—even with extremely large, headline type. You don't need to go to the extremes of our example (a single retinal ganglion cell for the whole eye) in order to discover that convergence is incompatible with good resolution. Generally, greater degrees of convergence lead to poorer resolution. In summary, convergence is the enemy of resolution. Look at the distribution of light within the ON and OFF regions of the two receptive fields shown in the bottom portion of Figure 3.17. Although the cell with the larger receptive field receives input from more receptors, its separate responses to dark and light bars would cancel one another. As a result, this cell would fail to respond to the pattern that is superimposed on the receptive field. The cell with the smaller receptive field—receiving input from fewer receptors—would give a vigorous response to the pattern, since the light and dark portions of the pattern "fit" within this cell's receptive field profile. The smaller receptive field has superior visual acuity because the convergence—the enemy of resolution—is limited.

Now for the good news about convergence. Going back to the hypothetical case, suppose again a single retinal ganglion cell collects information from all the receptors in an eye. Before the impulse rate of any ganglion cell can be changed, the cell must receive a certain amount of transmitter substance from the cells that feed information to it. The retinal ganglion cell weighs together all the neurochemical influence on it, without caring which particular cells contributed to that influence. What consequences does this have for the retinal ganglion cell's ability to tell the brain about the presence of light on the retina? Take a very dim light and use it to cast an image on the retina. If this image was very small, only a few receptors would be affected by it and each only weakly. The messages passed along to collector cells would also be weak. As a result, the retinal ganglion cell might not receive enough transmitter substance to alter the rate at which it generates action potentials. Because weak messages from very few cells may not be passed along, the brain might not be informed that light was present.

However, if the same dim light were to cast a larger image on the retina, more receptors and more collector cells would be affected. This in turn would increase the number of inputs to the single retinal ganglion cell, making it more likely that the cell would be activated. As a result, the brain *would* be informed that light was present.

Generally, increasing the number of receptors contributing input to a retinal ganglion cell allows weak signals to be summed, yielding a total input strong enough to change the activity of that ganglion cell. A retinal ganglion cell sums weak signals originating from a range of retinal locations, an ability known as **spatial summation.** Spatial summation enables you to see very dim light; in other words, it enhances the sensitivity of your eyes. Because summation depends on convergence, one can say that *convergence is the ally of sensitivity.*

Note the conflict. On the one hand, convergence is a prerequisite for high sensitivity; on the other, convergence interferes with good resolution. To design an eye that detects very dim lights *and* possesses good spatial resolution represents a real challenge.

The Duplex Solution. How do your eyes manage to resolve these two conflicting demands—resolution and sensitivity? To answer this question, let's return to an analogy we've already used, the analogy between the eye and a camera.

Cameras are faced with the kinds of problem we've been discussing. Some types of film have extremely high sensitivity to light, making them usable at very low light levels. These highly sensitive films usually have relatively poor resolution—they don't produce very sharp photographs. Other types of film—such as the microfilm used by librarians—produce very sharp photographs (even in huge enlargements) but work properly only at relatively high light levels. In film, then, as in the eye, there is a trade-off between resolution and sensitivity. The photographer can solve this dilemma simply by changing the film in the camera, matching the film to available light. The eye, however, doesn't allow the capability of loading and unloading different types of film as needed. In fact, this is unnecessary because the "film" in the eye is **duplex,** meaning that the eye contains two types of photosensitive elements (or "films"). One—associated with the rod photoreceptors—provides high sensitivity to light; the other—associated with the cone photoreceptors—provides high resolution. In the human eye, the two types of film occupy somewhat different locations along the back of the eye.

To see how this duplex arrangement works, think back to the convergence of receptors onto ganglion cells. Recall that the central region of

the eye (where cones predominate) has very little convergence. Hence it has excellent resolution but only average sensitivity to light. Peripheral regions of the retina (where rods predominate) have high degrees of convergence, hence poor resolution but good light sensitivity. (For further discussion of high sensitivity, see Box 3.3, p. 88–89.)

The preceding chapter pointed out that the center of the primate retina contains mainly cones and very few rods. As a result, activity of retinal ganglion cells with receptive fields near the center of the retina reflects mainly the responses of cones. Because of the predominance of rods in the retinal periphery, activity of ganglion cells with receptive fields in that region reflects mainly the influence of rods. Now as you are about to learn, rods and cones differ in numerous ways important to vision. This means that ganglion cells in the rod-dominated periphery make different contributions to vision than do ganglion cells in the cone-dominated central region of the retina.*

In particular, rod-dominated ganglion cells support vision even when light levels are several hundred times less than that demanded by their cone-dominated counterparts. This results from the rods' own greater sensitivity (Detwiler, Hodgkin, and McNaughton, 1980), as well as greater convergence on rod-dominated retinal ganglion cells. Vision under conditions of very little light is described as **scotopic** (from the Greek *skotos,* meaning "darkness," and *ops,* meaning "sight"). We'll use the term "scotopic vision" to signify vision that depends on rod-dominated ganglion cells.

The cone-dominated retinal ganglion cells require higher light levels in order to function properly. Hence vision using these ganglion cells is described as **photopic** (from the Greek stem *phot,* meaning "light" or "daylight"). Figure 3.18 indicates what levels of light are considered pho-

---

* Although some retinal ganglion cells receive inputs from both rods and cones (Enroth-Cugell, Hertz, and Lennie, 1977), for many ganglion cells the two influences are sufficiently unbalanced to justify our talking about "cone-dominated" and "rod-dominated" ganglion cells.

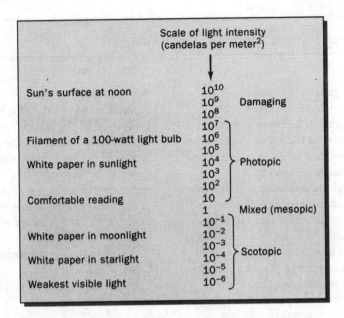

FIGURE 3.18 Scale of light intensity expressed in units called "candelas," a measure of light energy.

topic and what levels are considered scotopic. This is an important distinction because, as you'll see later, photopic and scotopic vision differ in a number of ways.

As noted earlier, the eyes must satisfy two competing goals, good resolution and good sensitivity. We now discuss each of these goals in turn.

RESOLUTION

Since convergence is the enemy of resolution, the photopic system, having less convergence, should have better resolution. In particular, resolution should be best in the center of the macula, where the ratio of cones to ganglion cells is about 1 to 1. We do not yet know precisely how the convergence of the cone system changes across the retina—the extensive physiological measurements required to answer that question have yet to be performed. Instead, we must infer the answer using related information: the density of cones at various places on the retina. The solid line in Figure 3.19, representing the "number of cones," shows how the number of cones per square mil-

FIGURE 3.19 Graph showing how visual acuity and number of cone photoreceptors covary with retinal eccentricity. In this graph, a visual acuity of 1.0 corresponds to an image of about 0.005 millimeters on the retina. Values less than 1.0 correspond to larger images on the retina and, hence, poorer acuity.

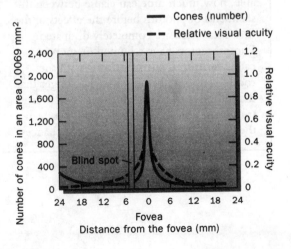

Box 3.3 *Adding Photons Over Time and Space*

Multiple factors govern the eye's sensitivity. Some have already been discussed—the wavelength of light, its intensity and spatial pattern, and where on the retina the stimulus falls. But there are two other, very important variables: its duration and its size.

To understand the importance of duration and size, we must consider exactly what events need to occur before one can detect a very weak stimulus. Suppose that seeing the stimulus requires that the photoreceptors absorb some small number of photons—a **photon** being the smallest unit of light energy. (The actual number of photons doesn't matter so long as it is greater than 1.) Imagine that we split the stimulus into two installments, each intense enough to cause the receptors to absorb exactly one-half the total number of photons needed for seeing. Now let's introduce one condition: allow 1 hour to elapse between delivery of the first and second installments of photons. Will you see the stimulus? No, because by the time the second installment of photons arrives, the effects of the first installment will have long since disappeared.

Granting that an hour's delay is unreasonable, how much time can elapse between installments of photons before the effects of the first installment are completely dissipated? Photoreceptors have a limited memory—called **temporal summation**—with the rods' "memory" being somewhat longer than that of the cones. But whichever system is stimulated, the shorter the interval between the two installments, the greater the chances

that the residue of the first installment will be available to add to the effects of the second. Delivering all the photons within a very short time of one another guarantees that effects produced by the earliest photons will add to those of the later ones. If the stimulus is stretched out in time, a greater *total* number of photons must be delivered to the eye, since losing the advantage of temporal summation makes each photon less efficient.

This fact has been formalized as **Bloch's Law,** which states that a constant product of light intensity and time will be equally detectable. Sometimes Bloch's Law is expressed as

$$I \times T = C$$

where I stands for intensity, T for time, and C for constant visual effect. Bloch's Law says that time can be traded for intensity. Lengthening the presentation of some relatively weak light makes it just as visible as another, more intense light that is presented only briefly. So long as each has the same product (of intensity and time), the two stimuli contain the same total energy and will be equally detectable. These relationships are depicted in the figure at the end of this Box. There, the vertical axis represents the stimulus intensity that is just barely detectable (I), and the horizontal axis represents the stimulus's duration (T). Two lines are shown on the graph, one representing the behavior of the scotopic system, the other representing the behavior of the photopic system. Bloch's Law predicts that data should fall on an oblique line, of 45 degrees slope. Note that in both lines, this prediction holds when the durations are relatively short.

For the rods, Bloch's Law breaks down at about one-tenth of a second; for cones, it breaks down much earlier, at about one-twentieth of a second or less (Hood and Finkelstein, 1986). These values reflect the temporal memories—temporal summation—of the two systems.

There is a *spatial* analog to the *temporal* law just discussed. We mentioned before that many photoreceptors will share a single collector cell. In other words, the collector cell adds together signals from spatially separate sources—two or more photoreceptors—a capacity referred to in the text as spatial summation.

Suppose we take a very small stimulus and by trial and error determine how intense it must be in order to be just detectable. This stimulus causes the absorption of a minimum, or threshold, number of photons. If we distribute that same number of photons widely over the retina, seeing will not result. The spatially dispersed photons stimulate photoreceptors that do not contribute to the same collector cells. As a result, the opportunity for cooperative effect is reduced.

Within certain limits, all stimuli having the same product of intensity *and* area will be equally detectable. This is not completely surprising since any two stimuli having the same product of area and intensity contain identical amounts of total light. This trade-off between intensity and area is known as **Ric-**

co's Law. Ricco's Law holds only in the fovea; and even there, it holds only for very small stimuli. Leo Hurvich and Dorothea Jameson (1966) give a particularly clear account of both Bloch's Law and Ricco's Law.

We don't want to leave you with the idea that the visual system responds *solely* to the number of photons gathered over time and space. If it did respond that way, you'd confuse long, weak flashes with brief, intense ones. This confusion would be particularly strong when flashes of different durations contained the same total number of photons, since according to Bloch's Law, they would be equally detectable. However, even when two flashes contain the same total number of photons (and hence are equally detectable), people can still discriminate between a long, weak flash and a brief, intense one (Zacks, 1970). In other words, the visual system registers more than just the total number of photons; it also discriminates how those photons are packaged over time. At present, though, it is not known how the visual system manages this discrimination.

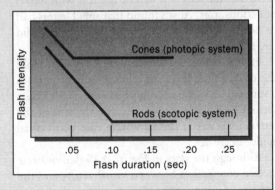

limeter decreases with distance from the fovea (eccentricity). The dotted curve in the same graph shows visual resolution measured for various regions of the retina. This second curve, representing "relative visual acuity," comes from measurements with humans who tried to read a well-lit eye chart while directing their gaze away from the center of the chart by various distances to the chart's side. Fixating this way causes the letters on the chart to be imaged at different, known places on the retina. Note the correspondence between the perceptual measurements of resolution (visual acuity) and the anatomical measurements (the number, or density, of cones).

You can see one consequence of the variation in acuity with eccentricity by gazing steadily at any letter on this page. You'll have little trouble recognizing that letter. However, if you're careful not to move your eyes, you'll notice that letters in the periphery appear less distinct.

Stuart Anstis was interested in how this ability to recognize letters varies depending on how far from the fovea the letters are imaged. With a person seated 57 centimeters (about 22 inches) from a bright, white screen, Anstis moved a letter inward from the edge of the screen. Starting far enough away from fixation so that the person could not identify the letter, Anstis brought the letter in, toward the fovea, until the person could recognize the letter. When he did this with letters of various sizes, Anstis found that small letters had to be brought much nearer to fixation than did larger letters (Anstis, 1974).

Figure 3.20 demonstrates Anstis's results. Hold the chart a little less than arm's length away from your eyes and stare steadily at its center. All letters should be equally legible, because the size of the letters increases at the same rate that your visual acuity decreases.

Although the data in Figure 3.19 demonstrate a close connection between visual acuity and the density of cones, cone density is not the entire explanation of visual acuity. Acuity decreases appreciably as the level of illumination drops (you probably already know this from your own difficulty reading a menu in a dimly lit restaurant).

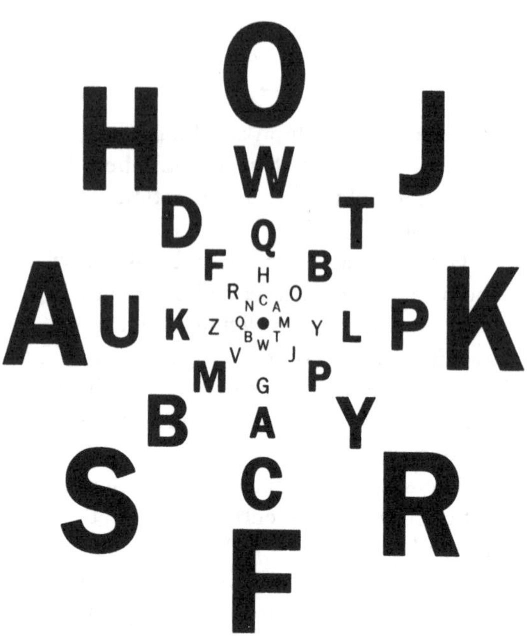

FIGURE 3.20 All letters in this chart should be equally legible when the small dot in the center of the chart is fixated.

Yet it's obviously not the number of cones that changes with light level. The reduction in acuity with decreasing illumination is probably caused by changes in the receptive fields of the ganglion cells. For instance, the relative contribution from the centers and the surrounds of ganglion cell receptive fields depends on the overall level of illumination (Barlow, Fitzhugh, and Kuffler, 1957; Maffei and Fiorentini, 1972). Box 3.4 (pp. 92–94) completes the story by describing additional influences on visual acuity.

SENSITIVITY

Scotopic Vision. A rod photoreceptor is at the theoretical limit of its sensitivity; it can respond even when just a single photon is absorbed by its photopigment (Lewis and Del Priore, 1988; Hecht, Shlaer, and Pirenne, 1942). But the capture of a single photon does not constitute seeing. In order for you to see—experience light—photons must be caught by more than one rod, though not by many more. For the small number of rods needed for seeing to be activated efficiently, conditions must be exactly right. The rods' own properties, together with those of the collector cells connected to the rods, define those right conditions. So enumerating some of the conditions gives a very good, quick introduction to scotopic vision in general. Let's consider the conditions, one at a time.

The first requirement is that the eye have a full supply of photopigment molecules. Exposure to light uses up these molecules, much as exposure to light consumes the light sensitivity of film. To restore the full supply of photopigments requires keeping the person you're going to test in complete darkness for some 35 minutes. This period of adapting to the dark suffices to build the rod photopigments to maximum level.

Second, the photons need to be imaged on an area of the retina where rods are plentiful. Thus it makes no sense to present the stimulus to the fovea, where there are no rods. Rods are most plentiful in a region slightly more than 3 millimeters away from the fovea. To stimulate this retinal region requires knowing where the person is actually looking. So the person is asked to fixate a small, continuously visible spot. As Figure 3.21 illustrates, knowing the position of fixation makes it possible to situate the test stimulus at the right distance from that fixation spot. The test stimulus must be fairly small so that it stimulates only the desired retinal region.

Remember that the goal is to determine the dimmest light necessary for detection. The fewer the photons that are needed for vision, the higher visual sensitivity is said to be. Not all wavelengths of light are equally effective in stimulating rods. Therefore, to find the wavelength to which the scotopic system is most sensitive, we must stimulate the eye with various wavelengths of light, noting how many photons are needed for detection of each wavelength.

When these procedures are carried out, the data take the form shown in Figure 3.22 (p. 94). The horizontal axis shows the wavelength of light used to stimulate the eye. The vertical axis shows sensitivity (the reciprocal of the number of photons needed for vision). The curve represents the sensitivity of the rod-based system and is usually called the scotopic sensitivity function. The scotopic sensitivity function peaks at 500 nanometers, with the eye being less sensitive when stimulated by either shorter or longer wavelengths of light. In daylight and at sufficient intensity, light of 500 nanometers appears blue-green. To the person whose scotopic vision is being tested, however, the faint test target will appear colorless (the explanation for this failure of color vision is given in Chapter 6).

Photopic Vision. Although sensitivity is not the specialty of photopic vision, it's worth considering photopic sensitivity so that we can compare with scotopic sensitivity. To measure *photopic* sensitivity requires imaging the target on a retinal area containing only cones; rods can play no role.

FIGURE 3.21 When fixating the X, the test spot falls in the periphery of the retina.

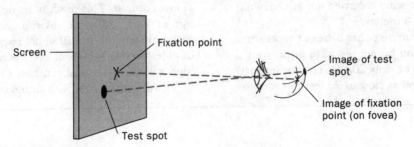

Box 3.4 *Visual Acuity: The Meaning of 20/20 Vision*

Visual acuity can be defined in several different ways. One common definition relates acuity to the smallest target—such as a letter—that can be correctly recognized. A person able to recognize smaller letters is said to have better acuity. You may have heard someone comment with pride about having 20/20 visual acuity. What exactly do these numbers mean?

When optometrists and ophthalmologists began quantifying acuity more than a century ago, they created eye charts containing letters of various sizes. Patients tried to read ever smaller letters, until they came to letters so small that reading was impossible. One Dutch doctor, Hermann Snellen, tested hundreds of people who had no eye diseases (so-called normals) and found that half these people were unable to see details smaller than a certain size. He designated this size—details whose images on the retina were about 0.005 millimeters high—as "normal." For any given detail, the viewing distance is crucial. If you move far enough away, even headlines become impossible to read. So visual acuity is expressed in relation to the distance at which the eye chart is read, usually 20 feet. Someone is said to be normal if, while standing 20 feet from the chart, that individual can read the same letters that the average healthy person can read at 20 feet. Hence the notation "20/20." The metric equivalent of 20/20 is 6/6, since testing is carried out at a viewing distance of 6 meters.

Acuity can be either better or worse than 20/20. If you cannot see small print, your acuity may be only 20/60. This means that you must get as close as 20 feet in order to read what the average person can read from 60 feet. Likewise, if you have really sharp eyes, your vision may be 20/15 or even 20/10. This means that you can read letters at a distance of 20 feet that the average person cannot; he or she has to move closer, to within 15 feet of the letters (in the first case) in order to be able to read them or 10 feet (in the second) to be able to read them.

But 20/20 is not good enough. A normal, healthy young person *should* be better than 20/20. This is shown in the graph at the end of this Box (see p. 84), which summarizes the variation in visual acuity with age. With young people, visual acuity is on average better than 20/20; with increasing age, acuity declines. Part of this decline is caused by the reduced light reaching the retina because the older person's pupils are reduced in size (Owsley, Sekuler, and Siemsen, 1983). Older people also have particular difficulty with eye charts whose letters are of low contrast. Such charts are made by substituting light gray letters for the traditional black ones (Pelli, Robson, and Wilkins, 1988). Tony Adams of the University of California's School of Optometry used a low-contrast eye chart to measure the acuities of young and old people, all of whom had 20/20 acuity when tested at normal, high contrast. Adams, Wang, Wong, and Gould (1988) found that the older observers showed a far greater decline in acuity at low contrast. This result bears on the design of work and home environments that accommodate the special visual requirements of older persons who will likely benefit from higher illumination and contrast.

Visual acuity varies with things other than

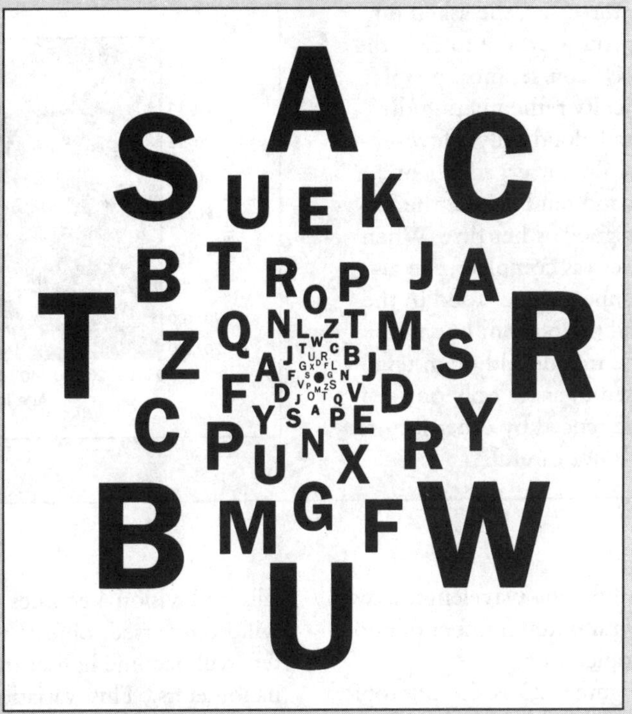

age and light level. Some people have particular trouble reading eye charts composed of letters bunched together. They'll be able to read smaller letters on a less crowded line of the eye chart, even though they fail with a line of larger letters that are crowded together. You can see this **crowding effect** in an eye chart prepared by Stuart Anstis, shown above. Compare the legibility of this crowded chart to the legibility of the chart in Figure 3.20. They are almost the same, except that Anstis has added many extra letters.

Visual acuity scores may also be affected by cognitive factors, including memorization of the eye chart (by someone who is particularly anxious to "pass" an eye test). Sometimes these cognitive factors play a role even though neither patient nor doctor intend them to. Erica, the youngest daughter of one of the authors (R.S.), was having her eyes examined by a well-meaning though inexperienced ophthalmologist who, to make matters worse, was in a hurry. Wanting to measure acuity separately for each eye, he asked her to close her left eye and read the five small letters at the bottom of the chart, using only her right eye. After she had finished a perfect rendition of the requested letters, she was told to switch eyes, now using her left eye to read the letters. Since the doctor had not

(continued)

bothered to change the chart, she asked him incredulously, "Do you want me to read the *same* letters again?" Of course, most people would have no difficulty remembering the five letters they'd read aloud only a few seconds before. But the doctor urged her on. No surprise: her second rendition of the letters was every bit as good as her first. When the testing procedure was complete, she almost—her good manners alone stood in the way—offered to read the bottom line with *both* eyes closed. The moral? Although tests of acuity are supposed to assess only one's vision, they can be influenced by other factors as well if the tester is not careful.

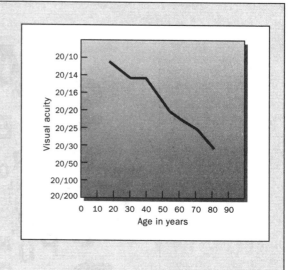

Again, for stimuli of different wavelengths, we want to determine the minimum number of photons required for photopic vision.

The solid line in Figure 3.23 is the photopic sensitivity curve, with sensitivity plotted as a function of stimulus wavelength. (Box 3.5, pp. 66–67, discusses one very practical implication of this curve's shape.) The dashed line replots the *scotopic* sensitivity function in Figure 3.22. Comparing the two curves, note that scotopic sensitivity is greater than photopic sensitivity at all except the longest wavelengths, the "red" end of the spectrum. Note also that the peaks of the two curves occur at different wavelengths; maximum scotopic sensitivity occurs at 500 nanometers, whereas photopic sensitivity peaks at 550 nanometers.

The Purkinje Shift. The difference between the wavelengths at which the photopic and scotopic curves peak has an important perceptual consequence, one that you may have experienced. This effect was first described by Johannes Evangelista von Purkinje, a Bohemian physiologist of the early nineteenth century (Kuthan, 1987). During the day, when vision is photopic, objects close to 550 nanometers wavelength will tend to appear lighter than objects of 500 nanometers. As night

falls and vision becomes scotopic, the situation will be reversed; objects reflecting 500 nanometers will become lighter than those reflecting 550 nanometers. This variation in relative lightness with time of day is known as the **Purkinje shift.**

Fortunately, the Purkinje shift can be easily seen under rather pleasant conditions. Get a com-

FIGURE 3.22 Visual sensitivity of rods (scotopic system) varies with wavelength of light.

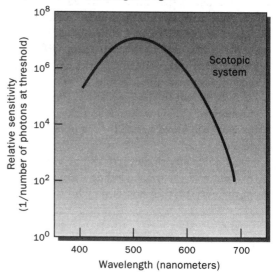

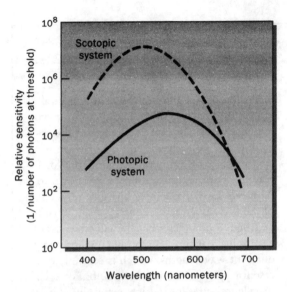

FIGURE 3.23 Visual sensitivity of cones (photopic system) varies with wavelength of light (solid line). For purposes of comparison, the scotopic curve from Figure 3.22 is included (dashed line).

fortable chair and a good book, and sit in a flower garden on a nice, warm day. Compare the lightness of yellow daisies with the lightness of the green foliage. During the day, the daisies will look lighter because their reflected wavelengths fall closer to the peak of the photopic sensitivity curve. But as twilight falls, the foliage will appear lighter, since it reflects wavelengths closer to the peak of the scotopic sensitivity curve. This is the Purkinje shift.

Dark Adaptation. The retina's duplex nature produces the differences between photopic and scotopic vision. We've already explored some of these differences. The retina's duplexity affects vision in another way, too—by controlling the recovery from exposure to light, a process called **dark adaptation.**

Everyone is already familiar with dark adaptation from common experience. Most people know about it from going to the movies. Upon first entering the darkened theater from the bright lobby, you have difficulty finding a seat or seeing the faces of people around you. After a while,

though, you "get used to" the dark and can see better. A small part of your improved vision can be traced to changes in your pupil. In darkness, the pupil dilates, allowing more light into the eye. But dark adaptation cannot be explained solely by pupillary dilation. For one thing, as you dark adapt, your sensitivity to light may improve by a factor of 100,000 or more, whereas the change in pupil area is relatively small, a factor of 16 at most. Moreover, your sensitivity may continue to improve for 30 to 40 minutes, whereas the pupil reaches its maximum size within a matter of seconds.

When dark adaptation is studied in the laboratory, it is possible to time the recovery of vision. Such experiments are numerous and have revealed a lot about vision's duplex nature. We'll present some of the highlights here; for a more extensive treatment, see Hood and Finkelstein (1986).

Studies of dark adaptation typically begin by exposing a subject to a strong light, called the *adaptation stimulus.* The idea is to determine how fast a person recovers from the effect of that strong light. After the adaptation stimulus has been extinguished, the person sits in complete darkness and looks for a very dim flashing light (the *test stimulus*), which is presented about once per second. The test light's intensity increases slowly until the light becomes visible to the person; then the intensity quickly decreases. This cycle is repeated over and over, perhaps for as long as 30 minutes. Each time the test stimulus becomes visible, two values are recorded: the *intensity* of that just visible stimulus and the *time* at which it was seen (that is, the time elapsed since the person entered into darkness). The general outcome can be described simply: the longer the person stays in the dark, the less intense the test stimulus need be in order to be seen. To put it another way, the longer the period in the dark, the more sensitive the person becomes.

Now suppose that you wanted to measure the recovery of rod sensitivity separately from the recovery of cone sensitivity. How might that be done? You could capitalize on the uneven distribution of these two types of photoreceptors to

Box 3.5 *Does the Electric Company Give You Your Money's Worth?*

The bill from your electric company has just arrived. Shocked by the numbers, you want to know whether you're getting your money's worth. A dollar value cannot be placed on the pleasure you may have gotten from playing your stereo and the like, so let's ignore those uses of electricity, sticking to one we can say something about—the use of electricity to produce light for reading.

Because it is the photopic system that affords reasonable resolution, we use that system when reading. So we can begin the analysis by looking at the photopic sensitivity curve (Figure 3.23). Since the photopic system is most sensitive to light whose wavelength is 550 nanometers, your electricity dollars would be most efficiently spent if they were used to produce radiation of only that wavelength. Electricity devoted to producing ultraviolet or infrared radiation is, of course, wasted, since you can't see either. Moreover, any electricity spent to produce visible radiation but at wavelengths other than 550 nanometers is not being used as efficiently as it could be.

Suppose you use only ordinary tengsten light bulbs for reading. How could you determine the effectiveness of each dollar spent to power one of these bulbs? The answer depends on the spectral distribution of the light emitted by these bulbs. If they emitted only at 550 nanometers, they'd be highly efficient—putting out light precisely at the wavelength that has the greatest impact on the human visual system. The left graph in

the accompanying figure shows the spectral distribution of the radiation emitted by a typical tungsten bulb. Note that most of the radiation that you pay for consists of wavelengths that you can't see, let alone use for reading. For quantification, we must turn to **Abney's Law** (named for a British physicist of the early twentieth century).

Abney's Law describes the effectiveness of a stimulus that simultaneously contains many different wavelengths, which is certainly the case for light from a tungsten bulb. For each wavelength present in such a stimulus, Abney's Law instructs one to take the product of two quantities: the amount of light present at that wavelength and how sensitive the photopic system is to that wavelength. The first of these quantities can be obtained from measuring devices (spectrum analyzers of various sorts); the second can be obtained from a table of the photopic sensitivity function's numerical value at various wavelengths (see Figure 3.23). After these products are obtained for each wavelength in the stimulus, Abney's Law requires that one sum up all the products. The resulting sum is a numerical statement of the visual effectiveness of the spectrally complex stimulus. Stated simply, Abney's Law says that one can predict the impact of a complex stimulus composed of many wavelengths by evaluating the effectiveness of each of its component wavelengths and then summing their separate effects.

To make quantitative sense of the out-

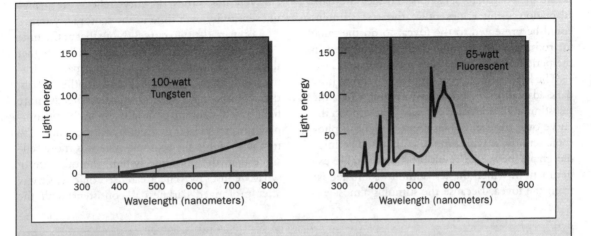

come, though, we need some reference—say, some stimulus that represents 100 percent efficiency, the maximum obtainable. Since that's the best you could achieve, let's say that such a stimulus gave you a full dollar's worth of light for each dollar spent on electricity. Compared to that standard, you get only 3 cents worth of light for each dollar put into electricity for a tungsten bulb. Some tungsten bulbs do a little better—5 cents return per dollar spent—but these lamps tend to burn out quickly.

We can apply the same analysis to another common type of light used for reading—fluorescent lamps. The spectrum of a typical fluorescent lamp is shown in the right graph in the accompanying figure. Compared with the tungsten bulb, the fluorescent lamp emits far more of its radiation within the visually effective band (400 to 700 nanometers) and far less in the infrared (which is experienced as

heat, not light). Applying Abney's Law to the spectrum of a fluorescent lamp, we find that you get 10 cents worth of reading light for each dollar's worth of electricity, a much better buy.

Oddly, the most efficient light source for reading is one that doesn't require any electricity at all. The distinguished French vision scientist Yves LeGrand (1968) pointed out that fireflies and glowworms emit light very near the peak wavelength of the photopic sensitivity curve (p. 82). Because fireflies achieve very high photopic efficiencies, a lamp full of fireflies would certainly give you your money's worth of reading light.

We don't usually tell you things that we don't want you to remember. But for your own peace of mind, the next time you have to pay an electric bill, maybe you should forget how few of your dollars are going for something you actually used.

isolate their separate behaviors. To measure dark adaptation using cones only, the test stimulus could be presented to the fovea; to do the same for rods, the test stimulus could be presented in the periphery where the rods predominate.

The left-hand graph of Figure 3.24 shows how dark adaptation experiments turn out when the test stimulus is presented foveally. The drop in the curve over time shows an improvement in photopic sensitivity with time in darkness. The middle graph shows the results of a comparable experiment in which the test stimulus is imaged far from the fovea. Because the stimulus almost ex-

clusively affects rods, the curve reflects the changing sensitivity over time of the scotopic system.

Compare the two curves. Note that at the time "0," the scotopic curve (middle panel) is higher than the photopic curve (left-hand panel). Immediately after entering darkness, in other words, the scotopic system is less sensitive (needs more light to see) than the photopic system. Now compare the curves later in time, say, at the points "20 minutes." Here the scotopic system is more sensitive than the photopic system, the opposite of what we just saw. The greater scotopic sensitivity after prolonged darkness is consistent with the

---

Box 3.6 *Recovering from Light*

When people compare the human eye to a camera, they liken the retina to the camera's film. But in one sense, the retina is more like videotape than film—both the retina and videotape are reusable. Even this analogy is inadequate, though, because unlike videotape, the retina can be used and reused millions of times. Wilhelm Kühne, a German physiologist and one of the first to study the retina's recovery, commented that

bound together with the pigment epithelium, the retina behaves not merely like a photographic plate, but like an entire photographic workshop in which the workman continually renews the plate by laying on new light-sensitive material, while simultaneously erasing the old image. (Translation in Wald, 1950, p. 33)

How does the retina renew itself, recovering sensitivity after being exposed to light? When a photopigment molecule breaks up, it is said to have become "bleached"—a most apt term. When Franz Boll first studied this process, he noticed that the retina of the frog was usually intensely red. But when the frog's eye was exposed to light, the color of the ret-

ina disappeared; that is, it was bleached. Now we know that this loss of color is associated with the splitting apart of the retina's photopigment molecules.

In the 1880s, Kühne was struck by the analogy between the retina and the photographic plate, then still a novelty. Kühne exploited this resemblance scientifically, using retinas to make "retinal photographs," or as he called them, "optograms." An optogram treats the retina as though it were a photographic plate or piece of film, actually developing and fixing the image on the retina using special chemicals (Kühne, 1879/1977). Kühne used this approach to examine the image that various objects cast on the retina.

To make one particularly imaginative but gruesome optogram, Kühne got the cooperation of a man sentenced to die on the guillotine. The man's eyes were shielded from light for several hours before the execution, allowing light-sensitive material to accumulate in the retina. Then, just before the beheading, his eyes were uncovered. Immediately after the execution, Kühne removed the eyes and chemically treated the retinas to preserve the image of the last thing the man had seen

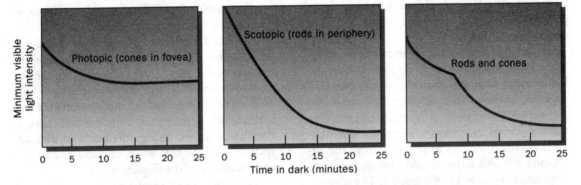

FIGURE 3.24 Graphs showing change in sensitivity with time in darkness.

(Wald, 1950). Unfortunately, the optogram was ambiguous, perhaps because instead of staring fixedly at just one object, the condemned man understandably moved his eyes around, taking his "last look" at one thing after another.

How does the retina manage to process millions of images over a lifetime? The secret lies in the retina's ability to restore its own sensitivity to light through a complex biochemical process (Stabell, Stabell, and Fugelli, 1992). Earlier we mentioned Boll's observation on bleaching in the frog's eye. He also noticed that the retina regained its normal, reddish color if the frog stayed in the dark for a short time (Boll, 1877/1977). We know now that the reddish color returns because new photopigment molecules have been created. This restoration is just as important for the visual process as is bleaching. If photopigment could not be restored, an animal would quickly become blind because all the available photopigment molecules would become bleached and thus unable to signal the presence of light.

To produce new photopigment after light has bleached part of the retina requires that a derivative of vitamin A diffuse through the retinal pigment epithelium and combine with protein available within the retina. Since all the body's vitamin A comes from the food one eats, a serious deficiency of vitamin A in the diet slows down the restoration of the photopigments. In vitamin A deficiency, once a photopigment molecule is bleached, its return to the unbleached state is slowed. A person with a vitamin A deficiency is described as "night blind" because he or she typically experiences difficulty seeing at night or in other dim illumination (Dowling, 1966). Such people might have extreme difficulty seeing after entering a darkened theater, be unable to recognize friends on the street in a dim light, or be unable to see clearly while driving at night.

The problem of vitamin A deficiency is common in developing countries, where diet is often inadequate and vitamin supplements rare. Even people in developed countries are not immune to poor diet and night vision problems. For example, some years ago, one-third of the medical students tested showed diminished night vision that was attributable to their diet (Jeghers, 1937). These medical students were simply too busy to eat proper quantities of carrots and leafy vegetables. We should also note that night blindness can come from other causes, too, including impairment at virtually any stage of the rods' response (Ripps, 1982).

large difference between the peak sensitivities of photopic (cone) and scotopic (rod) spectral sensitivity curves (Figure 3.23).

Returning to the dark adaptation curves in Figure 3.24, note that the scotopic system starts out less sensitive than the photopic system but ends up more sensitive. After an interval of about 8 to 10 minutes, their *relative* sensitivities reverse. One other point emerges from these curves. The photopic system completes its recovery from the adaptation stimulus rather quickly (since the curve stops declining after 5 to 6 minutes). The scotopic system takes a lot longer (the curve doesn't stop declining until about 15 minutes have elapsed).

Next, suppose we modify the previous study by imaging the test stimulus on a retinal region that contains both rods and cones. Measuring recovery from the same adaptation stimulus as before, the outcome will resemble the curve shown in the right-hand graph of Figure 3.24.

Compare the curve in this graph with the others, noting the kink in this new curve. Things seem to go along smoothly from time "0" until "8 minutes." In fact, recovery seems to have leveled off. Then all of a sudden, at the 8-minute mark, recovery starts over again, eventually subsiding once more at about the 15-minute mark. What is going on here? Note that the left-hand part of the kinked curve bears a striking resemblance to the early part of the photopic dark adaptation curve (left graph in Figure 3.24); the rest of the kinked curve resembles the late part of the scotopic curve (middle graph in Figure 3.24). The explanation of the kinked curve, then, is simple. Because in this case the test stimulus affects both cones and rods, we have measured both types of adaptation simultaneously. Early in dark adaptation, the photopic system is more sensitive, so it alone determines the threshold. Later in dark ad-

aptation, the scotopic system is more sensitive, so it alone determines the threshold.

The exact outcome of these studies depends on a number of experimental details, notably the strength of the initial adaptation stimulus, the size of the test stimulus, and the wavelength of light used in the test stimulus. All these variables as well as many others (including an individual's diet, as Box 3.6 indicates) change the curve of dark adaptation in ways that are predictable from one's understanding of the duplex retina.

You don't need special equipment to verify some of these observations. Pick a clear night, and just before going outside, stand for a few moments in a brightly lit room. Then quickly go outside and look at the sky. At this point you probably won't be able to see any stars. Keep looking, though, and after a while some will become visible. The first ones you'll be able to see will probably lie at the location you're fixating, because early in dark adaptation the photopic system is more sensitive than the scotopic. After a few minutes, your scotopic system will have caught up and will exceed the photopic system's sensitivity. Then you will be able to see very dim stars, using the rod-dominated periphery of your retina.

After you've dark adapted for some minutes, you can verify that the rod-dominated periphery of your retina is more sensitive than the cone-dominated central region. Glance slowly around the sky, stopping when you can just barely see some very dim star that lies away from the spot you're looking directly at. If the star is just barely visible using the most sensitive part of your retina (where rods are most numerous and convergence is greatest), that star will become invisible when you look directly at it (imaging it on a less sensitive part of the retina).

S U M M A R Y   A N D   P R E V I E W

This chapter outlined how various aspects of visual perception are shaped by the properties of the retina, notably the center/surround antagonism of

retinal ganglion cells and the differences between the photoreceptors that feed the ganglion cells. Clearly, though, not all vision is determined by the retina; there are lots of facts that defy explanation at this retinal level. To increase the number of explained perceptual phenomena, we have to push farther into the nervous system, following the messages generated by the retina back into the brain itself. There you'll see that these messages originating in the retina are further refined and reorganized in ways that account for still other properties of the way you see the world.

KEY TERMS

Abney's Law
action potentials
axon
Bloch's Law
crowding effect
dark adaptation
duplex
eccentricity
Hermann grid
intensity

lateral inhibition
lightness
lightness constancy
lightness contrast
M cells
Mach bands
microelectrode
P cells
photon
photopic

Purkinje shift
receptive field
resolution
retinal ganglion cells
Ricco's Law
scotopic
single cell recording
spatial summation
temporal summation
visual acuity

Central Visual Pathways

I n this chapter we continue tracing the flow of information within the visual nervous system. You'll learn how visual information about objects and events in the world is carried to the brain and distributed to different sets of neurons in the visual cortex. You'll also see how patterns of activity within these brain cells can be related to various aspects of visual perception. Let's begin by examining the **optic nerve,** the bundle of fibers carrying information from the eyes to various processing stages in the central nervous system.

THE OPTIC NERVE

Each eye's optic nerve comprises axons from all its retinal ganglion cells. Thus the optic nerve from each eye resembles a cable that contains roughly 1 million individual wires. Multiplied by two eyes, this means that the brain receives visual input from 2 million separate channels, each carrying information about a small region of the visual world. That may seem like a huge number of communication lines, but it is really quite modest compared with the hundreds of millions of neurons populating the visual areas of the brain. Keep in mind that all neural processing of visual information within the brain depends on the optic nerves for input data; the optic nerves provide the brain with the raw material for visual perception. Interruptions in the flow of that information to the brain destroy vision.

Within the eye itself, the axons of ganglion cells are not covered by **myelin;** as you may know, myelin is a membrane that both insulates the axon from activity in neighboring axons and speeds the conduction of nerve impulses. Presumably, axons within the eye remain unmyelinated in order to reduce the clutter through which light must pass to reach the receptors—a coating of myelin could double the diameter of an axon. Once outside the eye, though, this restriction is removed, and individual axons acquire a coating of myelin.

Within each optic nerve, fibers from different regions of the retina congregate in an orderly fashion, with fibers carrying information from neighboring regions of the retina running adjacent to one another within the nerve (Torrealba et al., 1982). From the point at which it leaves the eye, the optic nerve travels approximately 5 centimeters (2 inches) before rendezvousing with the optic nerve from the other eye.

The optic nerves from the two eyes converge at the **optic chiasm.** The term "chiasm" comes from the Greek word meaning "cross," and a glance at Figure 4.1 shows why this term is appropriate. At the chiasm there is a wholesale rearrangement of the constituent fibers. Using Figure 4.1, carefully trace the fibers from different regions of either eye as those fibers enter and leave the optic chiasm. Notice that some fibers always remain on the same side of the brain—these are called uncrossed fibers, or **ipsilateral fibers** ("ipsi" means "same" and "lateral" refers to side). Regardless of which eye they come from, these ipsilateral fibers originate from that eye's temporal

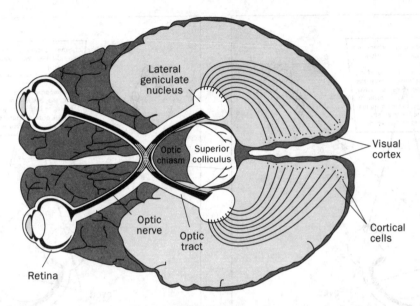

FIGURE 4.1 The projections of the optic fibers from the two eyes to the two hemispheres of the brain. The fibers represented by the solid black lines originate from the nasal retina of both eyes; they cross at the optic chiasm to the opposite hemisphere and are called contralateral fibers. The fibers represented by the hatch marks originate from the temporal retina of both eyes; they remain on the same side of the brain and are called ipsilateral fibers.

retina ("temporal" refers to that half of the retina nearest the temples). Other fibers cross to the opposite side of the brain at the optic chiasm. These are the crossed fibers, or **contralateral fibers,** and they come from the nasal retina of each eye ("contra" means "opposite"; "nasal" refers to the half of the retina closest to the nose). Thus the optic nerve from each eye branches into two segments—one crossed, the other uncrossed. Within the chiasm, crossed fibers from one eye join with uncrossed fibers from the other eye, yielding two new combinations of retinal axons. These new combinations, which run from the chiasm to structures deeper in the brain, are known as **optic tracts.** Don't be fooled by the terminology—an optic tract is still composed of axons from ganglion cells; the change in name from "nerve" to "tract" is simply a convention used by anatomists. The important thing to understand is that each optic tract contains fibers from *both* eyes, the temporal retina of one eye and the nasal retina of the other.

The proportion of crossed and uncrossed fibers in the optic tract varies among species. The percentages are not related to the species' position on the evolutionary scale; instead, they relate to the position of the animal's eyes within its head. For instance, in animals with laterally placed eyes, such as the rabbit, nearly all the axons cross to the opposite side of the brain. In humans, about 50 percent of the axons from each eye cross at the chiasm, while the other 50 percent remain uncrossed. This division between crossed and uncrossed occurs along an imaginary vertical seam bisecting the fovea.

But why should eye position in the head be related to the percentage of crossing fibers? To figure out the answer, think about the relation between the position of an object in space and the position of that object's image on the retina. The following exercise will help (see Figure 4.2). While looking at the center of this page, place your right thumb on the right-hand edge of the page. The image of your thumb will now fall on

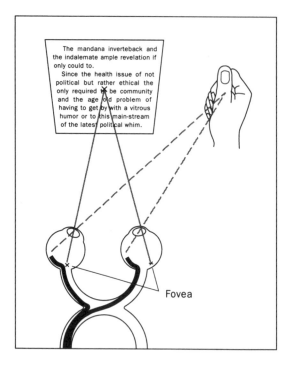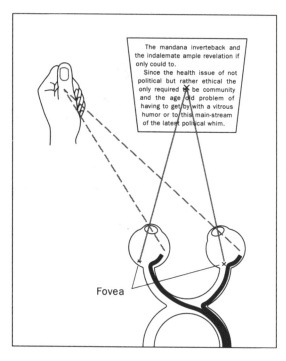

Fovea   Fovea

FIGURE 4.2 Objects to the right of the point of fixation cast images on the nasal retina of the right eye and the temporal retina of the left eye; fibers from these two retinal areas project to the left side of the brain (left drawing). Objects to the left of the point of fixation cast images on the nasal retina of the left eye and the temporal retina of the right eye; fibers from these two retinal areas project to the right side of the brain (right drawing).

the temporal retina of your left eye and nasal retina of your right eye. Looking at Figures 4.1 and 4.2, you will see that fibers from these regions of the two retinas wind up together in the optic tract on the left side of the brain. Keeping your gaze on the center of the page, place your left thumb on the page's left-hand edge. Now your thumb is imaged on the nasal retina of your left eye and the temporal retina of your right eye. Figures 4.1 and 4.2 show that these two regions end up sending fibers to the right side of the brain.

As this exercise demonstrates, there is a general rule to describe how information from the two halves of the visual field is distributed to the hemispheres of the brain: the right hemisphere processes information from the left visual field, while the left hemisphere processes information from the right visual field. Those portions of the left and right eyes that look at the *same* area of visual

space send their nerve fibers to the *same* region of the brain. The partial crossing of axons at the chiasm makes this possible. Rerouting the axons sets the stage for combining information from the two eyes, a process that we'll learn more about shortly.

In animals with eyes on the side of their heads, the two eyes look at *different* areas of visual space. For these animals, it would be extremely maladaptive to mix information from the two eyes because such information specifies different objects in the world. Consequently, mixing information from the two eyes could lead to serious confusion about the location of those objects. To avoid this potential for confusion, the optic fibers from the two eyes remain strictly segregated, crossing in their entirety at the optic chiasm. This serves to route information from the two laterally placed eyes to different halves of the brain.

Let's resume tracing the destination of the fibers of the optic tract. Remember, we're still talking about the axons of the ganglion cells originating in the retina. About 80 percent of the fibers project to a cluster of cell bodies known as the **lateral geniculate nucleus (LGN).** The remaining 20 percent of the optic tract projects to several neighboring structures in the midbrain, the most prominent being the **superior colliculus.** Since the superior colliculus and the lateral geniculate nucleus are both regions of the brain to which retinal axons project, these places are referred to as *projection areas.*

To make it easier to follow the flow of visual information from the optic tract, we'll discuss the two major branches of the optic tract separately. We'll first briefly describe the branch to the superior colliculus and then cover in more detail the other branch, to the lateral geniculate nucleus and its projection site, the visual cortex. But don't let our separate treatment of these areas of the brain mislead you. These visual centers are richly interconnected, and their functions can be carried out only when all the components work in harmony. Moreover, there are several other midbrain structures—thought to be involved in control of pupil size, registration of self-motion, and postural adjustments—omitted from our discussion.

THE SUPERIOR COLLICULUS

Tucked away at the top of the brain stem (see Figure 4.3), the superior colliculus is a phylogenetically older, more primitive visual area than the visual cortex. In many lower animals, such as frogs and fish, the superior colliculus represents *the* major brain center for visual processing. In human beings and other higher animals, however, the phylogenetically newer visual cortex has supplanted the superior colliculus as the more important visual area. Nonetheless, even in these higher animals, the superior colliculus plays a prominent role in visual orienting reflexes, including the initiation and guidance of eye movements (Wurtz, Goldberg, and Robinson, 1982;

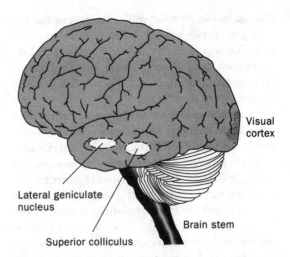

FIGURE 4.3 View of the left side of the brain showing the relative locations of several visual structures. The lateral geniculate nucleus and superior colliculus (drawn with dotted lines) are actually located within the brain and are not visible from its surface.

Sparks and Nelson, 1987). The evidence pointing to this conclusion comes from several sources.

For one thing, cells in the superior colliculus have receptive fields with rather ill-defined ON and OFF regions. These cells will respond to just about any visual stimulus—edges, bars of any orientation, light flashes—falling within their receptive fields, regardless of the shape or orientation of that stimulus (Goldberg and Wurtz, 1972). These properties suggest that the colliculus is not concerned with precisely "what" the stimulus is but rather with "where" it is. For another thing, cells in the superior colliculus clearly are involved in controlling eye movements. Many cells in the superior colliculus emit a vigorous burst of activity just before the eyes begin to move. This burst of activity occurs, however, only if the eyes move in order to fixate a light flashed in the visual periphery; eye movements made in darkness evoke no activity in these cells. So the *intention* to move the eyes toward some object seems to be critical for the cells' responsiveness. Besides initiating eye movements, the superior colliculus also plays some role in guiding the direction and extent of those eye movements (Carpenter, 1992). Thus, damage to the superior colliculus impairs the accuracy of visually guided eye movements in monkeys (Kurtz and Butter, 1980; Albano, Mishkin, Westbrook, and Wurtz, 1982) and in humans (Heywood and Ratcliff, 1975). At present, though, there is debate about the details of how the superior colliculus actually does guide eye movements (Schiller and Koerner, 1971; Wurtz and Goldberg, 1972). Moreover, the superior colliculus is just one of several brain areas playing a role in guidance of eye movements; other prominent areas include the visual cortex (Seagraves et al., 1987) and the frontal eye-field situated in the frontal lobe (see Schall, 1991, for an excellent review of this literature on neural control of eye movements). Eye movements themselves will be discussed in more detail in Chapter 8.

Besides receiving visual input, cells in the superior colliculus also receive auditory input from the ears, as evidenced by their responsiveness to sound stimulation (Gordon, 1972). Because they receive sensory input from the eyes *and* ears, these are called *multisensory cells*. In order for most multisensory cells to respond, auditory and visual stimulation has to originate from the same region of space. For example, if some multisensory cell responds to a light flash in the upper right portion of the visual field, that cell will respond to a sound only if it, too, comes from the same vicinity. Additionally, when visual and auditory inputs occur simultaneously, a multisensory cell responds more strongly than when either input occurs alone. Because of this property, a weak auditory input can amplify the effects of a weak visual input, producing a strong combined response. As a result, sight and sound can reinforce one another in these multisensory cells, enabling an animal to detect the location of feeble environmental events (Meredith and Stein, 1983).

In summary, the superior colliculus seems designed to detect objects located away from the point of fixation and to guide orienting movements of the eyes and head toward those objects (Sparks, 1988). The colliculus does not, however, contain the machinery necessary for a detailed visual analysis of such objects. That job, instead,

belongs to the other branch of the optic tract, the one projecting to the lateral geniculate nucleus and then on to the visual cortex. It is to those sites that we turn next.

THE LATERAL GENICULATE NUCLEUS

In this section we shall first consider the interesting structure of the lateral geniculate nucleus and the way in which retinal input is distributed throughout the structure. Then we'll describe the receptive field properties of geniculate neurons and speculate on the role of these neurons in vision. Figure 4.3 indicates the area of the brain where the LGN is located.

STRUCTURE OF THE LGN

The LGN has a very distinct, layered appearance, as you can see in panel A of Figure 4.4. The layers consist of cell bodies, and the number of layers in the LGN varies from one species to another. In humans, the LGN on each side of the brain contains six layers stacked on top of one another and bent in the middle. This bend gives the LGN its name: "geniculate" comes from a Latin word meaning "with bent knee," as in "genuflect." For purposes of discussion, let's number the successive layers 1, 2, 3, 4, 5, and 6, going from the bottom to the top of the structure. Note also in Figure 4.4 that cells in layers 1 and 2 are larger than those in layers 3 through 6. These two large-cell layers are termed the **magnocellular layers,** and the four small-cell layers are called the **parvocellular layers** (the prefixes come from the Latin words *magnus,* meaning "large," and *parvus,* meaning "small"). You will recall the P and M retinal ganglion cells from the previous chapter. The P ganglion cells provide the input to the parvocellular layers of the LGN, whereas the M cells feed into the magnocellular layers of the LGN. Recall also that the P cells and the M cells differed in the kinds of visual stimuli to which they respond best; those response differences are maintained at the level of the LGN, as we shall discuss in a moment.

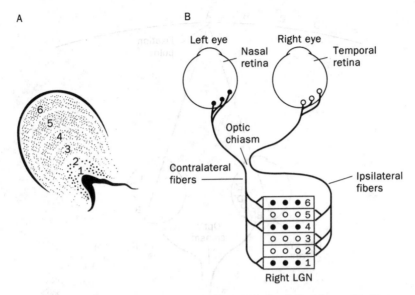

FIGURE 4.4 Cross section through the LGN showing its distinct layers (A). Diagram showing projections from both eyes to the right LGN (B); a corresponding diagram could be drawn for the projections to the left LGN.

First, however, let's consider some of the anatomical properties of this well-organized nucleus.

To begin, consider how fibers of the optic tract make contact with cells in the different layers of the lateral geniculate nucleus. Remember that each optic tract contains a mixture of fibers from both eyes, the temporal retina of the ipsilateral eye and the nasal retina of the contralateral eye. These fibers become very strictly segregated when they arrive at the lateral geniculate nucleus: the contralateral fibers contact only the cells in layers 1, 4, and 6, whereas the ipsilateral fibers contact only the cells in layers 2, 3, and 5. Take a moment to study panel B of Figure 4.4 to be sure you understand this pattern of input to the various layers. In sorting out these projections, keep in mind that the brain contains a pair of lateral geniculate nuclei, one residing in the left hemisphere and the other in the right hemisphere. This paired arrangement means that a single eye provides the contralateral input to one lateral geniculate nucleus and the ipsilateral input to the other. Now let's look at how retinal input is registered within these layers.

RETINAL MAPS IN THE LGN

Each layer of the LGN contains an orderly representation, or map, of the retina. This point is illustrated in Figure 4.5. As you can see, axons that carry information from neighboring regions of the retina connect with geniculate cells that are themselves neighbors. This way of distributing retinal information within any layer of the LGN creates a map of the retina within that layer. Since such a map preserves the topography of the retina, it is known as a **retinotopic map.** Each of the six layers contains its own complete retinotopic map, and these layers are stacked in such a way that comparable regions of the separate maps are aligned with each other. For instance, the foveal parts of adjacent layers are situated on top of one another.

RECEPTIVE FIELD PROPERTIES OF LGN CELLS

Just like their retinal counterparts, LGN cells have circular receptive fields, subdivided into concentric center and surround components. As in the

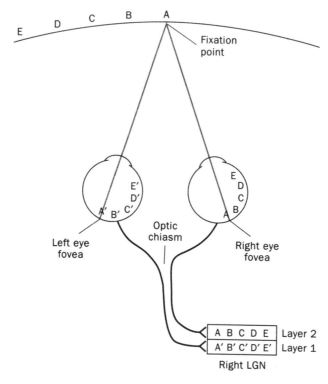

FIGURE 4.5 Drawing showing how different areas of the visual field are mapped onto the two retinas and then onto various layers of the right LGN. For simplicity, only two layers are shown.

retina, these two components interact antagonistically; some cells have ON centers paired with OFF surrounds, whereas others have exactly the opposite configuration. There is an important difference, though, between LGN and retina: the surround of an LGN receptive field exerts a stronger inhibitory effect on its center than does the surround of a retinal ganglion cell (Maffei and Fiorentini, 1972). This means the LGN cells amplify, or accentuate, differences in illumination between neighboring retinal regions even more than do retinal ganglion cells. Incidentally, because their fields are circular in shape, LGN cells, like their retinal counterparts, will respond to borders or contours of any orientation.

This center/surround layout of LGN receptive fields is characteristic of essentially all LGN cells, regardless of whether they are located in a parvocellular layer or a magnocellular layer. There

are, however, several major differences between cells in the magnocellular layers and cells in the parvocellular layers (Livingstone and Hubel, 1988; Schiller and Logothetis, 1990), differences that relate to the P versus M ganglion cell inputs to these layers. These differences strongly imply that the two subdivisions—magnocellular and parvocellular—make their own unique contributions to visual perception.

Color. Nearly all parvocellular cells (that is, the cells in layers 3 through 6) are differentially sensitive to the *color* of light imaged within their receptive fields (DeValois, Smith, Kitai, and Karoly, 1958; Wiesel and Hubel, 1966; Dreher, Fukada, and Rodieck, 1976). A vigorous response can be evoked from these cells only if the center of the field is illuminated by light of one particular color (for example, red); when the surround is illuminated by a different color (for example, green), the cell's activity is inhibited. Because of their unique response to the pairing of "opposite" colors, these cells are called *color opponent cells*. Some opponent cells exhibit red/green organization, whereas others exhibit blue/yellow organization. We'll consider these opponent cells in greater detail in Chapter 6. Just to reiterate: the opponent color cells in the parvocellular layers are thought to receive their inputs from the P cells in the retina.

Cells in the magnocellular layers (and a small fraction of cells in the parvocellular layers) respond to all colors. Their response depends solely on the relative intensity of light falling in the center and surround portions of their receptive fields. To reiterate: cells in the magnocellular layers are thought to receive their inputs from the M cells in the retina.

Acuity. Within each of the six layers of the LGN, receptive fields vary systematically in size, with the smallest fields devoted to representation of the fovea. For a given region of the retina, cells in the magnocellular layers have receptive fields that are 2 or 3 times larger than receptive fields for cells in the parvocellular layers. Hence parvocellular cells analyze spatial information at a finer level of detail than do magnocellular cells.

Speed of Motion. Magnocellular cells respond vigorously to fast, abrupt fluctuations of light intensity within their receptive fields, whereas parvocellular cells respond sluggishly—if at all—to such fluctuations. Rapid motion of an object generates such intensity fluctuations within a cell's receptive field, implying that magnocellular cells, but not parvocellular cells, are able to signal the presence of rapid movement.

* * *

These two distinct populations of LGN neurons—magnocellular cells and parvocellular cells—both send their axons to the visual cortex. As we will discover shortly, however, those axons terminate in different parts of the visual cortex, thus maintaining the functional segregation of in-

formation found within these different layer types. Before moving up to the cortex, though, let's spend a moment speculating about the importance of the LGN for vision.

POSSIBLE FUNCTIONS OF THE LGN

You now have a thumbnail sketch of the chief characteristics of the LGN, the relay station between the retina and higher visual areas in the brain. What do the various anatomical and physiological properties we've discussed suggest about the LGN's role in vision? As just described, cells in the LGN are primarily concerned with differences in intensity between neighboring regions of the retina, and in some instances with the color of light; these cells are unconcerned with the overall level of light. In other words, LGN cells are designed to register the presence of edges in the visual environment. This alone, however, does not represent a unique contribution to vision; retinal cells have already accomplished this job of signaling the presence of edges. So we are led to ask, does the LGN seem uniquely suited for some other role, or does it merely relay messages broadcast from the retina straight on to higher brain sites with no editing or censorship? There are several reasons for thinking the LGN is considerably more than just a relay station.

For one thing, the LGN receives input not only from the retina but from the **reticular activating system** as well (Burke and Cole, 1978). Buried in the brain stem, the reticular activating system governs an animal's general level of arousal. Hence the flow of visual information from the LGN to higher visual centers could be modified by the animal's state of arousal. The LGN may well operate like the volume control on a radio, modulating the intensity of retinal inputs according to the animal's current state of arousal. In support of this idea, Livingstone and Hubel (1981) found that when an animal was in a drowsy state (as evidenced behaviorally and by brain-wave recordings), the overall level of activity in the LGN was low. The reduced level of LGN activity meant that the higher visual centers of the drowsy animal were receiving signals that were attenuated compared with those they would have received had the animal been more alert. This interplay between arousal level and the strength of signals going to the higher visual centers could promote attentiveness to visual information.

In addition to input from the reticular activating system, the LGN receives a large input from the visual cortex. You may find this intriguing, since the visual cortex itself *receives* a substantial amount of its input from the LGN. In effect, the LGN formulates a message and transmits it to the cortex; the cortex, in turn, sends back a reply to the LGN, thereby allowing that message to be altered. This kind of arrangement is known as a *feedback loop,* and it is widely used in electronics to regulate electrical current within a circuit. At present, the biological purpose of the visual feedback between the cortex and the LGN is not known, although intriguing speculations have been advanced (Martin, 1988).

The highly organized arrangement of this structure and the distinct physiological differences between magnocellular and parvocellular layers strongly suggest that the LGN plays another crucial role in vision. Recall that information about color is processed exclusively in the parvocellular layers, while information about large, rapidly moving intensity contours falls within the domain of the magnocellular layers. This orderly sorting of visual information sets the stage for the next level of processing occurring in the visual cortex. An analogy may help clarify what we mean.

Think for a moment about the most efficient way to assemble a complex jigsaw puzzle. You usually begin by sorting the jumble of pieces into groups, according to some shared property. You might locate and place all the pieces that make up the border into one pile, the pieces of comparable color into another pile, and so on. In general, before assembling the puzzle pieces into a picture, you will organize them so that the solution emerges with minimal trial-and-error effort. The lateral geniculate nucleus may perform an analogous sorting operation. The orderly arrangement of information within the LGN could help the next stage of visual processing to begin piecing the puzzle together. This next stage takes place in the primary visual cortex, to which we now turn.

THE VISUAL CORTEX

The visual cortex is located at the very back of the cerebral hemispheres (see Figure 4.3), in a region called the **occipital lobe.** If you place your cupped hand on the back of your head just above the base of your skull, your hand will be resting over this region. The visual cortex receives input from the LGN, but it is anatomically more complex than the LGN. This anatomical complexity is paralleled by an increase in physiological complexity—particularly in the variety of receptive fields exhibited by cortical cells. But before tackling the anatomical and physiological details of this fascinating region of the brain, let's consider some important findings from clinical neurology that first pointed to the cortex as a major visual center.

CORTICAL BLINDNESS

By the middle of the last century, neurologists had developed a keen interest in how the brain was subdivided. To examine its subdivisions, they removed localized regions of tissue from animals' brains and noted the behavioral consequences (this is the lesion technique mentioned in Chapter 1). Using this technique, neurologists observed that an animal seemed to be blind after destruction of the posterior area of its cerebral hemispheres.

At about the same time, case records began appearing in the medical literature describing permanent loss of vision in humans who had suffered brain damage from injury (Glickstein, 1988). This evidence also established the occipital lobe as the visual center in humans. The most thorough set of case studies was published by the Irish neurologist Sir Gordon Holmes. Most of his patients were veterans of World War I with localized brain damage from gunshot wounds. Holmes (1918) measured areas of blindness within their visual fields by moving a small spot of light throughout the patient's field of view while the patient stared at a stationary point. The patient reported when the light was visible and when it was not. Holmes was thus able to locate patches of blindness, or **scotomas,** within the patient's visual field. (Recall from Chapter 2 the simple demonstration of the small scotoma in *your* visual field, associated with the optic disk; also, see Box 4.1, pp. 114–115.) Holmes compared the size and location of the scotoma with the extent and position of the damage within the occipital cortex.

His results showed that the visual field (and, by extension, the retina) is represented within the cortex in a very orderly, topographic fashion. The center of the visual field maps onto the posterior region of the occipital lobe, and the periphery of the field maps onto the anterior portion. The upper portion of the visual field is represented in the lower portion of the occipital lobe, and vice versa.

Holmes found that visual disturbances always appeared in the visual field contralateral to the damaged hemisphere of the brain. Thus a wound to the left occipital lobe would be accompanied by blindness somewhere within the right visual field. Holmes also observed that the cortical map of the visual field appeared greatly distorted. The amount of cortical tissue devoted to the central portion of the field far exceeded the amount devoted to the periphery. This distortion, in which representation of the center of the field is highly exaggerated, has come to be known as **cortical magnification** (Daniel and Whitteridge, 1961). From a retinal perspective, cortical magnification means that a large portion of the cortex is devoted to a very small area of the retina. That area of the retina is the *fovea,* on which the central portion of the visual field is imaged (see Figure 4.6). Thus the lion's share of the cortex is devoted to that region of the retina responsible for highly acute vision.

Holmes's clinical work provided the earliest description of the retinotopic map on the visual cortex. Since these pioneering studies, many other neurologists (for example, Teuber, Battersby, and Bender, 1960) have cataloged the visual deficits that result from damage to various brain centers. We shall describe some of these unusual and informative syndromes later in this and other chapters. In general, the victims of unfortunate accidents have greatly advanced scientific understanding of the anatomy of vision. And as Box 4.2 (p. 116–117) indicates, even the study of totally blind people has shed light on the neural basis of visual perception. Now let's look in more detail at the structures that are implicated in Holmes's clinical work.

STRUCTURE OF THE VISUAL CORTEX

The primary visual cortex is that portion of the occipital lobe receiving input from the lateral geniculate nucleus. It is sometimes referred to as Area 17, on the basis of a postal-codelike labeling scheme, whereby neighboring, anatomically defined areas of the brain are sequentially numbered. Other names for this area include V1 (in recognition of its being the first in a hierarchy of cortical visual areas) and striate cortex (owing to the region's faintly striped appearance when seen under a low-power microscope). But the terms "primary visual cortex," "Area 17," "V1," and "striate cortex" all refer to the same portion of the brain.

Like the rest of the cerebral cortex, the visual area consists of a layered array of cells about 2 millimeters thick. In all, there are approximately 100 million cells in the Area 17 of each hemisphere. Figure 4.7 is a magnified picture of a section of brain tissue from Area 17 of a monkey. Note that various layers differ in thickness and that the concentration of cells varies from layer to layer. The million or so axons arriving from the six layers of the LGN connect with cortical cells within layer 4 of the visual cortex. The axons of cells from the magnocellular layers of the LGN make their contacts within an upper subdivision of cortical layer 4, while LGN axons from the parvocellular LGN layers contact the lower subdivision of layer 4 (see Figure 4.7). From here, connections within the cortex carry information to neurons in other layers above and below layer 4 and, eventually, to other areas within the brain. Throughout this network of connections, the magnocellular pathway seems to remain segre-

A

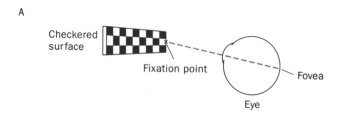

Checkered surface

Fixation point

Fovea

Eye

B

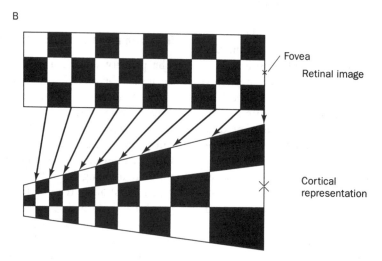

Fovea

Retinal image

Cortical representation

FIGURE 4.6 Imagine looking at the right-hand edge of a checkerboard pattern (A). The resulting retinal image will look something like the upper portion of panel B. Notice the position of the fovea in this image. By means of the processes described in Chapters 2 and 3, this retinal image is converted into neural signals and is conveyed to the visual cortex via the LGN (represented by arrows in B). The bottom portion of drawing B depicts how this retinal image is transcribed into neural activity within the visual cortex. The size of each square in the cortical representation is proportional to the *number* of cortical cells activated by any given square on the checkered surface being viewed. (This is not to imply, however, that a checkered pattern appears in the cortex.) Notice that the squares near the point of fixation are expanded in the cortical representation. This expansion reflects the disproportionately large number of cortical cells devoted to neural representation of information falling on and near the fovea. Conversely, squares located far from the point of fixation appear small in the cortical representation, reflecting the relatively small number of cortical cells devoted to the peripheral retina.

gated from the parvocellular pathway, reinforcing the idea that the two represent functionally distinct processing channels (Livingstone and Hubel, 1988).

What this picture cannot convey is the remarkable transformations of visual information occurring within this cortical area. To appreciate these transformations, you must know something about the visual stimuli necessary to activate these

cortical cells. This brings us to the research of David Hubel and Torsten Wiesel, neurobiologists whose pioneering studies of the visual cortex earned them a Nobel Prize in 1981. Their discoveries have had an enormous impact on several areas of brain science, and from their work a great deal is now known about the machinery of visual perception. The following paragraphs highlight some of their major findings. Interested students

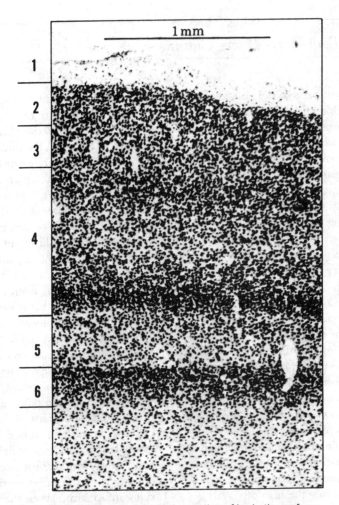

FIGURE 4.7 Magnified picture of a section of brain tissue from the visual cortex of a monkey (from Hubel & Wiesel, 1977). The top of the brain is situated just above layer 1. Below layer 6 lies the "white matter" of the brain, tissue consisting of the incoming axons from the LGN. Those LGN axons make connections with cortical neurons in layer 4.

will be rewarded by reading a more detailed account of their work (Hubel and Wiesel, 1977, 1979).

RETINAL MAPS IN THE CORTEX

The first notable property of cortical cells is that each cell responds to stimulation of a restricted area of the retina—this area constitutes that cell's receptive field. You will recognize this property as a continuation of the processing scheme inaugurated in the retina and carried forward in the lateral geniculate nucleus: at each of these processing stages, individual cells analyze information from a limited area on the retina.

Considered as a group, the receptive fields of

Box 4.1 *Look Both Ways Before Crossing*

Damage to different parts of the visual system produces predictable losses of vision within regions of the **visual field.** A visual field is easy to envision: while staring at some point straight ahead of you, your visual field is the entire region of space that is visible to you. Your attention is naturally focused on the center of the visual field, but you are aware of events occurring on the periphery as well.

Physicians and vision researchers use a routine procedure to measure a visual field; it is called **perimetry** (from the roots *peri*, meaning "around," and *meter*, meaning "to measure"). While an individual has one eye covered and the open eye staring at a fixed point, a small, dim exploring spot is moved around slowly in front of that person's open eye, and the individual reports when the spot disappears. The positions where the spot disappears are traced out on a map of visual space; the map shows areas of sight (unshaded regions) and areas of blindness (shaded regions). Keep in mind that a visual field map describes visual space, not the retina. To draw the map based on retinal geography requires inverting and reversing the map of visual space.

A normal visual field map for each eye looks like the pair numbered 1 in the accompanying figure (for simplicity, the blind spot has been omitted). Note that the nose obscures the right portion of the left eye's view and the left portion of the right eye's view. Now suppose that because of some accident the left optic nerve was completely severed. This would totally eliminate the left eye's field, leaving the right eye's field intact; this situation is shown by the pair of maps numbered 2.

Let's consider a more complicated visual field loss. In humans, the pituitary gland lies immediately behind the middle of the optic chiasm. A tumor in the pituitary gland can squeeze this structure against the chiasm, damaging the fibers that cross through the chiasm. These fibers, you will recall from Figure 4.1, originate from the nasal portion of each retina. The resulting visual field loss will resemble that shown in the pair of maps numbered 3; the lost regions of visual space are those that are normally represented within the fibers originating from the nasal retinas.

Consider a case that is virtually the opposite of the one just described. The internal carotid arteries, branches of the prominent arteries in the neck, pass very near to the sides of the chiasm. These arteries can develop an aneurysm, a balloonlike bulge of the arterial wall. This bulge can push against the fibers that form the outer margin of the chiasm; recall that these are *un*crossed fibers. Thus, for example, an aneurysm of the left internal carotid artery would affect uncrossed fibers coming from the left eye—that is, fibers carrying information about the right half of the left eye's field. In this case, the visual field map would resemble the fourth pair of maps. See whether you can determine the visual field loss produced when *both* left and right internal carotid arteries have developed aneurysms, a condition that does occur sometimes.

This close connection between visual field loss and disease makes perimetry a very useful diagnostic tool. But there's one surprising aspect to visual field loss, even severe cases such as those shown here: the person exhibiting the loss is often unaware of it! Apparently, by

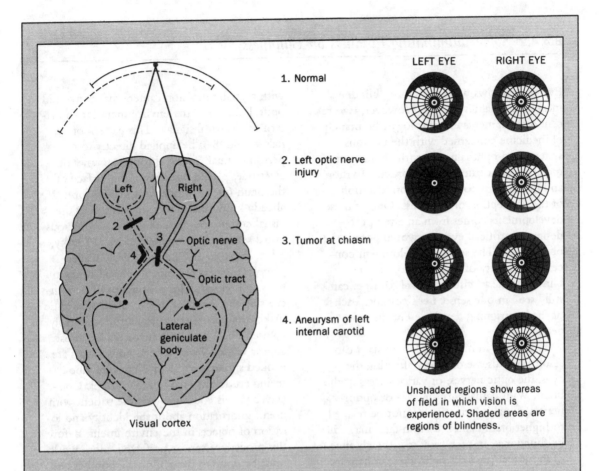

1. Normal

2. Left optic nerve injury

3. Tumor at chiasm

4. Aneurysm of left internal carotid

LEFT EYE   RIGHT EYE

Unshaded regions show areas of field in which vision is experienced. Shaded areas are regions of blindness.

Left

Right

Optic nerve

Optic tract

Lateral geniculate body

Visual cortex

moving the eyes around, a person's residual visual field can provide coverage that's adequate for most situations. But sometimes the coverage proves inadequate, as the following illustrates, and the outcome may by fatal.

Freytag and Sachs (1968) studied the records of certain traffic accidents in Baltimore. They were interested in pedestrians killed under circumstances suggesting that the victims should have seen the vehicle that struck and killed them. Autopsies revealed that the visual systems of some accident victims had been damaged *before* the accident. In these cases, the location and extent of that damage implied a visual field loss that explained the accident. In one case, for instance, a man was struck and killed by a car approaching from his right. Autopsy showed that his right optic nerve was completely atrophied. Consequently, if this man were looking straight ahead, a car approaching from his right would fall within the blind portion of his visual field. Thus while this man's vision was probably good enough for his activities at home, his unsuspected visual deficit proved lethal when he had to cross the street.

Box 4.2 *Some Illuminating Findings on Blindness*

Everyone knows what the word "blindness" means—an inability to see. However, two recent developments in neurology (the branch of medicine concerned with the nervous system) and ophthalmology (the branch of medicine concerned with disorders of vision and the eye) are forcing a reconsideration of the conception of blindness. One of these developments comes from an attempt to design an artificial eye that would permit the blind to see. The second development concerns the ability of people who, despite blindness due to visual cortical damage, can still "see" in one sense. Let's consider each of these intriguing developments in more detail.

First, keep in mind that loss of sight can result from disease or injury affecting the eyes, the optic nerves, or various areas of the brain. With damage to the eyes or optic nerves, visual information cannot be relayed to higher brain centers that, in fact, may still be functional. In such cases it is the absence of input that prevents sight. Researchers are now exploring the possibility of directly stimulating the visual cortex in these blind patients, thus bypassing the defective route to the cortex. The scheme, still early in the developmental stage, would work something like this. The blind person would be outfitted

with a small television camera that converted optical images of the environment into a pattern of electrical signals. This pattern of signals would then be applied directly to the person's visual cortex, through an array of electrodes placed directly on the surface of the brain (see accompanying illustration). We already know that direct stimulation of the visual cortex does indeed generate conscious visual sensations (Dobelle and Mladejovsky, 1974; Brindley and Lewin, 1968). Called *phosphenes*, these sensations are said to resemble small, glowing spots or grains of rice. Increasing the duration of the stimulating pulse makes the phosphenes brighter; occasionally, colored phosphenes are reported, but most appear white. When several phosphenes are evoked simultaneously, patients describe seeing crude but recognizable shapes. Conceivably, this could provide the patient with useful information about the identity and location of objects in the environment. Before this procedure can be perfected, more work must be done to determine the number and placement of electrodes necessary to convey useful pattern information. In the meantime, this research very clearly demonstrates that the visual cortex *can* generate conscious visual sensations in the absence of input from the eyes; these observations, incidentally, bear on

---

cells in each hemisphere of Area 17 form a topographic map of the contralateral visual field. This cortical map, like its counterpart in the LGN, is said to be *topographic* because adjacent regions of visual space are mapped onto adjacent groups of cells in the visual cortex. The map in each hemisphere is said to represent the *contralateral* visual field because the left half of the visual field is

represented in the right hemisphere, and vice versa.

Now let's consider *how* this map of the visual field is distributed over the cortex. Recall that Holmes's studies of brain-damaged people implied that a great deal of cortical area is devoted to representation of the fovea. This implication has since been confirmed by actually plotting the

the notion of cortical specialization discussed in Box 1.2 in Chapter 1.

Perhaps even more intriguing are the residual visual abilities of some cortically blind people. In these individuals, the eyes and optic nerves remain intact; their permanent loss of sight results from injury to the visual cortex. As you will recall from the text, the extent of the region of blindness (a region called a *scotoma*) depends on the size of the damaged area of cortex. Light flashed anywhere within this scotoma elicits no sensation of vision. Yet when asked to guess *where* a light is flashed within this blind region by *pointing* to it, these individuals can do so with reasonable accuracy. At the same time, they deny seeing any hint of the flash and describe the exercise as rather silly. Some patients can even direct their gaze toward an unseen light, can report the color or orientation of a visual stimulus, and can adjust their hands and fingers to grasp an object they cannot see! These puzzling abilities, summarized by Cowey and Stoerig (1991), are all instances of what is termed **blindsight.** The common denominator in all these studies is the use of **forced-choice** testing (see Appendix). With this procedure, an individual doesn't describe what is seen but rather judges where a stimulus is presented or when it was presented, guessing if necessary.

By what means can a blind person accurately "guess" the location of a flash she or he

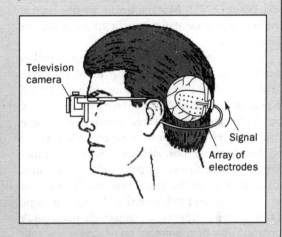

never saw? (For a thorough discussion of possible answers, see Campion, Latto, and Smith, 1983.) Recall that earlier in this chapter we discussed the superior colliculus, a subcortical area of the brain thought to be involved in visual orienting reflexes. Because it lies below the cerebral hemispheres, the superior colliculus should be unaffected by injury to the visual cortex and hence remain available to provide visual information for the guidance of hand or eye movements. Because in blindsight, behavior is divorced from awareness, we might conclude that subcortical brain regions process visual information at an unconscious level (see also Marshall and Halligan, 1988). Conscious perception may be a unique property of the phylogenetically newer cerebral cortex.

---

locations of receptive fields of cells sampled from throughout the primate visual cortex (Hubel and Wiesel, 1974a). It is estimated that about 80 percent of the cells in the visual cortex are devoted to representing the central 10 degrees or so of the visual field (Drasdo, 1977). Earlier we pointed out that this exaggerated cortical mapping of central vision is referred to as cortical magnification.

Much of this bias toward the central portion of the visual field is inherited from the retina and the LGN. Recall from our discussion of the retina that the number of ganglion cells subserving the fovea is considerably larger than the number devoted to the rest of the retina, even though in terms of area the periphery dwarfs the fovea. This foveal bias appears in the LGN's retinotopic map, too, where it is even further exaggerated (Malpelli and Baker, 1975). Moving on up to the cortex, the foveal representation swells to even greater proportions.

This magnified foveal representation makes sense when we consider the sizes of receptive fields of cortical cells representing different retinal eccentricities. Cells concerned with the fovea may be "looking at" a retinal area covered by no more than a few photoreceptors, whereas cells devoted to the periphery look at areas hundreds of times larger. Because foveal receptive fields are so small, it stands to reason that many cells may be required to cover a given patch of retina. In the representation of the periphery, a comparably sized patch of retina may be monitored by relatively few cells (recall Figure 4.6). This principle explains why local damage to visual cortex (from a bullet wound, for example) may produce scotomas of different size. Damage within the foveal representation will destroy cells with small receptive fields, yielding a small scotoma in the center of vision. Damage within the peripheral representation may destroy the same number of cells, but the scotoma will be considerably larger because those cells have bigger receptive fields. This large scotoma will also, of course, be located away from the center of gaze.

So, in effect, the bulk of the machinery in the visual cortex processes information about objects that are viewed directly. This is why head and eye movements play such a prominent role in seeing: such movements turn the eyes toward objects of current interest. These newly fixated objects then cast their images on the fovea, ensuring that those objects will receive the most detailed visual analysis possible by the visual cortex.

* * *

So far we've considered the orderly layout of cortical receptive fields and the resulting topographic map. Our discussion focused on *where* in the visual field different cortical cells are looking. Now let's ask *what* each cell is looking for. Exactly what kind of visual stimulus must be present within a cell's receptive field in order to evoke activity in that cell? On the basis of your knowledge of the

retina and the geniculate, you can probably anticipate one fact: cortical cells are unconcerned about overall levels of illumination. Simply increasing or decreasing the ambient illumination has no appreciable impact on a cortical cell's activity. Instead, cortical cells respond best to gradients in light intensity, such as those produced by borders, edges, and lines. In this respect, cortical cells behave like their retinal and geniculate relatives from whom they inherit input. But cortical cells exhibit several notable characteristics not present in their precortical relatives, characteristics described in the following section.

FUNCTIONAL PROPERTIES OF CORTICAL CELLS

Orientation, Direction, and Size Selectivity.

One of the most striking characteristics of cortical cells is their **orientation selectivity.** Recall that retinal and geniculate cells, because of their circular-shaped receptive fields, respond indiscriminately to all orientations. In marked contrast, most cortical cells are very fussy about the orientation of a stimulus. As shown in the left-hand portion of Figure 4.8, any particular cell will respond only if the orientation of an edge or line falls somewhere within a rather narrow range. Each cortical cell has a "preferred" orientation, one to which it is maximally responsive. If a line tilts a little away from this optimum, the cell's response decreases markedly; if the line tilts even more, the cell no longer responds at all. This behavior can be summarized by graphing a cell's response strength as a function of orientation; the resulting "tuning curve" resembles a tepee with its peak defining the cell's preferred orientation (see the right-hand portion of Figure 4.8).

The preferred orientation varies from cell to cell, such that within an ensemble of cells all orientations are represented (see Box 4.3, pp. 121–122). Usually the most effective orientation for a cell can be sharply defined. In many cells, a tilt of no more than 15 degrees away from the optimum orientation is sufficient to abolish that cell's response completely. An angular deviation this small corresponds to about the difference in position of

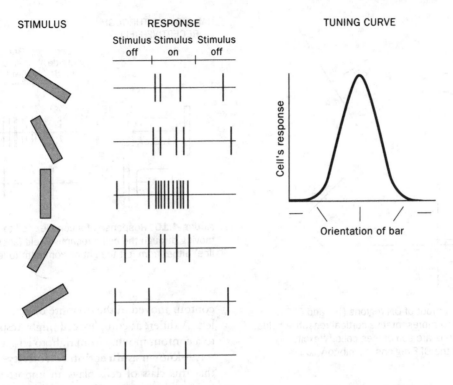

STIMULUS   RESPONSE   TUNING CURVE

FIGURE 4.8 Response of a single cortical cell to bars presented at various orientations.

a clock's hand at 12:00 and at 12:03! Just about all cortical cells are selective for orientation, with two notable exceptions. These unusual, nono-riented cells are found in the lower subdivision of cortical layer 4 and in regularly spaced patches of cells found near the cortical surface. Outside these restricted areas, in all other regions of visual cortex, orientation matters very greatly.

Let's take a look at the layout of ON regions and OFF regions constituting the receptive fields of some cortical cells; from these you should be able to see why these cells are selective for orientation. Some representative cortical receptive fields are shown in Figure 4.9. There you can see that receptive fields are elongated, not circular as in retinal and geniculate cells. Notice, too, that the discrete zones of ON and OFF activity are arranged differently depending on the particular cell. Simply by inspecting these various arrangements, you should be able to picture what kind

of oriented stimulus would evoke the best response from a given cell. For this reason, cortical cells within these well-delineated zones are called **simple cells:** there is a simple relation between their receptive field layout and their preferred stimulus. For cells of this type, a properly oriented bar or edge must be exactly positioned within the receptive field to yield a large neural response—changing either the orientation or the position of the stimulus will reduce the cell's response. This specificity of response means that simple cells are able to signal the orientation of a stimulus falling within a particular region of the visual field.

Other cortical cells do not have such well-defined ON and OFF zones, yet they also exhibit a preference for a particular orientation. These are called **complex cells,** because it is more complicated to predict just what stimulus will optimally activate them. Just looking at their responses to spots or bars of light does not give us a map of

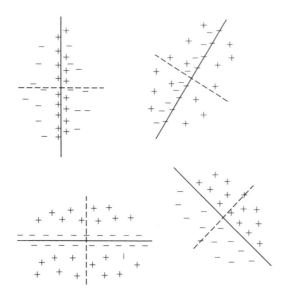

FIGURE 4.9 Layout of ON regions (+) and OFF regions (−) of several representative cortical receptive fields. The ON regions are sometimes called ''excitatory zones'' and the OFF regions, ''inhibitory zones.''

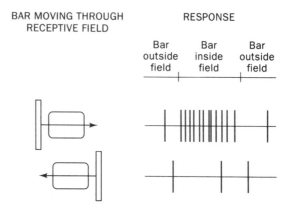

FIGURE 4.10 Response of a complex cell to a bar moving through the cell's receptive field (shown in outline) either from left to right or from right to left.

the best-shaped target. Unlike simple cells, complex ones will respond to an appropriately oriented stimulus falling anywhere within the boundaries of the receptive field—precise location is not nearly so important for a complex cell, so long as the stimulus falls somewhere within its receptive field and remains properly oriented. Incidentally, because a complex cell lacks clearly defined ON and OFF regions, it will respond quite vigorously to a bar or an edge that moves through the receptive field. In fact, most complex cells strongly prefer moving contours to stationary ones, even if the contour travels rapidly across the receptive field. Simple cells, on the other hand, respond only to stationary or slowly moving contours (Movshon, 1975).

Besides preferring contours that move, complex cells often respond to one *direction* of motion only. For instance, such a cell (like the one illustrated in Figure 4.10) might give a burst of activity when a vertical contour moved from left to right, but would remain unresponsive when that same contour moved in the opposite direction, right to left. A different complex cell might respond only to a contour moving from right to left. This property—known as **direction selectivity**—suggests that this class of cells plays an important role in motion perception (Regan, Beverley, and Cynader, 1979). We'll return to this idea when we discuss motion perception in Chapter 8.

We've already mentioned that receptive fields of cortical cells vary in size, being smallest in the fovea and larger in the periphery; this is true for both simple and complex cells. Moreover, at any given region of the visual field there is also some variation in field size. Thus some cells have receptive fields favoring, say, a narrow vertical bar whereas others prefer a wider bar. This is reminiscent of the situation in the retina (recall Figure 3.5) and LGN, but in the cortex, orientation selectivity is incorporated together with size selectivity.

There are other, more subtle distinctions between simple and complex cells (for example, see Hammond and MacKay, 1977), and there are other cell types with even more complicated receptive fields. But for the present, let's refocus our attention on a property that all these cell types seem to have in common, which is binocularity.

Box 4.3 *The Oblique Effect*

Nearly all cortical cells in Area 17 have a preferred orientation, one that elicits the best response from the cell. Among a large sample of visual cortical cells, all possible preferred orientations are encountered—the distribution of preferred orientations covers the entire range. However, the distribution of preferred orientations is not uniform. Recording from many cells in the visual cortex of the monkey, Mansfield (1974) observed a distinct bias in favor of the principal axes, vertical and horizontal. The accompanying figure (adapted from Mansfield, 1974) illustrates his findings. In this polar plot, each line represents the preferred orientation of a single cortical cell. As you can see, although all orientations are represented, there is a clustering of cells that prefer vertical and another clustering of cells that prefer horizontal. Mansfield found that the unevenness of this distribution was most pronounced among cells with receptive fields close to and within the fovea. His findings raise two intriguing questions. What are the perceptual consequences of this bias in favor of vertical and horizontal? And what factors produce this bias in the first place? Let's begin with the first question.

Long before Mansfield's physiological discoveries, scientists interested in vision had noted that horizontal and vertical lines can be detected more easily and identified more rapidly than can lines oriented obliquely. For instance, visual acuity is highest for vertical and horizontal lines, and lowest for lines oriented 45 degrees in either direction from vertical. Compared with horizontal or vertical lines, oblique lines are also more difficult to see when the contrast of the lines is faint.

You can experience the oblique effect by looking at the two bar patterns pictured here. Prop the book up so that you can view the pair of patterns from a distance. Backing away from the book, you should discover that at some distance the thin vertical bars remain visible while the diagonal ones blend together and are, thus, unresolvable. By turning the book sideways, you can repeat this exercise, now comparing horizontal to diagonal.

This general superiority in the visibility of horizontal and vertical is called the **oblique effect** (Appelle, 1972). Most people experience the oblique effect, but there are some individuals who do not. In fact, some people show just the opposite bias, a tendency to see oblique lines of a particular orientation *more* clearly. Usually, those people who fail to ex-

(continued)

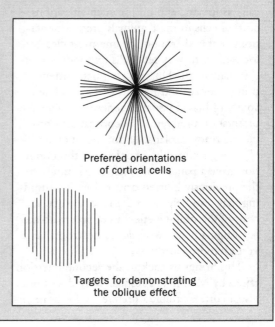

Preferred orientations
of cortical cells

Targets for demonstrating
the oblique effect

perience the oblique effect or who show a reverse oblique effect have some degree of astigmatism. Recall from Chapter 2 that astigmatism (an irregularly curved cornea) causes contours of certain orientations to appear blurred while other orientations appear sharply focused. Depending on the direction of the astigmatism, this condition can nullify the normal oblique effect, and it can also lead to a superiority in vision for oblique lines, a sort of reverse oblique effect. Interestingly, in cases where oblique is favored, the bias endures even when the astigmatism is optically corrected, thereby making all orientations equally sharp (Mitchell, Freeman, Millidot, and Haegerstrom, 1973); this condition is called **meridional amblyopia** ("amblyopia" literally means "dull vision" and refers to a visual loss that cannot be corrected optically). Apparently the astigmatism, prior to optical correction, altered the visual nervous system in a direction favoring oblique over horizontal and vertical. In fact, animals made artificially astigmatic exhibit just such alterations— cortical cells in these animals prefer orientations centered around the one most clearly focused, with very few cells responding preferentially to the blurred, astigmatic orientation (Freeman and Pettigrew, 1973). The ability of biased visual experience to alter the orientation preferences of cortical cells provides a ready explanation for meridional amblyopia: presumably, people with this condition have a paucity of cortical cells tuned to the previously blurred orientation. This finding may also help us understand the neural basis of the oblique effect in people who are *not* astigmatic but who *do* see horizontal and vertical more clearly.

This brings us back to the second question raised by Mansfield's results. Why does the visual cortex exhibit a preference for horizon-

tal and vertical over oblique? At present there are two general theories. One attributes the bias to the carpentered environment in which most people grow up (Annis and Frost, 1973). According to this idea, people receive more exposure to vertical and to horizontal contours than to oblique contours, because horizontal and vertical exist in abundance within an urban landscape of houses and buildings. This biased visual exposure, in turn, influences the development of orientation preferences among the cortical cells. This theory is supported by animal studies demonstrating that the brain *is* susceptible to biased visual experience early in life (Blakemore, 1976). The carpentered environment theory also receives support from studies testing the vision of people who grew up in noncarpentered, agrarian environments where no particular orientation predominates. These individuals *fail* to exhibit an oblique effect (Annis and Frost, 1973), presumably because their brains did not receive a heavy dose of vertical and horizontal contours. The opposing theory ascribes the neural bias for horizontal and vertical to unspecified genetic factors that operate to favor the development of cortical cells tuned to horizontal and vertical (Timney and Muir, 1976). Those who favor this genetic theory point to the fact that infants only a few months old exhibit an oblique effect (Leehey, Moskowitz-Cook, Brill, and Held, 1975). It is hard to imagine, this theory argues, how visual experience could already have shaped the brains of infants so young.

At present, this issue of the origins of the oblique effect remains unsettled. But regardless of how the issue is resolved, the oblique effect represents a strong link between visual pattern perception and cortical physiology (Orban, Vandenbussche, and Vogels, 1984).

Binocularity. Recall that information from the two eyes is distributed in separate layers of each lateral geniculate nucleus, with individual cells receiving input from either one eye or the other. Once information passes from the geniculate to the visual cortex, however, **monocular** (meaning "one eye") segregation gives way to **binocular** (meaning "two eyes") integration. At the cortical level, individual cells, with few exceptions, are innervated from both eyes. Figure 4.11 shows how a typical cortical cell responds to stimulation of the two eyes. This particular cell responds moderately well to a line presented to either eye alone, but its response is even stronger when both eyes are stimulated simultaneously. Some cells respond more vigorously to stimulation of the left eye, whereas other cells favor right-eye stimulation. This variation in the relative strength of the connection with the two eyes is called **ocular dominance.** Any cell that can be excited through both eyes, regardless of its ocular dominance, is called a **binocular cell.**

Because they can be excited by either eye, all

binocular cells really have two receptive fields, one for the left eye and one for the right eye. The two fields of a binocular cell are nearly always matched in type (simple or complex), preferred orientation, and preferred direction of motion. If, for instance, the cell responds best to a horizontal line moving upward in front of the left eye, then upward movement of a horizontal line will also evoke the largest response via the right eye.

The two receptive fields for any particular binocular cell also fall on approximately equivalent regions of the two eyes. Thus if one field is located to the right of the fovea in one eye, the other field will fall to the right of the fovea in the other eye. In general, binocular cortical cells respond most strongly when corresponding regions of each eye are stimulated by forms of corresponding size and orientation.

With this correspondence in mind, think for a moment about where a single object must be situated in the world in order to activate maximally the cell we've just described. To begin, suppose the two eyes fixate a point on the center of a viewing screen, as shown in Figure 4.12. For stimulation of the right eye to activate the binocular cell described above, an object has to be located within the area of the screen labeled "Right eye" (see panel A). Note, though, that at this position the image of that object does not fall within the cell's receptive field in the left eye; so at this position, stimulation of the left eye would not activate the binocular cell. To be imaged within the left eye's receptive field, and therefore activate this cell, the object must be displaced laterally on the screen, closer to the point of fixation (see panel B). Note, however, that in this location the image of the object no longer falls within the right eye's receptive field. In fact, there is no single position *on* the viewing screen where one object could simultaneously stimulate both the left and right eyes' receptive fields. But there is a position *in front of* the screen that could accomplish this—as shown in panel C: when the object is at a particular location in front of the screen (and hence closer to the eyes), both receptive fields are stimulated.

FIGURE 4.11 Response of a single cortical cell to stimulation of the left eye, right eye, and both eyes. The plus and minus signs show the receptive field layout for this cell.

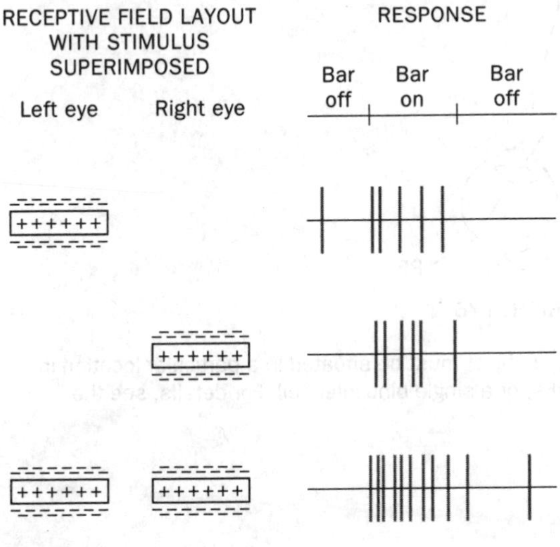

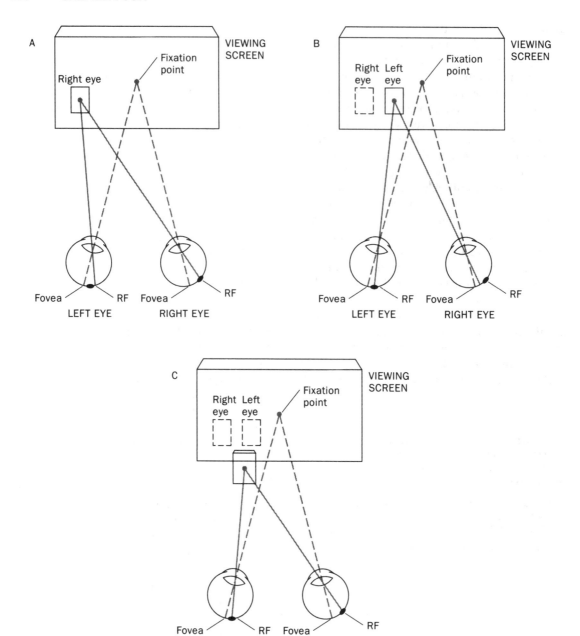

FIGURE 4.12 This series of drawings illustrates why a single object must be situated in a particular location in visual space to optimally stimulate both receptive fields (RFs) of a single binocular cell. For details, see the text.

Similarly, for each binocular cell there will be one position in three-dimensional space where the two receptive fields can be simultaneously stimulated. This position will vary, of course, from cell to cell, depending on the retinal placement of the pair of receptive fields for a given cell. Take a minute to be sure you understand why this is so. A little extra effort at this point will pay dividends when we talk about binocular depth perception in Chapter 7. As you will learn then, the layout of binocular receptive fields plays a fundamental role in one's ability to judge the distance from one object to another. For now, though, you should appreciate two properties of binocular cells: they respond preferentially to the same type of stimulus in both eyes, and the relative positions of the two receptive fields of a cell specify the location of the stimulus that will optimally excite the cell.

Color. Besides orientation, direction of motion, and binocularity, some cortical cells in Area 17 also register information about color. Most of these color-sensitive cells are concentrated in bloblike regions regularly spaced throughout the upper layers of visual cortex (Livingstone and Hubel, 1984), although some are found outside these regions (Lennie, Krauskopf, and Sclar, 1990). Each of these so-called **blobs** contains neurons that receive their inputs from the lower subdivision of layer 4, the one innervated by color-selective cells of the parvocellular pathway. Cells in the blobs constitute one of the unusual cortical groups that show no preference for contour orientation. Blob cells do, however, exhibit a complex form of color opponency, wherein the effect of a color (excitatory versus inhibitory) depends on whether that color falls within the center or the surround of the cell's receptive field.

Columns and Hypercolumns. Having summarized the major response properties of cortical cells, let's look at how two of these properties—orientation and binocularity—are arranged within the cortex. Earlier we mentioned that cortical cells vary in their preferred orientations, some responding best to vertical, others to horizontal, and

still others to orientations in between. These orientation-selective cells are not haphazardly arranged; they are grouped in a very orderly fashion within the cortex. To envision this grouping, imagine we are able to stretch out the visual cortex so that this thin, layered sheet of tissue (recall Figure 4.7) is lying flat. Now suppose we randomly select a position somewhere on the surface of this unfolded cortex. Starting here, we gradually move straight downward through the various layers in a direction perpendicular to the surface of the cortex. Throughout our short, 2-millimeter journey we carefully catalog the preferred orientation of each cell encountered. After penetrating all six cortical layers, we will discover that all cells along the path of this penetration have identical preferred orientations (except for cells in layer 4, which respond to *all* orientations). Along the way, there may be variation in the size of these cells' receptive fields, and some are likely to prefer edges while others prefer bars. But *all* cells will exhibit the same orientation preference.

Suppose we now repeat this sampling procedure, this time beginning at a position just a fraction of a millimeter away from our initial penetration. Now we will find that all cells prefer an orientation slightly different from the one encountered in the first sample. This is illustrated in Figure 4.13—note that the preferred orientation has changed by about 10 degrees from the first sample to the second one. If we repeat this sampling procedure over and over, always being careful to make the penetrations perpendicular to the cortical surface, we will uncover a regular sequence of preferred orientations. Each time we make a new penetration, spacing it about 0.05 millimeter from the last one, the preferred orientation will change by about 10 to 15 degrees. By the time we have sampled a strip of cortex less than a millimeter in width, the sequence of preferred orientations will have progressed through one complete rotation. This regular progression through a complete set of orientations is comparable to the range of positions assumed by the second hand of a clock as it advances from vertical (at 12 o'clock) to horizontal (at 3 o'clock) and back to vertical (at 6 o'clock). This tidy packaging

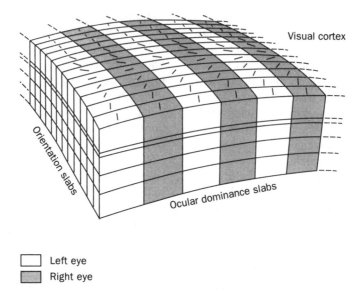

FIGURE 4.13 Orientation and ocular dominance columns in the visual cortex. All cells in a column have the same orientation preference and the same ocular dominance. An aggregate of columns representing a complete range of preferences is known as a hypercolumn.

of orientation-selective cells occurs throughout the visual cortex (Hubel and Wiesel, 1974b).

As we make these repeated samplings, another intriguing regularity emerges: within a given penetration perpendicular to the cortical surface, all cells have the same ocular dominance. If the first cell encountered responds strongest to stimulation of the right eye, all cells in that sequence will be right-eye dominant (with the exception of the monocular cells in layer 4). Moreover, if we now make another sampling penetration right next to the first one, the cells encountered will exhibit a different pattern of ocular dominance, perhaps responding equally well to stimulation of either eye. So ocular dominance—like preferred orientation—varies systematically as we move laterally over the cortex; this, too, is illustrated in Figure 4.13.

At first, all these facts may seem bewildering, but taken together, they produce an interesting and coherent picture. The visual cortex appears to be composed of columns of cells, with each column consisting of a stack of cells all preferring the same orientation and exhibiting the same ocular dominance. Altogether, it takes roughly eighteen to twenty neighboring columns to cover a complete range of stimulus orientations and ocular dominance. This aggregation of adjacent columns is collectively known as a **hypercolumn.** Each hypercolumn contains tens of thousands of cells whose receptive fields all overlap on the same retinal territory. The hypercolumns themselves are all uniform in size throughout the cortex, but the hypercolumns devoted to the central retina deal with a much smaller area of retina than do the hypercolumns concerned with the peripheral retina. This, of course, merely restates the principle of cortical magnification described in the previous section.

Hence each hypercolumn contains neural machinery for analyzing visual information within a local region of the retina. Throughout the entire visual cortex there are many such hypercolumns, each receiving input from different portions of the retina. Working simultaneously, the hypercolumns analyze multiple aspects of the retinal image—orientation, direction of motion, binocularity, size—in a local, piecemeal fashion. Each hypercolumn provides a "description" of that portion of the image falling within its own, restricted field of view. This description is embodied within the activity of cells in the constituent columns of the hypercolumn.

At the end of this chapter we shall consider how these cells might be involved in visual perception. For the moment, though, let's consider what might transpire within the visual cortex as a person stares with both eyes open at a very large picture composed exclusively of, say, vertical lines. This visual stimulus should maximally activate those cells in the cortex which prefer a vertical orientation, and since both eyes are open, ocular dominance preference should not matter. Cells signaling all other orientations would respond much less vigorously or not at all. Now suppose we could look directly at the person's cortex and visualize those cells activated by the vertical lines. On the basis of what you have just learned about the organization of the cortex, can you imagine what we would see?

Because the orientation and ocular dominance columns are more or less evenly spaced throughout the entire cortex, we should see a regular pattern of active cells interspersed among a set of inactive ones. And in fact, this is exactly what is seen. Hubel, Wiesel, and Stryker (1978) injected monkeys with a radioactive substance, 2-deoxy-

glucose, that is incorporated into neurally active cells but not into inactive ones. These monkeys were then exposed for 45 minutes to a visual display composed entirely of vertical bars of different widths. The display was large, and the bars moved back and forth to ensure that the visual cortex received a healthy dose of vertical visual stimulation. Following this exposure, each animal's visual cortex was viewed under a microscope, using a procedure that highlights cells containing the radioactive substance.

Figure 4.14 shows what those investigators saw when they took a sideways view of a slice of visual cortex from these animals. The regularly spaced, dark, vertical bands correspond to the columns of cortical cells activated by the vertical bars. The lighter bands in between denote regions of cortex containing very little of the radioactive chemical, indicating that cells in these regions were relatively inactive during the stimulation period. The uniformly dark stripe running through the middle of the bands corresponds to layer 4; in this layer, vertical contours activated all cells because these cells are not selective for orientation. Measuring the distance between the dark bands (points of maximum concentration of radioactivity) in the photograph gives a value close to half a millimeter. This corresponds nicely to the dimension of an individual hypercolumn estimated from physiological recordings from cortical cells.

These elegant anatomical experiments substan-

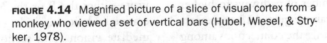

FIGURE 4.14 Magnified picture of a slice of visual cortex from a monkey who viewed a set of vertical bars (Hubel, Wiesel, & Stryker, 1978).

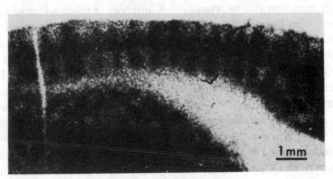

1 mm

tiate that orientation-selective neurons are packed in columns. To test your understanding of the material on hypercolumns, suppose these monkeys had been exposed to a set of lines that slowly rotated through all orientations. What would the distribution of radioactive substance have looked like? And what if while viewing all orientations, the monkey's vision had been confined to just one eye?

* * *

This completes our overview of the receptive field properties of cells and the architecture of hypercolumns in the visual receiving stage of the brain, Area 17. As mentioned at the outset of this section, our survey just hits the highlights of this stage in visual processing. Neurophysiologists have studied cortical cells in considerably greater detail than we've gone into here. They have also begun to unravel the neural circuitry (that is, the connections between cortical cells) underlying such receptive field properties as orientation selectivity. Although fascinating, that research is not immediately germane to the questions about visual perception that will occupy our attention in the next several chapters.

VISUAL PROCESSING BEYOND AREA 17

So far in this chapter, we have been focusing on cells in Area 17, a relatively early stage in visual processing. From this stage, neural information is distributed over a number of pathways to higher visual areas of the brain; Figure 4.15 represents one attempt to summarize the connections among the multitude of brain areas that can be visually activated (Felleman and Van Essen, 1991). Each labeled box represents a different visual area, starting with the retina (RGC), LGN, and V1 at the bottom (recall that V1 is another name for Area 17). These visual areas are distributed widely throughout the cerebral cortex.

Most of the details of this wiring diagram are not so important for our purposes; they simply underscore the large number and the hierarchical arrangement of these brain areas associated with

vision. However, the pathways denoted by thick lines are of interest, for they represent the neural pathways formed by the P and M systems. From our earlier discussion of inputs to V1 from LGN, you will recall that the P and M cells remain segregated within Area V1. This segregation remains in effect at least through the first several stages of processing following V1. Thus, the M pathway projects through V1 via certain parts of V2 to Area MT; the P pathway, in contrast, projects to an anatomically distinct area of V2 and then on to V4. There are also direct M projections from V1 to MT and direct P projections from V1 to V4. Within each of these Areas—V1, V2, V4, and MT—there exists an orderly retinotopic map.

Different visual areas appear to be concerned with different aspects of the visual world (Mishkin, Ungerleider, and Macko, 1983). Judging from the receptive field properties of cells in these various areas (Maunsell and Newsome, 1987), some areas appear specialized for analyzing information about color (for instance, Area V4), whereas others are more concerned with motion (Area MT). There is even a brain region (the two areas labeled STP in Figure 4.15) containing neurons responsive only to human faces viewed from particular angles (Perrett et al., 1991; Desimone, 1991).

P AND M CELL CONTRIBUTIONS TO VISION

Direct evidence for the role of P and M pathways in vision comes from studies in which one pathway—either the P or the M—is rendered inoperative by lesioning it, leaving only the other to mediate vision. This section summarizes consequences of those selective lesions.

To examine the contributions of P and M pathways in vision, Schiller and Logothetis (1990) created localized lesions in either parvocellular or magnocellular layers of the LGN of monkeys and then measured the perceptual consequences. (A lesion at this level of the LGN interrupts processing within this and subsequent stages of the pathways subserved by that cell type.) Schiller and Logothetis adapted a behavioral technique that was both sensitive and highly versatile, enabling

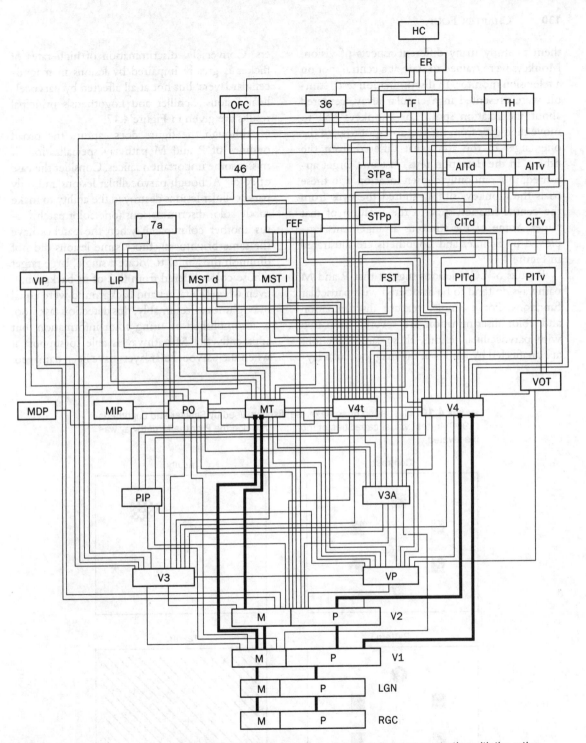

FIGURE 4.15 Diagram showing the hierarchical arrangement of visual processing stages, starting with the retina (bottom of diagram) and moving up through the multiple visual areas of the brain. The bold lines show the P and M pathways discussed in the text. (Adapted from Felleman and Van Essen, 1991.)

them to study many different aspects of vision. Monkeys were trained to stare at a central spot on a television monitor. In discrimination tests, stimuli were presented in a circular array, centered about the fixation spot. The monkeys had to move their eyes from the fixation spot toward the one target in the array that differed from the others. In the detection tests, just one target appeared, in a randomly chosen location. On these trials the monkeys simply shifted the eyes from the central fixation spot to the location of that target. Some of the stimulus arrangements employed by Schiller and Logothetis are illustrated in Figure 4.16.

Results of LGN lesions suggest that P and M pathways do tend to be associated with particular functions. For example, texture discrimination and color discrimination are severely impaired with parvocellular lesions; these same functions are unaffected by lesions of the magnocellular lay-

ers. Conversely, discrimination of high rates of flicker is greatly impaired by lesions in magnocellular layers, but not at all affected by parvocellular lesions. Schiller and Logothetis's principal results are given in Figure 4.17.

Although the figure does capture the broad outlines of P and M pathway specialization, it misses some important nuances. Consider the case of color. Although parvocellular lesions and only parvocellular lesions destroyed the ability to make subtle color discriminations (one color patch versus another color patch when the patches have the same brightness), those same lesions did not diminish the ability to locate a single, large target whose color differed from that of its background even when the target and background were equal in brightness. Presumably, this detection task, too, is accomplished by using color information, but apparently the M pathway is able to support it when the parvocellular layers have been damaged.

FIGURE 4.16 Illustration of some of the displays used by Schiller and Logothetis (1990) to test visual capacities of monkeys in which the P or the M pathway was inactivated.

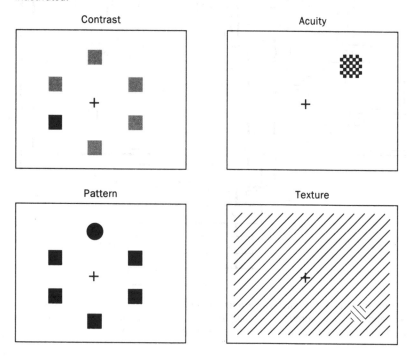

Function Tested	Result of Lesion in P-pathway	Result of Lesion in M-pathway
Color vision	Deficit	Normal
Texture perception	Deficit	Normal
Pattern perception	Deficit	Normal
Acuity	Deficit	Normal
Contrast perception	Deficit	Normal
Flicker perception	Normal	Deficit

FIGURE 4.17 Visual consequences of lesioning the P or the M cells in the LGN.

By the same token, consider the case of flicker. As Figure 4.17 shows, only magnocellular lesions impact the discrimination of flicker. But, if the flicker rate is low, the same lesion has no effect. Evidently the P pathway does have some capacity to process temporal modulation, so long as the modulation rate is not high.

These exceptions should not obscure the importance of the generalizations that can be made. First, under many conditions, the P pathway is primarily responsible for perception of color, spatial detail, and texture; second, under many conditions, the M pathway is primarily responsible for motion and flicker. Third, when the tests are made increasingly more subtle, by employing smaller details or lower contrast between the test object and its background, the division of specialization becomes sharper.

* * *

The anatomical diagram in Figure 4.15, the physiological measures of receptive field properties, and the lesion experiments described in the last few paragraphs all involved the study of nonhuman primates, principally the monkey. But several lines of evidence point to the existence of similarly organized, multiple visual areas in the human brain, too. We'll summarize just some of that evidence in the next section.

SPECIALIZED VISUAL AREAS IN HUMAN VISION?

One line of evidence is provided by some hitherto perplexing visual disorders described by people with lesions confined to specific areas of the brain. For instance, damage to Area V4 (an area in the occipital lobe) can produce a permanent loss of color vision (Pearlman, Birch, and Meadows, 1979; Rizzo, Nawrot, Blake, and Damasio, 1992); damage to the temporal lobe (which includes the visual areas in the upper right-hand portion of Figure 4.15) can produce **prosopagnosia**—the inability to recognize previously familiar faces even though visual acuity and general intellect remain intact (Damasio, Tranel, and Damasio, 1990); and selective lesions in the vicinity of Area MT can interfere just with motion perception (Zihl, von Cramon, and Mai, 1983). The selective nature of these visual disorders suggests, of course, that the damaged area was responsible for processing information relevant for the impaired ability. We shall return, incidentally, to each of these interesting disorders in subsequent chapters.

The tentative conclusions derived from studying people with brain damage are buttressed by investigations using the PET technique outlined in Chapter 1. Studies of brain regions metabolically active during different sorts of visual tasks also point to functional specialization (Zeki et al., 1991). Area V4 is highly active when one views multicolored displays, whereas activity in V5 (an area that is thought to include MT) is enhanced when animation displays are viewed. When one looks at pictures of faces, regions of the parietal and temporal lobes become especially active (Lu et al., 1991). In all conditions, V1 is highly active, confirming that it serves as the distribution center to other, more specialized visual areas.

There is another intriguing clue that suggests the involvement of specialized processing in different visual brain areas, a clue that you yourself may have experienced unwittingly. Imagine trying to identify the color *and* the shape of several objects while your attention is diverted to another task, such as recognizing briefly flashed numbers. When people are confronted with this kind of challenging task in the laboratory, they make what are termed **illusory conjunctions** (Treisman and Schmidt, 1982): upon being shown, say, a green square and a red circle, they confidently report the appearance of a red square. These errors suggest that information about color and information about shape were separately and accurately processed, but that the two bits of information were incorrectly conjoined. You can see how these illusory conjunctions might occur if color and shape were processed in different brain areas, making them liable to mistakes in combination. In the laboratory, illusory conjunctions seem to occur only when one must attend to multiple sources of visual information all at once. Attention, in other words, seems to provide the glue that promotes the unity of conscious visual perception; when that attentional glue is in great demand, errors of conjunction may result. Of course we are rarely aware of making illusory conjunctions in everyday life, although the conditions for their occurrence are surely present.

So we have seen converging lines of evidence for the existence of separate visual areas, each specialized for processing a particular aspect of the visual scene. But what is nature's reason for distributing visual processing among multiple areas of the brain? Research in computer science suggests one possible advantage:

Any large computation should be split up and implemented as a collection of small sub-parts that are as nearly independent of one another as the overall task allows. If a process is not designed in this way, a small change in one place will have consequences in many other places. This means that the process as a whole becomes extremely difficult to debug or to improve, whether by a human designer or in the course of natural evolution, because a small change to improve one part has to be accompanied by many simultaneous compensating changes elsewhere. (Marr, 1976, p. 485)

Just how many of these distinct visual areas exist remains a guess, and we certainly have no idea how activity in these separate areas is orchestrated to guide our actions in the world. An even more perplexing question remains unanswered: How does activity in visually activated neurons produce visual perception? In the next section we shall consider this question in more detail, for after all, it is a major concern of perception students.

RELATING VISUAL PERCEPTION TO NEUROPHYSIOLOGY

The previous sections outlined the receptive field properties of neurons in the visual cortex, with particular emphasis on Area 17. What can be said about the role these neurons play in visual perception? That is a question we take up in this section.

No one seriously doubts the visual cortex's crucial involvement in visual perception. This involvement is sadly evidenced by the blindness accompanying damage to this area of the brain. It is further underscored by the fact that visual sensations are evoked whenever the visual cortex is directly stimulated, either by the application of electrical current through a probe placed on the surface of the cortex (Dobelle et al., 1976; Brindley and Lewin, 1968) or by internally generated neural activity arising within the cortex during episodes of migraine headache (Richards, 1971). In these cases of direct brain stimulation, people see flashing spots and lines, sometimes colored, at various locations in their visual fields. Because they occur even with the eyes closed or in total darkness, these **phosphenes,** as the sensations are called, must arise entirely from within the person's visual system. Visual hallucinations experienced under the influence of psychoactive drugs may also reflect the abnormal discharge of cells in the visual cortex (Gregory, 1979).

But although these observations are intriguing, they merely demonstrate that certain areas of the brain are active during visual perception; they don't prove that these cells actually cause perception. What more can we say about the cellular events that actually mediate vision? How much of what you see can be explained by the activity of brain cells that "prefer" various kinds of visual stimuli? To answer these questions intelligently requires that you be familiar with the various aspects of visual perception—movement, color, form, and so on. Since you will read about these topics in the following chapters, it is premature for us to consider the above questions in specific detail now. However, it *is* worthwhile for us to consider several arguments that limit attempts to "explain" visual perception entirely on the basis of activity within a small set of brain cells.

WHAT INFORMATION DO CORTICAL CELLS REGISTER?

It is tempting to conclude that the activity of a cortical cell asserts something very specific about the nature of an object located at a particular region of visual space. This idea has been most thoroughly developed by Barlow (1972), who coined the term "feature detector" to characterize visual neurons with very specific stimulus requirements. According to this idea, feature-detecting neurons at higher and higher levels of visual processing become increasingly refined, to the point where they respond only to a very specific object or event (such as a red Miata sports car).

But this line of reasoning runs into a real stumbling block: it requires there to be as many feature detectors as there are unique, recognizable objects. These feature detectors would even have to be prepared to recognize novel objects that had never before been seen by anyone. Although enormously large, the number of brain cells available for this task hardly seems adequate to cover the repertoire of visual experiences that most people will enjoy in their lifetimes.

We run into another problem when talking about cortical cells as feature detectors. Ideally such a detector would respond only when the requisite feature was present in the visual image, and in the presence of any other feature it would remain completely silent. To behave otherwise would introduce ambiguity into the detector's message, for one could never be sure which feature had activated the cell. Yet real neurons suffer from exactly this **ambiguity problem.** Here is what we mean. As you learned earlier in this chapter, the responses of cortical cells may vary

depending on such stimulus features as orientation and direction of motion. A change in any one of those features would be sufficient to reduce the level of activity in such a cell. But purely on the basis of such a reduction in the level of activity of that cell, we could never be sure *which* stimulus feature, or features, had actually changed.

Let's illustrate this problem of ambiguity with an example. Suppose a single vertical line moves slowly from left to right in front of you. Presumably this event will produce a burst of activity in those cortical cells maximally responsive both to slow rates of movement and to vertically oriented contours. Panel A of Figure 4.18 illustrates how one such cell might respond to this stimulus. We can go so far as to presume that activity in cells such as the one illustrated *causes* you to see the moving line. But now suppose the same vertical line moves more rapidly from left to right. This increased speed will reduce the neural activity within your set of cortical cells, for they prefer slower motion. Such a reduction is illustrated in panel B of Figure 4.18. But an equivalent reduction in neural activity could be produced another way as well. We could present the line at the preferred, slow rate of movement but change the orientation of the line slightly, so that it was no

FIGURE 4.18 The response of one cortical cell to different combinations of speed and orientation of a moving bar.

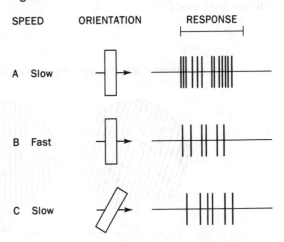

longer exactly vertical. As panel C of Figure 4.18 shows, this change in orientation also reduces the cell's response. Thus changing *either* orientation *or* speed of movement would diminish the level of activity in cells such as the one illustrated. Just looking at the activity level of a small set of cells, then, we cannot tell which stimulus event actually occurred. The activity level of a cell provides an ambiguous message.

Neurons in the visual cortex cannot really be called "feature detectors," then, because individual cells cannot signal the presence of a particular visual feature with certainty. The ambiguity inherent in the response of a single cell can be overcome, however, by *collaboration* among an ensemble of neurons (Regan, 1982). To illustrate, let's reconsider the example involving a moving line. When the line is tilted slightly away from vertical, neurons preferring vertical will show a drop in activity, just as we pointed out above. But at the same time neurons preferring the new orientation will show an increase in their level of firing. By comparing the levels of neural activity in these two sets of cells, each tuned to slightly different orientations, we could infer that the line had changed in orientation, not in speed. In other words, ambiguity within single neurons can be overcome by considering the pattern of activity within an ensemble of neurons tuned to different values along a stimulus dimension such as orientation. To amplify this idea of ensemble coding, let's apply it to a visual illusion of orientation that you can experience.

We start with the observation that cells in the visual system, like those in other sensory systems, undergo a process called **adaptation.** When stimulated intensely for a period of time, they become temporarily fatigued and are, therefore, less responsive (Maffei and Fiorentini, 1973; Movshon and Lennie, 1979). What might be the perceptual consequences of temporarily reducing the responsiveness of orientation-selective cells of the visual cortex? One consequence may be the **tilt aftereffect,** a temporary change in the perceived orientation of lines. First you should experience this intriguing illusion, and then we can consider how it might be explained in terms of neural fatigue, or adaptation, within an ensemble of cortical neurons.

To begin, look at the three sets of bar patterns shown in Figure 4.19. Note that the bars in the middle set (the "test" pattern) are oriented straight up and down. Now stare for a minute or so at the left-hand pattern, the one composed of bars tilted counterclockwise. Let your gaze wander around the circle within the pattern while you are "adapting" to it. Finally, after this period of adaptation, quickly look back at the test bars in the middle. You will see that the vertical bars now appear tilted slightly clockwise. This compelling illusion wears off rather quickly, so you can repeat this adaptation procedure as soon as the test bars once again look perfectly vertical. This time, adapt for a minute to the tilted bars in the right-hand pattern, again being careful to move your eyes around the circle. After you have adapted to

FIGURE 4.19 Displays for generating the tilt aftereffect. Follow the instructions in the text.

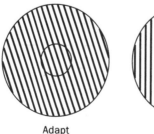
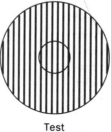
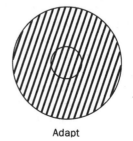

Adapt   Test   Adapt

this clockwise orientation, the bars of the test pattern will appear rotated in a counterclockwise direction.

So you have learned that the apparent orientation of the test bars deviates *away* from the orientation of the adapting bars. Now let's consider how this tilt aftereffect may be explained. Recall our discussion of the ambiguity inherent in the response of any single cell. We concluded that this problem could be circumvented if stimulus properties such as orientation were represented by the relative activity within an ensemble of orientation-selective cells. In the case of vertical lines, this activity profile might look like that shown in the left-hand portion of Figure 4.20. In the upper left part of the diagram, below the test pattern, each tepee-shaped curve represents the orientation tuning curve for a cortical cell with a particular preferred orientation (recall Figure 4.8). The preferred orientation for each of the cells shown is represented just above the peak of the cells' tuning curve. For example, the middle tun-

FIGURE 4.20 Possible explanation for the tilt aftereffect, based on the concept of ensemble coding of orientation information. The left-hand portion of the drawing shows neural activity evoked by vertical bars prior to adaptation; the right-hand portion shows activity evoked by vertical bars after adaptation to bars tilted slightly clockwise.

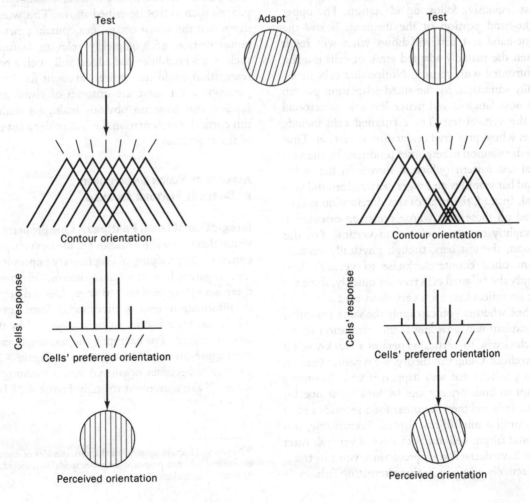

ing curve corresponds to a cell maximally responsive to vertical. When this ensemble of cells is stimulated by vertical test bars, the cells within the ensemble respond unequally. Cells with preferred orientations at vertical respond most vigorously, and those with preferred orientations removed from vertical respond less vigorously. This distribution of responses is depicted in the left-hand bar graph, just below the tuning curves. Because this distribution of activity peaks at vertical, this is the perceived orientation of the test pattern.

Suppose we now adapt this array of cells to bars tilted clockwise from vertical (the pattern labeled "Adapt"). With prolonged exposure, all cells activated by this orientation will be fatigued; the cells maximally responsive to the adapting orientation will be maximally fatigued and hence least responsive following adaptation. The upper right-hand portion of the diagram, below the right-hand test pattern, shows what will result when the partially adapted array of cells is again confronted with vertical. Notice that cells maximally stimulated by the tilted adaptation pattern are now fatigued and hence less able to respond to the vertical test. These fatigued cells include ones whose preferred orientation is vertical. Thus the distribution of responses produced by the vertical test pattern (which is shown in the right-hand bar graph) is no longer centered around vertical. Instead, the peak of this distribution is centered on those cells whose preferred orientation is slightly counterclockwise to vertical. For this reason, the test bars, though physically vertical, seem tilted counterclockwise to vertical. Evidently the fatigued cells recover quickly, since the tilt aftereffect lasts for a very short time.

See whether you can apply the same reasoning to explain why adapting to an orientation counterclockwise to vertical generates a clockwise tilt aftereffect. Using this theory, see whether you can also predict what will happen if you alternately adapt to both orientations by looking at one for 5 seconds and then the other for 5 seconds and so on, until a minute has elapsed. Presumably, this should fatigue cells on both sides of vertical. After you have derived your prediction, you can test it by actually adapting in that alternating fashion.

So according to this activity profile scheme of information coding, stimulus features are signaled within an ensemble of cells.* The ensemble, in effect, would inspect the contour information within a local region of the retinal image and "vote" on the most likely feature producing the activity profile within that ensemble. These local "elections" would be occurring among a large number of ensembles devoted to different regions of the retinal image. In fact, these ensembles could consist of the hypercolumns we described earlier. At the moment, however, we have no idea how votes would be tabulated within an ensemble, or hypercolumn.

For the sake of argument, let's assume that the ambiguity inherent in the responses of individual cells can be solved by some local collaboration process such as that described above. This would mean that the visual cortex *does* contain a neural representation of biologically relevant features, such as oriented lines and edges. Still, such a representation could not entirely account for visual perception, for there are qualities of visual perception that have no obvious analogues within this cortical representation. Let's consider a couple of these qualities.

ASPECTS OF VISION UNEXPLAINED BY CORTICAL FEATURE ANALYSIS

Integration of Local Features. One property of vision that you will learn about in the next chapter concerns the grouping of fragmentary impressions into organized, meaningful patterns. In vision there is a strong tendency to group bits and pieces of information into a meaningful form, even when that form is only vaguely suggested by the bits and pieces. For example, the seemingly random aggregation of black patches in Figure 4.21 eventually becomes organized into a meaningful scene. (Take a moment to study Figure 4.21 be-

---

* As you will learn in subsequent chapters, this idea of ensemble coding has been proposed for other modalities, including hearing, taste, and smell.

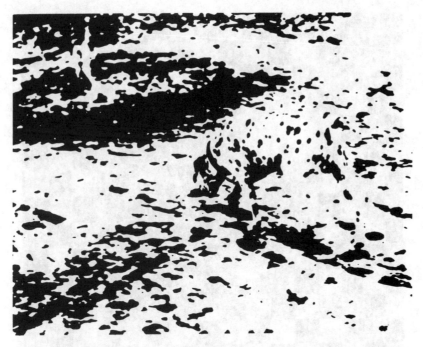

FIGURE 4.21 Differentiating the elements of this picture into meaningful objects is difficult at first and would probably be impossible if you had no previous knowledge of or experience with the objects depicted. If you cannot discern the composition of the picture after studying it, consult Figure 4.22's caption.

fore reading on.) This percept must result from the synthesis of contour information gathered from over a large portion of the picture. Looking at only local regions of the picture, as cortical cells do, would never lead to recognition of the scene and the central object within that scene. Rather, we see the scene and the object because of some more widespread, or global, comparison of local contour information. Moreover, knowledge of what to look for dramatically simplifies the job of realizing what you are looking at. (This role of knowledge in perception is discussed in great detail in Chapter 13.) How can knowledge and memory be incorporated into the activity of cortical feature detectors?

Another effective demonstration of the global nature of perception is shown in Figure 4.22. This computer-generated picture depicts two spheres— one opaque and the other transparent—resting on a textured surface; shown, too, are the shadows of those objects. As the creators of this picture point out:

A fundamental difficulty for analyzing the image of a complex scene is that the contours produced by opaque objects, transparent objects, texture, and shadows are completely indistinguishable within a single local region. To obtain reliable information from these higher-order properties, it would be necessary to adopt a method of analysis that makes use of the global organization of an image in addition to its locally defined gradients. (Todd and Mingolla, 1984, p. 394)

Visual perception is replete with examples like these, and they remind us that local feature analysis by the brain represents an early stage in the sequence of neural events underlying global perception.

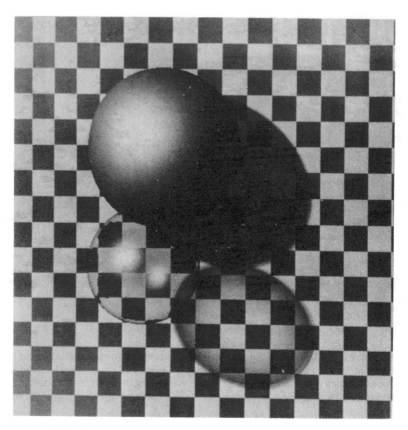

FIGURE 4.22 Computer-generated picture of two spheres resting on a textured surface (courtesy of Ennio Mingolla & James Todd). Incidentally, Figure 4.21 depicts a Dalmatian dog walking toward a tree.

Instability of Perception. Figure 4.23 illustrates another formidable challenge for theories of visual perception based solely on neural analyzing mechanisms in the visual cortex. Here the visual system is presented with a single figure that, although physically invariant, may be seen in two strikingly different ways. This well-known example was introduced into the scientific literature by E. G. Boring (1930).* If you look at the picture for a few moments, you will see why it is sometimes called the "Wife and Mother-in-Law" figure: sometimes the figure looks like a shy young woman and other times it appears to be an unattractive old woman. These fluctuations in the figure's appearance occur even though the stimulus information reaching your eyes remains unchanged. From what we know about the receptive field properties of cortical cells, the activity in the visual cortex should not be changing over time as one stares at this picture, because the contour information contained in the picture remains the same. Presumably the neural events responsible for the spontaneous changes in the appearance of the figure arise at some higher level of visual processing beyond the visual cortex. This supposition is bolstered by the fact that perceptual

_____

* For many years the creator of the figure was thought to be British cartoonist W. E. Hill, who published it in 1915. Recently, though, it was revealed that Hill almost certainly plagiarized from a French original published 15 years before (Wright, 1992).

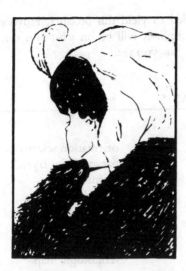

FIGURE 4.23 An ambiguous figure that can be seen in either of two ways.

reversals are far more frequent when observers have been alerted to the possibility of such reversals (Rock and Mitchener, 1992).

Externalization of the Visual World. Let's consider one final aspect of visual perception that has no obvious analogue within the activity of visual cortical cells—the externalization of sensed events (Prinz, 1992). One never feels that visual sensations are localized within the eyes or the brain, yet the requisite events for seeing occur entirely within the head. Why, then, are the objects and events one sees automatically referred to the world beyond one's eyes? "Objects are externalized," you might reply, "because in fact that's where they really are." But this merely restates the observation without explaining how this as-

pect of perception of externality is represented within the visual nervous system. Having accepted the idea that vision evolves from the pattern of activity within areas of the brain, one cannot now treat externality as a fundamentally different aspect of vision that supersedes this level of explanation. Instead, one is obliged to view externality as a property of perception that must eventually be included within any brain-based theory of perception. At present, however, it is not known why objects are visualized outside the body, and the reason may prove as elusive as the basis of conscious experience itself.

To sum up, it would be a mistake to make the visual cortex bear the entire burden of visual perception. The cortex is elegantly designed to derive information concerning the shapes and locations of boundaries in the retinal image—an important early step in the process of seeing (Marr, 1982). But seeing involves more than this. Rather than experiencing a conglomeration of unconnected contours scattered throughout the field of view, we see these contours organized into whole objects whose sizes and shapes remain constant. This organization in perception mirrors the organization of real objects as they actually exist. The correspondence between perceptual experience and the objects represented in that experience is not accidental (Campbell, 1974; Shepard, 1981). After all, the visual system did evolve for a purpose, namely, to inform one about the objects with which one needs to interact. Presumably, natural selection has sponsored this correspondence between perception and the physical world. William James (1892) put this idea succinctly: "Mind and world . . . have evolved together, and in consequence are something of a mutual fit" (p. 4).

SUMMARY   AND   PREVIEW

These last two chapters have provided an overview of some of the neural machinery of visual perception. We are now ready to shift the focus to perception itself. In the next several chapters,

we are going to examine different aspects, or qualities, of vision. These qualities of vision—shape, color, movement, and depth—serve to differentiate objects from one another. In discussing each of these qualities of vision, we shall treat them as the final product of the visual system's processing. We shall consider what sort of mechanism would be needed to yield this product. However, the major emphasis will be on *what* you see, rather than on *how* you see.

K E Y   T E R M S

adaptation
ambiguity problem
binocular
binocular cell
blindsight
blobs
complex cells
contralateral fibers
cortical magnification
direction selectivity
forced-choice
hypercolumn
illusory conjunctions

ipsilateral fibers
lateral geniculate nucleus
   (LGN)
magnocellular layers
meridional amblyopia
monocular
myelin
oblique effect
occipital lobe
ocular dominance
optic chiasm
optic nerve
optic tracts

orientation selectivity
parvocellular layers
perimetry
phosphenes
prosopagnosia
reticular activating
   system
retinotopic map
scotomas
simple cells
superior colliculus
tilt aftereffect
visual field

Spatial Vision and Pattern Perception

S ight serves many different purposes: reading street signs, telling when a friend has had a haircut, catching a football, flying an airplane, finding a pencil amid a desk's clutter, and many others. Though an enormous number of quite different tasks depend on vision, a key part of most involves picking out objects from their surroundings. We can call this process **detection.** Some tasks require that we go a step further, distinguishing one object from another. We can call this second, more refined process **discrimination.** In still other circumstances, we must know exactly what a particular object is or who a particular person is. This third process we may call **identification.** To deal with the environment successfully, people must be able to accomplish all three processes rapidly and accurately: detect, discriminate, and identify.

Detection discloses the presence of an object or objects; discrimination and identification serve more complicated purposes. For example, visual discrimination allows you to sort out important from unimportant information. Of course, what is important depends on your needs. Faced with a homework assignment, you must be able to distinguish one book from another; when famished, you need to distinguish the edible from the inedible; when you read, you have to distinguish one letter from another. Identification goes one step further—not only must one object be distinguished (discriminated) from among others, that object must also be recognized. To find your white car in a crowded parking lot, you must discriminate the white cars from all the rest *and*

then identify yours based on other familiar cues. Discrimination enables you to tell one car from another, but identification tags one specific car as the object of interest.

From the examples given above, it should be apparent that these three perceptual processes form a hierarchy: discrimination first requires detection, and identification must be preceded by discrimination. Of course, we do not consciously step through this sequence in the course of perception; the perceptual act of identifying a stimulus within a complex scene often occurs effortlessly in the blink of an eye. Nonetheless, the stimulus information required for the three processes differs, with each successive process requiring more refined information.

An object can differ in many ways from its surroundings. Specifically, the object can differ in color (a ripe, red berry against the green leaves of its bush), movement (a moving insect in a stationary environment), shape (a chocolate-covered cherry in the box of mixed chocolates), or depth (an aspirin tablet lying on a white tile floor). Usually, several of these sources of information are available simultaneously, facilitating detection. For example, a breeze causes some red berries to *move* relative to the green leaves, making the berries even more conspicuous. But having detected those berries, one must discriminate the ripe from the unripe, which often involves judging subtle color differences. And, of course, one must identify the type of berry, to ensure safe consumption; identification entails comparing the current environmental stimulus with stored knowledge about categories of berries. Because identification involves this extra step of knowledge consultation, we shall postpone further discussion of this process until Chapter 13 and focus here on detection and discrimination.

This chapter and the three that follow deal with the sources of visual information supporting detection and discrimination. These chapters also go into the details of how that information is registered and processed by the nervous system. Although each chapter emphasizes one source (such as movement), we shall also examine how these various sources interact. The present chapter examines how an object's spatial properties influence detection and discrimination. We use the term "spatial properties" to refer to those attributes of an object that jointly determine the perceived size and shape of the object. Defined in this way, the term "spatial properties" is more or less synonymous with the often-used terms "form" and "visual pattern." The material in this chapter focuses on what some experts would characterize as "early vision," meaning that the underlying processes represent the initial stages in an increasingly more refined analysis of a visual scene. On this view, we postpone discussion of those more refined aspects of perception until Chapter 13.

WHAT DEFINES AN OBJECT?

What are the requirements for recognizing that an object is present? To answer this question, let's imagine an object that appears within uniformly illuminated surroundings. Success in recognizing the object's presence depends not so much on the amount of light reflected by the object as on the *difference* between that amount of light and the light reflected by the object's surroundings. Recall from Chapters 3 and 4 that the nervous system is well suited to register such differences. In general, as the intensity of an object's background increases, the light reflected from that object must be even more intense in order for the object to be seen. This is why you cannot see the stars in the daytime sky even though they are present and no less intense than they are at night.*

The difference in intensity between an object and its immediate surroundings is termed "contrast." Although there are various definitions of contrast, for our purposes you need remember only that contrast grows with the difference between the intensity of an object and the intensity of its surroundings. It doesn't matter whether the object is lighter or darker than its surroundings; rather it is the *difference* between object and surround that influences whether the object's presence can be recognized. Sometimes, however, it's insufficient to know merely that an object is present; the object's shape must also be known. This requires information about more than just contrast. You need to know the spatial arrangement of the contrast, since that's what defines an object's shape. Therefore, both contrast and spatial arrangement are key elements in the perception of form.

WHAT DEFINES "FORM"?

You probably have some intuitive notion of what is meant by an object's "form"—the term typically refers to attributes such as size and shape. Form is an inherent property of all objects, including things as nebulous as clouds. Are there universal laws governing the perception of form? Is it useful to consider a visual form as the composite of more elementary features, and if so, what are those features? How does the visual system extract form information from the retinal image? These are questions we shall explore in the next several sections.

From the outset, keep in mind an important caveat about the study of form perception. Like other aspects of visual perception, form is the culmination of a series of processing steps, most of

---

* This is but one example of a more general principle known as Weber's Law, which is discussed in the Appendix.

which transpire at a preconscious level. Simply looking at an object tells you precious little about the steps involved in deriving your impression of that object's form (Snyder and Barlow, 1988). To understand what we mean, consider this analogy: the end product of cooking can be a sophisticated dish, but just tasting the dish discloses little about the steps involved in preparing it. Complete understanding of the cooking process requires knowing the ingredients as well as the recipe by which those ingredients were prepared and combined. The same requirement applies to our attempts to understand form perception.

The point stressed here is reminiscent of one raised in Chapter 1: perceiving is a biological process wherein the brain, using information gathered by the senses, derives descriptions of objects and events in the world. Those descriptions can be construed as symbolic representations of the visual scene (Frisby, 1980; Johnson-Laird, 1988), representations that themselves result from a series of ever more refined computations performed on the image of that scene (Marr, 1982). A complete theory of form perception must consider how form information is represented within the visual system, early on in the process as well as late.

In this chapter we emphasize one particular theory of form that explicitly deals with this issue of representation. This approach unifies results from many different experiments, both perceptual and physiological (DeValois and DeValois, 1988). Before learning about this approach, though, you should be familiar with two important earlier approaches that helped shape it. These views advocate diametrically opposed ideas about the nature of form perception. One view assumes that perceptual forms consist of elementary, punctate sensations. The opposing view assumes that form perception cannot be decomposed into elementary units of sensation; instead, forms must be considered as unitary structures with unique properties. The first approach could be described as atomistic or microscopic, and the second approach as global or macroscopic. The contemporary view emphasized in this chapter captures the best of both these extremes. We'll begin, then,

with an overview of these two older, conflicting approaches.

TRADITIONAL APPROACHES TO FORM PERCEPTION

STRUCTURALISM

The structuralist tradition in perception germinated in Europe during the late nineteenth century and flowered after being transplanted to the United States. Its main idea is simple and attractive: complex mental processes—ideas and perceptions—are created by combining fundamental components. According to this view, simple sensations constitute the building blocks of perceived form. Given this assumption, how does one identify these simple sensations? Edward Titchener, a leader of the structuralist movement, championed a very simple method, called **analytic introspection.** He trained people to ignore all aspects of an object except its immediate, primary qualities. By attending only to an object's appearance and nothing else, people tried to enumerate the various sensations evoked by that object. For example, a person looking at an apple might report seeing four different colors and seventy-three different levels of lightness, with both color and lightness distributed over the apple's surface in some particular way. According to the structuralists, these ingredients constituted the sensations from which the percept of the apple was built.

After analytic introspection had been in use for a while, the number of cataloged "elementary" sensations ballooned out of control, to more than 40,000 (Boring, 1942). Compared with the number of chemical elements in the periodic table (currently 109), 40,000 perceptual elements seemed excessive. To make matters worse, one person's reported elementary sensations often differed from those of another person. These disagreements were particularly striking because they involved people working in different laboratories. This suggests that the technique of introspection is susceptible to such nonperceptual influences as motivation and instruction. As you might imagine, what people *say* they saw depends partly on what they're encouraged to see ("Don't you think this apple has a slight tinge of green?").

Besides these problems, introspection suffers from a logical flaw, too. Even if someone can learn to recognize a particular sensation when it occurs all by itself, there's no guarantee that the person will be able to recognize it when that sensation occurs in combination with various other sensations. Taken together, these difficulties undermined the usefulness of analytic introspection. Nonetheless, one can embrace the structuralists' idea that perceptions are built from elementary units without subscribing to introspection as the method for isolating those units.

THE GESTALT SCHOOL

In Chapter 3 we saw that the neural response to even the simplest stimulus—a patch of light—depends on its surroundings. It has long been known that this dependence operates at the perceptual level. In 1920, the German psychologist Wolfgang Köhler (1920/1938) insisted, "We do not see individual fractions of a thing; instead, the mode of appearance of each part depends not only upon the stimulation arising at *that* point but upon the conditions prevailing at other points as well" (p. 20). Köhler's comment relates to the lightness illusions described in Chapter 3.

Köhler's view formed the basis of the second major theory of pattern perception—a theory which rejected the idea that perception is an aggregate of simple elements somehow knitted together. Instead, its adherents, called *Gestalt psychologists,* emphasized overall structure or pattern as the major determinant of form perception (*Gestalt* is a German word meaning "form"). Their credo is often summarized by the phrase "The whole is different from the sum of the individual parts." Here is an analogy. Perhaps you have seen the intricate and precise formations assumed by migrating geese (see Figure 5.1). Focusing on in-

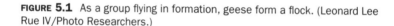

FIGURE 5.1 As a group flying in formation, geese form a flock. (Leonard Lee Rue IV/Photo Researchers.)

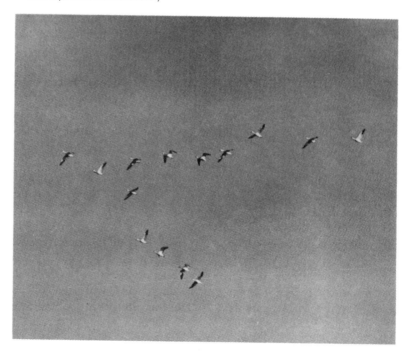

dividual members of the flock makes it impossible to capture the overall pattern of the formation. The formation itself emerges only from the coalescence of all the birds. In a similar vein, Gestalt psychologists assert that form cannot be comprehended by focusing on its discrete components.

Origins of the Gestalt Approach.

The birth of Gestalt psychology in 1912 was heralded by Max Wertheimer's ground-breaking monograph on illusory motion (discussed in Chapter 8). Wertheimer and his associates, notably Wolfgang Köhler and Kurt Koffka, went on to make important contributions to educational theory, social psychology, and other areas of psychology (Rock and Palmer, 1990). Arguably, though, their most important and lasting impact was on the area of perception, particularly their formulation of the **Gestalt principles of organization.** These principles identified factors that tend to encourage the emergence of perceptual forms and promote the grouping of those forms, segregated from their surroundings (Wertheimer, 1923/1958). Recall from Chapter 1 that grouping and segregation are crucial in the early stages of all perception, including vision.

When many elements are present simultaneously, Wertheimer observed that they tend to become grouped or organized perceptually into distinct patterns (1923/1958). Although various alternative organizations are possible for any set of elements, people do tend to see them as organized or patterned in a particular way. The Gestalt principles of organization describe how figural properties determine perceived pattern (Hochberg, 1971). Let's examine several of the principles that Wertheimer considered particularly important (for an extensive discussion, see Pomerantz and Kubovy, 1986).

The principle of **proximity** describes the tendency of objects near one another to group together as a perceptual unit. As you can see in panel A of Figure 5.2, no particular organization seems to predominate when the dots are equally spaced. Instead, the dots can be seen as forming rows, columns, diagonals, or simply as a collection with no pattern. None of these weak organizations per-

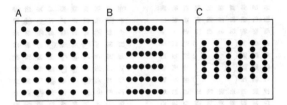

FIGURE 5.2 Objects close together tend to unite perceptually into groups.

sists, and none seems compelling. In fact, some effort is needed to see any of these organizations. Notice what happens, however, when the vertical distances among neighboring dots are made greater than the horizontal distances, as in panel B of the figure. With this simple modification, a strong organization emerges: the dots form horizontal strings, or rows. Panel C illustrates what happens when the horizontal distances are made greater than the vertical: dots group into vertical strings, or columns. Simply by varying the ratio of vertical to horizontal distances (that is, by varying the dots' proximity), we can bias the resulting percept in favor of one organization or the other. So proximity is one of the regularities used to organize a visual scene into distinct objects.

Wertheimer identified another major organizational tendency, known as the principle of **similarity.** "Other things being equal, if several stimuli are presented together, there is a tendency to see the form in such a way that the similar items are grouped together" (1923/1958, p. 119). The dimensions of similarity that control grouping include lightness, orientation, and size. Examples of these effects are illustrated in Figure 5.3. Notice in the left-hand panel how the circles form a perceptual group in the midst of the squares. Apparently the differences between circles and squares in both lightness and shape contribute to this grouping. In the right-hand panel, the disks form two diagonals crisscrossing the squares. Here shape alone promotes grouping.

A third, related grouping principle is called **closure.** Closure also tends to unite contours that are very close to one another; Figure 5.4 illustrates this tendency. At first the figure may look like a

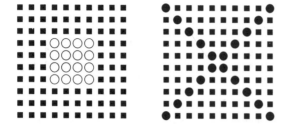

FIGURE 5.3 Objects similar in shape and size tend to group together.

meaningless row of heartlike forms. But actually the pattern contains a handwritten version of a simple and common word—"men." In fact, the pattern contains two copies of that word, each standing in mirror-image relation to the other. Closure causes the two mirror images to cohere into a single pattern, thereby obscuring the two components. Closely related to closure is the principle of **good continuation,** wherein neighboring elements are grouped together when they are potentially connected by straight or smoothly curving lines.

With these four factors—proximity, similarity, closure, and good continuation—in mind, consider Figure 5.5. Looking at the photograph, you have no trouble recognizing the face of a girl gazing through a window. That may seem simple, until you consider what the visual system must accomplish to arrive at this percept. Early on, vision had to identify regions that were likely to be neighboring parts of a single surface. Follow-

FIGURE 5.4 A demonstration of closure. (Adapted from Köhler, 1969.)

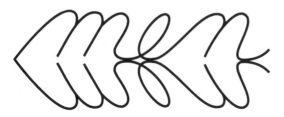

ing our four Gestalt principles, the visual system would tend to group regions that adjoined one another (proximity) and/or had similar attributes, such as lightness, texture, and so on (similarity). Extended contours, such as the window frame, would be seen to form a single object (closure, good continuation). The visual system also had to segregate *different* objects from one another, even though they overlapped; the Gestalt psychologists called this process **figure/ground organization,** that is, the tendency to see parts of a scene as solid, well-defined objects—the "figure"—standing out against a less distinct background—the "ground". Here, vision had to group the boundaries separating one object (such as the face) from others (such as the window). Note that within local regions of a scene, one Gestalt principle may conflict with another: in the photograph, for instance, proximity of the window frame to the girl's face would tend erroneously to group the two. Evidently, the ultimate force of any Gestalt principle is not governed by the properties of local regions of the image taken in isolation. Instead, potentially conflicting Gestalt principles are reconciled in accord with rules as yet not fully understood.

The Gestalt grouping processes capitalize on certain regularities that characterize our physical world. Recall the discussion on pages 21–22 in Chapter 1. The Gestalt principles of organization seem to embody many of the regularities that typify most natural objects. Natural objects tend to be compact; their parts, if there are parts, are connected rather than scattered hither and yon. As a result, perception of natural objects is well served by a tendency to group adjacent elements (principle of proximity) and to treat extended contours as a single form (good continuation). Also, the parts of natural objects tend to be made of a single material, which reflects light in a uniform and characteristic way. Changes in material (and hence light reflected from the material) usually signify the boundaries between parts or the boundaries between an object and its surroundings. So object perception is helped by the tendency to group elements that are similar and segregate ones that are dissimilar (principles of

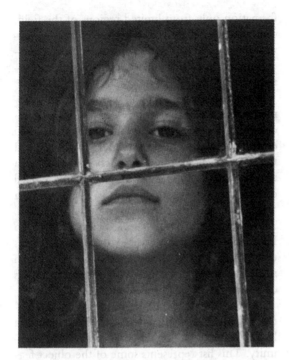

FIGURE 5.5 Seeing an object entails segregating contours into a meaningful whole. (R. Sekuler.)

similarity and closure). With these facts in mind, look again at Figure 5.5 and determine how these different principles contributed to perception of the objects in the scene.

The Gestalt psychologists embedded their principles of organization within a particular theory of how the brain worked. According to their theory, visual perception is determined by the pattern of electrical activity within the brain. To illustrate this concept, imagine that you are looking at an object—such as a bottle of soda—while someone else measures the distribution of electrical activity within your brain. The Gestalt psychologists, without benefit of modern neurophysiological insights, believed that this distribution would resemble the shape of the object you were seeing. This comparability between perception and brain activity is known as **isomorphism,** and it plays a prominent role in Gestalt theory. Note that "isomorphism" doesn't imply an exact correspondence, just an approximate one.* But as Chapter 4 explained, modern work has amply demonstrated that the visual world is not represented as a single, isomorphic picture within the brain. Also, although activity does spread across the cortex, both within and between cortical areas, the spread does not obey the principles that govern the distribution of forces within simple inorganic systems as the Gestalt theorists thought.

Extensions of the Gestalt Approach. Despite these limitations, today important research builds upon the Gestaltists' insights and shares some of their viewpoints. Some of this research aims to rectify a key deficiency in Gestalt psychology: though Gestalt demonstrations were interesting and impressive, they did not readily predict what would be seen in the case of other, novel stimuli. Now, as we shall see, the rules required for quantitative generalization are finally being worked out.

Figure 5.3 demonstrated that differences in elements' shapes can spawn perceptual grouping. But it's important to recognize that not all such differences do so. In Figure 5.6, the cluster of plus signs stands out in the midst of the little "L"s; it is very hard, though, to see the cluster of "T"s embedded in the "L"s in the right-hand side of the figure. Only by scrutinizing the elements individually can you discover the existence of a group of "T"s. Because only particular properties promote grouping, these properties may constitute the basic elements of perception. Using a term from mathematics, we call these visual elements or building blocks **primitives.**

On the assumption that knowledge of these primitives might reveal how grouping processes work, many researchers try to identify vision's

---

* *Iso* means "the same"; *morph* refers to "form." "One system is said to be isomorphic with another . . . if every point in one corresponds to a point in the other and the topological relations or spatial orders of the points are the same in the two. If a system of points is marked on a flat rubber membrane and the membrane is then stretched tightly over some irregular surface, then the points in the stretched membrane are isomorphic with the points in the flat membrane" (Boring, 1942, pp. 83–84).

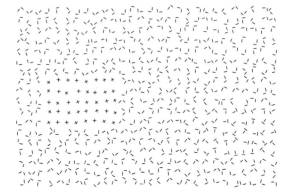

FIGURE 5.6 Demonstration of some limits on object segregation by shape. (From Julesz, 1984.)

primitives (Julesz, 1984, 1991; Beck, Prazdny, and Rosenfeld, 1983). The work of Anne Treisman (1986) is a good example of this effort. Her method assumes that at an early stage, vision extracts information from across the entire visual field all at once; at some later stage, which requires scrutiny of individual details, vision registers in-

formation only from limited regions of the field, one after the other. Drawing on computer terminology, we might describe early visual processing as "parallel" and later processing as "serial."

Treisman's method, then, seeks to identify elements that are detected very early in visual processing. These are elements that could be detected equally well, anywhere in the field, with no need for scrutiny. Phenomenally, such elements seem to pop out of their surroundings. Four typical displays are shown in Figure 5.7. Presenting a target at randomly chosen locations in the field, Treisman measured how long observers took to locate the target. In order to distinguish targets that pop out from those that do not, Treisman measured judgment times with varying numbers of nontarget, distractor elements.

Several dozen experiments showed that features that pop out include color, line curvature, line tilt, target contrast, length, number, and proximity. This list represents some of the object features that early vision uses in order to define ob-

FIGURE 5.7 Four displays typical of those in Treisman's work on target pop-out.

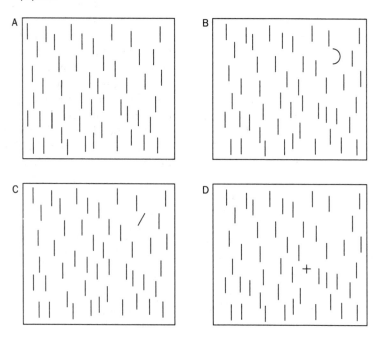

jects and surface boundaries, but the list is probably not complete. Bela Julesz (Rutgers University), who has also done important work in this area, has advocated that pop-out ought to be assessed with spatially dense displays (as in Figure 5.6). Such displays can give rise perceptually to an emergent property called texture. Differences between one texture and another can pop out just as differences between widely separated but highly distinctive elements do. Since perceptual textures exist only when displays are fairly dense, Julesz (1991) argues that displays that contain relatively few widely spaced elements foreclose possible interactions among adjacent elements. As a result, such displays may obscure the importance of texture as a primitive in early stages of vision.

* * *

Thus far this chapter has focused on two contrasting approaches to pattern perception. One, the structuralist approach, treated form perception as an analytical process, whereby complex forms were decomposed into small, simple elements. Although intuitively plausible, this approach floundered because of disagreement about what those simple elements might be. In part, this disagreement stemmed from the unreliability of the introspective technique. But the structuralist approach also could not account for the figural properties that the Gestaltists emphasized. The Gestaltist theorists, while discovering seemingly important principles of perceptual organization, were unable to develop a lasting theory of the neural origins of those principles. Interestingly, some of those influenced by the Gestalt approach are actually fostering the structuralist's original agenda, using objective and quantitative methods in order to identify and understand visual primitives.

A CONTEMPORARY APPROACH TO FORM PERCEPTION

We are now ready to consider the multiple spatial channels theory, a major contemporary theory of form perception that incorporates some of the good qualities of both the Gestalt and the structuralist approaches. To help you appreciate the novelty and power of this theory, we begin by pointing out an important function of form vision that this theory makes explicit.

Look at the photograph and three line drawings in Figure 5.8 (p. 150). By showing a tracing or an outline of different structures in the photo, each line drawing captures a different aspect of that photograph's information. These line drawings differ in what we shall call **scale**. Drawings captures the scene on the largest scale—the emphasis is on the proverbial "big picture," or overview of the scene. Drawing C portrays the scene on the smallest scale—this focuses on the scene's details. Drawing B emphasizes information on a scale intermediate to the other two. The photograph contains all the information that one sees in each drawing. Their differences in scale allow the three drawings to emphasize different aspects of the scene: A emphasizes the skyline, B highlights individual buildings, and C spotlights the architectural details.

Regardless of the distance from which a scene is viewed, images of naturally occurring scenes or objects (trees, rocks, bushes, etc.) tend to contain information at many different spatial scales, from very fine to very coarse (Field, 1987). The viewer's goals determine what component of this information is paramount. Because goals change, one scale may be more important than another now, but less important later. Sometimes it's important to see the forest; other times the trees, or the leaves, are essential. Ideally, then, your brain's neural representation of a scene would contain the information from all scales simultaneously. By having access to representations of scenes or objects at different spatial scales, the visual system can solve problems that would be intractable using a single representation (Hildreth, 1986). We will encounter some of those problems later in this and subsequent chapters. For now, though, let's consider how the visual system implements this multiple-scale representation.

The mammalian visual system is well suited to create neural representations of any visual scene simultaneously on several different scales. In prin-

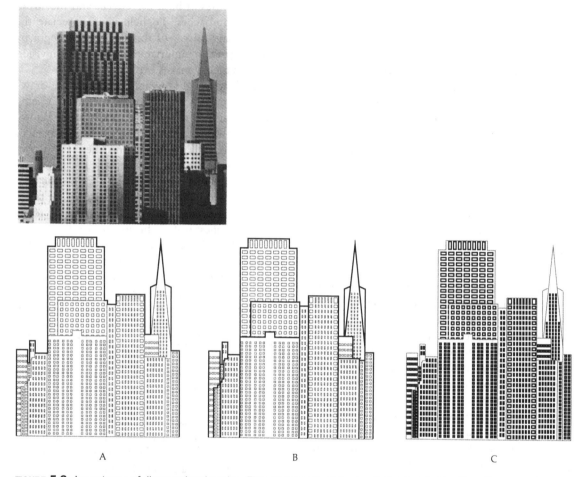

FIGURE 5.8 Importance of diverse visual scales. The photograph at the top left, taken in San Francisco, contains information on many different scales. The line drawings highlight three different scales of information: the skyline, or large scale (drawing A); individual buildings, or intermediate scale (B); and architectural details, or fine scale (C). (Photo: Judith Canty/Stock, Boston.)

ciple, neurons with different receptive field diameters could capture the presence of borders or edges at different scales (see Figure 3.7). In 1968, two British vision researchers, Fergus Campbell and John Robson, developed a theory of form perception in which the visual system would use neurons with different receptive field sizes to create a series of neural representations on different scales. Their theory, which has been subjected to numerous empirical tests, has been enormously influential.

Campbell and Robson (1968) hypothesized

that at different levels of the visual system, the responses of various neurons form a neural representation of the image falling on the retina. Because neurons' receptive fields vary in size, the responses of different subsets of neurons would constitute a neural representation at some particular scale. To test their hypothesis, Campbell and Robson needed stimuli whose orientation and size could be varied systematically. In addition, knowing that contrast is important in detection, they needed to specify and vary contrast as well. A stimulus such as the one shown in

Figure 5.9 satisfies all these requirements. Such patterns, called **gratings,** can be generated on a television display. The one in Figure 5.9 is called a **sinusoidal grating** because the intensity of its light and dark bars changes gradually, in a sinusoidal fashion. At sufficiently low contrast, the television screen would appear uniform and unpatterned; at higher contrasts, the pattern would be visible. For various gratings, Campbell and Robson determined the *minimum* contrast necessary to see the grating, a value called the **contrast threshold.**

Two types of gratings were used: *simple* and *compound.* Compound gratings were created by adding together several different simple sinusoidal gratings. Before describing the experiment itself, let's examine the process by which a compound grating is created. This process is illustrated in Figure 5.10, where a compound grating is constructed from three different simple sinusoidal components. The left column shows the simple components, labeled A through C. Note that as we go from top to bottom, gratings have thinner bars. Specifically, bars in grating A are 3 times as wide as those in grating B and 5 times as wide as those in grating C. All three patterns have the same contrast.

The middle column of Figure 5.10 portrays the creation of a compound grating from the three simple components shown in the left column. To make it easier to visualize, we have broken the process down into steps. Grating D is the starting point, a replica of grating A. When gratings A and B are added, the result is grating E. When C is

FIGURE 5.9 A sinusoidal grating pattern.

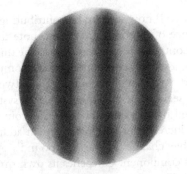

added to E, the result is grating F. Grating F exemplifies the compound gratings that Campbell and Robson worked with.

We'll now turn to the predictions Campbell and Robson made about the visibility and appearance of compound stimuli. According to their theory, the different components of a compound grating activate different sets of neurons in the visual cortex. Each set of neurons would be sensitive to bars of a particular size and, hence, to only one component in the compound. In other words, Campbell and Robson thought that perception of compound gratings, such as grating F, was mediated by several different sets of neurons and that each set of neurons responded to a different component in the compound. Thus, although the compound grating doesn't *look* like any of its components, its appearance nonetheless depends on all of them. Neurons activated by the separate components would have to be simultaneously activated in order for the compound to appear the way it does.

If this theory is correct, it should be possible to measure the contributions made by the separate components in a compound grating. How, though, can this be accomplished? Campbell and Robson reasoned that they could do this by comparing the contrast threshold for a compound grating to the contrast thresholds of its components. From measurements with simple gratings, they already knew that the various components had different thresholds—some components required more contrast to be seen, others less.

Imagine that we set the contrast of grating F at a value low enough to make the pattern invisible. We then begin increasing F's contrast until something *is* seen on the television display. At this point, the display does not look like a compound grating; instead, it looks like one of the simple components (though at low contrast). Specifically, it resembles that component which has the lowest contrast threshold (grating A). In fact, the contrast of that one component in the compound is precisely equivalent to the contrast threshold of that component alone. At this low contrast, only this one component produces activity in the visual system sufficient for the component to be seen

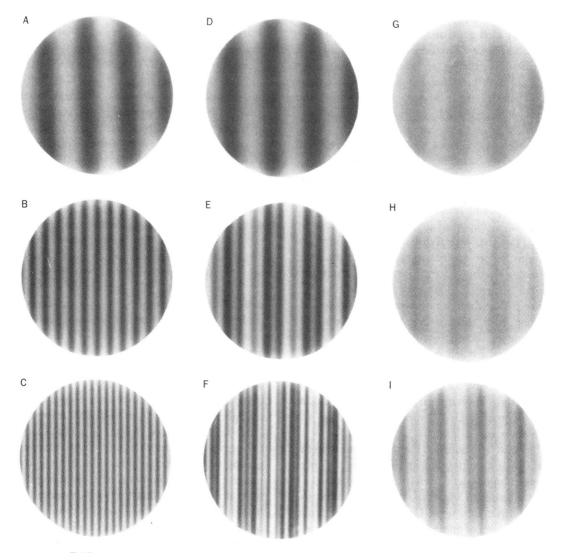

FIGURE 5.10 Steps involved in generating a compound grating from a set of simple sinusoidal gratings.

(grating G). Although physically present in the display, the remaining components are too weak to affect the appearance and visibility of the compound.

Now suppose we continue to increase the contrast of the compound grating. At some point, the display no longer looks like that one simple component (grating A) alone. Instead, the display looks like a low-contrast version of grating E. This is represented in grating H. Component A and

component B now seem to be contributing to the appearance of the display. We also note that this higher-contrast value corresponds to the threshold value for a second component of the compound, grating B. At this higher contrast, then, two components seem to be affecting the visual system, as evidenced by the appearance of the compound. Further increases in contrast bring an additional, predictable change in the compound's appearance. As component C reaches its own threshold contrast, the appearance of the compound is again altered (grating I).

This, then, is the essence of Campbell and Robson's classic study. Using various compound gratings, they showed that the visibility and appearance of a compound grating depends on the independent effects that each of its components has on the visual system. At high contrast, a compound grating doesn't resemble any of its components, but the visual system still treats that compound as an aggregation of several components. These results supported Campbell and Robson's hypothesis that the visual system contains sets of neurons tuned to different bar widths. They called these sets of neurons *channels,* and because their theory relates form perception to activity within many such channels, it is known as the **multichannel model.** Although it can account for Campbell and Robson's results, you may have some reservations about this model. When looking at complicated forms, you see no hint of simpler components consisting of bars of different sizes; your conscious experience doesn't point to any such process of decomposition. You might argue, therefore, that Campbell and Robson tested this model using highly artificial stimuli. We'll address this reservation by showing how the approach of Campbell and Robson can be extended to more natural, everyday scenes. To make this extension, though, we first need to consider grating patterns in greater detail.

GRATINGS AS TOOLS FOR EXPLORING FORM PERCEPTION

What Exactly Are Gratings? Gratings have four properties—**spatial frequency, contrast, orientation,** and **spatial phase.** These properties are independent of one another, in the sense that any one of them can be changed without affecting the others. Since Chapter 4 described what is meant by "orientation," that term needs no explanation here. But we will have to consider the other three.

"Spatial frequency" refers to the number of pairs of bars imaged within a given distance on the retina. One-third of a millimeter is a conve-

nient unit of retinal distance because an image this size is said to subtend 1 degree of visual angle. For example, your index fingernail casts an image of this size when that nail is viewed at arm's length; a typical human thumb, not just the nail, but the entire width, casts an image about twice as big, 2 degrees of visual angle (O'Shea, 1991). The size (or visual angle) of the retinal image cast by some object depends on the distance of that object from the eye; as the distance between the eye and an object decreases, the object's image subtends a greater visual angle. The unit employed to express spatial frequency is the number of cycles that fall within 1 degree of visual angle (each cycle is one dark and one light bar). A grating of high spatial frequency—many cycles within each degree of visual angle—contains narrow bars. A grating of low spatial frequency—few cycles within each degree of visual angle—contains wide bars. Because spatial frequency is defined in terms of visual angle, a grating's spatial frequency changes with viewing distance. As this distance decreases, each bar casts a larger image; as a result the grating's spatial frequency decreases as the distance decreases. For example, when held at arm's length, the grating in Figure 5.9 has a spatial frequency of about 1.0 cycle per degree of visual angle; when held closer, the grating's spatial frequency would be lower.

"Contrast" is related to the intensity difference between the light and dark bars of the grating. If this difference is great, the grating's contrast is high; a small difference means the contrast is low. If the contrast is low enough, the bars of the grating may not even be visible. In this case, the grating contrast is said to be "below the threshold for visibility." Quantitatively, contrast runs from 0 percent (when there is no difference at all between the intensity of the light and dark bars) to 100 percent (when the difference between light and dark bars is maximum).* The contrast of the

---

* There are several formulas for computing contrast. For gratings, though, contrast is equal to the difference between the light intensity of the lightest part of the grating and the light intensity of the dimmest part, divided by the sum of these two quantities.

print you are reading is about 70 percent; the contrast in the grating shown in Figure 5.9 is about 40 percent.

"Spatial phase" refers to a grating's position relative to some landmark (such as the edge of the television display). A convenient landmark is the left edge of the display. Looking at that edge, we can say that a grating "begins" with a dark bar, a light bar, or something in between. The gratings at the top and bottom of Figure 5.11 are in opposite phase; one begins with a light bar, the other with a dark one. The phase of the middle grating is midway between those at the top and bottom.

Grating F in Figure 5.10 showed that when we add gratings together, the appearance of the resulting compound depends on what spatial frequencies are in the mixture. The compound's appearance also depends on the phases of those components. As shown in Figure 5.12, two compounds composed of the same spatial frequencies will look rather different if those components are placed in different phases.

Manipulating these four properties of a grating—spatial frequency, contrast, orientation, and phase—we can construct any visual pattern, even a human face. To start, let's see how far we can get using just two orientations. Our plan is to start with a pair of gratings, one with bars oriented diagonally clockwise (CW) and the other with bars oriented diagonally counterclockwise (CCW), and add pairs of higher-frequency gratings, each additional pair consisting of a CW and a CCW component. Looking at Figure 5.13, in A you see the first two gratings superimposed. Adding in the next two components (1) results in B. Adding to this the next two components (2) produces the pattern shown in C. In each case, the added components are nothing more than a pair of obliquely oriented gratings of a particular frequency. Note two things about C's evolution. First, from A through C, the resemblance to a plaid grows. Here, interactions between components are creating visual structures (diamonds) that are not associated with individual components themselves (Kelly, 1976). Second, from A through C, the diamonds become more sharply defined, even though only unsharp, sinusoidal components

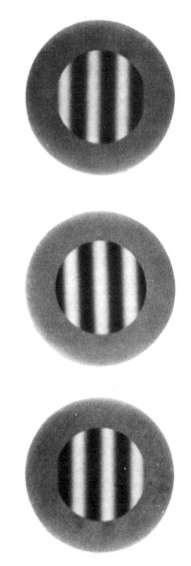

FIGURE 5.11 These three gratings differ in phase only.

were used. We remind you of a point made earlier: you cannot always tell what elementary components make up a pattern.

Now let's try to synthesize an even more complex figure, a photograph of a natural scene. This synthesis requires that we use more than just two orientations. Because it would take a great many frequency components to synthesize the natural scene, it would be tedious to show each individual

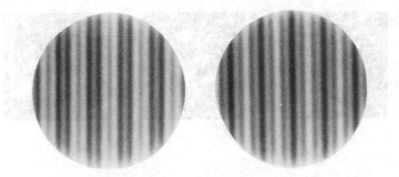

FIGURE 5.12 The same components added in different phases yield distinctly different compound gratings.

step of the process. Instead, at each stage we'll add whole clusters of frequencies. Looking at Figure 5.14, you will see that A shows the frequency and orientation cluster with which we start. From this point, we follow the same procedure used in Figure 5.13, successively adding the clusters shown in 1 and 2 to create B and C. Note how each cluster makes its unique contribution to the final product, C. Bear in mind that this complex scene results from adding various simple components that differ in frequency, contrast, orientation, and phase. Notice, incidentally, that A, 1, and 2 represent the low, medium, and high spatial frequency information of the final product.

FIGURE 5.13 Steps involved in generating a plaid.

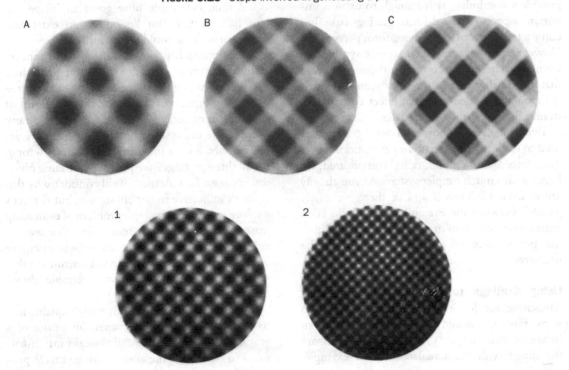

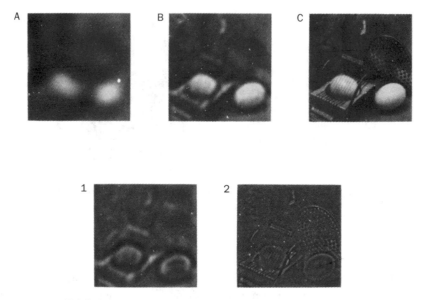

FIGURE 5.14 Steps involved in generating a natural scene, in this instance a photograph of objects commonly found in a kitchen.

As just shown, spatial frequency components can be used to create a visual scene. Because they provide a vocabulary rich enough to express important aspects of visual form, gratings have become a favorite tool for studying form perception. However, just because a scene can be synthesized from spatial frequency components does not mean that the visual system analyzes that scene into such components; evidence to that effect comes from studies that we shall consider later.

Eventually, we'll show you how gratings are used to explore human pattern perception. However, since *human* vision is rather complicated, we begin with a much simpler system. As you already know from Chapters 2 and 3, there are many parallels between the eye and a camera. So as an entrée to human pattern perception, let's see how the performance of a camera's lens might be measured.

Using Gratings to Measure Performance.

Measuring the lens's performance requires two steps. First, we would use the lens to create an image of some target; then we would compare the image with the actual target. For example,

using a lens, we would create an image of a grating of specified spatial frequency and contrast. We could then determine how good an image the lens had created. But "good" is an extremely vague term; how could we quantify it?

One approach is simply to judge the appearance of the image. But this subjective procedure can be misleading. To illustrate, look at the three gratings in Figure 5.15 and rank them in terms of their apparent contrast. Most people would rank them in the order shown, with the leftmost grating deemed lowest in contrast. But this is wrong, for all three gratings have precisely the same physical contrast. In a moment we'll consider why this error in subjective judgment occurs; but first let's explore in greater detail this problem of evaluating image quality. A better, more objective way to assess the quality of images such as those in Figure 5.15 is by means of some physical instrument that measures light. The following example shows how this can be accomplished.

Suppose we use an expensive, high-quality lens to cast, on a clean white paper, an image of a grating. We can use the light-measuring instrument to determine the contrast of the image pro-

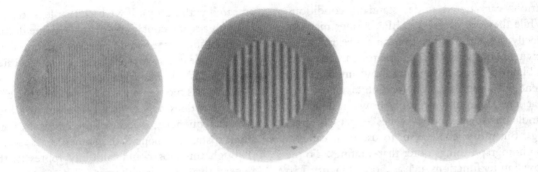

FIGURE 5.15 Which of these three gratings appears highest in contrast and which appears lowest in contrast?

duced by the lens. Let's repeat this for different spatial frequencies, always using gratings of the same contrast. We can graph the results in the following way. The horizontal axis of the graph will show spatial frequency; the vertical axis will show the image's contrast (as a percentage of the target's contrast). The resulting plot is often called a **transfer function,** because it specifies how contrast is transferred through the lens. A typical graph of this kind is shown in Figure 5.16.

Look first at the heavy line in the graph. Note that up to a certain spatial frequency the contrast in the image is identical to that of the target. For these frequencies, the lens faithfully reproduces

the target. However, for still higher spatial frequencies, the contrast in the image is reduced even though the contrast in the target is constant. For these spatial frequencies, the lens reproduces the target less faithfully. The frequency at which the image contrast falls to zero is called the **cutoff frequency;** once the frequency in an actual target exceeds this value, the image will no longer contain any contrast whatsoever—the target itself might as well have zero contrast.

Notice the second curve in Figure 5.16 (the thin line). This curve connects the points we would observe if we repeated the experiment after having made one modification: smearing the lens by running a buttery finger over its surface. At very low spatial frequencies, the smear makes little difference in the performance of the lens. However, at intermediate spatial frequencies, the contrast in the image is degraded by the butter on the lens. This is shown by the difference between the curves for the lens in its buttered and unbuttered states. Note also that the cutoff frequency for the buttered lens is lower than that for the clean lens. This difference between the curves makes intuitive sense: a high-quality lens excels at imaging fine spatial detail *and* coarse spatial detail, while a low-quality lens images only the latter.

So, the transfer function of a lens summarizes its performance, although in a rather abstract way. In this respect, the transfer function serves the same purpose as the United States Environmental Protection Agency's (EPA) mileage ratings for

FIGURE 5.16 Two transfer functions for a lens. The curves specify how contrast in the image formed by the lens is related to contrast in the object.

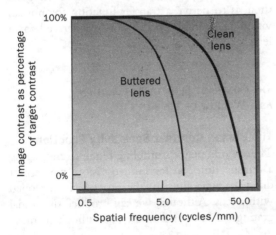

various cars tested under standard conditions. While they are useful, the EPA ratings may not specify the performance of a car under particular driving conditions. By the same token, the curves in Figure 5.16 do not indicate how any particular scene will appear on a photograph taken through that lens. They indicate only how the lens will handle one special set of "scenes"—namely, gratings. But most people want to use their cameras to photograph things other than gratings. To see how transfer functions such as those of Figure 5.16 can be applied to photographing some scene, we must relate that scene to gratings.

One method for doing exactly this comes from the work of Jean Baptiste Fourier, a nineteenth-century French mathematician who, incidentally, was also a friend and associate of Napoleon. As part of a prestigious mathematics contest, Fourier was required to develop equations expressing how heat is transferred from one body to another. He recognized that extremely complex equations would be needed and that those equations would have to be general enough to apply to a wide variety of different bodies. To satisfy these requirements, Fourier developed a powerful simplification. He showed that if some quantity (such as heat) changed in a complex manner over time, that complex function of time could be approximated by a series of simple sinusoidal functions. This simplification was an enormous advantage because it allowed Fourier to break a mathematically difficult function down into simpler, mathematically more tractable components. From here he could solve the problem by working with the simple components (incidentally, he won the contest). In recognition of his accomplishment, we now refer to this technique as **Fourier analysis** (Bracewell, 1989).

But how does Fourier's solution enable us to relate simple sinusoidal functions to a photograph of some scene taken through a lens? First, we can consider that scene as the sum of a series of simple sinusoidal components. Then, using the transfer function of the lens, we can evaluate how the lens would image each of those components.

Consider the lens whose transfer function is given by the lighter line in Figure 5.16 (the lens

smeared with butter). If we used that lens to photograph a scene containing many *very* fine details, the resulting image would be low in contrast and would appear *very* washed out. This is because "fine detail" is equivalent to "high spatial frequency." As the transfer function shows, the buttered lens does a poor job of transferring high spatial frequencies; it reduces the contrast of any high spatial frequencies contained in a scene. Though this lens could faithfully represent the general shape of a large target (such as a tree that is near the camera), it would not be adequate for fine details (such as the wrinkles in the tree's bark). This illustrates that sinusoidal targets can predict the quality of a photograph produced by a lens. To reiterate: Several steps are involved. First, we determine the transfer function of the lens. Second, we analyze the visual scene into its spatial frequency components. With these pieces of information in hand, we determine which spatial frequency components will be preserved in the image of that scene and which will not. The second of these steps is beyond the scope of this book; while not terribly complicated, the calculations are tedious (Weisstein, 1980; Rzeszotarski, Royer, and Gilmore, 1983). The first step, measuring the transfer function, is straightforward in the camera. But how easy is it to measure a transfer function for a visual system such as your own? If we did know your transfer function, we could better predict the visibility of scenes you might look at. As we'll describe later, these predictions confer some practical benefits. Our next goal, then, is to derive a transfer function for human vision comparable to the one we derived for a lens.

THE CONTRAST SENSITIVITY FUNCTION AS A WINDOW OF VISIBILITY

The Human Contrast Sensitivity Function.

There's one major stumbling block to measuring a transfer function for human vision: we cannot duplicate with humans the procedure employed with a lens. Although we can produce sinusoidal gratings of known contrast, it's difficult to measure the image such gratings produce because that image is inside the eye. Anyway, measuring this image would give only part of the visual system's complete transfer function. Although describing the eye's *optical* components, this transfer function would not reflect the *neural* components of the visual system. And since we are interested in visual perception, not just the image formed in the eye, we must be concerned with the *perceptual* transfer function, which depends on both the optical transfer function and the *neural* transfer function.

How then can we measure the *perceptual* transfer function? If your visual system (both its optical and its neural components) did a good job of transferring some spatial frequency, it stands to reason that you'd need little contrast to see a grating of that frequency—in other words, you'd be relatively sensitive to that frequency. However, if your visual system did a poor job of transferring that spatial frequency, you'd need more contrast to see it—you'd be relatively *in*sensitive to that frequency. In general, the sensitivity of the visual system determines the threshold contrast needed to detect a given spatial frequency. By measuring contrast thresholds for different spatial frequencies, we can derive a curve that describes the entire visual system's sensitivity to contrast. Let's call this curve the **contrast sensitivity function (CSF),** to distinguish it from the transfer function of a lens. The term "sensitivity" is a reminder that we are dealing with a property of the visual system, not just a property of the stimulus. As you'd expect from everyday usage of the term "sensitivity," someone is said to have high sensitivity if that person requires little contrast to see a pattern. By the same token, someone is said to have low sensitivity if that person requires considerable contrast to see a pattern. Defined in this way, sensitivity is inversely related to threshold contrast.

Figure 5.17 shows a CSF for a human adult; this curve defines the adult's **window of visibility.** Before explaining the importance and usefulness of the CSF, let's describe how it was measured. A test grating was created electronically on a specially designed and calibrated television screen. The screen displayed a grating of fixed

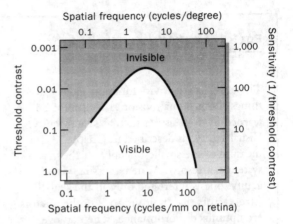

FIGURE 5.17 A contrast sensitivity function for an adult human. The upper horizontal axis is scaled in units specifying the number of pairs of light and dark bars of the grating falling within 1 degree of visual angle on the retina.

spatial frequency. Using a knob (like the contrast control on a television set), the contrast was adjusted until the grating was just visible. This threshold contrast was recorded by an experimenter. Typically, several estimates of the contrast threshold were measured for that spatial frequency and these estimates were averaged. This procedure was then repeated for other spatial frequencies, and the results were finally displayed as in Figure 5.17. This curve defines a window of visibility: the region below the curve represents combinations of contrast and spatial frequency that can be seen; the region above the curve represents combinations that cannot be seen. To clarify this idea, pick any point on the CSF curve. Because this point is the threshold contrast for seeing that pattern, decreasing the pattern's contrast (moving upward from the curve) renders the pattern invisible. Conversely, increasing the pattern's contrast (moving downward from the curve) makes the pattern more visible.

Note that in one respect the *shape* of the human CSF resembles the shape of the transfer function of a lens (Figure 5.16): each displays a high-frequency cutoff. However, in another respect the two are different. In particular, the CSF drops at low frequencies, whereas the lens's function does

Box 5.1 *Practical Uses of the CSF*

The contrast sensitivity function indicates things about human vision than cannot be learned from measures such as visual acuity. Visual acuity, as described in Chapter 3, is a measure of the smallest detail that the visual system can resolve. When assessing visual acuity, one is interested only in the spatial (size) factors that limit vision, so other factors are optimized. For instance, when an eye chart is printed with very light gray ink on a gray card stock—rather than with very black ink on a white card stock—the letters are harder to see (Regan, 1988). In this case, the letters' reduced contrast limits visual acuity, preventing one from assessing performance on the basis of size alone. When measuring

visual acuity, then, one tries to optimize contrast and illumination so that they do not limit performance.

When measuring visual acuity, one is interested in how size alone limits vision; when measuring the CSF, one is interested in how both contrast and size limit vision. In fact, two people can have exactly the same visual acuity but have different contrast sensitivities, as the following demonstrates. Arthur Ginsburg and his associates used the CSF to predict how well pilots would be able to see objects in the air and on the ground. At least under conditions of reduced visibility—twilight or fog, for example—visual acuity gives a poor account of a pilot's visually guided

not. The visual system, in other words, is less sensitive to very low spatial frequencies than it is to intermediate ones. As a result, there is a range of spatial frequencies, toward the center of the horizontal axis in Figure 5.17, where humans are maximally sensitive. Gratings are less visible if they lie on either side of this optimum spatial frequency; a person requires higher contrast in order to see them. The same line of reasoning can be applied to a visual scene or photograph of that scene. If the objects in a scene have most of their spatial frequency information around the optimum point on the CSF, those objects will be clearly visible even when they are of low contrast. If those objects contain only very low spatial frequencies (very large objects) or only very high spatial frequencies (very small objects or fine details), they will be less visible and their contrast will have to be high in order for those objects to be seen. This also explains why the gratings in Figure 5.15 *appear* different in contrast: their apparent contrast varies with your sensitivity to different spatial frequencies.

You know from experience that you are able to see better under some conditions than others. If the CSF and your ability to see are importantly related, conditions that change one should also change the other. In fact, this is precisely what happens. Let's consider one such condition.

As discussed in Chapter 3, resolution is poor under scotopic conditions. That is why it's hard to read in dim light. Since resolution involves seeing fine detail, we'd expect decreased light to affect particularly that portion of the CSF corresponding to fine detail. Indeed this happens, as the curves in Figure 5.18 illustrate. The upper curve shows a photopic (daytime) CSF; the middle curve shows a mesopic (twilight) CSF; the lowest curve represents a scotopic (nighttime) CSF. As the level of light decreases from daylight to twilight, visual sensitivity drops primarily at high spatial frequencies; lower frequencies are little affected. But when the light falls to extremely low levels (nighttime), sensitivity decreases even at low frequencies.

Think about what these curves imply for your

performance. In fact, very fine details that might normally be seen are invisible at twilight or in fog. Ginsburg found that under conditions of reduced visibility, the CSF of a pilot provided a very good account of his ability to see targets on the ground. He tested ten pilots in a sophisticated aircraft simulator that provided a panoramic (wraparound) view through the plane's widescreen. Pilots flew simulated missions and then "landed." On half their landings, an obstacle (another plane) blocked the runway, requiring them to abort the landing. Ginsburg determined how close each pilot came to the obstacle before aborting the landing. Even though all were experienced jet pilots, they varied in the distance at which they could spot the obstacle; the best pilots saw the obstacle 3 times farther away than did the worst. Significantly, the pilots

who saw the obstacle from the greatest distances were those who had the highest contrast sensitivities; pilots who had to get close to the obstacle before seeing it had the lowest contrast sensitivities. Finally, Ginsburg noted that acuity was unrelated to the performance of the pilots on this test (Ginsburg, Evans, Sekuler, and Harp, 1982).

This is just one example of the usefulness of the CSF in predicting visual performance in everyday settings. Other uses include predicting how well various visually impaired people can get around in their environments (Marron and Bailey, 1982), gauging the disabling effects of glare from various types of lighting sources (Carlsson, Knave, Lennerstrand, and Wibom, 1984), and enhancing printed materials for use by the visually impaired (Peli et al., 1991).

---

vision under changing conditions of illumination. Driving at night, you may be unable to see the fine details (high frequencies) of the shrubs alongside the road. At the same time, you probably will be able to see larger objects (low frequencies),

such as another car, just about as well as you do under daylight conditions. If you park your car in an unlit place and turn off your headlights, you will be operating under light conditions like those producing the scotopic curve. Under such conditions, even large objects will be difficult to see. Box 5.1 gives an example of a practical use of the CSF.

In summary, the CSF characterizes the ease with which people are able to detect objects of various sizes and perceive the structural detail, such as texture, of those objects. Conditions that alter the CSF, such as light level, change the visibility and appearance of objects. In a sense, these conditions thrust one into a different visual world. From this it follows that two creatures with different CSFs actually live in different visual worlds. The next two sections develop this intriguing possibility.

FIGURE 5.18 Contrast sensitivity functions measured at three light levels.

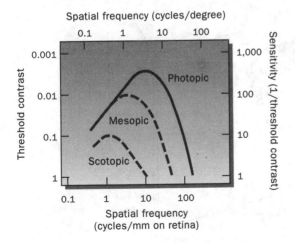

CSFs of Other Species. Cat owners sometimes notice that their pets seem to watch things their owners can't see, as if there were ghosts present.

Such inexplicable behavior enhances the cat's reputation for spookiness. While we don't deny that cats can be spooky, it may well be that under certain conditions they actually do see things that are real, though invisible to their owners (Blake, 1988a). We'll explain this and, in so doing, show how the CSF allows you to compare your vision with that of other animals.

Just as it does for humans, the CSF defines a window of visibility for other species. Provided they have sufficient contrast, objects producing retinal images composed of spatial frequencies falling within the range of a creature's CSF will be visible to that creature; objects producing images composed of frequencies outside that CSF will be invisible, regardless of their contrast. Thus by knowing an animal's CSF, one can predict what that animal will be able to see and what it won't be able to see. But how does one measure the CSF in a nonverbal animal such as the cat? The basic problem is to determine how little contrast a cat needs to distinguish a grating from a uniform

field of the same brightness. One setup for doing this is illustrated in Figure 5.19.

The cat faces two television screens, one displaying a grating, the second a uniformly bright field. The cat is rewarded with a morsel of food if it pushes against a small plastic switch located just in front of the television displaying the grating. The experimenter randomly presents the grating on the left or right television screen. When the contrast of the grating is above the cat's threshold, a hungry cat will respond correctly on virtually every trial. When the contrast falls below the cat's threshold, the animal will simply guess and will be correct only half the time. The cat's threshold, then, is defined as the contrast that allows it to respond correctly on 75 percent of the trials, a level of performance midway between chance and perfection. This threshold contrast can be measured for different spatial frequencies, and the cat's CSF can then be plotted in the same way as it is for humans. (This procedure, incidentally, constitutes a forced-choice threshold test and the

FIGURE 5.19 Apparatus for testing the cat's contrast sensitivity. (Drawing adapted by courtesy of Karin Boothroyd.)

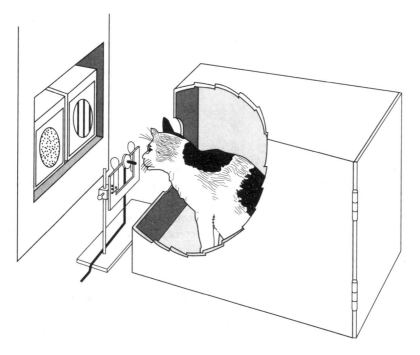

details of this method are covered in the Appendix.)

Figure 5.20 shows a typical CSF for a cat (solid line) and for a human (dashed line) tested under comparable conditions. Note first the area common to the two CSFs. This overlapping region defines combinations of spatial frequencies and contrasts that both you and a cat can see. Next, note the regions where the two CSFs do not overlap. Within these two regions one creature—you or the cat, depending on which one has the higher sensitivity—can see patterns that are invisible to the other. At high spatial frequencies, your sensitivity is better than the cat's; at low spatial frequencies, the reverse is true. Now suppose that a cat is sitting on your lap. If you are watching television there will be fine details in the picture that will be seen by you but not your cat (see Figure 5.21). This is because those fine details are composed of high spatial frequencies that fall outside the cat's window of visibility. But at the same time, if something large and very low-contrast appears in the room—say, an indistinct shadow on a wall—the cat may see it even though you cannot. In this instance, the shadow falls outside your window of visibility. These large, low-contrast objects could be the invisible "ghosts" that enhance the cat's reputation for spookiness.

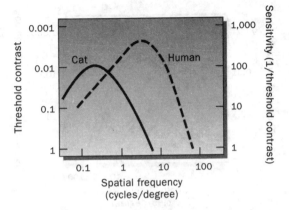

FIGURE 5.20 Contrast sensitivity functions for the cat and for the human being.

To date, CSFs have been measured for nearly a dozen species, and it's instructive to compare them. Figure 5.22 shows several representative curves. Look first at the curve labeled "Human"; this is the human adult CSF that you've seen in several previous figures. Next note the curve labeled "Rhesus monkey." Like several other nonhuman primates that have been studied, the rhesus monkey's CSF is highly similar to that of a human—suggesting that the world would probably appear very similar to you and to a monkey sitting

FIGURE 5.21 The two photographs are identical except that frequencies falling above the cat's high-frequency cutoff have been eliminated from the right-hand photograph. (Courtesy of Gregory Phillips.)

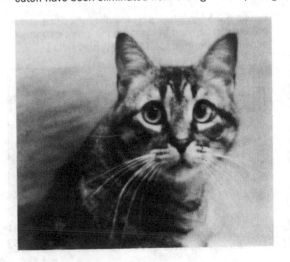
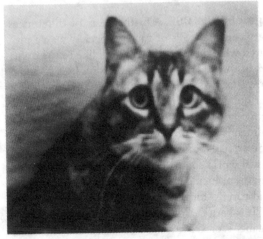

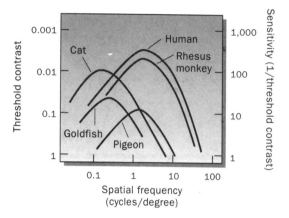

FIGURE 5.22 Contrast sensitivity functions for five species. (Adapted from Uhlrich, Essock, & Lehmkuhle, 1981.)

on your lap. It is certainly unlikely that you'd see things that the monkey could not, or vice versa. Next note that the goldfish's CSF is displaced toward lower spatial frequencies, a fact that makes sense considering where the goldfish lives. Its aquatic environment prevents high spatial frequencies from ever reaching the fish's eye (Uhlrich, Essock, and Lehmkuhle, 1981; Lythgoe, 1979). Like the cat, the goldfish is equipped for seeing either very large objects or smaller ones that are quite nearby. In general, there seems to be a good fit between what an animal uses its eyes for and where its CSF lies along the spatial frequency scale.

Age and the CSF. On the basis of differences between the CSFs of various species, we've pictured what the world might look like to the owners of these CSFs. In the same way, let's consider how the world might appear to individuals at various points in their lifetimes. To begin, suppose while you are reading this book, someone puts a human infant on your lap (where previously you've had a cat and a monkey). How does your visual world compare with that of the infant? This question, incidentally, has intrigued philosophers and parents for centuries.

It is hard to know what very young, preverbal infants see. Obviously, you can't use the same

methods to study infant vision that you use with cooperative, attentive adults. To get around this limitation, researchers have exploited a naturally occurring tendency exhibited by infants. It has been known for some time that an infant prefers to look at complex rather than dull scenes (Fantz, 1961). Several research groups have exploited preferential looking to measure the infant's ability to see gratings (Atkinson, Braddick, and Moar, 1977; Banks and Salapatek, 1978; Teller, 1979; Held, 1979).

Confronted with a patch of grating and a patch of uniform brightness, an infant will prefer to look at the grating (see Figure 5.23). If the infant shows no preference for the grating over the uniform field, it is inferred that the infant cannot see the grating. This could happen for one of two reasons: either the contrast of the grating is too low or the spatial frequency of the grating falls outside the range visible to the infant.

The basic findings are summarized in Figure 5.24, which shows CSFs for an infant somewhere between 3 to 6 months old and for a typical adult. Note that the infant's window of visibility is very different from the adult's. An infant held on your lap will not be able to see fine spatial details visible to you (see Figure 5.25). In this respect, the infant more closely resembles a cat. But unlike a cat, the infant does not have an advantage over you at low frequencies: you should be able to see everything

FIGURE 5.23 An infant's preference for looking at a pattern can be used to measure the infant's contrast sensitivity. (Drawing courtesy of Richard Held.)

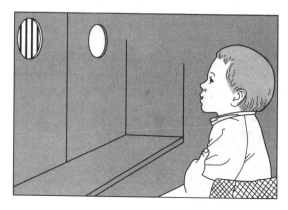

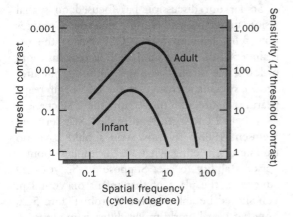

FIGURE 5.24 Contrast sensitivity functions for an infant and for an adult. (Infant data redrawn from Banks, 1982.)

that the infant can see. Also, even for spatial frequencies visible to both of you, the infant will require more contrast than you do. In a sense, these CSFs confirm what some parents have noticed: their very young infants seem oblivious to everything except very large, high-contrast objects (Banks, 1982). Incidentally, the lack of sensitivity to high frequencies does not stem from

optical causes but from the fact that the infant's immature visual nervous system fails to encode high frequencies. In effect, infants are best suited for seeing objects located close to them (recall that spatial frequency is distance-dependent), which makes sense from a behavioral standpoint.

The infant's CSF improves gradually over the first year or so of its life. The improvement may be arrested, though, at an immature level if the infant does not receive normal visual experiences (Jacobsen, Mohindra, and Held, 1983). There are several visual disorders that can alter the quality of visual experiences received by an infant and hence keep spatial vision from its normal course of development. First of all, any condition that chronically blurs the images reaching the infant's retina will limit the information available to the visual system. Optical blur of this sort can result from myopia or hyperopia and from congenital cataracts or corneal scars (see Chapter 2). Misalignment of an infant's two eyes can also retard the development of good spatial vision. When its eyes are not properly aligned, an infant must suppress or ignore visual input from one eye in order to avoid seeing double. For reasons unknown, continuous suppression of one eye can lead to a

FIGURE 5.25 An infant looking at these two pictures from a distance of 2 meters (about 6 feet) would be unable to tell them apart. The two photographs are identical except that frequencies falling above the infant's high-frequency cutoff have been eliminated from the right-hand photograph (1984 Muppets, Inc., courtesy of Children's Television Workshop; computer-processed pictures by Gregory Phillips.)

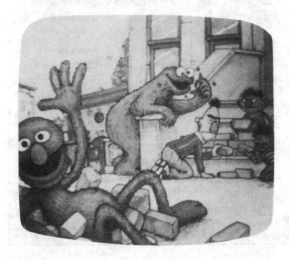
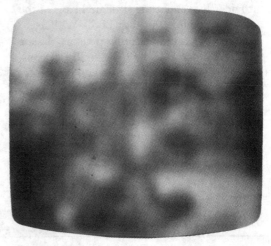

loss in spatial vision, a condition called *amblyopia* (recall Box 4.3).

Fortunately, infants afflicted with any of these disorders can recover normal spatial vision, providing that the disorder is corrected sometime during the first few years of life (von Noorden, 1981). But if correction is postponed until the child reaches school age, the prognosis for full recovery is much poorer. Apparently there is a critical period early in life when the visual nervous system requires normal input to mature properly. During this period, neural connections are still being formed (Hickey, 1977). This critical period of neural development ends by the time a child reaches 3 or 4 years of age. If the visual nervous system arrives at this stage not completely developed because of inadequate visual experience, any neural abnormalities are irrevocably preserved throughout the remainder of life. In view of this critical role of early visual experience, you can appreciate the importance of detecting and correcting visual disorders in infants as early as possible. One important reason for studying infant vision is to develop and refine techniques allowing early diagnosis of such disorders.

So far our discussion has focused on spatial vision in infants and young children. Consider now what happens to the CSF during the remainder of the life span. The CSF remains more or less stable through young adulthood; but after age 30, systematic changes in the CSF begin reappearing. Figure 5.26 shows how the CSF changes from age 20 to age 80 (Owsley, Sekuler, and Siemsen, 1983). By now you should have no trouble interpreting what a CSF implies about a person's ability to see. Suppose an 80-year-old aunt takes the place of that infant on your lap; you should be able to predict from Figure 5.26 how her visual world might differ from yours.

Very likely, much of the loss in your aunt's sensitivity to high frequencies results from optical changes in her eyes. For example, as she has grown older, her pupil has become smaller, which means that her retina now receives considerably less light than it did earlier in life (Weale, 1982). This reduced illumination of her retina mimics changes that would be seen in a young adult's CSF as testing conditions changed from photopic to mesopic (see Figure 5.18). But whatever its origins, the variation in the CSF from birth to old

---

Box 5.2 *When Things Go Wrong with Pattern Vision*

The way in which diseases affect vision can provide clues about the structural basis of the CSF. The neurologist Ivan Bodis-Wollner has noted that in some of his patients, disease produces a notch in the CSF—a loss of contrast sensitivity limited to a certain range of target sizes. Moreover, the location and severity of loss of sensitivity varies from one patient to the next (Bodis-Wollner, 1972).

The loss in sensitivity was produced by damage to the visual cortex from a stroke. Other diseases can produce similar losses. The most common of these diseases is *multiple sclerosis*, a disease that attacks the insulation on nerve fibers, including fibers that make up

the optic nerve. Even though their visual acuity is good, some multiple sclerosis patients complain that the world appears "washed out." Presumably, this washed-out appearance is related to the nervous system's diminished capacity to code contrast.

In addition, about 30 percent of all people who have multiple sclerosis experience *Uhthoff's symptom,* a condition first described by Wilhelm Uhthoff, an eminent turn-of-the-century ophthalmologist. For individuals with Uhthoff's symptom, exercise or emotional strain heightens their visual problems for several minutes. No one yet understands how emotional or physical strain or exercise causes

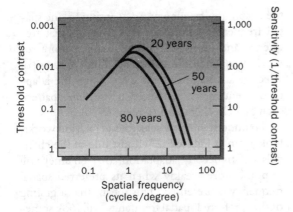

FIGURE 5.26 Contrast sensitivity functions for three age groups.

This range of "preferred" frequencies varies from one set of neurons to another. According to this hypothesis, the sensitivities of these frequency-tuned neurons, or channels, together determine the overall CSF (see Figure 5.27). Some of Campbell and Robson's own experiments (1968) support this view. But there is other evidence as well.

One reason for believing that the CSF depends on several different channels is the fact that certain conditions can alter one portion of the CSF without affecting others. As Box 5.2 explains, diseases attacking the visual system can produce this frequency-selective change in the CSF—implying that only certain neurons are affected by the disease. But we need not wait for disease to change the CSF; we can change it intentionally, using a technique called **selective adaptation.** This procedure, mentioned in Chapter 4, produces a temporary loss of sensitivity to particular spatial frequencies.

Selective adaptation involves several stages. First you assess the person's CSF; then you have the person view a high-contrast grating for a minute or so, thereby adapting to one spatial frequency. As you might imagine, steady viewing of

age means that people experience very different visual worlds at different stages of their lives.

The Structural Basis of the CSF. Campbell and Robson, whose work we described earlier, proposed that the human visual system contains sets of neurons, each capable of responding to targets over only a narrow range of spatial frequencies.

these effects. But these conditions offer a unique opportunity to study the visual system under conditions of transient impairment. In one study (Sekuler, Owsley, and Berenberg, 1986) a 30-year-old accountant with Uhthoff's symptom reported that when he was emotionally upset his vision grew hazy and objects lost much of their apparent contrast. For example, during a confrontation at work, his boss's face appeared totally washed out and featureless. Surprisingly, during these episodes the patient retained his ability to read columns of small numbers, an important part of his job. Thus he seemed to suffer a size-selective loss, retaining the ability to see fine details while losing the ability to see larger objects.

This strange set of symptoms was con-

firmed by comparing the patient's contrast sensitivity before and immediately after he exercised. Contrast sensitivity for high spatial frequencies was unchanged by exercise, but sensitivity for intermediate frequencies dropped. Longer periods of exercise produced an even greater loss of vision: not only was contrast sensitivity drastically reduced at all frequencies, but visual acuity was seriously impaired as well.

We do not yet understand the specific physiological basis for these restricted losses in the CSF. But such losses do imply that the CSF—and the ability to see patterns of different sizes—depends on the coordinated responses of different sets of visual cells, any one of which may be attacked and damaged by disease.

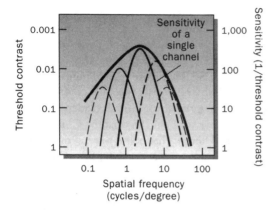

FIGURE 5.27 The overall contrast sensitivity function is determined by the individual sensitivities of neurons responsive to limited ranges of spatial frequency.

this adaptation grating fatigues those visual neurons that respond to its frequency (Movshon and Lennie, 1979; Albrecht, Farrar, and Hamilton, 1984). After the person has adapted to this grating for a minute or two, you redetermine his or her CSF (interspersing threshold measurements with additional adaptation to keep the level of adaptation high). The typical outcome of such experiments (for example, Blakemore and Campbell, 1969) is shown in Figure 5.28. In each panel, the arrow on the horizontal axis indicates the frequency to which the person adapted. Note that the notch carved in each CSF is centered about

the adaptation frequency. So adapting to one spatial frequency diminishes sensitivity to that frequency and neighboring ones, leaving more remote frequencies unaffected. This process of selective adaptation works even when the adaptation frequency is contained in a complex pattern such as a checkerboard (Green, 1980).

To understand how selective adaptation works, look again at Figure 5.27. If just one of the channels is fatigued by adaptation, that channel will respond more weakly when its preferred spatial frequency is presented. This means that a grating of that preferred spatial frequency will look somewhat washed out compared with its normal appearance (Blakemore, Muncey, and Ridley, 1973). A low-contrast grating that is normally visible will stimulate the adapted channel so weakly that the grating will be below threshold. In order to attain visibility, this grating's contrast will have to be boosted—resulting in a dip in the CSF. The width of this dip depends on the selectivity of the fatigued channel. Presumably, unaffected regions of the CSF depend on channels that were not fatigued by the adaptation grating.

You can demonstrate selective adaptation for yourself. Figure 5.29 shows several different low-contrast test gratings and one high-contrast adaptation grating. Before looking at the adaptation grating (in the center of the figure), note the apparent contrast of the test gratings surrounding it.

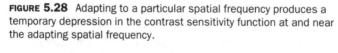

FIGURE 5.28 Adapting to a particular spatial frequency produces a temporary depression in the contrast sensitivity function at and near the adapting spatial frequency.

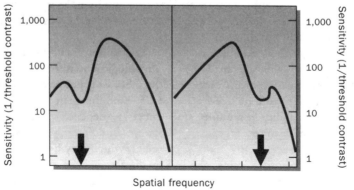

Spatial frequency

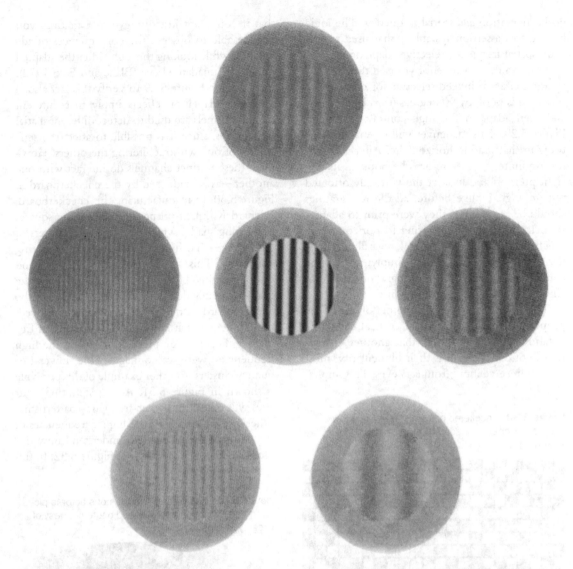

FIGURE 5.29 By following the instructions in the text, you can experience the consequences of selective adaptation.

Now inspect the high-contrast grating for about a minute; don't stare fixedly, but allow your eyes to roam around the circle in the grating's center. Then, without delay, look at one test grating and note its apparent contrast. After looking back at the adaptation grating for another minute, note the apparent contrast of another test grating. By adapting and then examining each test grating in turn, you'll find adapting alters the appearance of only some test gratings. Now you've seen for yourself that spatial frequency adaptation is selective.

Selective adaptation probably occurs in visual cortical cells (Albrecht, Farrar, and Hamilton, 1984). Such cells are indeed selective for spatial frequency (size); but as Chapter 4 showed, they are also selective for orientation. As a result, you might expect grating adaptation to be selective for both orientation *and* spatial frequency. The logic behind this assertion resembles that used to explain spatial frequency selective adaptation.

You can demonstrate for yourself that this adaptation effect is indeed selective for orientation. Rotate this book by 90 degrees (turn it sideways) and then adapt to the high-contrast grating in Figure 5.29. This maneuver will orient the contours in that grating horizontally. After adapting for a minute, quickly return the book to its upright position and look at the vertically oriented test gratings. Unlike before, *all* the test gratings should be as visible as they were prior to adaptation. In other words, adapting to horizontal has no effect whatsoever on vertical, regardless of similarities in spatial frequency—implying that the cells fatigued by the horizontal grating are not at all involved in seeing vertical contours.

This demonstration is a reminder of one of the properties exhibited by visual cortical cells: orientation selectivity. Recall that another characteristic of cortical cells is their binocularity: most of them receive input from *both* eyes. This implies

that if you adapt just one eye to a grating, you will be able to observe the consequences of adaptation while looking through either the adapted eye or the unadapted eye (Blake and Fox, 1972). You can use Figure 5.29 to verify this fact also.

These adaptation effects imply that different neural channels are used to detect different spatial frequencies, since it is possible to affect the sensitivity of one without altering the others. However, these distinct channels do interact with one another—as is evidenced by the checkerboard in Figure 5.30. In manufacturing this checkerboard, Richard Kirkham purposely made some squares the wrong shade, which creates some clusters of dark squares. To find these clusters, try squinting your eyes. This should make the clusters stand out. Squinting blurs your vision, reducing the high-frequency details in the retinal image of the checkerboard. Once those details are removed, the clusters, which constitute a lower spatial frequency, become conspicuous. In effect, the high frequencies were camouflaging the lower-frequency clusters. Another example of this principle is shown in Figure 5.31. Again, squinting your eyes will reveal the lower-frequency pattern that otherwise is masked by the higher frequencies of the edges of the blocks. To understand how this block portrait was created, see Figure 5.32. In this

FIGURE 5.30 Checkered pattern containing a few squares incorrectly shaded. (Courtesy of Richard Kirkham.)

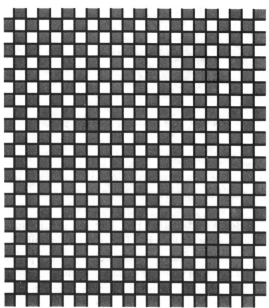

FIGURE 5.31 Can you tell what famous actor is pictured here? (Computer-processed photo courtesy of Gregory Phillips.)

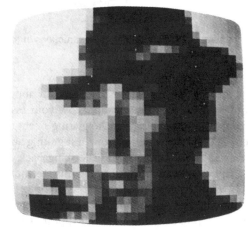

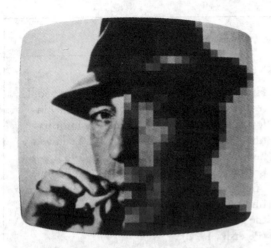

FIGURE 5.32 The picture in the previous figure was constructed by setting the light level of each block so that it was the average intensity of the region covered by the block. Squinting (thus blurring the high frequencies) should make the detail in the two photographs equivalent. (Computer-processed photo courtesy of Gregory Phillips.)

instance, strong high-frequency information camouflages and weakens low-frequency information. But when all frequencies are more nearly equal in strength, they can interact more cooperatively (see Box 5.3, pp. 172–173).

In summary, recent studies of detection and pattern visibility converge on a common view of the human visual system. In this view, detection of any spatial target depends on responses generated in a set of visual cells tuned to contours of a particular size and orientation. Each set of cells is responsible for the ability to see targets over some range of sizes and orientations. In the next section, we'll see how this view provides an explanation of other aspects of form perception as well.

FORM DISCRIMINATION

So far we've described how the CSF defines a window of visibility within which objects can be seen. Our emphasis was on form detection, as determined by an observer's sensitivity to contrast and spatial frequency. Now we are ready to extend our analysis of spatial vision to form discrim-

ination, the ability to tell one object from another. Before getting into details, though, it will be useful to specify what must go on within the visual system to make discrimination possible.

The perception of pattern, or spatial structure, depends on the responses of cells in the visual system. This dependence sets some limits on what stimuli will appear different and what stimuli will look alike. All stimuli that produce *identical* effects within the visual system will be indistinguishable from one another. But if stimuli produce different effects, potentially you have the information for telling them apart. Whether you actually can tell them apart depends on how different the neural responses are (Brindley, 1970, pp. 132–134). In Chapter 4 you learned that the response of any one cell—say, a "simple" cell in the visual cortex—provides ambiguous messages about the characteristics of stimuli in the visual world. As a result, the visual appearance of objects probably depends on the pattern of activity within an *ensemble* of cells, not just one cell alone.

Metamers. If you look at two exact duplicates of the same object, each will produce precisely the same effects on your visual system and they will look identical. But two objects that are physically different can also have identical neural effects and, therefore, appear identical. In other words, things need not *be* identical to *look* identical. Two objects that are perceptually indistinguishable from one another, despite their physical differences, are called **metamers.**

We can learn much about human vision by determining which stimuli are metamers and which are not. Metamers exist because of a "blindness" to certain stimulus characteristics—characteristics that the visual nervous system fails to register. If the human visual system generates identical responses to two objects, the objects will appear identical, even if they are physically different. This might happen when two objects are identical except for one physical attribute too small or too dim to be detected.

But the fact that two stimuli are metameric for *your* visual system does not mean that they will be metameric for all visual systems. In Figure 5.21,

Box 5.3 *Not Seeing the Forest for the Trees*

In this chapter we have been developing the idea that certain mechanisms process information about fine spatial detail while others process information about coarser structure. Let's think what this idea means in terms of an everyday situation where form information is simultaneously present at several different scales (recall Figure 5.8). If you were standing near a forest, one set of visual mechanisms would be responsible for allowing you to see the overall forest while another set would be responsible for your seeing individual trees. How might this neural specialization of function be helpful? According to one view (Broadbent, 1977), after the low-frequency mechanisms have defined the global structure of some object, it becomes easier to make sense of the detailed information provided by the high-frequency mechanisms. In the example at hand, once you see that you're standing in front of a forest, it's easier to see its individual components.

This view is attractive for several reasons.

First, it is consistent with the idea that people respond more quickly to low-frequency information than to high-frequency information (Breitmeyer, 1975; Calis and Leeuwenberg, 1981; Navon and Norman, 1983). Second, when stimuli are presented very briefly, only their low-frequency components find their way into perceptual experience—the stimuli appear like "blobs" or "blotches" (Petersik, 1978).

Normally, then, perception depends on cooperative interaction between the processing of global (low-frequency) and local (high-frequency) information. To study these interactions requires stimuli that contain both kinds of information. Kinchla and Wolfe (1979) used stimuli in which the relation between high and low spatial frequencies could be easily varied. Their stimuli, devised by Navon (1977), were large letters made up of small letters; the small letters were always different from the large letter that they defined. An example is shown in the accompanying

the two photographs are identical except for the presence of high spatial frequency information in the left-hand photograph. You are probably able to tell the two photos apart because from this reading distance, these high spatial frequencies are visible to you—in other words, the two photographs are not metameric for you. However, if a cat were to view this same pair of photographs from your viewing distance, the high frequencies in the left-hand photograph would be outside its window of visibility. Thus the two photographs would be indistinguishable to a cat, meaning the pair would be metamers for the cat.

Moreover, two stimuli that are not metameric for you under one condition (say, intense light or close viewing) might become metameric under

another condition (say, dim light or distant viewing). For example, if you move away from Figure 5.21, the high frequencies in the left-hand photograph will fall beyond the limits of your acuity, rendering the two photographs metameric.

But it's not only light level or distance that determines whether two stimuli are metameric; any condition that alters the response of the nervous system influences whether stimuli are metameric. One good example derives from the work of Campbell and Robson, discussed earlier. We've already seen that the appearance of a compound grating depends on the responses it evokes in visual channels tuned to different spatial frequencies. If these responses could be temporarily altered, the appearance of the grating should

figure, where the global structure creates the letter "H" (large letter) while the local structure consists of the letter "E" (small letters).

On each trial, the observer first heard the name of a letter; then, several seconds later, one of the stimuli was briefly presented. The observer had to judge whether the stimulus contained the letter whose name had been spoken. If *either* the global or the local structure matched that spoken name, the observer was to respond yes; otherwise, no. Kinchla and Wolfe compared how long people took

to respond yes when the spoken letter matched the *global* structure and how long people took to say yes when the spoken letter matched the *local* structure. They made these comparisons for stimuli of various overall size.

When the overall stimulus was very large (about the size of the retinal image cast by this book seen at arm's length), observers were quicker at detecting a match between the spoken letter and the local structure. However, when the overall stimulus was 5 times smaller, observers were quicker at detecting a match between the spoken letter and the global structure. To Kinchla and Wolfe, this result demonstrates that neither the lowest spatial frequencies nor the highest spatial frequencies enjoy guaranteed priority in processing. Instead, the tendency is initially to process information represented by some intermediate band of frequencies.

Returning to the example at hand, we could say that when you're standing close to a very large forest, it's easier to see the trees than the entire forest, but when the forest is small, it's easier to see the forest than the trees.

change. As Box 5.4 (pp. 174–176) demonstrates, this is exactly what happens.

Perceived Similarity. Even when objects do not appear to be identical, they may still resemble one another to varying degrees. For instance, you may be able to judge whether the baby in the carriage looks more like its mother or its father. But how do you make these judgments? You might compare the baby's features with those of its mother and father and decide which parent looks more like the baby on the basis of which parent shares the greater number of features with the baby.

This description of how resemblance might be judged has much commonsense appeal. It relates such judgments to a checklist of features. For ex-

ample, if two people share many features, they are said to look alike (such as identical twins). Presumably, the more features in common, the greater the similarity. But do people really judge the similarity of complex forms in this way? To answer, consider one class of complex forms that you are constantly judging, letters of the English alphabet. Reading would be very difficult indeed if all letters of the alphabet looked very much alike. And in fact, sone letters do bear a strong resemblance to one another. Did you notice the substitution of one such letter for another in the preceding sentence? Since correctly recognizing letters is so important in daily life, it would be particularly interesting to know how this recognition succeeds and when it fails. To understand

Box 5.4 *The Size Aftereffect*

One popular theory explains perceived size in terms of the responses in channels tuned to different spatial frequencies (Blakemore, Nachmias, and Sutton, 1970). This theory is depicted in the illustration below. In the two upper panels, the horizontal axes represent spatial frequency and the vertical axes represent sensitivity. To make the argument easier to follow, we show only three channels. As the upper left panel indicates, channel A prefers the lowest frequency of the three, B pre-

fers an intermediate frequency, and C prefers the highest frequency.

Suppose we present a test grating whose frequency falls halfway between the preferred frequencies of A and B. (This condition is not crucial for the argument; it merely simplifies the description.) Note that the test grating produces equal responses within channels A and B (bottom left panel). According to the theory, this neural code—equal activity in A and B—determines the

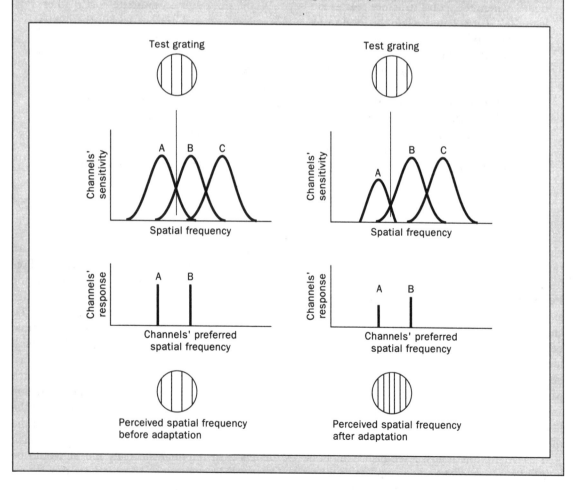

way the grating looks. But if we did something to change the distribution of activity produced by that same grating, the grating's appearance would be altered. This idea was tested using an adaptation procedure much like that described in the text. First, a person looked at a grating and judged its spatial frequency. We'll refer to this as the test grating. Next, the person adapted to a high-contrast grating whose spatial frequency was lower than that of the test grating. We'll call this the adaptation grating. Finally, after 1 minute of adaptation, the person looked back at the test grating and again judged its spatial frequency. Did the test grating still look the same? To answer this question, let's consider how adaptation would have affected the neural code described before.

Suppose that prior to adaptation, the test grating produced equal responses in channels A and B. Suppose also that the adaptation grating is one to which A is highly sensitive and to which B is relatively less sensitive. Prolonged adaptation will thus fatigue A considerably but B very little (upper right panel). When presented again, the test grating will evoke a nearly normal response from B but a weakened response from A (lower right panel). This pattern of responses—a greater response in B than in A—is not usually produced by the test grating. Instead, this pattern of responses is usually evoked by a spatial frequency *higher* than that of the test grating. As a result, after adaptation, the spatial frequency of the test grating should *appear* higher than usual. This was the effect that Blakemore, Nachmias, and Sutton (1970) found. On the basis of the theory, can you predict what will happen if the person has adapted to a spatial frequency *higher* than that of the test grating?

You can experience this so-called **size aftereffect** for yourself. To prove that this aftereffect is not peculiar to gratings, we've borrowed from Stuart Anstis a demonstration using more familiar patterns. Still, the outcome is the same—a temporary change in apparent size. So that the effect is easier to see, this demonstration simultaneously produces two size aftereffects in opposite directions. Here's how to use the figure below. Look at the small black dot between the upper and lower panels of the left side of the figure. With your eyes fixed on the black dot, verify that the letters in the text above look the same size as the letters below.

We'll now explain what you must do to alter the apparent size of these letters. Because timing is important, finish reading the instructions before you execute them. First adapt, using the right side of the figure. The patch of small, tightly packed letters corresponds to high spatial frequencies, while the

(continued)

mountains to the perate business of ssenia. It was not ansion but land-gr l brought its neme ne a garrison in the omitted to the rigid gus," their legenda ame the most form

ry camp, artistically and in ren. The part Spartans pla airs became, oftener than those who were internation nded to be treacherous, stup home, the ownership of l e qualification for being a concentrated in fewer t so that from the fourth c s the effective population ations supervened, and Spa the miserable inheritor

mountains to the perate business of ssenia. It was not ansion but land-gr l brought its neme ne a garrison in the omitted to the rigid gus," their legenda ame the most form

which was the citizen, was fewer hands, tury onwards clined, revolu became only treat name ar

patch of larger, more spread out letters corresponds to low spatial frequencies. To adapt, slowly move your eyes back and forth along the bar between the two patches of letters. Keep this up for about 90 seconds. *Caution:* Do not look directly at either patch; keep your gaze on the horizontal bar between the two. Otherwise, you'll intermix the two types of adaptation. Finally, at the end of adaptation, look back at the dot between the patches in the left side of the figure. Keeping your eyes on the dot, note the sizes of the letters above and below. You will see that letters in the upper patch look smaller than those in the lower patch. Here, then, is a situation where stimuli that were initially metamers are rendered temporarily nonmetameric by altering your visual nervous system.

the process of recognition, let's consider two different accounts.

One account, the *feature* theory, uses a checklist approach—it claims that letters are represented in the nervous system as a set of features, lines, and contours of various orientations (Gibson, 1965). The other account uses a spatial frequency approach derived from the work of Campbell and Robson. Lewis Harvey and his associates at the University of Colorado Jonathon Roberts and Martin Gervais (1983) compared how well these two approaches explain the discrimination of one letter from another. Harvey and his colleagues were interested in the number of times that people confuse one letter with another. The perceptual similarity of letters was defined by their tendency to be confused. The basic idea is that if two letters look a lot alike, they will often be confused with one another. A good theory of perceptual similarity should, therefore, predict which pairs of letters re confused and which are not.

In the features approach, it is necessary first to compile a checklist of features—that is, to decide *what* features should make up the list. In other words, how might the nervous system represent a letter of the alphabet? One such set of features is listed in the left-hand column of Figure 5.33. For each letter, the number of horizontal, vertical, and oblique lines, as well as the number of curves, can be counted. These and other features formed the checklist that Harvey worked with, and each letter was evaluated against the list. The feature theory makes a very clear prediction: if two letters have many features in common, they will tend to be confused; letters that have few features in common will not be. The alternative approach hypothesizes that the spatial frequencies of various letters account for confusions. (It should be noted that two letters can have similar spatial frequencies but differ widely in features.)

To test the two approaches, Harvey briefly flashed randomly chosen letters and asked people to name them. The flash was so short that people could correctly name the letter only half the time. When he tallied the confusions, Harvey found that some letters having several features in common, such as "K" and "N," were not confused with one another—which contradicts the feature theory. Instead, the letters that were confused tended to be those with similar spatial frequencies—which suggests that letters may be represented in the visual system in terms of their frequency content.

However, you should not conclude from Harvey's work that spatial frequency is the *only* way to describe the basis for perceived similarity. Suppose that one aspect of a complex stimulus is so striking or conspicuous that it dominates your perception of the object. In this case, you might judge the resemblance between that and other objects solely or primarily on the basis of that feature (Harmon, 1973). Not only do alternative ways exist for utilizing pattern information, but quite likely the alternatives available increase as people mature. When recognizing people's faces, young children base their judgments on isolated

	A	B	C	D	E	F	G	H	I	J	K	L	M	N	O	P	Q	R	S	T	U	V	W	X	Y	Z
EXTERNAL																										
1. Horizontal					2	1				1								1								2
2. Vertical		1		1	1	1		2	1	1	1	1		2		1		1		1	2					
3. Slant (/)	1										2										1	1		1		
4. Slant (\)	1																				1	1		1		
5. Convex segment		2	3	2			3		1						4	1	4	1	2		1					
OPEN																										
6. Horizontal			1			1										2										
7. Vertical								1								1										
8. Wedged, horizontal		1								1				1		1								2	1	2
9. Wedged, vertical									2			1		2		1		1				1	1	2	1	
10. Internal protrusion										1											1					
11. Intersection, internal	2	1			1	1		2		1						1		1								
12. Bar-horizontal	1				1	1	1	1																		
13. Bar-slant, crossing																	1									
14. Symmetry, vertical	1							1	1				1		1					1	1	1	1	1		
15. Symmetry, horizontal		1	1	1	1			1	1		1				1									1		

FIGURE 5.33 A list of the features distinguishing letters of the alphabet. (Adapted from Geyer & DeWald, 1973.)

characteristics, such as bushy eyebrows or a large mouth; adults can base their judgments either on isolated characteristics *or* on the face's overall configuration, without reference to particular features (Carey and Diamond, 1977). As a result, children are more likely than adults to be thrown off by a change in hairdo or by a new hat.

LIMITATIONS OF THE MULTICHANNEL MODEL

The multichannel model provides a good account of the early stages of visual processing of form information, and it explains several phenomena associated with visual form. However, it by no means represents a complete theory, for there are aspects of form perception that remain unexplained. Let's take an example. When you look at an object from different perspectives, the dimensions of the retinal image of that object dif-fer—for instance, a coin casts a circular image when viewed head-on but an ellipsoidal image when viewed at an angle. Now, changes in image dimensions are going to alter the spatial frequency content of the retinal images associated with viewing that object from different perspectives. Yet, you tend to perceive the true, unchanging shape of the object. This constancy of perception in the face of an altered retinal image is called **shape constancy,** and its occurrence implies that form perception transcends spatial frequency information contained in the retinal image (Hochberg, 1971). In Chapter 13, we'll describe one recent attempt to understand shape constancy, particularly the constancy of three-dimensional objects.

Other phenomena also seem to lie beyond the grasp of the multichannel model. Some of these involve an interplay between your knowledge about the world and what your eyes tell you. A simple example of this interaction between cognition and vision was given in Figure 4.21 (page 137). Recall that at first the illustration appeared merely as a random collection of light and dark regions. However, when informed that a Dalmatian was pictured in the illustration, you were able to see the dog. Suddenly, the figure's randomness was abolished. Because they are so familiar, naturalistic scenes are particularly effective in influencing the perceived form of objects. Chapter 13 takes up these and other phenomena in which both cognition and vision are partners.

Some prior knowledge of the world is indispensable for making good use of sensory information. The more you *know* about some object ahead of time, the less your senses must tell you. This principle is illustrated by work on **computer vision** (Rosenfeld, 1988). Equipped with television cameras, computers can "see" their surroundings. Such computers act as models for human vision and help test speculations about human sight. A key question in this research concerns how much prior information the computer must be given before it can interpret what it is seeing. The television camera gives the computer a two-dimensional record of the intensities of light at various points in the scene. But with no information about the world from which the scene came, the computer would not "know"

even that contiguous areas of similar intensity tend to belong together. As a result, the computer could not even distinguish objects from their background, let alone develop detailed representations of the objects. Unable to segment the video information correctly (Marr, 1982; Poggio, 1984), the computer would be like you were before you learned that there was a Dalmatian in Figure 4.21.

These are just some aspects of form perception that defy explanation by the multichannel model. It's not surprising that the model is unable to explain everything. After all, the model is based on information about only one stage in the visual system, the visual cortex. And as Chapter 4 pointed out, the primary visual cortex is not the only place in the brain where visual information is processed. Trying to explain all pattern perception with concepts relating to just the visual cortex is like trying to comprehend a novel by reading only a small part of it. If you pick the right part, of course, you can learn a lot, but certainly not everything. The contributions of other neural centers and the interactions among centers are now being actively studied. Perhaps as those centers are explored and their interactions better understood, satisfactory explanations will develop for currently inexplicable phenomena.

S U M M A R Y   A N D   P R E V I E W

This chapter emphasized that visual information is used to distinguish objects from their backgrounds and to discriminate objects from one another. After presenting two traditional views of form perception, structuralism and Gestalt psychology, we described the multichannel model derived from measurements of the CSF. This model is an attempt to relate human form perception to what is known about the visual cortex. The model can account for many aspects of human and animal vision, including detection, discrimination, and certain visual illusions, but it, too, has its limitations.

As a prelude to the next three chapters, it's worth noting that the visual system uses basically the same scheme to represent many different kinds of visual information. As we've seen, pattern information is analyzed into various components and is then represented as a distribution of activity across a set of channels. As outlined in the next chapter, this same type of arrangement is used to represent information about color.

KEY TERMS

analytic introspection
closure
computer vision
contrast
contrast sensitivity function (CSF)
contrast threshold
cutoff frequency
detection
discrimination
figure/ground organization

Fourier analysis
Gestalt principles of organization
good continuation
gratings
identification
isomorphism
metamers
multichannel model
orientation
primitives

proximity
scale
selective adaptation
shape constancy
similarity
sinusoidal grating
size aftereffect
spatial frequency
spatial phase
transfer function
window of visibility

Color Perception

S taying up all night studying for an examination is not much fun. There is one small consolation, though—a chance to see the beauty of sunrise. As you stare at the horizon through half-shut eyes, you realize that all through the dark night the world outdoors has been a drab, colorless collection of blacks, whites, and various grays. Then just before the sun itself becomes visible, you see a marvelous transformation. A world that had been colorless now springs to life as objects don their daytime colors. When the world puts on its colors, you realize how bland it would appear without them.

But color gives you more than unending wonder and beauty; in fact, it influences many facets of your life. For example, color can alter the "taste" of the food and drink you consume (Duncker, 1939). You can prove this to yourself by using food coloring to create red milk or green orange juice. In addition, some people believe that the world's colors ebb and flow with mood—that envy can make you "green," infuriation makes you "see red," and all too many circumstances make you "blue." These are merely figures of speech, but some people believe that the connection between emotions and color is more than just figurative (Sharpe, 1974). Although the evidence is unclear, some people do try to exploit the behavioral effects attributed to particular colors (Birren, 1978; Kunishima and Yanase, 1985). For example, some tavern owners cover their walls with colors that they expect will stimulate greater consumption of alcoholic beverages. Also, certain shades of pink are reputed to calm

prisoners in jail and quiet the irate fans of hapless football teams. It has been said that Knute Rockne, the legendary Notre Dame football coach, has his team's locker room painted red to excite his players and the opposing team's locker room painted blue to induce calm and relaxation.

People are selective not only about the colors of their walls, but about the colors they wear. In fact, it's been claimed that you can tell a lot about people—perhaps even about an entire nation—just from the colors of their clothing. One person who made such a claim was Johann Wolfgang von Goethe, the German poet-philosopher of the nineteenth century. Goethe wrote:

Lively nations, the French for instance, love intense colours . . . ; sedate nations, like the English and Germans, wear straw-coloured or leather-coloured yellow accompanied with dark blue. Nations aiming at dignity of appearance, the Spaniards and Italians, for instance, suffer the red colour of their mantles to incline to the passive side. (1840/1970, p. 328)

But all these effects, whether real or fanciful, are simply by-products of color's real purpose, to which we turn now.

WHY IS IT IMPORTANT TO SEE COLORS?

The ability to see color makes detection and discrimination possible for us. In fact, this is undoubtedly why color vision has evolved. Color makes it easier to pick out an object from its background **(detection).** Manufacturers of sporting equipment exploit this fact by producing yellow tennis balls that are easier to see on the court and orange golf balls that are hard to lose on the fairway. Nature also exploits the conspicuity color affords. Many animals call attention to themselves by means of color, especially for purposes of mating. Plants, too, announce their availability for pollination with color. At the same time, however, nature uses color to make some creatures and plants inconspicuous (Owen, 1980). For example, the color of a praying mantis blends in so well with that of the leaves it frequents that unless the insect moves, it is invisible. Similarly, the arctic fox's white pelt provides excellent camouflage when it hunts on snow-packed land, thus giving the fox a considerable advantage over its prey.

Besides affecting your ability to see objects against a background, color helps you distinguish among various objects in the environment **(discrimination).** One shade of red tells you instantly that a vehicle is a fire truck; another tells you that an apple or tomato is ripe and ready to eat (Gibson, 1966, p. 183). One shade of yellow tells you that a vehicle is a taxi rather than a police car; another shade of yellow ensures that Kodak's photographic products will be recognized everywhere in the world merely from the color of the box. Farmers use color to identify rich soil and to tell when their crops are ready for harvest. Doctors routinely rely on color to make diagnoses: blood that is pale red indicates anemia, and a yellowish skin pallor suggests a liver disorder (Birren, 1941, p. 191). Government meat inspectors pay attention to the color of animal tissue when judging its fitness for human consumption (Collins and Worthey, 1984).

Our general point, then, is that although color does have emotional and aesthetic impact, the main purpose of color perception—as with the perception of form, motion, and depth—is to help creatures detect and discriminate objects. To explain how color serves these goals, this chapter describes the important characteristics of color perception. The chapter also explains how human color experiences depend on two factors: the light reflected from objects and the properties of the eyes and nervous system.

WHAT ARE THE UNITS OF COLOR PERCEPTION?

A MULTITUDE OF COLOR NAMES

The preceding chapter started out by asking about the *units* of form perception. We'll begin our discussion of color perception the same way. Most people tie their experiences of color to the names used to describe those colors. So we might expect to get some idea of the units of color perception by asking this simple question: How many color names are there? Some dictionaries list hundreds of color names, and new names are created by advertisers every year. However, in many cultures, everyday language manages to get along with just under a dozen different color names (Berlin and Kay, 1969; Ratliff, 1976). In our own culture, when people are asked to assign names to various color samples, there is good agreement on names for only those few basic colors (Boynton and Olson, 1987).

Since people don't always agree on color names, perhaps it would be more useful to concentrate instead on experiences of color. One could ask: How many different colors can people see? Unfortunately, this simple question yields not just one answer but a whole series of them. If color samples are placed side by side, most people can distinguish more than a thousand different colors. You can try this for yourself the next time you're in a paint store. However, if samples are presented one at a time, performance declines (Newall, Burnham, and Clark, 1957; Nilsson and Nelson, 1981). In fact, when samples are seen one at a time—with several seconds elapsing between samples—most people can reliably recognize fewer than a dozen different colors (Halsey and Chapanis, 1951; Boyce, 1981). So how many colors *can* people see—thousands or just a dozen? The difficulty in answering this question suggests that we need to examine what people actually mean by the term "color." To do this, let's look at early attempts to understand the nature of color.

WHAT IS COLOR? THE INSIGHTS OF ISAAC NEWTON

Not even the briefest discussion of color perception can ignore the contributions of Isaac Newton, undoubtedly one of the greatest geniuses who ever lived. During a brief retreat to his mother's farm while a plague was raging at home in Cambridge, England, Newton discovered the binomial theorem, invented the calculus, and devised a theory of gravitation. He also bought a prism that he used later to study the nature of light and color (Westfall, 1980). These studies led Newton to draw a distinction that remains fundamental to this day, a distinction between physical phenomena and perceptual phenomena. In particular, Newton observed that

the rays, to speak properly, are not coloured. In them there is nothing else than a certain Power and Disposition to stir up a Sensation of this or that Colour. (1704/1952, pp. 124–125)

These two sentences imply that even the most compelling intuitions can be wrong—objects themselves have no color; nor is the light reflected from those objects colored. Instead, color is a psychological phenomenon, an entirely subjective experience. Objects *appear* colored because they reflect light from particular regions of the visible spectrum. But even that is not enough. In order for an object to appear colored, light reflected from that object must be picked by the right sort of eye or nervous system. Because some people have abnormal eyes and nervous systems, their experiences of color differ radically from those that most people enjoy.

Actually, waves in that portion of the electromagnetic spectrum that is called "light" are no more colored than waves in any other portion of the spectrum—for example, radio waves. Color arises from the capacity of particular light rays to evoke certain responses in the nervous system. To illustrate, imagine seeing someone who is wearing a red sweater. According to Newton, there is nothing inherently red about the light reflected from that sweater. No matter how firmly rooted in the sweater it may *seem,* the redness ultimately depends on your eyes and nervous system.

So to refer to a "red sweater" is incorrect, strictly speaking. To be correct, you should describe it as a "sweater that when seen in daylight can evoke a sensation most humans call 'red.'" However, we don't advise going into a clothing store and using this description to ask whether the store has any red sweaters. Nor will this chapter use such cumbersome language to describe the colors evoked by objects.

While on the subject of terminology, we should further clarify the term "color." Our dictionary offers nineteen different meanings of "color" in its noun form alone. If you've ever sorted objects such as crayons or "orphan" socks, you know that colors differ from one another in various ways. Blue and green socks differ from one another but not in the same way that two green socks do—say, one brand new and another that's been washed many times. In the study of perception, the single word "color" covers three different qualities. So that one quality can be distinguished from another, each quality is given a particular name—"hue," "brightness," and "saturation."

Hue refers to the quality that distinguishes among red, yellow, green, blue, orange, and so on. Incidentally, the word "color" is not an acceptable synonym for "hue." In fact, technically, you should refer to the "hues of the rainbow" and to Joseph's "coat of many hues" (Genesis 37:3). The second quality of color, **brightness,** is related to the amount, or intensity, of light. This quality enables you to describe an object (like a star in the sky) as "bright" or "dim." Or suppose you're dining by candlelight and find that it's hard to see with just one candle. If you increase the illumination by lighting additional candles, you'll increase the brightness of your surroundings. The third quality, **saturation,** characterizes a color as "pale," "vivid," or something between the two. After your jeans have been laundered with some bleach in the wash water, their blueness will be less saturated than when you first got them. Color Plate 1 will help you visualize more easily what is meant by "hue," "brightness," and "saturation."

Since your color experiences vary along these three dimensions, describing a color completely requires that you specify its hue, its brightness, *and* its saturation. Moreover, an adequate theory of color perception must explain the origin of these dimensions of color experience. Having clarified what we mean by "color," we're now ready to return to the units of color perception. Let's look at the observations that led Newton to propose that color resides within oneself, not within the light rays.

What a Prism Reveals About Color. In one experiment, Newton allowed a beam of sunlight to pass through a small circular hole in a shutter and then through a glass prism (see Figure 6.1). After passing through the prism, the light fanned out into a rainbow of **spectral colors,** or spectrum. Newton described the spectrum as consisting of seven different colors—red, orange, yellow, green, blue, indigo, and violet. These seven colors are indicated in the spectrum shown in Color Plate 2. In this plate, the upper scale defines the spectrum in terms of color experiences, a psychological dimension. The lower scale defines the spectrum in terms of wavelength of light, a physical dimension. The latter dimension, wavelength, was not known to Newton, which is why he had

to describe color solely in psychological terms (color names).

Actually, it was known long before Newton that a prism could decompose sunlight into a spectrum of colors (Ronchi, 1970). For centuries, people had seen spectra created by glass chandeliers, soap bubbles, and diamond jewelry. Newton's contribution lay not in the observation but in the uses to which he put that observation. Two experimental techniques were particularly important in this regard. First, he developed a simple scheme for selectively blocking out or reducing the intensity of various colors in the spectrum; second, by means of a convex lens, Newton was able to collect this modified spectrum and pass it through another prism (see Figure 6.2). The combination of these two techniques allowed him to distinguish between **pure light** and light that is made up of several different components—**composite light.** For instance, if he blocked out all the colors of the spectrum except for green and then passed the green through a second prism, the resulting light continued to be green. Because the second prism could not break green into further components, Newton deemed the green to be pure light.

To Newton these observations suggested that light from the sun was *not* pure but consisted of seven different colors that could not be decomposed. Though the first conclusion (that sunlight is not pure) is correct, the second (that sunlight

FIGURE 6.1 Newton's basic experiment.

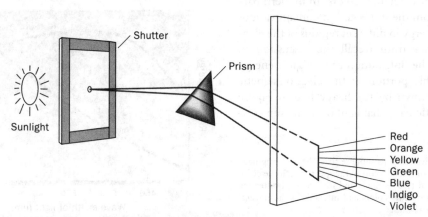

Shutter
Prism
Sunlight
Red
Orange
Yellow
Green
Blue
Indigo
Violet

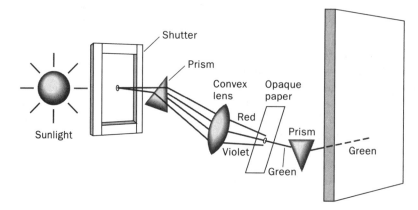

FIGURE 6.2 A modification of Newton's basic experiment.

contains only seven pure components) is not. Since the mistakes of geniuses can be as enlightening as their successes, let's see why Newton went wrong.

Like anyone else, scientists must be alert to the possibility that their observations can be influenced by expectation. Newton's conclusion that there were seven colors in the spectrum was influenced by just such an expectation, one based on his belief that seeing and hearing were closely related (Gouk, 1988). In particular, he thought that since the musical scale included seven tones and semitones within each octave, the spectrum had to contain seven colors (Boring, 1942).*

But this error should not diminish the fact that Newton's main idea was right—light from the sun, sometimes called white light, can be decomposed into many different colors. In modern parlance, light from the sun is said to contain various amounts of energy in different regions of the electromagnetic spectrum (recall the discussion in Chapter 2). The distribution of sunlight's energy over the visible portion of the electromagnetic spectrum is shown by the heavy line in Figure 6.3. Note particularly that light from the sun con-

sists of nearly equal amounts of energy at all the wavelengths shown. Contrast this with the distribution of energy from an ordinary light bulb. As shown by the dashed line, a typical light bulb emits more energy at longer wavelengths than it does at shorter ones. This is why photographs taken with indoor lighting can have a slightly more yellowish tint than do those taken with natural light.

The idea that white light is decomposable into elementary components is universally accepted today. However, when Newton first suggested the idea, it aroused passionate disagreement that continued well after Newton's own lifetime (see

FIGURE 6.3 Energy distribution of sunlight (heavy line) and of light from an ordinary light bulb (dashed line).

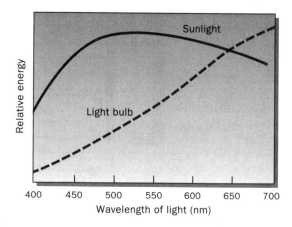

---

* There is actually reason to suppose that Newton originally noticed only five different colors in the spectrum. Some claim that he later added two—orange and indigo—to bolster the analogy between spectral colors and intervals in the musical scale (Houston, 1917).

Box 6.1). For example, many people were upset that their eyes couldn't be trusted—what appeared to be innocent white light actually consisted of a host of components. In reality, the situation is even worse than people imagined: using far fewer than seven components you can fool the eye into seeing white. We now know that humans experience as white a light that consists of a mixture of just two, properly chosen spectral components. Because this does not work with all pairs of components, we give a special name to those pairs for which it does work. Any two spectral components which when added together appear white are said to be **complementary.** A mixture of one component that appears blue and one that appears yellow would look just like white. Moreover, a person would find this mixture indistinguishable from another that included orange light and greenish-blue light, which would also look like sunlight. So in effect, complementary components cancel one another, yielding a colorless, or achromatic, sensation.

We should stress that simple measuring instruments *can* distinguish among these various mixtures even though the human eye cannot. Hence the act of mixing components of light does not obliterate the individual spectral components; these components are still present in the mixture. These mixtures appear equivalent because of the way the visual nervous system processes spectral information.

What Metamers Reveal About Color. As we've just seen, various sets of physically different distributions of energy can produce identical color experiences. Members of such sets are said to be metameric, a concept introduced in Chapter 5. For example, Newton found that orange light, alone, was metameric to a mixture of red light and yellow light. In addition, pairs of complementary colors (that yield white) are also metameric to one another. Also, those two pairs of mixtures are metameric to a mixture of Newton's seven spectral colors, which as you know, also yields the perception of white light.

Recall that metamers imply that the visual system is "blind" to certain aspects of the physical

world. By identifying metamers, one learns what those aspects are. For example, suppose you have two objects that are physically identical in all respects but one. If you can't tell them apart by looking at them, your visual system must be ignoring whatever it is that makes the objects physically different. Conversely, if you can tell the two objects apart, your visual system cannot be ignoring that one distinguishing feature. The information that the system retains and the information that it discards say a lot about the workings of color perception. As a result, much of the understanding of color perception comes from the study of metameric matches. We'll turn to that topic now.

Newton's Color Circle. Newton did not have the degree of control over light that scientists enjoy today. Still, he managed to explore the perceptual results of various mixtures of light. For instance, to see what happens when two pure lights are combined, he blocked out all the other spectral components and used a convex lens to combine the remaining two. Examining the appearance of various mixtures of light, Newton developed the basic ideas of color mixture and expressed them in a graphic model of color perception. The model, known as **Newton's color circle,** is depicted in Figure 6.4. Although modest in appearance, this circle represents an incredible insight on Newton's part, namely that a simple geometric form could represent the properties of something as complex as color vision (Wasser-

FIGURE 6.4 Newton's color circle.

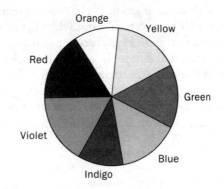

Box 6.1 *Newton Stirs Up a Hornet's Nest*

Newton first presented his work on light and color in 1672, when he was 29 years old. His ideas were greeted with such fury and disdain that Newton waited more than 30 years before publishing his complete work on these topics in *Opticks*. By that time, 1704, Newton's genius was nearly universally acknowledged. Despite his eminence, his ideas about light and color continued to provoke angry rebuttals for more than a century. None of these rebuttals was more impassioned than that advanced by German poet Goethe.

Goethe believed that he would be remembered not so much for his poetry as for his refutation of Newton (Pirenne, 1967, p. 153). Being a strong believer in the power of intuition and common sense, Goethe was shocked at the patent absurdity of Newton's prism demonstration. Goethe considered Newton a "Cossack" for denying the purity of white light (Southall, in Helmholtz, 1909/1962, vol. 2, p. 115). Since the time of Aristotle, white light had been regarded as the very essence of purity. According to this view, color represented the contamination of white by less exalted, worldly substances. Newton's decomposition of white into colors implied that white was no more special than any other color.

In addition to these aesthetic considerations, Goethe also objected to Newton's ideas on philosophical grounds. He believed that to accept Newton's claim about white light was tantamount to treating *all* sense perception as subjective and unreliable, an idea he detested. Feeling absolutely certain that white light could *not* be a mixture of other colors, Goethe urged people to disregard the experiments performed by Newton in a darkened room in Cambridge:

> *Friends, escape the dark enclosure,*
> *where they tear the light apart*
> *and in wretched bleak exposure*
> *twist and cripple Nature's heart.*
> *Superstitions and confusions*
> *are with us since ancient times—*
> *leave the specters and delusions*
> *in the heads of narrow minds.*
> *(Weisskopf and Worth, Trans.,*
> *in Weisskopf, 1976)*

To combat Newton further, Goethe got a prism and attempted to verify some of Newton's claims. Although he did use the prism for many different experiments, Goethe never correctly repeated what Newton had done. For example, Goethe looked directly through the prism but failed to see a spectrum of colors, leading him to believe that Newton, in addition to being a Cossack, was a charlatan. Goethe went further. He enlisted the services of a young man, Arthur Schopenhauer, who would later become a distinguished philosopher in his own right. Goethe interested Schopenhauer in his ideas about light and color, and persuaded him to continue the assault on Newton. Using Goethe's own optical equipment, the younger man began to do experiments with light (Birren, 1941, p. 214). Unfortunately for Goethe, though, these experiments convinced Schopenhauer that Newton had been right after all: sunlight *does* consist of many different colors.

man, 1978). Each of the seven wedge-shaped sectors represents one of the spectral colors—as Newton put it, "the Circumference representing the whole series of colours from one end of the Sun's colour'd image to the other" (1704/1952, p. 154). The circle, though, is only part of the model; Newton also devised several rules that relate colors and mixtures of colors to locations on and within the circle. Let's see how the appearance of various mixtures might be predicted by this geometric model.

Suppose we were to add equal intensities of red light and yellow light. These two equal-intensity lights are represented by two equal-sized triangles in Figure 6.5. One triangle is located on the circle, in the middle of the arc for yellow; the other triangle is also located on the circle, but in the middle of the arc for red. To find the color that results from the mixture of these two, you connect the two triangles with a straight line. The color of the mixture corresponds to the line's center of gravity. (You might imagine this line as a seesaw, and the triangles as people on either end; the sizes of the triangles signify how much the people weigh.) The location of the line's center of gravity gives the predicted color of the mixture. In this case, the center of gravity lies in the middle of the orange sector. In fact, orange is what you see when equal amounts of red and yellow light are mixed. Consider what happens when unequal amounts are mixed, say, a large quantity of red

and a small quantity of yellow. This case is shown in Figure 6.6. The center of gravity of the line connecting the two unequal-sized triangles lies close to the border of the red and orange sectors, signifying that the mixture will look reddish-orange, which it does. Adding two colors near one another on the color circle yields a mixture whose color is a compromise between the components. In fact, as one varies the portions of the colors in the mixture, the appearance of the mixture changes correspondingly.

Combining the appropriate components of light, Newton also discovered he could produce a color whose appearance was not like any of his seven pure lights. For example, if you add long-wavelength light (from the red end of the spectrum) and short-wavelength light (from the blue end of the spectrum) the result is purple. Today we call such colors, including purple, **nonspectral colors.** The existence of nonspectral colors reinforces the distinction between light's physical properties and its perceptual consequences. From the perceptual point of view, the physical spectrum has a gap—it does not contain all colors that can be perceived by the human eye.

When he examined the seven colors in his spectrum, Newton noticed that they were very vivid (today we would describe them as "saturated"). But when he added these vivid components together, the resulting mixtures appeared less vivid (today we would say "washed out" or

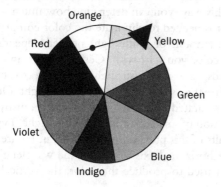

FIGURE 6.5 Newton's color circle can be used to predict the color produced by mixing equal amounts of yellow and red light.

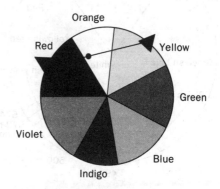

FIGURE 6.6 Newton's color circle can be used to predict the color produced by mixing unequal amounts of yellow and red light.

"desaturated"). This perceptual fact, that mixtures appear desaturated, is also represented in Newton's color circle. The most vivid colors lie along the circumference; less vivid colors lie away from the circumference. At the extreme, a completely desaturated color (white) is represented at the center of the circle.

As mentioned earlier, the seven pie-shaped wedges in Newton's color circle reflect his belief that there should be seven discrete pure colors. A color circle designed in this arbitrary way makes incorrect predictions about some mixtures involving colors widely separated on the color circle. In order to make correct predictions, Newton's color circle must be adjusted in two ways. First, the boundaries that divide the circle into discrete sectors must be erased, since those sectors could imply the existence of seven discrete pure colors. A circle without sectors correctly reflects the fact that color varies continuously. Second, some rational scheme for spacing the color names (or wavelengths) around the circle's circumference must be used. Complementary colors should be placed opposite each other on the circle, so that when they are connected, their balance point falls at the circle's center—white. A circle satisfying both these requirements is shown in Figure 6.7.

FIGURE 6.7 A revised color circle. (Adapted from Southall, 1937/1961.)

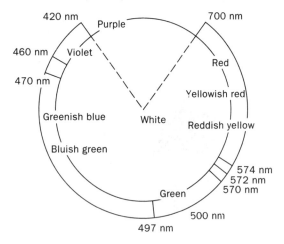

The circumference of the larger interrupted circle indicates the position of various spectral lights from 420 nanometers to 700 nanometers. Note that the wavelengths are not spaced uniformly; the wavelengths from 500 to 700 nanometers occupy less of the circumference than do those from 420 to 500 nanometers. In fact, the wavelengths have been positioned on the circle so that along any diameter, complementary colors stand directly opposite each other. Note that some wavelengths, such as 497 nanometers, have no single wavelength that is complementary. The inner complete circle indicates the color names an observer would give.

Although this revised color circle is far more satisfactory than Newton's original, it still fails to capture some elementary facts about color. For example, Newton (1704/1952) noted that "some colours affect the senses more strongly" (p. 97). He meant that yellows and greens are brighter (that is, more visible) than reds or blues. We now know that the visibility of various wavelengths of light defines the photopic sensitivity function (see Chapter 3), with maximum brightness at 550 nanometers.

There's another important fact that Newton's original circle doesn't capture: bright colors tend to look washed out or desaturated. You can see this for yourself in Color Plate 2 by comparing the colors in the middle of the spectrum (which appear relatively bright but desaturated) to those at either end (which appear less bright but more saturated). Moreover, how strongly saturated a color appears can be quantified. While someone looks at a light of a particular color, you can add white light to it, thereby desaturating that color. In this way, you can determine how much white light is needed to eliminate the color completely. The amount of white light needed depends on the color you start with. Certain colors, in other words, are more strongly saturated to begin with—they stand up better to white light. Other, less saturated colors are easily washed out by the addition of small quantities of white light. Typical results of this procedure are shown in Figure 6.8. The horizontal axis represents the wavelength of light used to produce the color; the vertical axis

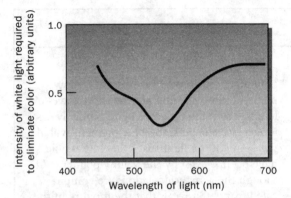

FIGURE 6.8 Intensity of white light needed to desaturate colors of various wavelengths.

shows the intensity of white light needed to desaturate the color completely. This V-shaped curve shows that lights at the middle of the spectrum (yellow) appear less saturated than do lights toward the ends of the spectrum (blue or red). Adding white light to light of a given wavelength can also alter the hue produced by that wavelength. For instance, adding white to long-wavelength light (red) shifts its hue slightly toward yellow (Kurtenbach, Sternheim, and Spillmann, 1984).

The dependence of hue, brightness, and saturation on wavelength is not a consequence of some physical property of light. Rather, it results from the way the visual system processes information about light's wavelength. A full explanation of color experiences, therefore, must account for brightness and saturation as well as hue.

In developing the concepts of color perception, we have given examples that utilized simple spectral lights and their mixtures. Such lights consist of a small band of wavelengths. However, light containing only a restricted range of wavelengths is rare outside the laboratory. Ordinarily, vision depends on white light (sunlight or artificial light) that illuminates the objects one sees. But, despite the fact that the illuminating light is white, one sees most objects as colored, not white, because those objects absorb certain wavelengths in the white light and reflect the rest. The wavelengths absorbed depend on the pigments contained in

the surface of those objects. For instance, "green" grass reflects a band of wavelengths more than 100 nanometers wide, nearly one-third the width of the entire visible spectrum. This distribution of reflected wavelengths reaches the eyes, and initiates the perception of color (see Box 6.2). Surfaces containing different pigments will reflect different distributions of wavelengths and, therefore, will appear different in color. The light reflected from a surface depends also on the wavelengths with which the surface is illuminated. However, even though the wavelength distribution of illuminating light changes—thereby changing the wavelengths reflected to the eyes—the colors of objects tend to remain constant. This fact is puzzling, since it means that one's perceptions are constant even though the light stimulating the eyes is not. Let's consider how this remarkable constancy of color perception is achieved.

COLOR CONSTANCY

The light reflected from a surface depends not only on the pigments in the surface but also on the light illuminating the surface. If the spectral composition of that illumination varies, so too will the spectral distribution of the reflected light. The composition of sunlight varies with the time of day—late afternoon sunlight contains more long-wavelength light than does noonday sun. As a result, the light reflected outdoors by any object will vary from one time of day to another. Moreover, the spectral composition of ordinary indoor lights (tungsten light bulbs) differs from the spectral composition of sunlight—the indoor light contains less short-wavelength light. Thus the light reflected by objects changes when you move the objects indoors. Even though the light reaching your eye changes, you usually don't notice any change in the perceived color of objects: green grass nearly always looks green, and yellow roses yellow. **Color constancy** is the name given to the fact that an object's color tends to remain constant even though the spectrum of light falling on that object, and thus the light reflected toward the viewer from the object, changes (Jameson and Hurvich, 1989). To achieve color constancy, the

Box 6.2 *Mixing Colors*

Every schoolchild knows it is possible to create a variety of shades of colors using just a few so-called primaries. Various shades of green, for example, are readily achieved simply by mixing blue and yellow inks in various proportions. This is called **subtractive color mixture,** since the component primaries each subtract a portion of the incident light, keeping that portion from reaching your eye. To understand this point, consider the curve in panel A of the accompanying figure (adapted from Pirenne, 1967), which shows the reflectance spectrum of a typical blue ink. The curve indicates that the ink reflects lots of light from the short-wavelength portion of the spectrum but less from the longer-wavelength portion. This happens because the ink contains a pigment that selectively absorbs light of particular wavelengths. Now look at panel B, which shows the reflectance spectrum for a typical yellow ink. Note that it reflects mainly wavelengths longer than 500 nanometers—hence its yellow appearance. Again, this is because the ink contains a pigment that absorbs light in a characteristic way. The curve in panel C shows the distribution of wavelengths reflected by a mixture of equal amounts of the two inks. How does this distribution come about, and why does it appear green?

When you mix the yellow and blue inks together, the mixture contains pigments from both components. Now suppose you view a surface that is coated with the mixture and illuminated by sunlight. The yellow pigment in the mixture will *absorb* part of the light that otherwise would have been *reflected* by the

blue pigment. In other words, the yellow pigment removes much of the short wavelengths from the reflected light. Similarly, at longer wavelengths, the blue pigment will *absorb* some of the light that otherwise would have been *reflected* by the yellow pigment. Although the actual calculations are complicated, panel C reveals that the mixture of the two inks reflects light mainly around the middle of the spectrum, the only region of the spectrum at which *both* pigments reflect appreciable amounts of light. As a result, the mixture will look neither yellow nor blue, but instead, greenish.

The principles of subtractive color mixture were employed 25,000 years ago by the prehistoric artists who worked in the caves around Lascaux (in what is today western France). These principles have been used ever since by people to color objects in their environment; but it was nature who devised the technique: plants and animals contain pigments that selectively absorb, or subtract, certain wavelengths. This selective absorption gives rise to the characteristic colors one associates with those plants and animals. Color can also be produced by a process of **additive color mixture.** This additive process is almost never used by nature and has been used by people only very recently, mainly for purposes of entertainment or research. We'll illustrate additive mixture using a familiar example, color television. The tube in a color television set contains hundreds of thousands of small spots packed very closely together. These spots light up when they are struck by an electron beam inside the set. A spot will

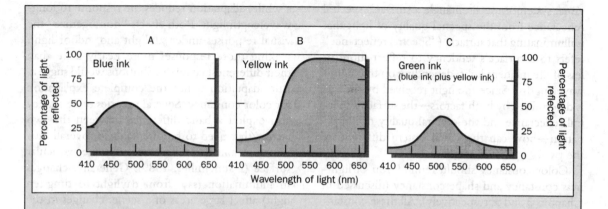

appear red or blue or green, depending on the material of which the spot is made. Each small section of the television tube contains many closely packed spots of each type. You can verify this by putting your eye very close to the screen of a color television set. At normal viewing distances, however, the spots are too small to be seen separately and instead are blended, or added together, by your eye. The resulting color, then, is produced by an additive process. Because the strength of the blue, red, or green glow varies with the intensity of the electron beam at any spot, the relative proportions of the three colors in the mixture also vary. As a result, although the tube itself produces only the three colors, the properties of your own nervous system generate perceptions of a wide range of different colors according to the laws of additive color mixture.

Color Plate 3 demonstrates the power of additive mixture. The plate is a portrait ("Susan") painted by the contemporary American artist Chuck Close. As you can see, the portrait consists of spots of various color and size, each surrounded by another color or colors. At normal viewing distance the portrait's individual elements stand in clear isolation from one another. From a great distance, though, your eye blends the individual elements, producing an additive mixture of their colors. With the book propped open to Color Plate 3, try viewing the portrait from 3–4 meters. Notice the blending of colors and the emergence of features that were hidden when the portrait was viewed up close. For example, from far away one not only discovers Susan's eyeglasses, but one also sees the reflections in their lenses. (Incidentally, when Newton superimposed lights of different wavelengths, he too was employing a form of additive mixture.)

We've seen, then, that there are two different techniques for color mixture. In one technique, the color is produced by the addition of wavelengths; in the other, by the subtraction (absorption) of wavelengths. The difference between these techniques of color mixture has nothing to do with the nature of color vision. It shows only that light is absorbed or reflected differently under different circumstances. For both types of mixtures, the color of a surface depends on the distribution of wavelengths reaching your eye.

visual system must disentangle a surface's spectral reflectance from the spectral quality of light that is illuminating that surface. ("Spectral reflectance" refers to a surface's tendency to reflect more or less of the incident light, depending on that light's wavelengths.) Since the light received by the eye is determined by both factors—the surface's spectral reflectance and the spectral quality of illumination—how can the visual system differentiate the two?

Color constancy should remind you of lightness constancy and shape constancy (discussed in Chapters 3 and 5, respectively). All these constancies make important contributions to the stability of the environment's appearance. If visual perception changed with every change in the light reaching their eyes, people would be hopelessly confused. Color constancy allows objects to be recognized regardless of the time of day, and indoors as well as outdoors.

Suppose, for example, you are sitting outside, reading this book. It gets chilly and you go inside to read, using a lamp containing an ordinary 150-watt tungsten bulb. The light outdoors contains relatively more short-wavelength energy (blue) than the light indoors. Because it has relatively more of its energy at medium and long wavelengths, the indoor light is yellower than the light outdoors. If your color perception depended only on the light coming from a page of this book, the surface would appear somewhat yellow indoors (since indoors the page reflects more light that is normally called yellow than it does outdoors). Yet you notice no such change, for the following reason.

When any stimulus is viewed for some time, the visual mechanisms it affects lose some of their sensitivity. This process, discussed in Chapters 4 and 5, is called adaptation. Adaptation promotes color constancy by reducing the effects of small differences among the physiological effects of various spectral distributions. After you've been exposed to the blue-rich outdoor light for a while, adaptation diminishes the visual system's response to short-wavelength light. After you've been exposed to the red- and green-rich indoor light for

a while, adaptation reduces the response to long-wavelength light. Both effects "homogenize" the visual responses under sunlight and indoor light, making those responses more nearly alike than their different spectral distributions would suggest. But adaptation is not the complete explanation for color constancy. Several theories of constancy also exploit a basic difference between the two factors that need to be disentangled, overall illumination and the reflectance of some particular surface (Dannemiller, 1989). Generally, changes in illumination (say, from daylight to tungsten light) affect large areas of a scene; changes in the spectral reflectance of an object (say, from an unripe to a ripe apple) are restricted to small regions of space. So, low spatial frequencies in the retinal image could convey information about overall spectral illumination, while higher spatial frequencies could convey information about the reflectances of individual objects. Note that this scheme would be defeated—and color constancy would fail—under exactly the same conditions that brightness constancy fails: when the illumination does not cover a large area of the field. This and other aspects of the scheme can be expressed as mathematical rules that would allow a television camera to exhibit color constancy much like our own (Wandell, 1987).

Finally, we should emphasize that this process of color constancy probably evolved in order to compensate for small variations in the broad wavelength distributions of *natural* light. As a result, when objects are illuminated by light with a restricted wavelength distribution, the compensation fails and color constancy is defeated. Color Plate 4 shows some common objects illuminated by natural sunlight and by two different lights of restricted wavelength distributions. Note how, in the latter cases, the objects take on highly unnatural colors, showing that color constancy works only under conditions of broadband illumination. Be warned that unscrupulous supermarkets exploit this limitation on color constancy. They can make their meat products look extra fresh (red) by illuminating them with light biased toward long wavelengths.

THE TRICHROMACY OF HUMAN VISION

The preceding sections reinforce the idea that color (a psychological experience) and light (a physical quantity) are connected in complex ways. Among the complexities is the fact that different combinations of wavelengths can yield the same color experience. Such psychologically equivalent combinations, so-called **metamers,** indicate that the visual system confuses certain combinations of wavelengths with one another. The number and kinds of confusions indicate how the eye analyzes the wavelength composition of the light it receives. Since this analysis is initiated by the photosensitive pigments in the cone visual receptors, color confusions depend on the number of different types of cone photopigments an eye has.* To see this connection, consider the color confusions made by an eye that possesses only one type of cone photopigment.

A DESIGN DECISION: HOW MANY CONE PIGMENTS?

What If Eyes Had Only One Cone Pigment?

Every photopigment absorbs some wavelengths of light more efficiently than others. However, once absorbed, light of any wavelength initiates exactly the same train of events in the visual receptor. Thus the receptor makes no distinction as to the wavelength of the light absorbed. The response of the receptor conveys information about how much light is absorbed, but the response conveys no information about the wavelength of the absorbed light. This is called the **univariance principle,** since a receptor's response can be summarized by a single number (one variable) that specifies the amount of light absorbed (Naka and Rushton, 1966). The univariance principle is the key to understanding the photoreceptors' role in

---

* We are focusing on cone receptors, since color experience requires that the eyes receive sufficient light to stimulate cones.

color perception. (Incidentally, the univariance principle also represents another case of the ambiguity inherent in the response of a single neuron, an issue discussed in Chapters 4 and 5.)

According to the univariance principle, an eye containing only one photopigment type is not able to see color. Such an eye is unable to distinguish one wavelength from another because, with the proper adjustment of intensities, all wavelengths could be made to affect the receptor in exactly the same way. This is illustrated in Figure 6.9, which shows the absorption spectrum of a single, hypothetical photopigment type. The curve's height represents the amount of incident light that the pigment would absorb at each wavelength. Note, for example, that the pigment absorbs twice as much light (50 percent) at wavelength B as it does at wavelength A (25 percent). So, if equal amounts of A and B were incident on the photopigment, more B would be absorbed. However, equal amounts of A and B would be absorbed if twice as much A were incident on the photopigment, relative to B. In fact, the intensities of many different wavelengths could be adjusted such that the amount of light actually absorbed by this pigment would be the same regardless of which wavelength was incident. This means, in other words, that many wavelengths would be metameric to one another. In addition, with

FIGURE 6.9 A one-pigment system.

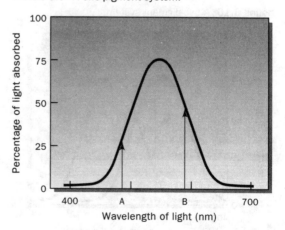

proper adjustment of intensities, any combination of wavelengths, including white light, could be perfectly matched by any other wavelength or combination of wavelengths. So an eye with only one type of photopigment would treat all sorts of light mixtures as metameric, including many that the normal eye does not. A person with just one cone pigment is unable to discriminate color. Everything appears various shades of gray; hence such a person is called a **monochromat** (meaning "one-colored"). Incidentally, everyone is a monochromat under conditions of dim light, because then they are forced to rely on the rods, which contain just one type of photopigment.

What If Eyes Had Two Cone Pigments? An eye with two different photopigments would be more discriminating that the one-pigment eye just described. Consider the consequences of having two photopigments such as those whose absorption spectra are shown in Figure 6.10. Again, since each photopigment obeys the univariance principle, *on its own* a pigment cannot convey information about what wavelengths of light are present. However, when two different types of pigments act *in concert,* they do provide some information about the wavelengths that are present. Let's see how. First, note that when stimulated by light, a two-pigment system makes two statements, not one, about the amount of light en-

ergy absorbed. For any given wavelength, the statement (or response) of either pigment depends on how well that pigment absorbs light of that wavelength. Now by definition, two types of photopigments differ in how well they absorb light of various wavelengths, as summarized by their different absorption spectra (Figure 6.10). As a result, any single wavelength (for example, A in Figure 6.10) will generate a *pair* of responses, one from each pigment. Note in the example shown that pigment 1 generates a larger response to A than does pigment 2. Of course, the magnitude of each pigment's response will also vary with light intensity, since more intense lights make more energy available for absorption. However, when light gets more intense but wavelength does not change, the two responses will grow proportionately. Consequently, so long as wavelength is unchanged, the *relative* strengths of the two pigments' responses will remain constant. In summary, because the two pigment types have different absorption spectra, an eye with two pigment types extracts some usable wavelength information from light.

This two-pigment system can nonetheless be confused about wavelength, as the following example shows. Consider the response produced by the wavelength represented in the left panel of Figure 6.11 (see arrow). Note that this wavelength stimulates both pigments 1 and 2, yielding a small response in pigment 1 and a larger response in pigment 2. We shall express this pair of responses as a ratio, which for this wavelength would be 4 to 1. Now, the ratio for this pair of responses to a single wavelength can be duplicated by an appropriate combination of two wavelengths. This is illustrated in the right panel of Figure 6.11, where the effects of a mixture of two wavelengths are shown. Note that the resulting pair of responses, one from each pigment, stands in the same ratio—4 to 1—as the pair of responses elicited by the single wavelength in the left panel. The owner of this eye, therefore, would confuse that single wavelength (left panel) with the mixture (right panel).

This eye would suffer many other color confusions as well. Any wavelength or mixture of

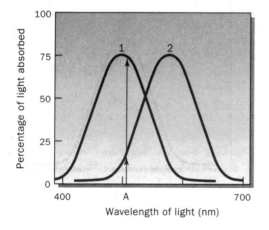

FIGURE 6.10 A two-pigment system.

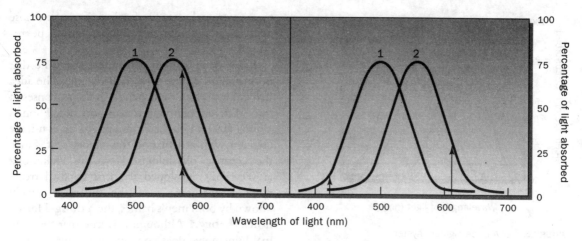

FIGURE 6.11 A two-pigment system can be confused.

wavelengths (no matter how complex) will be represented by just a pair of signals. As a result, the effect of any wavelength or mixture of wavelengths can always be matched by just two wavelengths, provided that the two are presented in the right proportions. Moreover, such matches can be produced using any of a large number of different pairs of wavelengths. An eye exhibiting these kinds of confusions is said to be **dichromatic** (meaning "two-colored"). However, note that not all wavelengths are confused. Unlike the one-pigment eye, a dichromatic eye retains certain information about the wavelength composition of light, and this information provides a basis for color vision.

An eye with only two types of cone pigments would make one particularly interesting color confusion involving sunlight—which, as you know, consists of nearly equal amounts of all wavelengths within the visible portion of the spectrum. Like any other complex mixture of wavelengths, sunlight will be represented in this eye by a pair of responses, one from each pigment type. There also exists a single, particular wavelength of light that will produce exactly the same pair of responses. Therefore that one wavelength will be confused with sunlight. Since all other wavelengths will produce different pairs of responses, they will not be confused with sunlight. We can call the one wavelength that is confused

the **neutral point** of the eye's spectral response. The existence of a single neutral point is the hallmark of a two-pigment eye. For most people, such a neutral point cannot be found, indicating that their eyes contain more than two cone pigments.

What If Eyes Had Three Cone Pigments? So far we've seen that a one-pigment eye can match any complex combination of wavelengths using just a single wavelength. Such an eye would be wholly color-blind. We've also seen that a two-pigment eye can match any complex combination of wavelengths using two properly selected wavelengths. Such an eye would have some ability to discriminate the wavelength composition of light. Now you should be able to anticipate what happens if an eye contains three pigments, like those represented in Figure 6.12. Note that any wavelength (such as A) will produce a trio of responses, one from each photopigment. Moreover, this trio of responses cannot be mimicked by any other single wavelength. To mimic these responses would require the ability to vary the intensities of up to three different wavelengths (with some exceptions, to be explained in the next paragraph). Hence an eye containing a trio of photopigments is said to be **trichromatic** (meaning "three-colored"). Color Plate 5 illustrates the variety of colors that can be produced by mixing just three

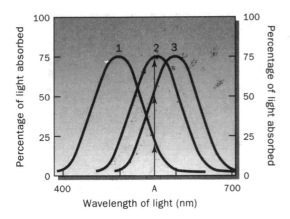

FIGURE 6.12 A three-pigment system.

colors. Note that each projector contains a transparency that creates a beam of a different color—one blue, one red, and one green. In the center, where all the beams overlap, your eye receives the reflected light from all three, and the result is white. Where only the red and green beams overlap, the light appears yellow. If the relative intensities of each beam could be adjusted, other, intermediate colors would appear.

The demonstration in Color Plate 5 does not require the particular trio of lights used there; many others would work equally well. But why *three* lights? If an eye contains three different cone photopigments, its response to any complex mixture of light can be represented by a trio of signals, one generated by each type of cone. To mimic this trio of signals, three independently adjustable lights are needed. Although any single wavelength will stimulate more than just one cone type, certain wavelengths do stimulate one type particularly well and the other types less well. A trio of wavelengths can be chosen so that each member of the trio determines *mainly* the response of one pigment. We noted earlier that there are limitations to the matches that are possible with any set of three lights. To match any light, you need independent control of the response in each cone type. Because any single wavelength will stimulate all types of cones, three lights that have been chosen to match most colors will not be able to match

many extremely saturated colors. To make those matches, a different set of lights would be required.

It has been known for quite some time that normal human vision is trichromatic. The idea that color perception depends on the responses of three different pigments is also quite old. Thomas Young (1801/1948), a British physician, is usually credited with articulating this theory first. Since the German physiologist Hermann Helmholtz (1909/1962) developed the first detailed treatment of the same idea, the theory is usually known by both men's names, the **Young-Helmholtz theory.*** Although it is true that the normal human eye does contain three types of cone pigments, it is instructive to consider the consequences of having even more types.

What If Eyes Had 300 Cone Pigments? Suppose an eye contained 300 different types of photopigments. Suppose further that each pigment type responded to only a very narrow band of wavelengths—one nanometer wide—with each pigment's response signaling the presence of one particular wavelength. Whenever the pigment sensitive to 462 nanometers signaled the capture of light energy, it would be a sure sign that the light contained that wavelength. This degree of pigment selectivity would make metamers difficult to produce, since most combinations of wavelengths would produce unique sets of responses among the 300 photopigments. Very few combinations of wavelengths would produce the same set of responses.

Since increasing the number of pigment types decreases the number of confusions (metamers), why does the visual system use only three? Actually, an eye with lots of different types of cone pigments would be at a disadvantage compared with one with only a few. In order to preserve the wavelength information generated by the

---

* In fairness to Thomas Young's genius it must be acknowledged that Helmholtz originally rejected Young's theory and came only grudgingly to accept its validity (Hurvich and Jameson, 1949).

cones, each cone type would require its own set of collector cells. Otherwise, if different cone types shared collector cells, wavelength information would be lost (Brindley, 1970). Producing the right connections between cones and collector cells would be a nightmare for the developing visual system, like 300 mothers (collector cells) each trying to find her particular child among a mob of 300 children (the cone types).

Although it may be hard to justify three cone types rather than four (Bowmaker, 1983), a very much larger number would not offer much more advantage (Barlow, 1982). Actually, color vision is remarkably keen with just three types of cones. For example, most people can appreciate extremely subtle hue differences among stimuli: they are able to discriminate more than 100 different hues on the basis of wavelength information alone. And if stimuli vary in brightness and saturation as well as hue, the number of discriminable colors grows to over 1,000. Of course there are some wavelength combinations that the human eye cannot discriminate from one another, as laboratory studies of metamers show. You should realize, though, that although metamers are vital for understanding color vision, they can be produced only if one has strict control over the wavelength composition of light. This kind of control never occurs in the natural environment, in which the visual system evolved, and it rarely occurs in everyday situations involving artificial illumination. In fact, mathematical analyses of natural surfaces and the wavelength distributions of typical illuminants reveal that trichromacy represents a very good solution to the problem of color vision: it provides an accurate description of surface colors under most conditions (Lennie and D'Zmura, 1988).

WHAT ARE THE THREE CONE TYPES?

Psychophysical studies of color vision point to the existence of three different cone pigment types (Brindley, 1970). This conclusion is consistent with the absorption spectra of cone types measured directly.

The technique of directly measuring the light absorption of photopigments is aptly named **microspectrophotometry.** Consider each part of the term: "photometry" involves the measurement *(metry)* of light *(photo)*; "spectro" indicates the spectrum (determining which wavelengths of light are present); and "micro" means "small." Hence, in the application to cone pigments, microspectrophotometry involves shining a small spot of light onto a single cone and determining, for various wavelengths, how much of that light is absorbed (MacNichol, 1964). The results obtained by studying cones in several human retinas are shown in Figure 6.13 (Dartnall, Bowmaker, and Mollon, 1983). The vertical axis portrays the amount of light absorbed, expressed as a percentage of the light shone on the cone; the horizontal axis indicates the light's wavelength. To facilitate comparisons among pigments, each one's maximum absorption has been arbitrarily set equal to unity.

These absorption curves have several notable features. First of all, there are three different cone pigment types (one type per cone), as one would expect from experiments on color metamers. Each pigment type is most sensitive to light of a particular wavelength—approximately 420, 530, and 560 nanometers, respectively. Because of

FIGURE 6.13 Microspectrophotometric records from three cone types in the human eye. (Redrawn from Dartnall, Bowmaker, & Mollon, 1983.)

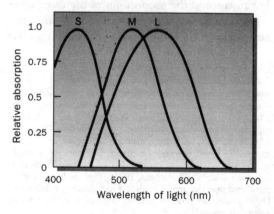

their peak sensitivities, these three cone types are referred to as short-wavelength sensitive (S cones), medium-wavelength sensitive (M cones), and long-wavelength sensitive (L cones).* Notice also that each cone pigment absorbs a broad range of wavelengths. As a result of this breadth, most lights—even those of only a single wavelength—stimulate more than just one class of cones. For example, stimulation in the region of 475 nanometers affects all three types. This breadth also means that the response of a single cone type provides no information about the wavelength(s) of light being absorbed. By itself, each pigment type is "color blind" (recall the univariance principle described earlier).

You may be struck by the odd way that the pigment absorption spectra distribute themselves along the wavelength continuum. Pairs of absorption spectra overlap substantially, particularly in the case of the spectra for M and L cones. Later, we'll see that this substantial and asymmetrical overlap reflects the evolutionary history of these pigments.

THE GEOGRAPHY OF THE CONES

We've been considering the connection between color perception and the cones' absorption spectra. Let's focus now on other perceptually important facts about cone receptors. Knowing that the signals coming from three cone types are important in color perception, we need to consider how the three types are distributed across the retina. For instance, if the proportions of the three cone types varied from one retinal region to another, color perception would vary correspondingly. To ascertain the distribution of cone types, one can apply a certain chemical to a retina that has been exposed to light. This chemical stains stimulated cones, causing them to appear dark when viewed under a microscope (unstimulated cones do not appear dark). Imagine viewing a retina that had been stimulated by a weak light of a single wavelength. Simply by noting the number and location of dark spots, you can visualize the distribution of cones that had responded to that wavelength (Marc, 1982). By appropriate choice of stimulating wavelength, you can selectively stain any one of the three cone types. These measurements confirm something long suspected from psychophysical studies of color perception, namely, that S cones are far less numerous than the other two types. Each of your eyes has fewer than 1 million S cones. Of the remaining 7 million cones, about two-thirds are L cones and one-third are M cones (Cicerone and Nerger, 1989).

This chemical staining technique confirms something else long suspected from psychophysical studies: the three types of cones are unevenly distributed across the retina. S cones are scarce at the fovea (the center of the retina), sharply increase to a maximum concentration just outside the fovea, and then decline in number with increasing eccentricity. In contrast, M and L cones are most numerous *at* the fovea and decline gradually with increasing eccentricity. Color Plate 6 is a computer-graphic idealization of the very center of the cone mosaic (Williams, 1991). For ease of visualization, cones are portrayed end-on and they have been color-coded by the computer (S cones are shown in blue, M cones are in green, and L cones are in red).[†] Because it shows only

---

* Recent biochemical and psychophysical studies reveal a somewhat more complicated picture. These complementary studies confirm that normal trichromatic humans may have either of two slightly different alternative types of L cone pigment. Approximately two-thirds of people tested have one type of pigment, with the remainder having the other. This genetically based diversity reflects a difference of a single amino acid in the protein structures of the two kinds of L pigments (Merbs and Nathans, 1992). The result is a shift in peak absorption of approximately 4 nanometers, a difference large enough to produce reliable individual differences in color matching (Winderick et al., 1992).

[†] The colors in the plate have been chosen arbitrarily as aids to visualization and memory. It is not intended to suggest that L cones are actually red, that M cones are green, or that S cones are blue. We agree with Mollon (1990) that "Whatever its mnemonic convenience, the use of colour names for the different cone types has been one of the most pernicious obstacles to the proper understanding of colour vision" (p. 64). Also note that the details remain to be established about how various cone types are actually interleaved in the human retina. The regular arrangement within the schematic mosaic shown is just one possible scheme.

the very central retina, this mosaic cannot convey all the geographical variations described earlier. As you examine the mosaic, though, you should find a region from which S cones are absent; this is the fovea. The mosaic will also help you appreciate the numerical advantage that L cones enjoy over M cones. With all the geographical variations in mind, it is time to inquire into their possible impact on your experience of color.

Since color appearance depends on the signals generated by a trio of cone types, color appearance should vary from one part of your retina to another. Indeed, this variation has long been known. To study this regional variation in color appearance requires that different, restricted regions of the retina be stimulated. When this is done, color appearance varies with the region stimulated. For example, a small light that appears greenish-blue when imaged slightly away from the fovea will appear green when imaged directly *on* the fovea. This change reflects the diminished contribution of S cones at the center of the retina. In addition, as that same light is moved into the periphery of the retina—where cones are less numerous—the light's color becomes less conspicuous. To sustain color perception in the periphery requires enlarging the size of the stimulus, to compensate for the reduced density of cones. Far into the periphery, where cones are essentially absent, vision becomes achromatic, meaning "without color." Thus, when an object is seen out of the corner of your eye, you may recognize its shape, but it will appear colorless. You can see this for yourself using Color Plate 7. Looking directly at the plate, you can see that the square is yellow and the disk blue. As you fixate at points farther and farther away from the plate, however, notice how the colors become less saturated. Although the composition of the light remains constant, the subjective experience of color changes. This happens because of regional variations in the machinery of color vision.

You can also use Color Plate 7 to see the consequence of having so few S cones in your fovea. Look at the center of the blue disk. At normal reading distance, the image of the blue disk not only will cover the region free of S cones (your fovea) but also will extend into regions that do contain S cones (around your fovea). Now, while continuing to fixate the blue disk, back away from the book. As you get farther from the book, the image of the blue disk will get smaller, eventually shrinking so that it falls entirely within your fovea. As this image shrinks, the disk will cease to appear blue. Notice that at the same distance, though, the square will continue to look yellow. This demonstration raises a paradox: when viewed from normal reading distance, why doesn't the blue disk appear less blue in its center? We have no ready answer for this paradoxical uniformity of perceptual experience, though it may be related to the "filling-in" process noted in Chapter 2 and discussed by Ramachandran (1992).

The variation in color appearance with retinal region or image size has practical consequences. For example, if two stimuli containing precisely the same wavelengths differ in size or in retinal location, their color appearances will also differ. As one result, even the most faithful photographic reproduction of a scene is bound to look different from the scene itself (Hurvich, 1981).

WHAT IS SPECIAL ABOUT SHORT-WAVELENGTH (S) CONES?

The S cones differ from the M and L types in several ways (Mollon, 1982). Geographically, the S cones are special, having a geographical distribution that is unlike those of the other types. The sparseness of S cones creates large gaps between neighboring S cones (Marc, 1982). What do these gaps mean for perception? Recall from Chapter 3 that the distance between receptors limits the eye's resolving power (acuity). The large separations between S cones help explain why acuity with blue targets is much poorer than acuity with targets of other colors (Pokorny, Graham, and Lanson, 1968; Williams, MacLeod, and Hayhoe, 1981).

Because the S cones are few and far between, you may wonder why you don't see holes or gaps when looking at a large, blue-colored region. One reason is that early on, the visual system integrates signals from many different cones of the same type. Since the S cones are relatively far apart, this integration covers relatively large distances. As a result the S cones not only give poor acuity but also can distort your perception of boundaries. And since boundaries contribute to the perceived shape of an object, the S cones can distort that perceived shape. Robert Boynton (1982) devised a strong demonstration of this fact. One version of this demonstration is given in Color Plate 8. Note first the pale yellow rectangle at the left of the plate. The ink used to print the rectangle absorbs short-wavelength light and reflects longer wavelengths. This reflected light stimulates primarily M and L cones, hence its yellow appearance. However, the white paper around the rectangle reflects light more or less uniformly, thereby stimulating S as well as M and L cones. As a result, then, one side of the yellow-white boundary excites S cones while the other side does not. To show how poorly the S cones register contour information, we've taken the same rectangle and drawn a squiggly black line around the outline of the rectangle. This is shown at the right of Color Plate 8. Prop the book open so that you can see the color plate; then walk slowly backward. You'll reach a distance at which the yellow-white boundary of the right-hand figure will appear squiggly rather than straight. The region outside the squiggly boundary appears white, while the region inside appears yellow. This means that some portions in and around the boundary that used to look white now look yellow, and vice versa. It is as if the yellow had spread outward toward the black squiggly line, and the white had spread inward. This spreading does not occur for all colors, only those differentially stimulating S cones on either side of a boundary. Fortunately, the demonstration you've just experienced is a very special case. Ordinarily the two sides of a boundary do not differ only in their effect on cones of the S type. The normal involvement of M and L cones ensures that shape information is accurately registered.

As we've said, under normal conditions, there is no direct perceptual trace of the sparseness of S cones. For one thing, ordinary stimuli affect more than just a single class of cones; for another thing,

most stimuli are sufficiently large that many different cones would be stimulated simultaneously. David Williams of the University of Rochester and his colleagues developed special conditions that overcame both these limitations, allowing them to measure the response of individual S cones (Williams, MacLeod, and Hayhoe, 1981). Using tiny, brief, violet test stimuli on a yellow background, so as to stimulate only S cones, Williams measured psychophysical thresholds at many different closely spaced spots on the retina. The data show remarkable variation in sensitivity from one spot, presumably where an S cone lay, to one immediately adjacent, where presumably there was no S cone. These very sharp variations in threshold mimic the distribution of S cones as revealed by chemical stain (Marc, 1982). Moreover, these variations were quite repeatable, even over a period of more than a year. Williams's perceptual data, then, confirm that single S cones are separated by fairly large stretches of retina in which there are no S cones at all.

THE EVOLUTION OF COLOR VISION

At the beginning of this chapter we asked, "Why is it important to see colors?" Let's revisit that question now, drawing on insights from recent work on how color vision evolved over millions of years. This historical perspective frames some intriguing possibilities about the purpose of color vision.

The normal human eye contains four types of photopigments, rhodopsin (in the rods) and three different cone photopigments. Genes, which are the basic units of inheritance, carry molecular instructions that guide a cell's manufacture of proteins, the building blocks of every living cell. Each gene is a chain of several thousand units of deoxyribonucleic acid (DNA); these are the instructions for protein manufacture. Using molecular biological techniques, Jeremy Nathans (Johns Hopkins University) isolated the genes responsible for instructing visual cells in the proper manufacture of S, M, and L pigments. Nathans (1989) showed that the gene for S pigment is carried on chromosome pair number 7, while the genes for M and L pigments lie right next to one another on the X-chromosome. Various photopigments differ from one another because structurally different genes, and hence different instructions, control their manufacture. By analyzing the structural similarities among various genes, one can create an evolutionary family. Because genes tend to mutate over time, two genes that are highly similar in structure are more likely to have been formed closer together in time than are two genes whose structures differ markedly.

Structural resemblances among all four genes (those for rhodopsin and the three cone pigments) suggest all four evolved from some common ancestor (Nathans, 1989). Ninety-six percent of the DNA sequence in the M pigment gene is identical to that in the L pigment gene. Interestingly, the S pigment gene shares 42 percent of its sequence with rhodopsin, and almost exactly the same proportion with each of the L and M pigment genes. This pattern of structural resemblances, supplemented by information on the variations in color vision in humans, in nonhuman primates, and in nonprimate mammals, suggests that long ago a single ancestor gene gave rise to all the modern photopigment genes. John Mollon argues that the original cone pigment probably had an absorption peak in the range 510 to 570 nanometers (Mollon, 1989). This would harmonize the pigment's peak absorption with the spectral peak of light from the sun. But, with just one cone, as we've already discussed, vision cannot be said to be color vision. Much later, about 500 million years ago, the S cone came into existence. Its addition to retinas already possessing the original 510- to 570-nanometer pigment gave birth to color vision. The relative responses of two different cone types made it possible to extract some wavelength information from the incoming light. Note though that S cones conferred color vision that was only dichromatic. Finally, only 40 million years ago, the original type of cone, with its peak between 510 and 570 nanometers, is thought to have duplicated and differentiated, giving rise to both the L pigment and the M pigment found in certain monkeys and in humans. With the ad-

dition of this third cone type, color vision in primates attained trichromacy.

Mollon (1989) put these evolutionary facts together with various creatures' food preferences in order to refine an intriguing account of color vision's utility. He proposed that a preference for particular kinds of fruit contributed to the development of trichromatic color vision in primates. Certain fruits, especially ones that are orange or yellow, may be specialized for attracting monkeys. Those monkeys, in turn, promote the survival of those fruit species by dispersing the seeds of their fruit. On this theory, the monkey needs trichromatic color vision in order to find the orange and yellow fruit hidden among the tree's foliage. It is intriguing to imagine that the world's colors appear as they do to us today because, tens of millions of years ago, our primate ancestors received the gift of trichromacy as part of an implicit bargain with banana and citrus trees.

COLOR'S OPPONENT CHARACTER

We saw in Chapters 3 and 4 that information from the photoreceptors is transformed as it travels to the visual cortex. Messages from neighboring receptors are antagonistically organized into ON and OFF regions, which together constitute a neuron's receptive field. The characteristics of these receptive fields significantly affect the perception of visual form and brightness. So far in this chapter, we have concentrated on the initial stage of analysis of color information, an analysis performed by the three cone types. We now need to consider how messages from these three cone types are organized or linked at subsequent stages of the visual system. We can get some idea of this organization by considering several phenomena of color vision, all of which point to an opponent linkage pitting one color against another.

WHAT IS THE EVIDENCE FOR COLOR OPPONENCY?

One phenomenon that suggests some kind of opponent connection between colors is **color con-**

Box 6.3 *Color Contrast*

You've probably had the experience of purchasing an article of clothing, such as a tie or a scarf, to go with an outfit in your closet. In the store, the tie or scarf looks neutral gray; but when you get home and try on the outfit, the article acquires a distinct color other than gray. Moreover, that distinct color seems to vary, depending on what outfit you wear it with. In other words, the color of the tie or scarf depends on what color is adjacent to it. This effect, demonstrated in Color Plate 9, is called *color contrast*, and it is a powerful influence in many everyday settings. The two small colored disks on the left and right sides of the Color Plate are the same, though color contrast with the surrounds makes them appear different.

Some people have been able to capitalize on color contrast to enhance color perception. One such person was Michel Chevreul,

director of the Gobelin tapestry works in Paris. Chevreul knew that interweaving just gray and red yarns could create tapestries that appeared to contain other colors as well—including distinct blue-green stripes—produced in the viewer's brain by color contrast. Chevreul developed a set of rules for ensuring that color contrast would have the effect his designers and weavers wanted. He went further, though, publishing a huge volume (1839/ 1967) that set out the basic rules of color harmony and contrast as they related to painting, interior decoration, printing, flower gardening, and dressmaking. In fact, the French Impressionist painters of the nineteenth century used Chevreul's book as a guide.

These principles were unwittingly rediscovered by Edwin Land, the inventor of the Polaroid camera, whose published papers contain many interesting demonstrations of

---

trast. Just as lightness contrast (described in Chapter 3) exaggerates lightness differences between adjacent objects, *color* contrast exaggerates their color differences (see Box 6.3). The major facts of color contrast have been known for a very long time. More than 400 years ago, Leonardo da Vinci, a painter, scientist, and engineer, discussed color contrast in his *Treatise on Painting:*

Of different colors equally perfect, that will appear most excellent which is seen near its direct contrary . . . blue near yellow; green near red: because each color is more distinctly seen, when opposed to its contrary, than to any other similar to it. (Quoted in Birren, 1941, p. 135)

Strong interaction between the color of an object and the color of its surround suggests some

sort of antagonistic linkages within the visual machinery that processes color information.

You can use Color Plate 10 to experience another phenomenon that suggests color opponency. Stare at the left fixation point (in the center of the four colored patches) for about 60 seconds; then look at the right fixation point. The illusory colors you'll experience are called **afterimages.** Note that the afterimage produced by the yellow patch appears blue, whereas the one produced by blue appears yellow. By the same token, the afterimage of the red patch appears green, and vice versa. These color afterimages are consistent with the idea that the visual system treats certain colors as opponent pairs.

In color experience, blue and yellow are mutually exclusive: an object may appear blue; an object may appear yellow; but an object cannot appear *both* blue and yellow at the same time.

color contrast. Let's consider a typical one here (Land, 1959). Land took two black and white slides of the same scene. One slide (the "red record") was taken with a red filter in front of the camera, the other (the "green record") with a green filter. Using a pair of slide projectors, Land superimposed the two black and white slides on a screen. Not surprisingly, since the slides were black and white, the result was a black and white image of the original scene. The surprise came when Land placed a red filter in front of the projector containing the red record. The image on the screen now consisted of various amounts of red light (from the projector with the red filter) mixed with various amounts of white light (from the other projector). One might expect that the only colors perceptible would be white, grays, blacks, and various shades of red. However, the image on the screen produced a wide range of colors—for example, a blond-haired girl with pale blue

eyes, a red coat, blue-green collar, and natural flesh tones. Where had all these colors come from?

The major source of Land's colors was color contrast (Walls, 1960). For instance, the girl's collar appeared blue-green because it was surrounded by the red of her coat. This could be verified by examining the image of the collar through a narrow tube. When the tube blocked the surrounding region from view, the collar appeared colorless, rather than blue-green. Though Land's color demonstrations were surprising, perhaps they should not have been. More than 60 years earlier, the French photographer Ducos du Hauron had demonstrated basically the same phenomenon (Judd, 1960). Although not entirely novel, Land's color demonstrations serve one very useful purpose. They are a vivid reminder of how important contrast is in the everyday experience of the colors of objects.

Similarly, red and green are mutually exclusive: an object never can appear *both* red and green. Of course, other combinations of these four colors are not mutually exclusive: objects can be bluish-green or reddish-yellow. These observations suggest that the nervous system may treat red and green as one mutually antagonistic pair and blue and yellow as another such pair. These views were first articulated by Ewald Hering, a German physician. In the nineteenth century, Hering made important contributions to nerve physiology, binocular vision, the anatomy of the liver, and color vision. Unfortunately, Hering was often so far ahead of his time that his contributions could not be properly assimilated into then current scientific thought and were therefore either dismissed outright or misinterpreted (Hurvich, 1969). But Hering's views on color vision have been largely vindicated by later discoveries.

CHROMATIC AND ACHROMATIC SYSTEMS

A combination of psychophysical and physiological studies has now established that signals from the three cone types are processed by one **achromatic system** and a pair of **chromatic systems.** The neural connections thought to underlie these three systems are sketched out in Figure 6.14. For diagrammatic simplicity, the schematic designs of the various systems are shown separately, one in each panel of the figure. The boxes labeled "S cones," "M cones," and "L cones" represent the three cone types. Arrows emerging from any one of the boxes represent neural signals generated when cones of that type absorb light. Two different kinds of arrows are meant to suggest that the nervous system treats signals in two different ways, either adding them or taking their difference. When two signals are represented by

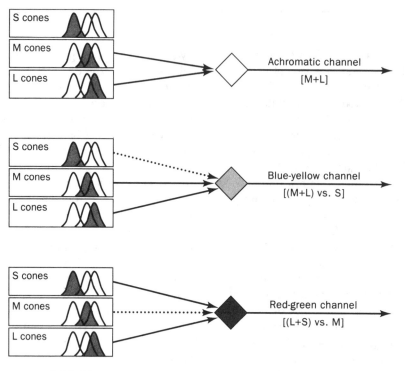

FIGURE 6.14 Chromatic and achromatic channels generated by combining the signals from three cone types. The achromatic channel is represented in the top diagram, the blue-yellow chromatic channel in the middle diagram, and the red-green chromatic channel in the bottom diagram.

solid arrows, the system adds those two signals together; when one signal is shown as a solid arrow and another is shown as a dashed arrow, the system takes the difference between those two signals. Before going further into the details of this figure, we should remind you how the nervous system adds and subtracts. Recall, from Chapter 3, that addition is accomplished via spatial summation. This operation is carried out when one neuron sums the messages from other neurons. Recall also that subtraction can be accomplished via an antagonism between ON and OFF signals. This operation is carried out when one neuron takes the difference between messages received from other neurons. So although the nervous system doesn't have access to a calculator, it can certainly add and subtract signals.

Return now to the discussion of Figure 6.14,

seeing first how the achromatic system is constructed. In the top panel, solid arrows indicate that the signals generated by M and L cones are added together. We can refer to the pathway carrying this sum to the brain as a *channel* (a set of nerve fibers bearing a common message). Activity in this *achromatic channel* depends on the total excitation of M and L cones. There are various reasons for imagining that activity in this channel determines an object's visibility. For example, the shape of the photopic sensitivity curve (closely related to visibility) can be predicted by taking a sum of M and L cone responses (Werner, Cicerone, Kliegl, and DellaRosa, 1984). Note that by adding together M and L cone signals, this achromatic channel actually discards the wavelength information that it rece ves.

Turn now to the two chromatic channels in

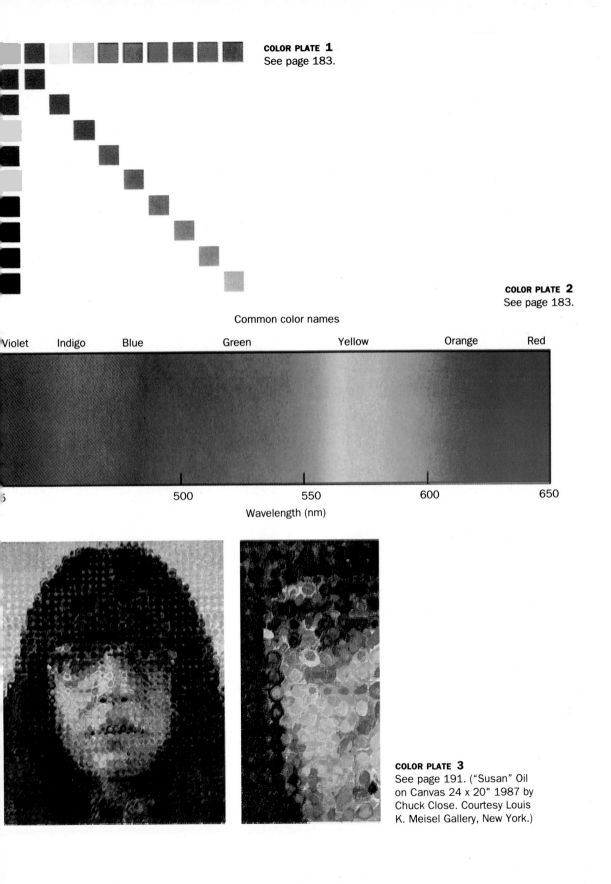

COLOR PLATE **1**
See page 183.

COLOR PLATE **2**
See page 183.

Common color names

Violet   Indigo   Blue   Green   Yellow   Orange   Red

500   550   600   650

Wavelength (nm)

COLOR PLATE **3**
See page 191. ("Susan" Oil
on Canvas 24 x 20" 1987 by
Chuck Close. Courtesy Louis
K. Meisel Gallery, New York.)

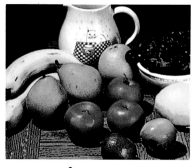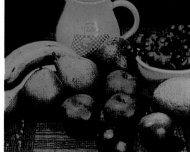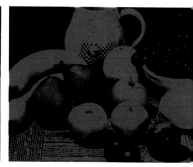

COLOR PLATE 4
See page 192. (Glen Cloyd)

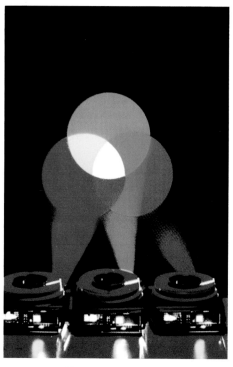

COLOR PLATE 5
See page 195.

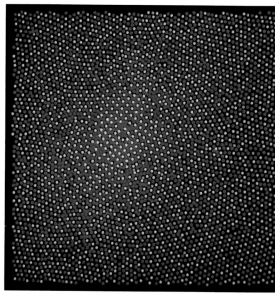

COLOR PLATE 6
See page 198. (Courtesy of David Williams.)

COLOR PLATE 7
See page 199.

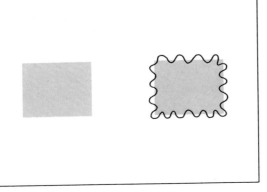

COLOR PLATE 8
See page 200.

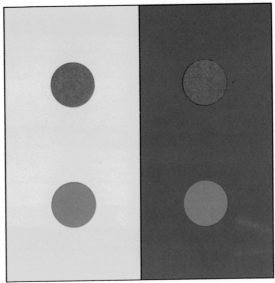

COLOR PLATE 9
See page 202.

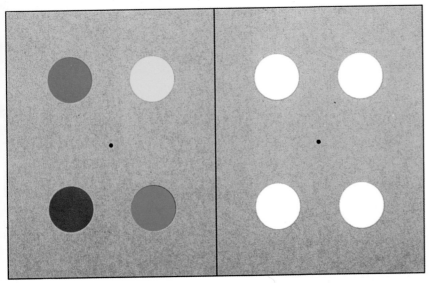

COLOR PLATE 10
See page 202.

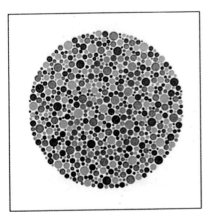
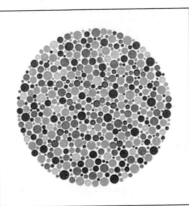

COLOR PLATE 11
See page 210. (Ishihara
Color Blindness Test
Charts. Exclusively
distributed by Graham
Field, Inc. Hauppauge,
New York.)

COLOR PLATE **12**
See page 210.

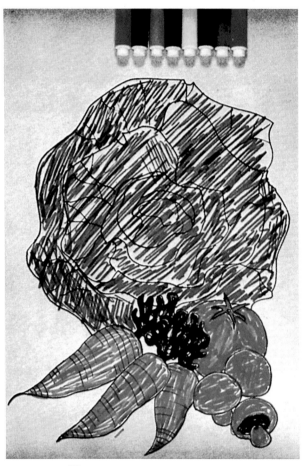

COLOR PLATE **13**
See page 213. (Courtesy of Alan J. Pearlman, M.D.)

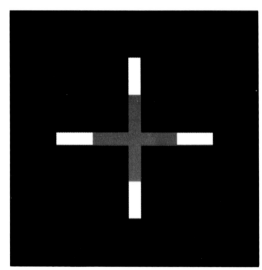

COLOR PLATE **14**
See page 233.

Figure 6.14. According to the diagram, one of these channels represents the *difference* between S cone signals, on the one hand, and the *sum* of M and L cone signals, on the other. This channel is referred to as the *blue-yellow channel* because it signals the difference between short-wavelength stimulation and stimulation throughout the rest of the spectrum. The other chromatic channel, the *red-green channel,* signals the *difference* between stimulation of the M cones, on one hand, and stimulation of both S and L cones, on the other hand.

To appreciate the implications of Figure 6.14, consider how the various channels might respond when an eye is stimulated by white light, which, as you know, contains a broad spectrum of wavelengths. Such light could stimulate M and L cones to the same degree. As a result, the difference between their signals would be zero, resulting in no signal in the red-green channel. This would be true regardless of the intensity of the light. White light would be similarly ineffective for the blue-yellow channel, because such light excites both of its contributors equally well. Note, however, that the achromatic channel, which adds responses from M and L cones, would be excited by white light. In fact, the more intense this light, the greater the response in that achromatic channel.

The scheme outlined in Figure 6.14 gives a straightforward explanation of a puzzling observation mentioned earlier in this chapter. Recall that hues drawn from the region near the middle of the spectrum (yellow) appear less saturated than hues drawn from the ends of the spectrum (blue and red). But why should one hue look more saturated than another? The scheme in Figure 6.14 gives a simple answer. A hue will appear desaturated (washed out) if it produces a strong response in the achromatic channel and at least some response in one of the chromatic channels. Note that if light produces a response in the achromatic channel but none in either chromatic channel, it will appear completely desaturated— white or some shade of gray. In contrast, a highly saturated hue results when a strong chromatic response is accompanied by a weak achromatic re-sponse. In general, the perceived saturation produced by light of any wavelength can be predicted straightforwardly by taking the ratio of the chromatic response it evokes to the achromatic response it evokes. For example, yellow will be relatively desaturated, because it elicits only a weak chromatic response while at the same time eliciting a strong achromatic response.

OPPONENT PROCESSES AND EFFICIENCY OF CODING

Many lines of evidence—behavioral, physiological, and anatomical—show that key attributes of color vision flow from its opponent-process organization. But one wonders what purpose is served by such a complex scheme. Although questions about the purpose of biological processes can never be truly answered, it is worth at least speculating about the possible advantage vision gains from sorting signals into opponent streams.

Think first about the relations among the three types of cones found in the normal human eye. Because their absorption spectra overlap so much (see Figure 6.13), the cones will yield similar, though not identical, responses under many conditions. Computing the theoretical response of each cone to various representative natural objects, one discovers that responses of the cones are very highly correlated. The correlation is especially strong between the responses of M and L cones. So, under most circumstances, the nervous system gets little more information from analyzing both M and L cone signals than it would have gotten from analyzing just one. Because the nervous system has limited transmission and processing capacity, this considerable redundancy represents significant waste. But what are the alternatives? Theoretically, how could the redundancy be reduced?

To answer this question, Buchsbaum and Gottschalk (1983) analyzed statistically the responses generated by human cones in an eye viewing various natural scenes. From the responses, the analysis derived a scheme that would minimize redundancy and allow the fibers in the optic nerve to carry as much color information as possible from retina to the brain. The analysis revealed that a truly efficient arrangement would take the responses of the three cone types and convert those responses into three others; the converted signals, rather than the original ones, would be fed to the brain. The best possible scheme turned out to be very much like the opponent-process system that we've been describing. When alternative designs are compared, the scheme illustrated in Figure 6.14, however complex it may seem, actually does make the best possible use of the biological hardware available.

THE PHYSIOLOGICAL BASIS OF OPPONENCY

Various details of the scheme in Figure 6.14 have been established by careful psychophysical studies (see Boynton, 1979, for a good summary). But how does the nervous system accomplish the adding and subtracting implied by opponency? To seek an answer to this question, let's return to the LGN, described in Chapter 4.

Russell DeValois studied cells in the lateral geniculate nucleus. Working with monkeys, he found that cells in the LGN could be divided into two major groups: nonopponent and opponent (DeValois aand DeValois, 1975). Let's consider each group in turn, starting with the nonopponent.*

When light was shown on the retina, some nonopponent LGN cells responded by increasing their activity (ON cells), while others responded by decreasing their activity (OFF cells). Cells of the ON type gave ON responses to all wavelengths, though more strongly to some wavelengths than to others. Similarly, OFF cells gave OFF responses to all wavelengths, but again in varying strengths. Together, such cells could constitute the achromatic channel represented in Figure 6.14.

Cells of the opponent type behaved differently.

In this group, any cell could give either an ON response *or* an OFF response, depending on the wavelength of light. For example, some of these cells would increase their responses when long-wavelength light was present but decrease their responses when short-wavelength light was present. The opposite pattern was also found: reduced response with long-wavelength light and increased response with short-wavelength light. When light contained *both* long and short wavelengths, the ON and OFF responses tended to cancel each other and the cell gave little response. As far as the cell was concerned, the light never appeared.

If a cell gives an ON response in one portion of the spectrum and an OFF response in the other portion, there must be some transition wavelength at which the response changes from ON to OFF. DeValois found that opponent cells could be divided roughly into two groups, according to their transition wavelengths. For one group the transition occurred between the portion of the spectrum called green and the portion called red. Hence DeValois called these cells **red-green cells.** For the other group, the transition occurred between the portion of the spectrum called blue and the portion called yellow. DeValois called these **blue-yellow cells.** Note that these two groups of cells link different regions of the spectrum in an opponent fashion. Such linkages could be the realization of the red-green and blue-yellow opponent channels schematized in Figure 6.14.[†]

---

* Primate retinas also contain both spectrally opponent and spectrally nonopponent cells (Gouras and Zrenner, 1981). Presumably these retinal ganglion cells are the origin of the opponent and nonopponent LGN cells studied by DeValois.

† Some researchers question whether all opponent cells can be put into just two distinct categories (Zrenner, 1983). Moreover, you should note that DeValois's experiments were performed by uniformly illuminating an LGN cell's receptive field with lights of different wavelength. Recall from Chapter 4, though, that each LGN receptive field is divisible into spatially distinct center and surround regions. More recently, physiologists have discovered that in some LGN cells, the center region of the receptive field responds best to one wavelength of light, while the surround region responds to a very different wavelength. So the color opponency derived by DeValois is really combined with the spatial opponency defined by the center/surround layout of the receptive field. Their spatially organized color opponency makes these cells ideal contributors to color contrast (Lennie, 1984).

We've already seen that the interplay between opponent and nonopponent channels can account for the way in which wavelength controls brightness and saturation. The interplay between these channels can account for other important phenomena of color perception, too (DeValois and DeValois, 1975). Using DeValois's results, consider some of these in detail. The curves in Figure 6.15 summarize some of DeValois's data. The curve labeled R represents the average response of red-green opponent cells to longer-wavelength light. Note that in such cells the response begins at about 600 nanometers and grows with increasing wavelength. The G curve represents the average response of these same red-green opponent cells to shorter-wavelength light. Curves Y and B represent the responses of yellow-blue opponent cells to longer and shorter wavelengths, respectively. How might these curves relate to color perception?

The simplest idea is that each curve corresponds to one particular color experience. For example, the G curve might correspond to the greenness evoked by various wavelengths. To examine the possible correspondence between the curves and color experience, let's consider the results of a color-naming experiment. Boynton and Gordon (1965) asked people to name the color of briefly flashed lights whose wavelength varied randomly across the spectrum. To help quantify these color names, people were asked to use only the names "blue," "green," "yellow," "red," and various combinations of these names—such as "yellow-red" (meaning a red that was tinged with yellow). The results are shown in Figure 6.16. The horizontal axis shows the wavelength of light, and the vertical axis shows the tendency to use a given color name in describing that wavelength. For example, the "green" curve reflects the use of the term "green" to describe color experience. Note that "green" is used to describe wavelengths ranging from about 470 to 600 nanometers. Toward the shorter-wavelength portion of this range, "green" is modified by the term "blue"; in the longer-wavelength portion of the range, "green" is modified by the term "yellow." At about 510 nanometers, the light is described solely as "green" (the "green" curve reaches its maximum at 510 nanometers). The use of "yellow" peaks at about 580 nanometers, and the use of "blue" at about 460. Note that the "red" curve consists of two segments—one at the right (longer wavelengths) and one at the left (shorter wavelengths). This is quite understandable, since very short wavelength light appears violet, a hue that can be produced by mixing blue and red.

Note the general correspondence between Boynton and Gordon's color-naming results (Figure 6.16) and DeValois's physiological results from opponent cells in the monkey (Figure 6.15).

FIGURE 6.15 Responses of different LGN cells to light of various wavelengths. (Adapted from DeValois & DeValois, 1975.)

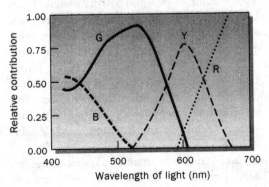

FIGURE 6.16 Proportion of trials on which different color names are assigned to various wavelengths.

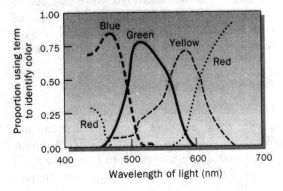

The use of the name "green" by humans seems to correspond quite well to the response of the red-green opponent cells to shorter-wavelength light—the G curve in Figure 6.15. Similarly, the use of the name "yellow" resembles the Y curve in that figure. The correspondence is suggestive, but less satisfactory, between the use of the name "blue" and the B curve. Finally, at long wavelengths, the name "red" corresponds quite well to the R curve. However, the occasional use of the name "red" at short wavelengths has no counterpart in the way DeValois's cells responded. Nevertheless, there is, overall, a suggestive correspondence between color naming and the responses of opponent cells. Remember, though, that the LGN represents an intermediate stage in the neural pathways signaling color information (recall the P pathway discussed in Chapters 3 and 4), so it would be incorrect to conclude that color naming is handled exclusively by the LGN. Rather, the LGN imposes an opponent organization on color processing that is passed on to higher stages and eventually reflected in our responses on perceptual tasks.

The general correspondence that we've just seen between physiology and color naming suggests that the major color categories—blue, green, yellow, and red—may be defined by the visual nervous system. If this were true, all people with normal visual systems would agree on these four color categories. Alternatively, the correspondence between physiology and color naming could be coincidental. According to this view, the consistency of color naming might simply reflect how people learn to use the words "blue," "green," "yellow," and "red." We can decide which view is correct by examining the use of color categories by infants not old enough to have learned the association between colors and names.

COLOR "NAMING" BY INFANTS

Do infants categorize colors, and if so, how? To answer these questions Bornstein, Kessen, and Weiskopf (1976) determined whether 4-month old infants divide the spectrum into color categories. As we've seen before, special techniques are needed to study perception in preverbal infants. The technique Bornstein and his colleagues devised capitalized on the fact that infants, like adults, get tired of looking at the same thing. When first shown some color, an infant looks at it intently. But when the same color is repeatedly presented, **habituation** occurs—the infant loses interest and looks away. Bornstein assumed that an infant would habituate not only to the very color it had been looking at but to other, similar colors as well. With this assumption in hand, Bornstein used habituation to infer whether infants categorize colors in the same way adults do.

Each of Bornstein's tests used three different wavelengths, for example 480, 450, and 510 nanometers. In this case, the infant would first see the 480-nanometer light. After an initial period of fascination with the light, the infant would lose interest. Once the infant had habituated to this 480-nanometer light, Bornstein determined whether the infant's interest could be rekindled by either the 450- or the 510-nanometer wavelength. Note that in *physical* terms, both of these lights are equally different from the 480-nanometer habituation light. However, in *perceptual* terms, they are not equally different. When viewed by adults, the 450-nanometer light falls in the same color category (blue) as the 480-nanometer habituation light, whereas the 510-nanometer light (green) does not. Evidently infants have the same blue-green categories as adults: the infants showed renewed interest in the 510-nanometer light but ignored the 450-nanometer light. In other words, the infants reacted as if the 450- and 480-nanometer lights fell in the same category, and the 480- and 510-nanometer lights fell in different categories. Similar tests were made for the other color categories. In all cases, these preverbal infants categorized colors in the same way that adults do, separating colors into "blue," "green," "yellow," and "red." Recent studies of adults and children in other cultures agree: these same four hue categories are of paramount importance (Uchikawa and Boynton, 1987; Zollinger, 1988). So, Japanese's "ao," "midori," "ki," and "aka" do not merely translate English's "blue," "green," "yellow," and "red"; terms in each set represent principal categories of hue. These cross-cultural results plus Bornstein's findings with preverbal infants make one believe that color categories *are* determined by the inherent nature of the nervous system, not by some arbitrary, learned scheme (Lumsden and Wilson, 1983).

ABNORMALITIES OF COLOR PERCEPTION

COLOR DEFICIENCY

Not everyone sees color in the same way. Tests of color vision expose individual variations in color perception, which take several forms, including some that are considered normal variations—subtle, functionally insignificant differences among individuals. More striking, though, are variations in which color vision deviates dramatically from the norm. People with such variations are described as "color deficient" (popularly called "color blind"). Consideration of color deficiency enhances understanding of normal color vision and also reinforces Newton's idea, mentioned earlier, that "the rays . . . are not coloured."

Color deficiency takes many different forms and can be either congenital or acquired during an individual's lifetime. The prevalence of congenital color deficiency varies among populations. For example, 8 out of every 100 Caucasian males, 5 out of every 100 Asiatic males, and only 3 out of every 100 black and Native American males are color deficient. In addition, within these groups the incidence of color deficiency is much lower in females than in males—for instance, Caucasian females are 10 times less likely to be color deficient than are males (Hurvich, 1981, p. 267).

Although color deficiency has probably been around for millions of years, the first recorded descriptions of the problem do not appear until the end of the eighteenth century. Among the first reports of color deficiency was one made by the English scientist John Dalton late in the eighteenth century. You may recognize Dalton's name—because he developed atomic theory, the unit of molecular weight is named in his honor. Since he was a person of considerable distinction, his description of his own "shortcoming" was all the more interesting. Dalton wrote of himself:

I was always of the opinion, though I might not mention it, that several colours were injudiciously named. . . . All crimsons appear to me to consist chiefly of dark blue: but many of them seem to have a tinge of dark brown. I have seen specimens of crimson, claret, and mud, which were very nearly alike. Crimson has a grave appearance, being the reverse of every shewy and splendid colour. Woolen yarn dyed crimson or dark blue is the same to me. (1798/1948, p. 102)

Although a keen observer of his own experiences, Dalton had a very mistaken idea of the origin of his abnormality. He reckoned that the vitreous humor of his eye was the wrong color, thus tinting his vision. A postmortem dissection of Dalton's eyes was performed on his instructions. Sadly, the results demolished Dalton's own theory posthumously (Sharpe and Nordby, 1990).

There are several reasons why color deficiency such as Dalton's went unnoticed for so long. First, the common forms of color deficiency are not dramatic. Rarely are people completely colorblind—in the sense that they can't see colors at all.* Rather, they do see color but in a way that differs from the norm. Second, many people simply don't notice that their use of color names differs from that of other people. Third, most color-deficient people manage to compensate for their deficiency. For example, people who cannot distinguish reds from greens may still know when to stop or go on the basis of which light—top or bottom—is lit in a traffic signal. Also, a person who confuses reds and greens may be able to distinguish a red shirt from a green one because they differ in lightness (Jameson and Hurvich, 1978). Sometimes, though, lightness differences

---

* One vision scientist, Knut Nordby (1990), with no color vision whatever gives an excellent personal account of his experiences and attempts to cope with a world devoid of color.

are not adequate substitutes for color. John Dalton, in fact, learned this to his dismay. A Quaker, Dalton was supposed to wear subdued clothing, preferably black. As a result, his friends were shocked when he paraded around in his crimson academic robes, believing that they were black.

Because color and lightness normally covary, special test materials must be designed so that lightness does not provide a clue to color. These tests consist of several sets of dots that differ only in hue, not in brightness. As a result, unless a person can distinguish the color of the numeral from the color of the background, the numeral will be invisible. For example, when the numeral is red and the surround is green, people with normal color vision will be able to identify the numeral but people who confuse reds and greens will not. This set of colors would detect only people who had one particular kind of color deficiency, one involving red-green confusions. To detect forms of color deficiency involving other confusions, the numeral and its surround would have to be made of some colors other than red and green.

Color Plate 11 shows a selection from one common type of test of color deficiency. Look at the Plate and note the digit or digits that you see. In the left panel of the Color Plate, people with normal color vision see the numeral 8; people with red-green deficiency see the numeral 3. In the right panel of the Color Plate, normal observers see "16" while most people with red-green deficiency see dots but no digits.

Now let's consider the origins of the color deficiencies themselves.

CONGENITAL COLOR DEFICIENCY

In most forms of congenital color deficiency, the eye has the normal number of cones, but it behaves as though it had fewer than three *types* of cone pigments. In fact this is exactly how Helmholtz explained color deficiency. We've already noted that an eye containing just two types of cones would be *dichromatic*. This means that the eye would require just two different wavelengths

to match the appearance of virtually any other wavelength. Since the normal, trichromatic eye—one with three types of cones—requires three different wavelengths to make such matches, many matches that are satisfactory to the dichromatic eye are unsatisfactory to a trichromatic one. For example, to a dichromat who is missing L cones, all three rectangles in Color Plate 12 appear to be of the same color. Unless you are that same type of dichromat, the rectangles won't look even vaguely alike.

Although genetic mistakes can eliminate any one of the three cone types, they more typically eliminate either M or L cones, not the S cones. When either M or L cones are missing, the red-green channel (see Figure 6.14) is also eliminated. As a result, middle and long wavelengths will tend to be confused with each other. However, all these wavelengths will be distinguishable from short wavelengths, since a modified form of the blue-yellow system remains functional. Dichromatic color deficiencies caused by the absence of either M or L cones are lumped together under the title *red-green deficiency*. This, incidentally, is the form of dichromacy John Dalton had. In the rarer form of dichromacy, S cones are missing. This disturbs only the blue-yellow chromatic channel, leaving the red-green channel intact. The scheme in Figure 6.14 implies, and data confirm, that in this rare deficiency, lightness perception is unaffected (since S cones make no contribution to perceived lightness anyway), and discriminations among middle and long wavelengths are normal (since the red-green channel is unaffected).

People categorized as dichromats make another kind of color confusion suggestive of a two-cone eye. We pointed out earlier that eyes with only two cone types should experience a neutral point in the spectrum, a single wavelength that looks white. People with dichromatic color vision show precisely such neutral points. However, the wavelength at which the neutral point occurs varies with their form of dichromacy. For example, the spectral location of the neutral point for an eye missing L cones differs from the neutral point for an eye missing S cones.

Besides these relatively rare color deficiencies, there are more common color abnormalities that we haven't mentioned yet. People with one of these common abnormalities have color vision that is an unusual form of trichromacy. These people are not dichromats; their spectrum shows no neutral point, and matches that satisfy dichromats fail to satisfy them. Since they require three separate lights to match virtually any hue they can see, their color perception is trichromatic. However, their color matches will not look satisfactory to someone with normal trichromatic vision. Because here color vision is trichromatic but anomalous, the condition is termed *anomalous trichromacy*. The anomaly probably stems from the fact that one of their three cone types has a decidedly abnormal absorption curve (Dartnall, Bowmaker, and Mollon, 1983).

Figure 6.17 summarizes the discussion to this point, giving the technical names for various forms of color abnormality, the color confusions associated with each, and prevalence rates in North America and Western Europe (Alpern, 1981).*

CONGENITAL SUPERNORMALITY?

The relative rarity of color-blind females is an important clue to the genetics of color vision, both normal and abnormal. Sex-linked inheritance, such as we find in color vision defects, implicates the X–chromosome. Molecular biological studies, mentioned earlier, confirmed this idea and have filled in many details. This same work raises an intriguing possibility, namely that some among us may actually possess color vision that is superior to the normal trichromatic variety.

---

* There are other forms of color deficiency, too. In a few rare cases, a person seems to lack two or even all three classes of cones. Since they don't illuminate the basis of color perception any more than the cases we've already considered, we'll say no more about them. Nordby (1990) provides an autobiographical account of the everyday challenges created by such a condition.

FIGURE 6.17 Major genetic color deficiencies.

NAME	CAUSE	CONSEQUENCES	PREVALENCE
DICHROMACIES			
Protanopia	Missing L-type pigment	Confuses 520–700 Has neutral point	M: 1.0% F: 0.02%
Deuteranopia	Missing M-type pigment	Confuses 530–700 Has neutral point	M: 1.1% F: 0.1%
Tritanopia	Missing S-type pigment	Confuses 445–480 Has neutral point	Very rare
ANOMALOUS TRICHROMACIES			
Protanomaly	Abnormal L-type pigment	Abnormal matches Poor discrimination*	M: 1.0% F: 0.02%
Deuteranomaly	Missing M-type pigment	Abnormal matches Poor discrimination*	M: 4.9% F: 0.04%

Note: "M" indicates males; "F" females. Wavelengths that are confused are given in nanometers. An asterisk (*) means that only some members of this group exhibit this problem.

Although a female has two X-chromosomes, one inherited from each parent, a male has only one X-chromosome, which he inherits from his female parent. Earlier we noted that anomalous trichromacy involves errors in the production of photopigments that are coded by genes on the X-chromosome. As a result, a male anomalous trichromat had to inherit the anomaly from his mother, who must have had an abnormal gene on one of her X-chromosomes. Suppose that her other X-chromosome was normal, in other words, that it instructed the manufacture of normal M and L pigments. What can we say about the color vision of this female, who has one normal and one anomalous X-chromosome?

Early in any female's embryonic development, half her X-chromosomes are permanently inactivated (Gardner and Sutherland, 1989). Which X-chromosomes get shut off in any cell seems to be random. But once an X-chromosome is inactivated, throughout the female's life that same X-chromosome is mute in every descendant cell. Inactivation serves an important developmental function. With twice as many X-chromosomes as males, females also have twice as many X-linked genes—and, potentially, instructions to produce twice as many X-linked proteins. Inactivation of half the X-chromosomes, then, maintains parity between the sexes.

Let's return to the mother of the anomalous trichromat. Random inactivation would, in different cells, turn off half her normal X-chromosomes and half her anomalous ones. Because different embryonic cells give rise to photoreceptors in disparate retinal regions, her retina would resemble a mosaic of different tiles, with normal regions interspersed among anomalous regions. Taking account of both normal and anomalous patches, overall her retina has four different photopigments: S, M, L, and an anomalous pigment whose absorption peak was some compromise between M and L cone peaks.

To date, no truly appropriate psychophysical technique exists for studying the color vision of females who may have four cone pigments. But Mollon (1990) has speculated on the visual and evolutionary significance of such color vision.

Quite possibly, their color vision is as superior to the "normal" variety as the "normal" variety is to the color vision of a dichromat. Four-pigment color vision, described as *tetra*chromatic, might give certain females a real biological advantage, making it possible for them to recognize subtle color differences that so-called normals, male or female, could not. These tetrachromatic females might even be supernormal mothers because their extra-good color vision might enable them to spot subtle complexion changes when their children were becoming ill. But, Mollon conjectures, tetrachromatic vision's real evolutionary advantage would have come when our ancestors hunted for food. On such hunts, their superior color vision might have made valuable tribal leaders of these tetrachromatic females. It would have been they who guided the tribe toward sought-after ripening fruit on the trees of those prehistoric forests.*

ACQUIRED COLOR ABNORMALITIES

All the color abnormalities considered so far are genetic in origin. But not all color vision problems are genetic; some fairly common ones are *acquired*. Since normal color perception depends on a whole series of neural events—starting in the retina and continuing back to the brain—disturbance in any part of the chain can alter color perception. We'll consider just a few kinds of acquired color abnormalities here; for a full discussion, see Birch et al. (1979).

Ocular Disorders. Some diseases—such as glaucoma and diabetes—affect the integrity of S cones, thereby disturbing color vision (Adams, Zisman, Rodic, and Cavender, 1982). Diabetes often changes the structure of the eye in ways that can be seen using an ophthalmoscope. Abnormalities of color vision usually precede these structural changes in the eye. Consequently, color

---

* Thompson, Palacios, and Varela (1992) give an excellent treatment to several issues in color vision, including differences among color vision in various species and how evolution has shaped those differences.

vision tests may be helpful in the diagnosis and treatment of glaucoma (Sample, Boynton, and Weinreb, 1988) or diabetes (Zisman and Adams, 1982).

In both diseases, changes in color vision are retinal in origin. In other cases, however, acquired abnormalities of color vision can be caused by disturbances in the optic nerve rather than in the retina. For example, alcoholics frequently exhibit a reduced sensitivity to long wavelengths, causing reds to appear dark and desaturated. This change in color vision reflects a dietary deficiency—the typical alcoholic doesn't get sufficient vitamin B_{12} in his or her diet to ensure proper optic nerve function. Supplements of B_{12} restore normal color vision. Besides alcohol, certain toxins such as carbon disulfide (a substance used in the manufacture of insecticides and rubber) can disturb color vision. In each of these conditions, the onset of abnormal color vision can serve as an early warning of a threat to health.

Though the above forms of acquired color deficiency are relatively rare, there is another form that affects nearly everyone sooner or later. Once people reach about 50 years of age, the crystalline lens of the eye begins to accumulate a yellow pigment. The pigment in the lens tends to absorb short-wavelength (blue) light and transmit the rest. It may well be that this pigment serves a useful function by screening out ultraviolet radiation that could damage the already fragile retinas of older people. However, because short wavelengths have been filtered out, the color of the world appears different when seen through an older, more yellow lens. Blues look darker and they tend to be confused with greens (Weale, 1982). The tendency of older people to confuse some blues and greens can have serious consequences. For example, a yellowed crystalline lens could cause someone to mistake one type of medicine tablet or capsule for another (Hurd and Blevins, 1984).

Cortical Color Blindness. Recall from Chapter 4 that different cortical areas are thought to be concerned with specific aspects of vision, such as color and movement. Selective damage to just one of those areas produces an equally selective visual dysfunction. What follows is an abbreviated history of one individual in whom damage to the cerebral cortex produced substantial color vision deficiency. This case is particularly interesting because the damaged region has been pinpointed using modern brain-scan techniques. (A detailed description of this case has been given by Pearlman, Birch, and Meadows, 1979.)

The patient was a man in his mid-fifties who prior to his illness had been a customs inspector. To get that job, he had taken a color vision test, which he had passed without difficulty. Following a stroke, he was examined on several occasions, each time complaining that he couldn't see colors. He likened the problem to watching a black and white movie. Although his general health and cognitive abilities remained sound, he was forced to take another job that did not require color judgments. In addition, his deficient color vision interfered with his daily routine. For instance, he had to rely on his wife to select his clothes, so as to avoid wearing weird color combinations, and he was unable to distinguish ripe from unripe fruit.

Following his stroke, this man retained good memory for colors, as evidenced by his ability to associate objects and colors. When shown a black and white outline drawing of familiar objects, he could readily say what color each *should* be. But when he attempted to color the outline drawing using felt-tip pens, he was unable to select the appropriate colors. An example of his results is shown in Color Plate 13. This page from a children's coloring book was colored (8 years after his stroke) using the pens shown in the upper part of the picture. He needed 30 minutes to complete this effort, with most of his time spent comparing the various pens before selecting one. Despite the obvious color confusions evidenced in this picture, the man confidently stated that tomatoes should be red, carrots orange, and so on. He wasn't sure, though, whether he had actually selected the appropriate colors.

Other, more formal tests confirmed that this person possessed very poor color discrimination over the whole spectrum. In this respect, his performance differed from that of people with congenitally defective color vision. Congenital color blindness usually involves color confusions within a restricted region of the spectrum; in all likelihood, these forms of color blindness stem from a deficiency in a particular cone photopigment. Because it is congenital, the condition is present throughout an individual's lifetime. In contrast, the person described here had perfectly normal color vision prior to his stroke. Moreover, the stroke affected only his perception of color—acuity and depth perception remained normal. This indicates that the brain damage resulting from the stroke occurred within a region specialized for analyzing color information. Brain-scan pictures from this patient reveal damage within a region just in front of the primary visual cortex. In monkeys, the prestriate cortex includes a physiologically identified area containing a large number of cells that can be activated only if stimulated by lines or edges of particular colors (Zeki et al., 1991).

S U M M A R Y   A N D   P R E V I E W

In this chapter we noted how ideas about color vision have developed over the past 300 years. We described the mechanisms of color vision, emphasizing that wavelength of light is first analyzed by three spectrally broad and widely overlapping cone photopigments and that the outcome of that analysis is then fed into chromatic and achromatic visual channels.

Unfortunately, science's success in explaining *how* people see color tends to obscure *why* they see color. Probably, the ability to perceive color developed to help creatures detect and discriminate objects in their environment. Because objects—artificial as well as natural—have characteristic pigments, they absorb and reflect light in characteristic ways. These patterns of spectral reflection make it advantageous to have color vision. An animal whose visual system retains information about the wavelength distribution of reflected light can usually tell where one object begins and another ends. Moreover, that wavelength information enables the animal to recognize what sort of object it has encountered and what action is called for. In the next chapter we discuss depth perception, still another property of vision that helps creatures appreciate the objects around them.

K E Y   T E R M S

achromatic system	composite light	Newton's color circle
additive color mixture	detection	nonspectral colors
afterimages	dichromatic	pure light
blue-yellow cells	discrimination	red-green cells
brightness	habituation	saturation
chromatic systems	hue	spectral colors
color constancy	metamers	subtractive color mixture
color contrast	microspectrophotometry	trichromatic
color deficiency	monochromat	univariance principle
complementary	neutral point	Young-Helmholtz theory

Depth Perception

T he previous two chapters dealt with aspects of visual perception—form and color—that define *what* an object is. In many instances, though, you need to do more than just identify an object. Often you must react to it in a specific way, such as reaching for it or avoiding it. Every time you drive a car, you're judging the distances from you to other vehicles. These judgments must be made rapidly and automatically; usually you cannot take the time to calculate these locations and distances consciously. The same type of judgment is required numerous times a day—for instance, when crossing a street in traffic or reaching for a pen on the desk. Reacting quickly and accurately requires knowing *where* the object is located in three-dimensional space. In other words, you need to know how far the object is from you, an ability usually referred to as **depth perception,** and the direction in which it is located relative to yourself, which is called **egocentric direction.** Some creatures, such as bats, can use their ears to pick up information about direction and distance (Griffin, 1959), but for humans, the most reliable sources for this information are visual ones.

EGOCENTRIC DIRECTION

Egocentric direction refers to the location of an object in the environment relative to the perceiver's current position; it can be specified in a two-dimensional coordinate system, where the two dimensions refer to up/down and left/right. Be-

cause this coordinate system is referenced to a person, the center of the coordinate system corresponds to the line of sight. Thus when you stare at, or fixate, an object, that object's location defines "straight ahead" (see Figure 7.1). Now, this two-dimensional layout of objects in the world is maintained in the images those objects form on the back of the eye—images of objects maintain their locations relative to one another.* In other words, all the up/down and left/right information in the two-dimensional egocentric coordinate system is preserved in the two-dimensional retinal image.

Now, recall from Chapter 4 that the mapping of the retina onto the cortex is topographic, meaning that neighboring regions on the retina are represented in neighboring regions of the cortex. As a result, the two-dimensional relations among objects in the world are maintained in the neural representations of objects in the visual cortex. Thus neural activity among cortical neurons devoted to the fovea specifies the direction "straight ahead," and other egocentric directions are simply registered by activity among neurons whose receptive fields are displaced in the topographic cortical map relative to the foveal representation. Of course, objects situated to the left of the center of gaze create neural activity in the

---

* In fact, the retinal image is inverted, with objects in the upper part of the visual field forming images on the lower part of the retina, and vice versa. But relative positions are strictly maintained—the inverted image maintains all the two-dimensional positional information present in the real world.

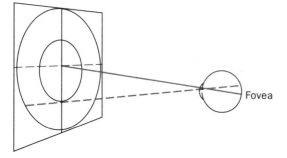

Fovea

FIGURE 7.1 Egocentric direction can be specified in a two-dimensional coordinate system, with the observer's center of gaze defining the center of the system.

right hemisphere, and vice versa (recall Figures 4.1 and 4.2).

So registering the egocentric directions of objects—up/down and left/right—relative to the current object of regard seems fairly straightforward. This two-dimensional information about direction is inherent in the topographic cortical map. But as you will now learn, representing information about the third dimension—depth—is far from simple.

DEPTH PERCEPTION: THE THIRD DIMENSION

It is remarkable that human beings are able to make distance judgments at all, let alone accurate ones. The retinal images from which depth information is extracted are two-dimensional, as we just discussed; they are inherently depthless. To dramatize this idea, imagine that we could take a photograph of the image falling on the back of the eye at a single instant in time. Like an individual frame in a motion picture, this photograph would consist of a complex distribution of contour and color. But all this information would be constrained to lie within the two-dimensional boundaries of the retinal image—depth is absent.

Fortunately for us, this photographic analogy is misleading. Unlike a photograph, the retinal

image is continuously changing, because of the observer's movements and because of movements of objects in the environment. These changes provide a rich source of depth information missing in a static snapshot. The photographic analogy also ignores the fact that the brain acquires depth information from *two* sources, the left eye and the right eye. Binocular vision affords another useful source of depth information.

Sources of information about depth are sometimes referred to as *cues* to depth. Following convention, we too shall speak of "cues" to depth, but don't misunderstand what we mean by this term. It does not mean that depth perception results from conscious deliberation on your part; to see objects in depth, you don't use cues like a detective trying to solve a mystery. On the contrary, despite its origins in a two-dimensional image on the retina, depth perception occurs automatically and effortlessly.

Accurate judgments of distance arise from the coordination of several different sources of information. In the normal environment, these various sources of depth information usually operate in harmony, yielding an unambiguous impression of three-dimensional space. But in the laboratory, it is possible to place cues in conflict, to study the relative potency of some cues relative to others. And in some instances, conflicting cues yield interesting visual illusions which provide insight into the normal operation of depth perception.

Before surveying the depth cues, we need to clarify precisely what is meant by "depth perception," because this term can be used in two quite different ways. In one case, the term refers to the distance from an observer to an object. This is sometimes called **absolute distance.** Consider an example drawn from the sport of baseball: an outfielder attempting to throw out a base runner must judge the distance between himself and the base where the runner is headed. Shooting a basketball also entails judgments of absolute distance. Alternatively, the term "depth perception" may refer to the distance between one object and another or between different parts of a single object. This is known as **relative distance.** When you place the cap on a ballpoint pen, you make a judgment involving relative distance. Distinguishing between these two types of depth perception is important because they differ markedly; the ability to judge absolute distance, while behaviorally useful (Rieser, Ashmead, Taylor, and Youngquist, 1990), is much less precise than the ability to make judgments about relative depth (Graham, 1965).

With this distinction in mind, we are now ready to explore the various cues to depth that are used by the visual system. We have divided these into two broad categories, **oculomotor cues** and **visual cues.** The oculomotor cues are actually *kinesthetic* in nature, meaning that the cue itself derives from the sensation of muscular contraction; this cue would be something like the feeling experienced when you tighten your fist. The visual cues, so called because they are genuinely visual in nature, are subdivided into those that are available only when two eyes are used (*binocular cues*) and those that are available when just one eye is used (*monocular cues*). Figure 7.2 summarizes the ways in which these types of cues to depth are related. As you will see, oculomotor cues are the only ones that provide unambiguous information about absolute distance, meaning that an oculomotor cue does not require supplementation by other cues. In contrast, any of the visual cues can provide good relative depth information, but they must be supplemented with other information in order to specify absolute distance.

OCULOMOTOR CUES TO DEPTH

As described in Chapter 2, whenever you are looking at, or fixating, an object, your eyes are focused and converged by an amount dependent on the distance between you and that object. To be seen clearly, close objects require more accommodation and convergence than do objects farther away from you. Now suppose we were able to attach tiny gauges to the two sets of muscles involved in these two reflexes, strain gauges that could tell us how much the muscles were contracted (see panel A of Figure 7.3). By monitoring the degree of muscular contraction, we could compute either of two values: your angle of **convergence** or the amount of **accommodation** of your eyes. And because these two values are related to the distance between your eyes and the object you are viewing, we would then have a useful index of absolute distance. In other words, by monitoring your eye muscles, *we* could compute the distance from you to the object of regard. But before this same information could serve as a cue to depth for *you,* your visual nervous system would have to be able to sense the contractions of your eye muscles.

It is simple to show that convergence is accompanied by a sense of muscle strain. Starting with your index finger held up at arm's length, steadily move it toward your nose while keeping both eyes focused on it. As your finger moves closer to

FIGURE 7.2 Major sources of depth information.

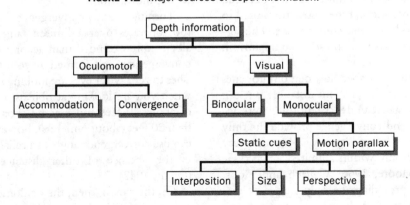

A

Accommodation
strain gauge

Convergence
strain gauge

B

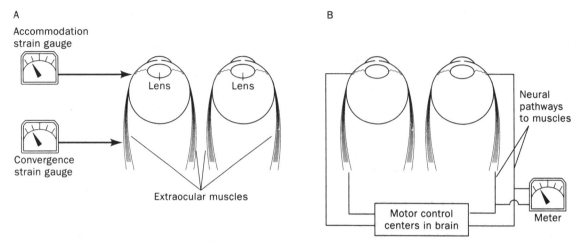

Neural
pathways
to muscles

Extraocular muscles

Motor control
centers in brain

Meter

FIGURE 7.3 Two possible schemes for registering oculomotor information.

your nose, you can feel the increased strain as your eyes turn inward to maintain fixation. At the same time, your accommodation is increasing too; the lens attempts to keep the image of your finger in sharp focus on your retina. In fact, these two motor responses—accommodation and convergence—usually operate in a yoked fashion, such that changes in one are accompanied by changes in the other.

There is potentially another source of information about the degree of accommodation and convergence. We could insert some measuring instrument along the neural pathway leading to the eye muscles (see panel B of Figure 7.3). Now we would be recording the strength of the command signals being *sent* to those muscles. In effect, we would be monitoring the instructions used to steer accommodation and convergence. The signals flowing out to your muscles could furnish information about distance.

So far we have described how oculomotor cues *could* furnish information about distance. But can people judge distance under conditions where accommodation and convergence provide the only cues to depth? The answer is yes, but not very accurately and only within a limited range (Leibowitz and Moore, 1966; Wallach and Floor, 1971). When providing the only source of distance information, do *both* cues—accommodation

and convergence—contribute equally? To answer this question, let's consider the two cues individually, starting with accommodation.

In accommodation, you have a cue whose potential effective range is necessarily limited. Whenever you focus on an object more than a few meters from you, the muscle controlling accommodation assumes its most relaxed state. So as a potential depth cue, accommodation would be useful only within the region of space immediately in front of you. Even within this small range, distance judgments based solely on accommodation are inaccurate (Heinemann, Tulving, and Nachmias, 1959; Künnapas, 1968). So we can dismiss accommodation as an effective source of depth information.

Turning next to convergence, we find that it, too, operates over a limited range of distance, albeit more extended than accommodation. The convergence angle formed by your two eyes vanishes to zero (your eyes are looking straight ahead) when you are looking at objects from a distance of about 20 feet and beyond. For distances less than 20 feet (about 6 meters), however, observers can use convergence angle as a reliable depth cue, in the absence of other distance information (Grant, 1942).

On their own, then, the oculomotor cues play only a restricted role in depth perception. In fact, people rely much more heavily on the so-called visual cues to depth. It is to those cues that we now turn, beginning with the cue provided by looking at the world through two separate eyes.

BINOCULAR VISUAL DEPTH INFORMATION: STEREOPSIS

Chapter 2 pointed out that in humans, the two eyes look at much the same region of visual space; only near the margins of the visual field do the two eyes provide exclusive monocular coverage. This overlapping binocular field of view comes about because the two eyes are located in the front of the head. Within this region of binocular overlap, the two eyes view objects from slightly different vantage points, owing to the lateral separation of the two eyes within the head. We are now ready to consider the perceptual consequences of this binocular arrangement.

To begin, why did nature position human eyes in such a way as to provide two views of the world, thereby duplicating a significant portion of those views? The answer seems clear. By virtue of the slight differences, or *disparities,* between the view seen by the left eye and the view seen by the right eye, humans are able to discriminate extremely small differences in relative depth, differences that are very difficult to discriminate using either eye alone. You can demonstrate this for yourself by performing the following simple experiment.

Take two sharp pencils, one in each hand, and hold them at arm's length. Their tips should be separated by 10 centimeters or so (about 4 inches) and pointed toward each other. Now slowly bring the two pencils together in such a way that the two points are touching. First try this several times with one eye closed, each time noting by how much, if any, the two miss each other. Next, repeat the exercise with both eyes open. You will probably find your accuracy much improved with binocular viewing. However, not *all* individuals benefit from using both eyes—some 5 to 10 percent of the general population do no better with

two eyes than they do with one. Why? The answer is given later in this chapter.

The perception of relative depth from binocular vision is called **stereopsis:** this word is derived from a Greek term meaning "seeing solid." Besides allowing you to judge relative depth with great accuracy, stereopsis also makes it possible for you to see objects that are invisible to either eye alone. This aspect of stereopsis is described in Box 7.1 (pp. 222–223). We are now prepared to consider two issues concerning stereopsis: the nature of the stimulus information specifying stereopsis and the nature of brain process responsible for registering that information. Let's consider each problem separately.

RETINAL DISPARITY

The two eyes look at objects in the world from slightly different angles. As a result, those objects, particularly those relatively close to you, do not appear exactly the same to your left eye and to your right eye. Ordinarily, however, you are unaware of any differences between the left eye's view and the right eye's view. This is because the brain combines information from the two eyes in a way that obscures these differences. Only by looking at something alternately with one eye and then the other can you actually notice the differences between the two eyes' views. You should take a moment to perform this simple exercise. Choose some object in front of you and look at it steadily using one eye and then the other. You should be able to see more of the left side of the object with your left eye while seeing more of the right side with your right eye.

While looking alternately through your two eyes, also pay special attention to the position of the object you are looking at and compare it with the position of another, neighboring object that is located a little closer to you than the one you are looking at. To make this comparison, you may want to arrange some objects on a table. Alternatively, you can simply hold up your two index fingers in front of you at different distances from your nose. Either way, you will now see that the lateral separation between the two objects appears to change when you switch eyes. Figure 7.4 illustrates this observation. These two photographs mimic the views seen by two eyes looking at a real scene from slightly different vantage points. These photographs were taken in succession, shifting the camera sideways by 65 millimeters (the typical distance between the two eyes) before taking the second photograph. Note that the separation between the two bottles is larger in the left-hand picture than it is in the right-hand picture. This comes about because the two bottles were located at different distances from the camera at the time these pictures were taken. The difference in lateral separation between objects as seen by the left eye and by the right eye is called **retinal disparity;** it provides information for stereoscopic depth perception.

The magnitude of the disparity, expressed in terms of lateral separation on the retina, depends on the distance between objects. If one object is much closer to the observer than the other, the resulting retinal disparity will be large. If one object is only slightly closer to the observer than the other, the disparity will be small. Figure 7.5 illustrates this geometrical principle.

This cue to depth, retinal disparity, arises whenever objects are located in front of *or* behind the object you are looking at. Of course, you can tell visually whether an object is nearer or farther than your point of fixation, which means that your visual nervous system distinguishes between the disparities produced by these two possibilities—objects nearer versus objects farther away. If an object lies farther from you than the object you're fixating, the disparity between the two is said to be *uncrossed*. If an object is located closer to you than the one you are looking at, the disparity is said to be *crossed*. To remember this distinction easily, just keep in mind that with crossed disparity you would need to converge, or *cross*, your eyes in order to look directly at the nearer object. By the same token, you would diverge, or *uncross*, your eyes to shift your fixation to a more distant object.

So the type of disparity, crossed versus uncrossed, specifies whether objects are in front of or behind the point of fixation, while the magnitude of the disparity specifies the amount by which objects are separated in depth. It is important to remember that retinal disparity specifies

FIGURE 7.4 The lateral separation between two objects as it might appear to the left eye and to the right eye. (McGraw-Hill photo.)

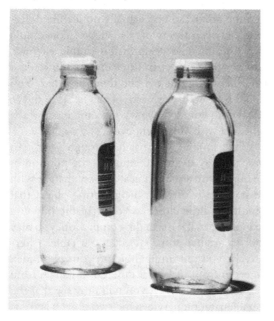
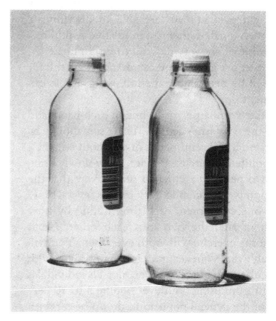

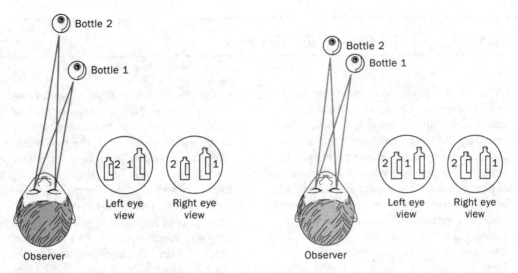

FIGURE 7.5 Retinal disparity increases with the distance, in depth, between two objects.

the *relative* depth between two or more objects; it does not provide information about absolute depth. When you fixate a single small spot in an otherwise empty field of view (such as the glow of a cigarette in a dark room), there is no disparity information to be used—only the convergence angle of your eyes (an oculomotor cue) provides binocular information.

Objects in the visual field can also be situated so that they give rise to zero disparity—a disparity that is neither crossed nor uncrossed. In other words, the lateral separation between the objects seen through the left eye will be identical to the separation between those objects seen through the right eye. As you should be able to deduce, zero disparity occurs when two or more objects are located at the same distance from the observer. An example of this situation is illustrated in Figure 7.6. In this case, the two bottles were located at the *same* distance from the observer. Images from such equidistant objects are said to fall on corresponding areas of the two eyes.*

* There are actually several alternative ways to specify retinal correspondence, but for our purposes, the definition based on depth is the most appropriate.

The foveas of the two eyes represent one set of corresponding retinal areas. Whenever you look directly at an object, an image of that object will be formed on the fovea of your left eye and on the fovea of your right eye; in this case, we say that the images fall on corresponding retinal areas. In addition, there are numerous other sets

FIGURE 7.6 Zero disparity occurs when two objects are located at equal distances from the observer.

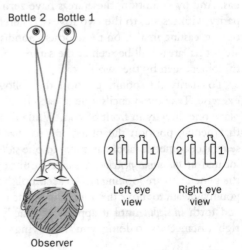

Box 7.1 *Cooperation Between the Two Eyes*

Of all visual abilities, none excels the keenness of stereopsis. Using binocular disparity information, humans are able to make exceedingly fine depth judgments that are simply impossible when using just one eye. To illustrate, imagine that you are viewing a pair of pencils oriented vertically and placed side by side 1 meter away from you. At that distance, stereopsis would make it possible for you to tell whether one pencil was as little as 1 millimeter closer to you than its neighbor. From a distance of 1 meter, a 1-millimeter difference corresponds to a judgment accuracy of one-tenth of 1 percent. In this case, the resulting disparity between the two eyes' views is less than 0.0004 millimeter. This distance is many times smaller than the diameter of a single visual receptor in your eye!

Because of this extraordinary resolving power, stereopsis provides a very effective means for uncovering slight differences between a pair of pictures presented separately

to the two eyes. For instance, imagine viewing a pair of $1 bills in a stereoscope (the familiar device used for presenting two pictures, one to each eye). If the two bills are identical down to the smallest detail, the resulting percept will be a single, absolutely flat bill; there will exist no disparity to differentiate the two. But if the two bills differ, even slightly, portions of the single, combined percept will appear to stand out in relief, as a result of retinal disparity produced by the slight differences. This stereoscopic technique has been used for identifying counterfeit currency, as well as for comparing small details in such things as the electronic circuits in computers.

Stereopsis also provides an effective means for detecting camouflaged objects. Two views of a visual scene taken from different vantage points can reveal the presence of forms that are invisible from either vantage point alone. As an example, aerial photogra-

of corresponding retinal areas. Whenever you nas. And by definition, these areas have zero disparity with respect to the two foveas. Therefore, objects casting images on these other, nondisparate retinal areas will be seen at the same depth as the object seen by the two foveas.

To clarify this point, perform the following exercise. Take two pencils, one in each hand, and place one directly in front of you. While fixating that pencil, position the other one so that it is several centimeters (about an inch) to one side but located *at the same perceived distance* from you as the pencil you are looking at. To accomplish this, you may want to move the nonfixated pencil back and forth *in depth* until it appears at exactly the right distance. By so doing, you are varying retinal

disparity between uncrossed and crossed until you settle on what amounts to zero disparity. If you are very careful, the second pencil will be placed so that it, too, casts left and right eye images on corresponding retinal areas. If you were to repeat this exercise, now repositioning the nonfixated pencil farther to one side of the point of fixation, you could generate another point at which the nonfixated pencil appeared to lie the same distance from you as the fixated pencil. In so doing, you would have established another zero-disparity location. If you repeated this exercise a number of times, all the resulting zero-disparity locations could be connected to form an imaginary plane called the **horopter** (see Figure 7.7). So long as you maintain fixation on some point in this plane,

phy of a landscape from two positions can disclose the presence and location of objects (such as military hardware) on the ground. Stereopsis can also help a predatory animal spot its next meal even when the color and texture of the meal blend into the environment.

A most dramatic example of the sleuthlike powers of stereopsis is provided by random-dot stereograms (an example of which can be seen in Figure 7.8). Each eye's view consists of a random array of dots, with no hint of an object hidden therein. Yet, when the brain combines the two views, a figure in depth emerges. The technique used to create this kind of stereogram is simple (it is described in the text). In contrast, the technique used by your brain to extract depth from such a stereogram must be quite complex. For this reason, you may be surprised to learn that infants as young as 4 months of age can see the depth in random-dot stereograms (Fox, Aslin, Shea, and Dumais, 1980). Moreover, this form of stereopsis is not unique to humans.

Monkeys (Bough, 1970), cats (Lehmkuhle and Fox, 1977), and falcons (Fox, Lehmkuhle, and Bush, 1977) show evidence of being able to discriminate the depth portrayed in random-dot stereograms.

If you are interested in experiencing this illusion of depth for yourself, several books provide stereograms as well as special glasses to help you view the stereograms (Julesz, 1971; Frisby, 1980). The visual system seems to have to learn to see depth in these random-dot stereograms, particularly those portraying complicated surfaces, with many hills, valleys, and curlicues. Upon first viewing a stereogram, you may need several minutes of concentrated viewing to see depth. During this time, the previously hidden surfaces appear to grow, slowly rising out of the page. Moreover, it is impossible to speed up this process by telling or showing a person what to look for (Frisby and Clatworthy, 1975). However, just as with riding a bicycle, once you learn to see depth in one of these stereograms, you never completely forget how.

all objects located anywhere in the plane produce images on corresponding, or nondisparate, retinal areas. Objects closer to you than this plane yield crossed disparities, whereas objects farther from you than this plane yield uncrossed disparities.

This, then, is how retinal correspondence and retinal disparity are related to binocular depth perception. Considering that the geometry of this situation is relatively straightforward, it is surprising that it took so long before anyone fully appreciated that disparity supplied information about depth. From his writings, it is clear that Leonardo da Vinci realized that the two eyes see slightly different portions of a solid, three-dimensional object, but he offered no descriptions of the detailed geometry of crossed and uncrossed dis-

parity and no demonstrations of stereopsis. It remained for a British physicist, Charles Wheatstone (1838/1964), to provide the first perceptual proof that a vivid impression of stereoscopic depth could be created from two flat pictures (Wade, 1988). His demonstration took the following form. On two cards Wheatstone sketched a pair of outline drawings of a three-dimensional object. One drawing depicted the view of the object as seen by the left eye and the other drawing depicted the view of the object as seen by the right eye. He then looked at this pair of two-dimensional drawings using a **stereoscope,** a device Wheatstone invented to present the two drawings (which together constitute a *stereogram*) separately to the two eyes. He observed that the two drawings of the

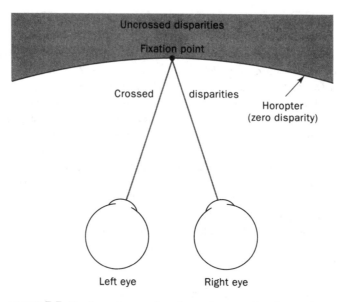

FIGURE 7.7 The horopter—an imaginary plane marking the positions of all objects located at the same perceived distance from the observer. Objects more distant than the point of fixation are said to produce uncrossed disparities (shaded area), whereas objects nearer than the point of fixation are said to produce crossed disparities (unshaded area). (The degree of curvature of the horopter plane varies somewhat with absolute viewing distance, for technical reasons we need not go into.)

object were seen as one. In addition, that one drawing conveyed an amazing sense of relief, or three-dimensionality. Thus by incorporating retinal disparity into his drawings, Wheatstone was able to re-create the three-dimensional appearance of an object—an effect that is lost in a single, two-dimensional picture. Wheatstone's novel observations demonstrated the potency of retinal disparity in producing depth perception.

So far, we have focused on stereopsis from a geometrical perspective. You have learned that objects nearer or farther than the plane of fixation project their retinal images on disparate regions of the two eyes. You have also learned that by mimicking these disparities in a stereogram (a pair of pictures), it is possible to create realistic stereoscopic depth artificially. Having defined the cues from which stereopsis *might* arise, let's consider what the visual system would have to do in order to utilize this depth cue of retinal disparity.

MATCHING THE LEFT AND RIGHT EYES' VIEWS

Imagine for a moment that you are a machine, facing the same predicament that your brain normally encounters. Handed two slightly different pictures (retinal images) portraying various objects, you must re-create the way in which those objects are actually laid out in depth. To do this, you must use only the information contained in the two pictures. How would you proceed? Since there is a connection between objects' relative distances from one another and their disparate positions in the two pictures, you might first compute these disparities. This computation requires that you compare the two pictures, noting in each where particular objects are located. Before you could perform that computation, you would have to figure out which portion of one picture matched which portion of the other. Only then would it be possible to measure the positional disparities between the two pictures.

This exercise indicates that stereopsis really involves two steps: first, matched features must be identified in the two eyes; second, the magnitude and direction (crossed versus uncrossed) of the retinal disparities between those features must be calculated. Let's consider these two steps in turn.

First, to match features in the two retinal images, you must decide what constitutes a feature. On the basis of intuition, the most plausible candidate would seem to be some recognizable form, or pattern, appearing in both of the pictures. For instance, if one's view included your roommate's face, it would be a simple matter to locate that face in the other eye's view. According to this idea, each eye's image is analyzed separately, and the two are then brought together for purposes of matching recognizable features. However, this idea cannot be entirely correct, for there are instances where stereoscopic depth can be perceived from stereograms that contain no recognizable objects whatsoever. An example of one of these **random-dot stereograms** is shown in Figure 7.8. These intriguing stereograms were first developed by Bela Julesz (1971).

Both halves of this stereogram consist of nothing more than an array of black and white dots. The two halves are identical with one exception. In one of the halves of the stereogram, a central subset of dots has been shifted laterally by several rows, as is illustrated schematically in the middle panel of Figure 7.8. This lateral displacement creates a retinal disparity between the two halves, in much the same way as would a speckled square held in front of an identically speckled background, as depicted in the bottom panel of Figure 7.8. Because the texture in the stereogram is completely random, it is impossible to pick out from either half of the stereogram alone which area will appear in depth when the two halves are viewed simultaneously.

Think for a moment about the confusing job confronting the brain in trying to sort out the depth in this jumble of dots. Because each half of the stereogram is made up of nothing more than a random array of tiny dots, there are numerous dots in one eye's view that would match up with any single dot in the other eye's view. Yet the brain does manage to find a satisfactory match between the two pictures, as is evidenced by the vivid illusion of depth produced by these pairs of random textures.

Thus random-dot stereograms disprove the theory that stereopsis results from an analysis of monocularly recognizable forms such as your roommate's face. But if not monocular forms, then what monocular features *does* the visual system match in order to compute disparity? Think back to Chapter 5, where you learned that form perception initially involves analyzing a figure's orientation and size, or spatial frequency. The same features are involved in stereopsis, too. The evidence favoring this idea is rather complicated, so we are going to mention just a couple of relevant studies here. More thorough discussions of feature matching and stereopsis can be found in Blake and Wilson (1991).

It is possibe to remove certain spatial frequencies from random-dot stereograms such as the one shown at the top of Figure 7.8; this process of removal is called *filtering*. When high spatial frequencies are removed from both halves of a stereogram, the dots are no longer sharply defined but instead appear blurred. Still, the phantom figure is easily seen to stand out in depth. By the same token, if just low spatial frequencies are removed from both halves of a stereogram, depth may still be experienced. But if high spatial frequencies are removed from one half of the stereogram while low spatial frequencies are removed from the other, stereopsis is abolished. Instead, the two halves undergo **binocular rivalry,** such that only one picture or the other is visible at any one moment (see Box 7.2, pp. 228–229). John Frisby and John Mayhew (1976) have devised several filtered stereograms of this sort, and the demonstrations are conclusive: for stereopsis to be experienced, the spatial-frequency content of the two halves of a stereogram must overlap at least partially.

These and similar findings (Julesz and Miller, 1975) indicate that the brain, to match the two eyes' views, relies on channels that are responsive to limited bands of spatial frequencies. Recall from Chapter 5 that the brain relies on similar

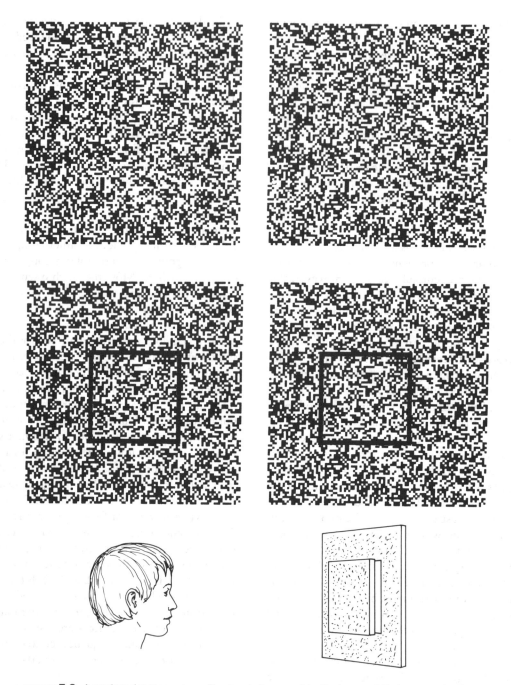

FIGURE 7.8 A random-dot stereogram. The two halves are identical, except that a central subset of dots has been shifted laterally. (The middle panel outlines the section of shifted dots.) This lateral displacement creates retinal disparity and, thus, stereoscopic depth (bottom panel).

channels in form perception. It is not surprising that form perception and stereopsis should utilize the same machinery, since both form perception and stereopsis are designed to distinguish objects from their backgrounds (Marr, 1982). Because of the remarkable human ability to resolve small depth differences stereoscopically, the two eyes together can unearth objects buried in complex visual environments, objects that when viewed monocularly remain hidden from sight. In this respect, stereopsis effectively adds another dimension to form perception.

THE NEURAL BASIS OF STEREOPSIS

So far we have considered the geometry of retinal disparity (the cue for stereopsis) and the matching features that seem to be used in the analysis of retinal disparity. But how does the brain actually do its feature matching and disparity computation? Certainly the entire process is not yet understood, but something is known about the neurobiological hardware involved in the initial stages of stereoscopic vision. Let's take a look at this hardware.

Recall from Chapter 4 that most visual cortical neurons receive input from both eyes, left and right. Each of these binocular neurons gives its largest response when the two eyes view the same stimulus. For instance, a particular binocular neuron that gives its most vigorous response when the left eye sees a vertical contour will respond best when the right eye sees a vertical contour too. The same holds for contour width, or size, as well as for the direction and speed of movement of a contour. In general, binocular neurons respond best when the two eyes view matched features (Hubel and Wiesel, 1962, 1970; Nelson, Kato, and Bishop, 1977; Poggio and Fischer, 1978). This property, then, satisfies one of the requirements for the analysis of disparity information, namely, the matching of monocular features.

Binocular neurons have another property, one that satisfies the second requirement for stereopsis: these neurons are sensitive to retinal disparity. In particular, some binocular cells respond only when their preferred features appear at the *same*

depth plane as the point of fixation. This is because the receptive fields for these binocular neurons are located on *corresponding* areas of the two eyes. These cells, in other words, would respond best to objects giving rise to zero disparity. Activity in such cells would serve to signal the presence of stimuli located *on* the horopter. Other binocular cells respond best to stimuli that are imaged on noncorresponding, or disparate, areas of the two eyes. Cells of this type would be activated by stimuli located at depth planes other than the plane of fixation (Poggio and Fischer, 1978; Ferster, 1981). Refer back to Figure 4.12 to see the layout of the receptive field of one of these so-called **disparity-selective cells.** As noted in Chapter 4, some cells prefer crossed disparities, whereas others prefer uncrossed disparities. Also, the amount of depth (disparity) giving the best response varies from cell to cell.

So it appears that these binocular neurons perform two of the operations necessary for stereopsis, feature matching and disparity computation. But can we be sure that these binocular neurons actually play a role in stereoscopic depth perception? One piece of evidence favoring such a role comes from studying cats who, while kittens, were allowed to see with only one eye at a time; the eyes were stimulated alternately by placing an opaque contact lens in one eye on one day and in the other eye on the next day. This rearing procedure effectively turns binocular neurons into monocular ones (Blakemore, 1976). When tested as adults, these animals were unable to perform binocular depth discriminations that were simple for normally reared cats (Blake and Hirsch, 1975; Packwood and Gordon, 1975). Because they lacked a normal array of binocular neurons, these cats were "blind" for stereopsis.

Recall our earlier comment that some people are stereoblind—unable to perceive depth from retinal disparity. By analogy with the stereoblind cats, we assume that this condition in humans stems from a lack of binocular neurons. Again, there is evidence to back up this assumption. For instance, when tested on the tilt aftereffect described in Chapter 4, stereoblind people show very little interocular transfer—adapting one eye

Box 7.2 *Competition Between the Two Eyes*

Charles Wheatstone, the discoverer of stereopsis, described another intriguing aspect of binocular vision. This second discovery concerned the perceptual outcome when one eye's view differs radically from its partner's view. Wheatstone's interesting observation can best be described by reference to the figure below.

Suppose you were to view these two dissimilar patterns separately with your two eyes in such a way that your left eye saw one set of diagonal lines while your right eye saw the other set. What would be the outcome? If

the two were combined by simply superimposing one on the other, the result would be a sort of checkerboard pattern. Yet when these figures are viewed stereoscopically, thereby allowing your brain to perform the combination, the two certainly do not blend into a single, stable pattern resembling a checkerboard. Instead, a person sees portions of one pattern and portions of the other, the net result resembling a mosaic of the two. Moreover, this mosaic changes over time, as regions of one eye's view replace regions of the other eye's view.

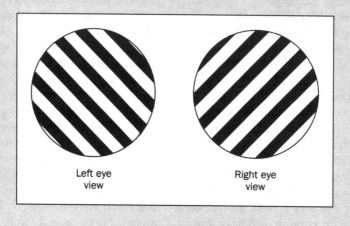

Left eye
view

Right eye
view

has very little effect on judgments of line orientation when the nonadapted eye is tested (Mitchell and Ware, 1974). In contrast, people with good stereopsis show a substantial degree of interocular transfer, which, we assume, results from adaptation of binocular neurons. The meager degree of interocular transfer in the stereoblind individual, then, probably reflects the paucity of binocular neurons in that person's brain.

It has been estimated that the incidence of **stereoblindness** may be as high as 5 to 10 percent in the general population. As a rule, stereoblindness is associated with the presence of certain vi-

sual disorders during early childhood. The most common of these disorders is misalignment of the two eyes, a condition known as **strabismus.** People with this condition are unable to look at, or fixate, the same object simultaneously with both eyes. Consequently, one eye's view rarely corresponds with the other eye's view. To deal with this potentially confusing situation, the brain eventually suppresses one eye's view from visual consciousness, an outcome reminiscent of binocular rivalry. Box 7.3 describes this and similar conditions in more detail.

If left uncorrected, strabismus can lead not

The resulting phenomenon is known as binocular rivalry, an appropriate term in view of the evident breakdown in cooperation between the two eyes. The occurrence of binocular rivalry indicates that the brain, in attempting to put together information from the two eyes, seeks to establish matches between features in the two eyes. When such matches are found, stable single vision and stereopsis result. But when satisfactory matches are impossible, the brain attends to portions of one eye's view at a time, ignoring or suppressing the corresponding portions of the other eye's view as though they were not there.

But how complete is this suppression of information during binocular rivalry? Is a person completely oblivious to new information presented to a region of the eye that is temporarily suppressed? To study this question, investigators have employed a "probe" technique whereby small visual targets (such as a word) are briefly flashed to a suppressed region; the observer's task is to report whether or not the probe target was noticed. The results are conclusive—during suppression, people fail to see targets that would normally be quite visible, including, for example, familiar names (Wales and Fox, 1970; Blake, 1988b). However, the eye is not completely blind to all visual stimulation during suppression. Abruptly increasing the brightness of a suppressed stimulus or suddenly moving it will cause the stimulus to become visible (Fox and Check, 1968; Wiesenfelder and Blake, 1991). Apparently during suppression an eye's overall sensitivity, though reduced, is not totally abolished. Although vision in the suppressed eye is erased from consciousness, some processing of information from that eye continues.

You might wonder what binocular rivalry has to do with normal vision, since ordinarily the two eyes view the same visual scene. Even then, however, the conditions for rivalry can arise. Specifically, when one object partially occludes a more distant object, one eye sees portions of that object that are screened from the other eye's view—there can be, in other words, unmatched image regions in the two eyes' views. As mentioned in the text, this is the geometrical principle first deduced by Leonardo da Vinci, and it has been studied in the laboratory by Nakayama and Shimojo (1990). These investigators provide clever demonstrations that the binocular visual system actually relies on information about interocular mismatches to figure out depth relations among objects.

only to stereoblindness but also to amblyopia—which as you will recall from Box 4.3 is defined as a permanent reduction in the acuity of the eye. Both amblyopia and stereoblindness can be prevented if eye misalignment is surgically corrected early in life. If correction is postponed until school age, the chances for the attainment of normal vision are significantly reduced (von Noorden, 1981; Banks, Aslin, and Letson, 1975).

The discovery of disparity-sensitive cells two decades ago was an exciting first step toward an understanding of the neural basis of stereopsis (Barlow, Blakemore, and Pettigrew, 1967). But, as Nelson (1986) and Blake and Wilson (1991) have pointed out, the existence of disparity detectors leaves a number of questions about stereopsis unanswered. For one thing, the perceived depth resulting from a given disparity depends on the absolute distance from your eyes to the object you are looking at. This can be demonstrated when an observer views a random-dot stereogram, such as the one in Figure 7.8, from different distances. The central square in the stereogram appears to move farther and farther in front of its background as viewing distance increases. This observation indicates that disparity must be sup-

Box 7.3 *Coordination Between the Two Eyes*

Like any other partners, our two eyes have to share the same viewpoint in order to get along. This means that movements of the eyes must be coordinated so that both eyes are always looking in the same direction. As you learned in Chapter 2, the eyes are guided in their movements by twelve extraocular muscles—six for each eye. Because the eye movement system is complex and dependent on fallible parts, things can and do go wrong. Here, we shall consider some of the most common errors and their remedies, emphasizing extraocular dysfunctions that affect perception.

When most people look at an object, the two eyes both end up aimed at that object. For these people, the two eyes fixate together. This binocular fixation depends on the coordinated responses of the extraocular muscles that guide the two eyes. For various reasons, however, some people lack this coordination. For example, if one extraocular muscle is too short, it can exert too much pull on the eyeball, turning that eye in (toward the nose) or out (toward the ear). Chronic deviation of an eye is called *strabismus,* or *squint.* Often this is a congenital condition, which means that an infant may lack coordinated binocular vision early in life. Because strabismic eyes look in different directions, they give the brain conflicting messages, which may result in double vision, or **diplopia** as it is called. Alternatively, the brain may simply ignore, or suppress, one eye's view altogether; in this case, only one eye contributes to vision even though both are open. This latter condition resembles a chronic form of binocular rivalry (see Box 7.2).

Various therapies have been developed for strabismus. In cases where the deviation between the positions of the two eyes is relatively small, visual exercises may help recoordinate the eyes. In more severe cases, surgical

---

plemented by other depth information (Ritter, 1984), perhaps accommodation and/or convergence angle (Foley, 1980). This idea was strengthened recently by a study of disparity-sensitive neurons in Area V1 monkeys. Using random-dot stereograms that monkeys fixated at different viewing distances, Trotter and his colleagues (1992) found that for most individual neurons, disparity-tuning was modulated by the viewing distance at which the stereograms were shown. The precise source of this modulation remains to be identified. We also know that depth from stereopsis can be influenced by other visual cues, such as perceived slant specified by perspective or texture (Stevens and Brookes, 1988), two monocular sources of information about depth discussed later in this chapter.

* * *

This completes our survey of stereopsis, the major source of binocular depth information. Keen as it is, though, stereopsis certainly is not the sole source of depth information. People can successfully perform visually guided tasks, such as landing an airplane (Grosslight, Fletcher, Masterton, and Hagen, 1978), while using just one eye. And you can easily confirm that the world retains a real sense of depth even when one eye is closed. Rather than collapsing into a single, depthless plane, objects in the visual field continue to appear three-dimensional. This is possible because the monocular view of the world contains many sources of information about depth. Let's consider these monocular cues.

correction may be required. This usually involves removing a small portion of one or more of the extraocular muscles and then reattaching the muscles to the eyeball, so that the eyes now line up. This procedure requires a high degree of skill, for altering the muscle by the wrong amount will leave the eyes still misaligned.

Other extraocular dysfunctions are less debilitating and less noticeable. When you do close work such as reading, your eyes must converge—each turns inward by the proper amount. Strong, constant convergence strains the muscles of the eye (Guth, 1981). Some people have difficulty converging their eyes, as you can discover for yourself. Stand facing a friend and ask him or her to keep both eyes on your finger as you move it slowly but directly toward a point between the eyes. Note how well your friend's eyes follow; some people will be able to keep both eyes fixated on the finger until it is within 1 or 2 centimeters of the nose. Others will not be able to follow the finger after it is within 5 or 6 centimeters of the nose. As the finger ap-

proaches, one of their eyes may wander off. If you try this small experiment with several people, you'll be amazed at the individual differences. In addition, when someone is tired or has consumed too much alcohol (Scott, 1979), that person's eyes may be unable to converge normally.

People who have trouble binocularly fixating close objects may experience eyestrain during prolonged reading. Eyestrain, in turn, can cause dizziness, headaches, and nausea, leading to reduced studying and hence poorer grades. Occasionally, college students suffer this kind of problem, called **convergence insufficiency,** while studying for final examinations. Amateur "psychologists" can do great harm by misdiagnosing this condition, thinking it is an aversion to studying or "a need to fail." In fact, the proper treatment is straightforward: spectacles, possibly supplemented with appropriate eye exercises. Reading will then become less of a strain, and higher grades may follow.

MONOCULAR VISUAL DEPTH INFORMATION

Some monocular depth cues are based on principles of geometry; others are based on conditions of atmosphere and illumination. In thinking about these various monocular cues, keep in mind that several of them were initially discovered by artists in their attempts to represent depth pictorially. By the fifteenth century, artists had learned how to create an amazing impression of depth in their works using just a handful of optical tricks. These artists managed to create two-dimensional representations that act upon the visual nervous system in much the same way as would the three-dimensional scenes being depicted. In developing the techniques of pictorial representation, artists ac-

tually discovered the cues of static monocular depth perception. The cues are called *static* because they are available to a stationary observer viewing a motionless scene.

STATIC CUES TO DEPTH

Interposition. When one object occludes, or obscures, part of another from view, as in Figure 7.9, the partially occluded object is automatically perceived as the more distant one. This cue is called **interposition,** and from the standpoint of pictorial representation, it is probably the most primitive. Young children often use interposition in their simple drawings, even though unable to reproduce any other pictorial depth cues. Ac-

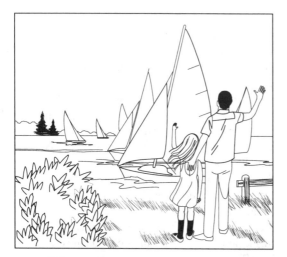

FIGURE 7.9 Interposition: When one object obscures part of another, the obscured object is perceived as the more distant one.

tually, there is evidence that by 7 months of age human infants can judge relative distance solely on the basis of interposition (Yonas, 1984). On the other hand, brain damage during adulthood can abolish a person's ability to judge depth from interposition without affecting the ability to use other depth cues (Stevens, 1983). Interposition is such a strong depth cue that it can override retinal disparity when the two cues conflict (Kaufman, 1974). Moreover, the effectiveness of interposition is amplified when the surface of the occluding object contains high spatial frequency information (Brown and Weisstein, 1988).

Perhaps the most compelling evidence for the potency of interposition are the so-called Kanizsa figures mentioned in Chapter 1; Figure 1.6 showed one example of a Kanizsa figure, and another version is shown in drawing A in Figure 7.10. As you can tell, these are drawings in which one object appears to partially occlude several others even though the boundaries of the nearer object are invisible. In drawing A, an illusory bar appears to have distinct edges where, in fact, none exist, and the entire bar is seen in front of objects that seem to be partially occluded. Descriptively

speaking, the visual system seems to employ a kind of interpolation process whereby separate edges or contours in the same spatial neighborhood are connected *if* this connection can be formed by a simple line or curve and *if* the operation is consistent with the principle of interposition. But how does the visual system make the seemingly complex decision to interpolate an object? There is evidence (Peterhans and von der Heydt, 1991) that this process of interpolation is accomplished by neurons in Area V2 of the visual cortex (recall Figure 4.15). These neurons, unlike those in Area V1, respond not only to real contours (like the bar in drawing B in Figure 7.10) but also to interpolated, illusory contours (like the one in drawing A in Figure 7.10). These V2 neurons perform an interesting new operation—interpolation—not evident in V1 neurons, and this operation involves not only boundary completion but also depth ordering. The illusory figure appears in front of the real figures.

It is also worth noting that objects being occluded by a nearer figure are themselves perceived to be complete, even though we are unable to see

FIGURE 7.10 An illusory bar (drawing A) and a real bar (drawing B), both of which activate neurons in Area V2 of the visual cortex.

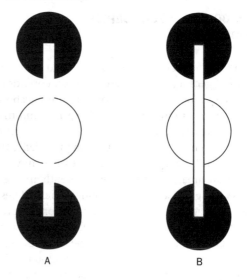

A   B

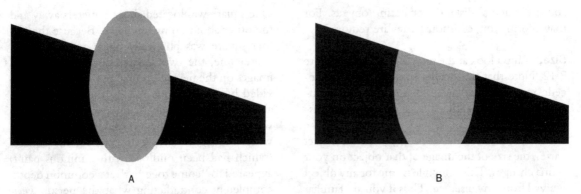

FIGURE 7.11 The drawing on the left (A) looks like a white object partially occluding a darker one. The drawing on the right (B) looks like a dark object with a light region in the middle.

those portions of their surfaces obscured by the nearer object. Thus in Figure 7.10, drawing A, we perceive the pair of black circles as complete, not notched. And in Figure 5.5, we see the girl's entire face uninterrupted by horizontal and vertical gaps. The perception of occluded areas of an object is termed **amodal completion.** How we are able to perceive parts of objects that are occluded is a challenging question (Kellman and Shipley, 1991). Here again the visual system seems to employ an interpolation process to complete the portions of the figure missing in the image.

In discussing interposition, we should touch on **transparency,** the special case where a nonopaque object partially occludes another object. Under these conditions, we perceive the occluded object in its entirety (see drawing A in Figure 7.11). This unitary percept is not really surprising, you might think, because all boundary information associated with the occluded object is physically represented in the image. Yet a perplexing question remains to be answered. Why don't we perceive the more distant object in drawing A in Figure 7.11 like the one in drawing B in Figure 7.11? Why in the left-hand drawing does the lighter area get assigned to the surface of the nearer, semitransparent object? The visual system seems to be assigning surface color based on something like the principle of good continuation, the Gestalt law discussed in Chapter 5. Once

this assignment is made, the arrangement of objects in depth is automatically specified by interposition.

Finally, take a look at Color Plate 14. Here the semicircular red portions at the center of the white cross seem to spread out into the black background, creating a circular, semitransparent "cloud" resting in front of the cross. This illusory migration of color into neighboring regions is called **neon spreading,** since it resembles the glow one experiences when viewing neon light. Neon spreading represents a form of interposition since one perceives a faintly colored surface resting in front of an object (the cross, in this example). Moreover, neon spreading is related to illusory figures, because the spreading color is confined to an area whose shape is insinuated by the semicircular red regions. The boundaries of the shape, in other words, are defined by illusory contours.

All these phenomena—occlusion, amodal completion, illusory figures, transparency, and neon spreading—entail the perception of depth relations among partially overlapping objects (Nakayama, Shimojo, and Ramachandran, 1990). They testify to the role of interposition in depth perception. Despite being a very strong depth cue, however, interposition by itself only specifies whether one object is nearer or more distant than another; it provides no quantitative information about the actual distance separating objects. For that information, additional cues are required.

Size. Take a look at the series of squares in Figure 7.12. Note that the smaller squares appear to recede into the distance, implying that size influences perceived depth. Why should size and distance be related?

As the distance between you and an object varies, the size of the image of that object on your retina changes. This principle is true for any object viewed from any distance. Thus if you are familiar with the size of an object, you can judge from the size of its retinal image how far away the object is. In fact, *familiar size* has been shown to be an effective cue to distance in the absence of other information (Ittelson, 1951). But the cue of retinal image size depends crucially on knowing the correct size of the object. When you are confronted with an unfamiliar object and are provided with no clues as to its true physical size, retinal image size gives you no clear sense of the distance from you to that object. For instance, you may have trouble judging the size of the sculpture pictured in Figure 7.13 and therefore its distance from the camera. But if something familiar appears in the vicinity of that object (such as the dog in Figure 7.14), the perceived size of the unfamiliar object becomes obvious. You are also now able to judge its distance from the camera.

Interestingly, even prior knowledge about the true distance to an object may not be sufficient to support the perception of relative depth. In one study (Gruber and Dinnerstein, 1965), a person was shown a pair of squares in a lighted corridor. One square was located about 8 meters away and the other about 16 meters away. Because the farther square was physically twice as large as the nearer one, the two squares cast the same-sized images on the person's retina, but depth cues provided by the corridor and by the apparatus enabled the person to see clearly that the two squares were located at different distances. However, when the lights were extinguished, the squares (which had been outlined with luminous paint) appeared to "come together" at a common depth, completely contradicting what the person *knew* about their real locations. This demonstration underscores the point made earlier, that depth cues are registered automatically, without conscious deliberation.

So far we have considered size as a determinant of perceived distance. It is just as easy for perceived distance to influence apparent size. When you look at panel A of Figure 7.15 (p. 236), the girl on the right appears to be almost twice as big as the boy on the left. But in fact the two are really equal in size. This compelling illusion stems from the unusual construction of the room. As shown in panel B of Figure 7.15, the left corner of the room is much farther away from the observer than the right corner. The floor-to-ceiling height as well as the sizes and shapes of the windows have been distorted to make the room appear rectangular, and hence normal, when viewed from a location directly in front of the room. The back wall looks perpendicular to the line of sight, with left and right corners appearing equidistant from the viewer. Actually, though, the person on the left is farther away than the one on the right;

FIGURE 7.12 Size alone can influence perceived depth.

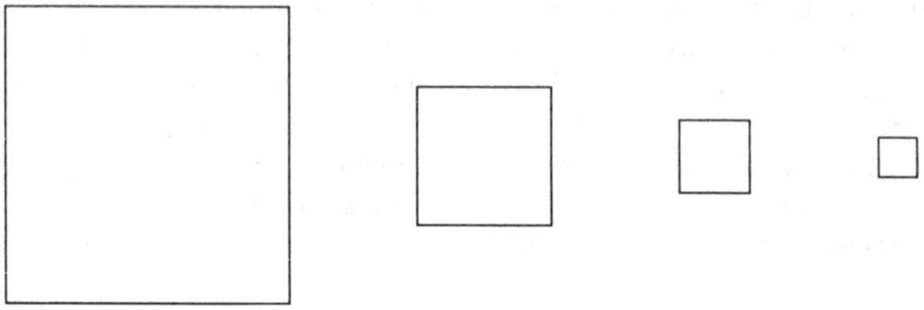

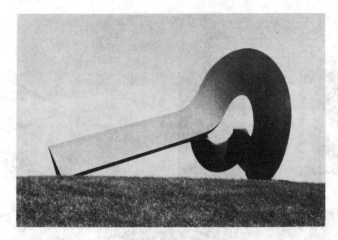

FIGURE 7.13 It is difficult to judge the size of an unfamiliar object in the absence of supporting cues.

the visual angles subtended by the two children are therefore quite different. From your perspective, this must mean that the girl on the right is larger, since you have been fooled into believing that the difference in visual angles is *not* due to a difference in distance. Adelbert Ames, a lawyer turned scientist, devised this clever demonstration of perceived distance's influence on apparent size; in his honor, this sort of distorted structure is called an **Ames room** (Ittelson, 1952/1968).

Besides the Ames room, another visual phenomenon, the moon illusion, vividly demonstrates the interdependence of size and distance. You will have noticed that the moon, especially when full, appears much larger when on the horizon than it does when overhead at its zenith. Of course, the actual size of the moon remains constant, as does its distance from the earth: the moon is 2,160 miles in diameter and 239,000 miles away. This means that regardless of its position in

FIGURE 7.14 The size of an unfamiliar object—and therefore its distance from you—becomes obvious when you see it in the vicinity of a familiar one.

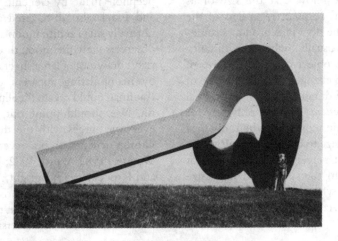

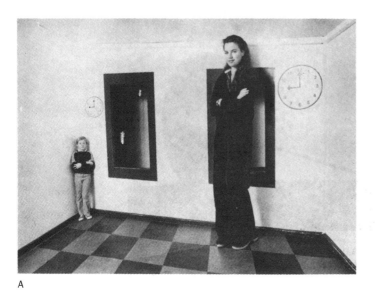

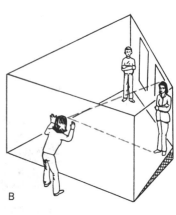

B

A

FIGURE 7.15 The Ames room: A demonstration that perceived distance influences apparent size. (Baron Wolman/Woodfin Camp & Associates.)

the sky, the full moon casts a circular image about one-sixth of a millimeter in diameter on your retina. Why, then, does the apparent size of the moon change so strikingly?

One possible answer is that the moon's **perceived distance** varies with its heavenly position. Near the horizon, where there are many depth cues, the moon seems to be farther away than when it is at its zenith. This idea is illustrated in Figure 7.16. But we know that the size of its retinal image remains constant regardless of the moon's position in the sky. This produces something of a conflict: usually, when the distance from you to a single object changes, the size of the retinal image also changes. Yet, in the case of the moon, perceived distance *changes,* but retinal image size *remains constant.* And the only way for image size to remain constant when distance changes is for object size to change, too. With the moon illusion, when perceived distance is great (moon on the horizon), then perceived object size must be large. But when perceived distance is reduced (moon at its zenith), perceived object size is smaller.

Support for this idea comes from some classic experiments by Lloyd Kaufman and Irvin Rock (1962). They found that the normally large horizon moon shrank as soon as it was viewed through a small hole in a piece of opaque material. Looking at the moon through such a tiny hole eliminated distance cues provided by the horizon. You can easily replicate this finding by viewing the horizon moon monocularly through a small peephole made by clenching your fist. Kaufman and Rock also discovered a way to make the normally small zenith moon appear large: they had observers view the moon through an artificial horizon drawn on a large sheet of clear plastic. Thus by manipulating apparent distance, Rock and Kaufman could create the illusion or make it vanish. We should point out, however, that not everyone agrees with the theory that the moon illusion depends on perceived distance (Baird and Wagner, 1982; Baird, 1982; Iavecchia, Iavecchia, and Roscoe, 1983; Enright, 1989). Perhaps these disagreements are not surprising; after all, people have been speculating about the moon illusion for more than 2,000 years (Hershenson, 1989).

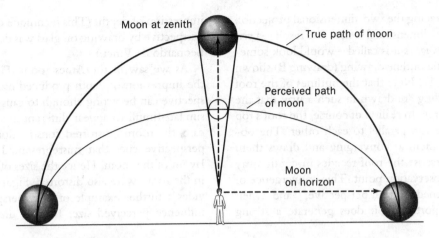

Moon at zenith

True path of moon

Perceived path of moon

Moon on horizon

FIGURE 7.16 Explanation of the moon illusion based on perceived distance.

The Ames room and the moon illusion are just two of many visual illusions involving errors in perceived distance and size. After completing the roster of monocular depth cues, we shall consider these other visual illusions in greater detail.

Perspective. The term "perspective" refers to changes in the appearance of surfaces or objects as they recede in distance away from an observer. The geometry of visual perspective was developed during the fifteenth century by Italian artists, most notably Leonardo da Vinci. Here we are con-

cerned primarily with perspective from the perceptual, not the geometrical, standpoint, so it will not be necessary to discuss the geometry of perspective in any detail. Pirenne (1970) offers a well-illustrated account of that topic.

Let's begin with **linear perspective,** which we shall illustrate with an example. Suppose you were to look out a window at a neighboring building, as depicted in drawing A in Figure 7.17. Now imagine using a marking pen to trace the outline of the building onto the glass windowpane, being careful to hold your head still. You

FIGURE 7.17 A method for generating a perspective drawing.

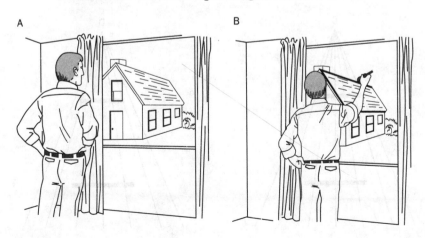

A

B

would be tracing the two-dimensional projection of this three-dimensional scene. The result—a *perspective drawing,* as it is called—would look something like the outline drawing (drawing B) shown in Figure 7.17. Note that the outlines of the roof of the building are drawn in such a way that the lines converge. In reality, of course, the roof's top and bottom run parallel to each other. The observer sees them as converging and draws them this way because the roof recedes in depth away from the observation point. This convergence of lines is termed "linear perspective," and when pictorially portrayed, it does generate a strong impression of depth. (This technique of depicting perspective by drawing on glass was developed by Leonardo da Vinci.)

As we saw in the Ames room (Figure 7.15), the impression of depth produced by linear perspective can be strong enough to cause physically similar stimuli to appear different in size. In that case, the room's distorted construction furnished perspective cues that misrepresented the actual layout of the room. Hence the sizes of the people in the room were also distorted. Figure 7.18 provides a further example of how perspective can influence perceived size. In fact, the perceived

FIGURE 7.18 Linear perspective. In which one of the four perspective drawings (A, B, C, or D) do the two thick horizontal lines appear equal in size? Use a ruler to discover the correct answer. This figure illustrates that linear perspective can cause objects whose sizes are really different to appear identical in size.

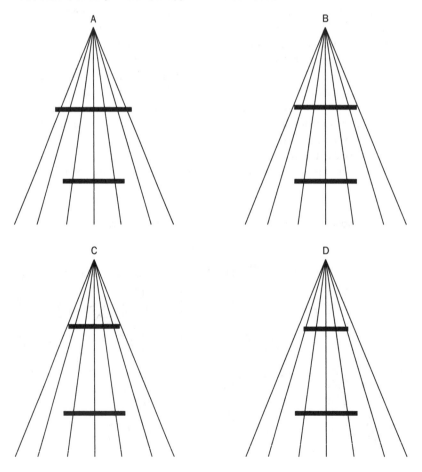

depth implied by linear perspective can be sufficiently robust to contradict depth information conveyed by retinal disparity (Stevens and Brookes, 1988), as mentioned earlier.

There is another consequence of viewing surfaces or planes that recede in depth. Most surfaces have a visible texture, such as the grain in wood or the irregularities in a sidewalk. And so long as a surface is not perpendicular to your line of sight, the density of the surface's texture will appear to vary with distance. Examples of this are shown in Figure 7.19. This form of perspective has been called **texture gradient** by James J. Gibson, the

first individual to underscore the saliency of this source of depth information.

According to Gibson (1950), texture gradients provide precise and unambiguous information about the distances and slants of surfaces, as well as about the sizes of objects located on those surfaces. Gibson also proposed that abrupt changes in texture gradient signal the presence of edges or corners. In Figure 7.20, note that the texture discontinuity implies the presence of a bend, or corner, in a continuous surface. Stevens (1981) provides a detailed description of the geometrical basis for determining distances from texture gra-

FIGURE 7.19 Texture gradients provide information about depth. (Frank Siteman/Stock, Boston.)

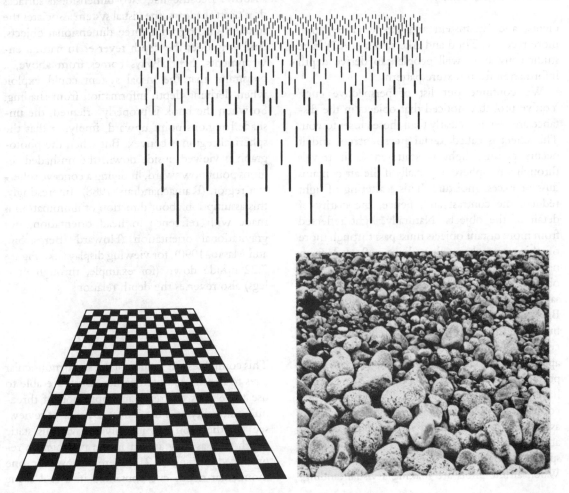

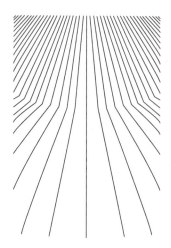

FIGURE 7.20 Texture discontinuity signals the presence of an edge or corner.

dients, and Braunstein and Payne (1969) and, more recently, Todd and Akerstrom (1987) have studied just how well people can derive depth information from texture patterns.

We continue our list of perspective cues. You've probably noticed that objects in the distance are seen less clearly than those closer to you. This effect is called **aerial perspective,** and it occurs because light is scattered as it travels through atmosphere, especially if the air contains dust or excess moisture. This scattering of light reduces the contrast and, hence, the clarity of detail of the objects. Naturally, light reflected from more distant objects must pass through more of this atmosphere than light reflected from nearby objects. As a consequence, more distant objects appear less distinct, or "hazy" as you might say (see Figure 7.21). Laboratory studies (Fry, Bridgman, and Ellerbrock, 1949; O'Shea, Blackburn, and Ono, 1993) show that reductions in the contrast of visual objects cause those objects to appear more distant—reduced contrast from aerial perspective is an effective depth cue. This cue can have perceptual consequences. Upon initially encountering conditions of extremely clean air (such as in the mountains), city dwellers used to looking at the environment through congested atmosphere may seriously underestimate distances. When airline pilots are making a visual landing,

they must constantly take into account the contribution of aerial perspective when judging distance because atmospheric conditions vary greatly.

Last in our list of perspective cues is **shading.** Look at the set of spherical regions in Figure 7.22 (p. 242); you probably see some of them as bumps rising from the background and others as scooped out cavities. When you turn the book upside down, bumps change into cavities and vice versa. This demonstration raises two questions: What gives the spherical regions this three-dimensional quality, and why does the perceived depth reverse when the book is upside down? We'll start with the first question. Depth is perceived because the intensity gradient across each region resembles a shadow. Because flat, two-dimensional surfaces don't cast shadows, the visual system associates the implied shading with three-dimensional objects. And why does the depth reverse? In natural environments, light always comes from above, a constraint that the visual system could exploit when deriving depth information from shading. So when the book is properly oriented, the unshaded regions point upward, implying that the spherical region is convex. But when the photograph is viewed upside down, the unshaded regions point downward, implying a concave spherical region (Ramachandran, 1988). Interestingly, this assumption about direction of illumination is made with reference to head orientation, not gravitational orientation (Howard, Bergström, and Masao, 1990), for viewing displays like Figure 7.22 upside down (for example, through your legs) also reverses the depth relations.

* * *

This completes our catalog of the static monocular cues to depth. As noted earlier, artists are able to use these cues to create an impression of three-dimensionality on a flat canvas. By way of review, see whether you can identify the various static depth cues as they appear in the photograph reproduced in Figure 7.21. There is, however, one monocular depth cue contained in a real scene

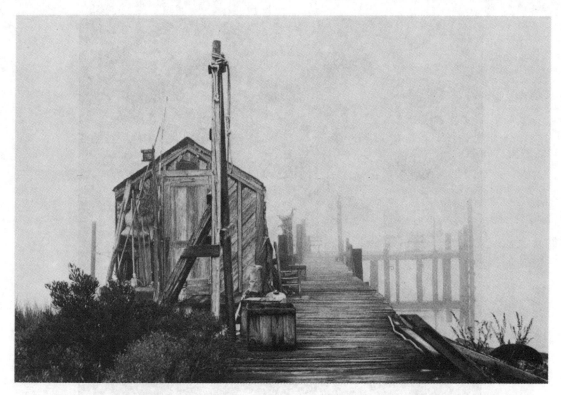

FIGURE 7.21 Try to identify the various depth cues in this photograph, "Relative Depth" by Dennis Markley. (Courtesy of Dennis Markley.)

that an artist can never capture on canvas. We shall consider that cue now.

MOTION PARALLAX

As indicated earlier, depth from static cues can be sufficiently convincing to distort the perceived size of objects. However, these distortions are experienced only so long as you are perfectly motionless. If you are allowed to move your head, the real layout of a distorted room becomes immediately apparent. Motion very quickly dispels any misperceptions that may be conveyed by static cues. This occurs because motion introduces another, very potent source of depth information.

As you move about in the world, objects constantly shift position within your field of view. This happens whenever you are walking, traveling in a car, or simply turning your head to look

at something. Next time you are a passenger in a car, notice how the world appears as you look out the window. Objects closer to you than the spot you're fixating will appear to stream past in a direction *opposite* to the car's movement. More distant objects also seem to move, but at a more gradual speed and in the *same* direction as you are traveling. This complex flow of motion, illustrated in Figure 7.23 (p. 243), is an example of **motion parallax**—the relative apparent motion of objects within your field of view whenever you move—which provides a very effective cue to the relative depth of objects.

To take advantage of this cue, you do not have to move your entire body: you can perceive depth from motion parallax by moving just your head. Take a moment to demonstrate this fact to yourself. Pick out an object in front of you and look at it with one eye closed, thus eliminating the cue

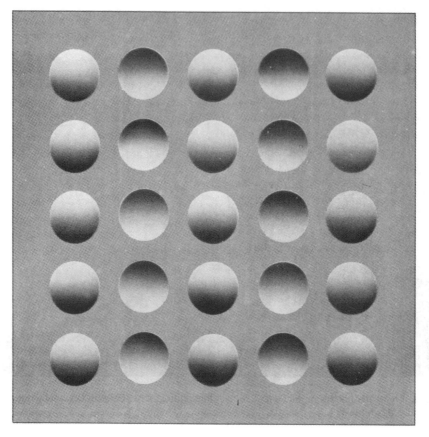

FIGURE 7.22 Shading as a cue to depth. Elements in the left, middle, and right columns appear to bulge out of the background; elements in the remaining columns appear to be cavities. When the book is turned upside down, the bulges become cavities and vice versa. Note that whatever the page's orientation, top-to-bottom shading within an element determines its depth.

of retinal disparity. Now, while continuing to look at this object, move your head back and forth in a sideways direction. Notice how other objects at different distances appear to move in relation to the one you are looking at. To dramatize this effect, hold your two index fingers at different distances in front of you and perform this exercise: again with one eye closed, stare first at the nearer finger and then at the farther one, all the while moving your head back and forth. Again you will see that objects appear to move relative to your point of fixation. The direction and speed of this

motion depends on the distance of those objects from the finger you are looking at.

So far we have discussed situations in which the observer moves and objects in the world remain still. However, motion parallax is also effective in the reverse situation, when a *stationary* observer views a scene in which objects themselves move. For instance, imagine looking with only one eye open at the leaves of a tree. When there is no wind, the still leaves seem to blend into a confusing array. But when stirred to life by a breeze, different groups of leaves stand out clearly

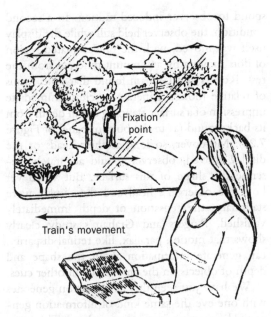

FIGURE 7.23 One situation in which motion parallax provides potent depth information. The arrows indicate the direction of relative apparent motion.

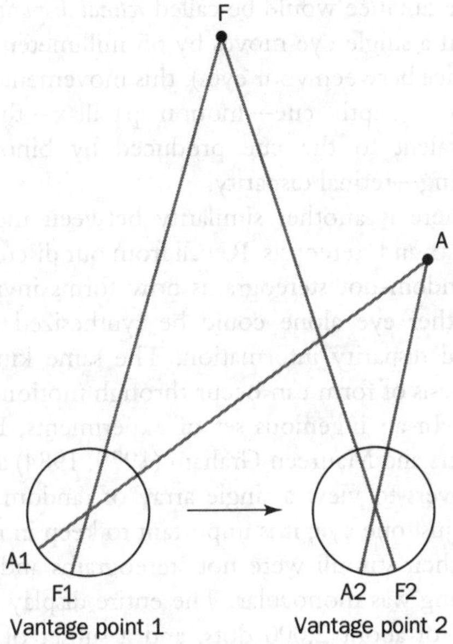

FIGURE **7.24** An illustration of the equivalence of retinal disparity and motion parallax.

in depth from one another. The movement of the leaves creates motion parallax information in the same way that movement of your head would. This creation of depth from motion has been exploited beautifully in some motion pictures. For example, many of the special effects in the *Star Wars* trilogy rely heavily on the cue of motion parallax. Myron Braunstein (1976) has described the various ways in which depth perception can be generated from displays containing movement.

Using motion parallax, observers are quite good at judging whether one object is situated in front of or behind another one. In fact, relative depth judgments based on motion parallax are almost as accurate as those made using binocular disparity (Graham, 1965). This makes sense when you compare the geometrical bases of motion parallax and binocular disparity. Figure 7.24 shows two objects, A and F, being viewed from two vantage points, 1 and 2. Let's assume that fixation is always maintained on object F (for "fixation"). This means that at both vantage points the image

of F will fall on the fovea. Because A is closer than F, the image of A will fall on one retinal area, A1, when A is viewed from vantage point 1; however, when A is viewed from vantage point 2, the image of A will fall on a different retinal area, A2. The distance between the retinal images produced by A and F varies from one vantage point to the other. At vantage point 1, the retinal images are separated by the distance between F1 and A1; at vantage point 2, they are separated by a different amount, the distance between F2 and A2. This variation in the retinal image distance between the images provides information about the distance between objects A and F.

There are two ways the situation shown in Figure 7.24 could arise. Vantage points 1 and 2 could represent the successive positions of a single eye as it moves from 1 to 2. In this case, the resulting variation in retinal image distance would be called *motion parallax*. Alternatively, vantage points 1 and 2 could represent the positions of left and right eyes. In this case, the variation in retinal image distance would be called *retinal disparity*. In fact, if a single eye moves by 65 millimeters (the distance between your eyes), this movement produces a depth cue—motion parallax—that is equivalent to the cue produced by binocular viewing—retinal disparity.

There is another similarity between motion parallax and stereopsis. Recall from our discussion of random-dot stereograms how forms invisible to either eye alone could be synthesized from retinal disparity information. The same kind of synthesis of form can occur through motion parallax. In an ingenious set of experiments, Brian Rogers and Maureen Graham (1979, 1984) asked observers to view a single array of random dots with just one eye; it is important to keep in mind that their stimuli were not stereograms and that viewing was monocular. The entire display consisted of about 2,000 dots, and a subset of dots could be displaced while the rest maintained their same positions. Figure 7.25 depicts one such display. In one condition, the displacement occurred whenever just the observer's head moved. In other words, moving the head from side to side caused the predesignated subset of dots to move relative to the rest. This condition would corre-

spond to observer-induced motion. In a second condition, the observer held still while the display itself was moved, with the predesignated region of dots moving by an amount different from the rest. Rogers and Graham found that both forms of relative motion generated a clear, immediate impression of a surface standing out in depth from its background (as in the bottom panel of Figure 7.25). Moreover, so long their heads or the display moved, observers could accurately describe the shape of this surface. But whenever both the observer's head and the display were stationary, the sensation of depth immediately vanished. Rogers and Graham's study clearly shows that motion parallax, like retinal disparity, can generate information about the shape and depth of objects, in the absence of all other cues.

We have just seen that head motion generates with one eye the same kind of information generated by two eyes in a stationary head. This raises an interesting question: Why is the visual system designed in such a way as to provide two equally sensitive mechanisms for seeing objects in depth, one monocular and one binocular? Wouldn't it be safer to relocate the eyes on the side of the head, thereby achieving a panoramic view of the

FIGURE 7.25 Motion parallax, like stereopsis, can generate information about object form. The five panels in the top row depict changes over time in the position of a subset of dots in the display. These changes are produced either by the observer's head movements or by movement of the display itself. The bottom panel depicts the stable percept produced by either of these maneuvers. (Adapted from Rogers & Graham, 1979.)

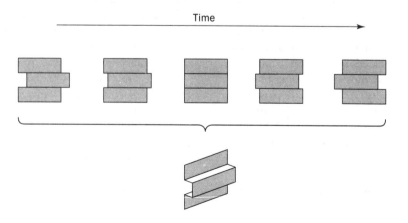

Time

world? The consequent loss of disparity information could be compensated for by relying on the equally effective cue of motion parallax.

The key to this puzzle may have something to do with the type of animals who possess well-developed binocular vision. As a rule, these frontal-eyed animals are predators, who rely on stealth to capture their prey. Movements of the hunter's head or body could forewarn an intended victim, thereby costing the hunter a meal. So it may have been advantageous for predators to develop the capacity for stereopsis, a quieter but equally accurate means of depth perception. For humans whose hunting is confined to the supermarket, where there is no real concern about giving away one's whereabouts, motion parallax and stereopsis provide largely redundant information.

INTEGRATION OF DEPTH INFORMATION

The previous sections have described various sources of information specifying depth relations among objects and distances from a perceiver to those objects. As you should now be able to appreciate, the visual world is rich with depth information. How, then, are these multiple cues combined? Do we rely only on the most salient? Do some work better than others in particular circumstances? How are other aspects of vision influenced by depth information? Investigators are now beginning to address these questions, and this section provides an overview of some of the emerging answers.

One strategy for studying depth interactions entails varying the number of depth cues present in a display and asking how depth perception is affected. An excellent example of the application of this strategy comes from the work of Bruno and Cutting (1988). They tested all different combinations of four sources of depth information—size, interposition, motion, and perspective—and measured for each combination the quality and the accuracy of depth. The results showed that these sources interacted additively, as if each source were processed separately and made its own unique contribution to depth perception.

Bruno and Cutting speculate that the visual system is composed of different "minimodules," as they were termed, each devoted to one source of depth information. Conceivably, these minimodules might relate to the multiplicity of specialized visual areas in the brain.

In their studies, Bruno and Cutting varied the number of available cues, but these cues were never placed in conflict. The strategy of pitting cues against one another has been employed in many other experiments (see, for example, Braunstein and Stern, 1980; Stevens and Brookes, 1988; Rogers and Collett, 1989). In essentially all cases, depth perception is degraded when cues conflict, implying that no single source of information dominates. In a related vein, it is possible to create displays in which one source of information (for example, perspective) generates ambiguous depth, meaning that the shape or configuration of a three-dimensional object can be seen in multiple, mutually exclusive ways. A classic example of an ambiguous figure, the Necker cube, was shown in Chapter 1 (see Figure 1.2). The cube's configuration changes over time, depending on which square is perceived as the front face of the cube. Either interpretation is consistent with the available perspective information specifying depth, so perception is unstable. However, the introduction of unambiguous disparity information stabilizes perception: the cube is seen in one perspective only. This strategy of disambiguating one source of depth information with another has been successfully applied to study other combinations of information, too (Dosher, Sperling, and Wurst, 1986; Nawrot and Blake, 1991).

Finally, another strategy involves determining how depth information influences other aspects of vision, such as object recognition. For example, Nakayama, Shimojo, and Silverman (1989) measured how well people could recognize faces when portions of the faces were obscured by blank, horizontal strips (Figure 7.26). Nakayama and colleagues created stereoscopic displays where the segments of face appeared either behind the horizontal strips (left drawing in Figure 7.26) or in front of the horizontal strips (right drawing in Figure 7.26). The first case (left) simply looks like

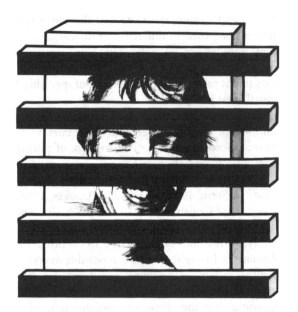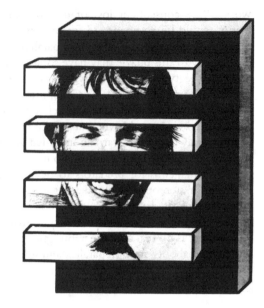

FIGURE 7.26 A partially visible face as it would appear behind (left) or in front of (right) a surface. In Nakayama, Shimojo, and Silverman (1989) stereopsis was used to place the face segments in depth relative to the surface.

the head of a person partially occluded by venetian blinds; observers had no difficulty recognizing the faces. But in the second case (right drawing), recognition performance was seriously impaired, even though the number of face segments and the quality of the image remained the same. The fragments made no sense, because the face no longer looked partially occluded. So the depth interpretation—occluded versus nonoccluded—influenced the perceptual organization of the face fragments.

DEPTH, ILLUSIONS, AND SIZE CONSTANCY

During our discussion of depth perception, we noted several perceptual errors that occur when people are confronted with misleading depth information. These errors involved some distortion in perceived size, such as the moon's unusually large appearance when it is on the horizon. Many

other visual illusions are also characterized by misperceptions of size. Examples of two of the better-known size illusions are given in Figure 7.27. In each case, one portion of the figure appears larger than its partner, even though both are really identical in size. Almost everyone experiences these size illusions and always in the same way. For over a century, psychologists have been fascinated by these illusions and have focused a great deal of research on testing various theories concerning their origins. (A good summary of these theories is Coren and Girgus, 1978.) Let's conclude this chapter by considering a particular theory that, although not universally accepted, has endured over the years.

The most popular theory of size illusions attributes errors in perceived size to the operation of monocular depth cues (Gregory, 1970). We'll call this the *depth theory*. Consider, for example, the left-hand illusion in Figure 7.27, the so-called *Müller-Lyer illusion*. According to the depth theory, the arrowheads on the ends of the vertical

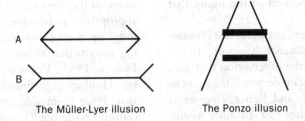

The Müller-Lyer illusion   The Ponzo illusion

FIGURE 7.27 Two size illusions.

lines can be seen as angles formed by two intersecting surfaces. An example of this idea is shown in Figure 7.28. In both drawings, the vertical line represents the point of intersection, or the corner, formed by two surfaces. When the arrowheads point outward (as in A), the two surfaces are seen as slanted toward you; when they point inward (as in B), the surfaces are seen as receding away from you. Why should the "corner" formed by the receding surfaces (inward-pointing arrowheads) appear longer than the one formed by the approaching surfaces (outward-pointing arrowheads)? According to the depth theory, the answer is simple: because of the perspective cues supplied by the arrowheads, the receding corner appears farther away than the approaching corner. At the same time, the retinal images of the two corners

are identical in size. Now there is only one way objects at *different* distances can cast images of *equal* size: the farther object must actually be larger. In the case of the two vertical lines, the height of the corner formed by the receding surfaces (inward-pointing arrowheads) would have to be longer than the height of the one that is formed by the approaching surfaces (outward-pointing arrowheads). And this is exactly how it is seen.

The same line of reasoning applies to the other size illusion illustrated in Figure 7.27, the so-called *Ponzo illusion*. In this case, too, perspective cues imply that one region of the figure is located farther away than another. According to the depth theory, this distance information enters into judgments of the sizes of objects occupying these different regions. Note that the apparently larger ob-

FIGURE 7.28 The Müller-Lyer illusion could arise from implied depth information.

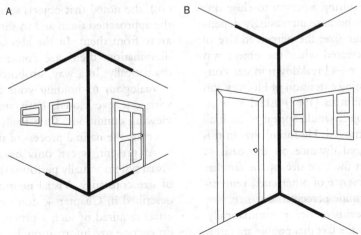

A   B

ject is situated in that portion of the figure that appears farther away.

The depth theory, then, attributes size illusions to errors in perceived distance (Gregory, 1970). The theory is based on the observation that perceived size remains constant despite differences in distance from the viewer and, hence, changes in the size of the retinal image cast. In other words, perceived size is *scaled* in terms of perceived distance, a process known as **size constancy.** We call size constancy a scaling process because one unit of measure (retinal image size) is converted, or scaled, into another (perceived size). Road maps typically include scales that transform centimeters into kilometers (or inches into miles); the visual system contains a mechanism that scales image size into object size. It's crucial that retinal image size be scaled, since the size of the image of an object depends on how far away that object is. As a result, *un*scaled *retinal* image size would be a poor index of *object* size. Without size scaling, one would always be confused about the height of people, the width of doorways, the size of cars, and so on. The fact that one rarely errs in these kinds of judgments means that the visual system uses depth information in making size judgments.

Just how good is the visual system at estimating the true sizes of objects? In a classic study, Holway and Boring (1941) found that an observer's accuracy at judging a circle's size was almost flawless under conditions rich with depth information. But as depth cues were progressively eliminated (for example, by requiring a person to close one eye), size judgments became increasingly dependent on retinal image size; the perceived size of the same object increased when the object was closer to the observer—a breakdown in size constancy. In an interesting extension of Holway and Boring's study, Schiffman (1967) asked at what *distance* a familiar object would appear to be if all depth cues were removed. He found that in this case, observers judged distance on the basis of their memory about the true size of the familiar object. So, in the absence of other cues, remembered size can determine perceived distance.

Size constancy seems to occur automatically. This is evidenced by the fact that people are rarely aware of the size of their retinal images. Yet with appropriate instruction people can accurately judge the retinal size of an object, in effect ignoring information about distance (Gilinsky, 1955; Epstein, 1963). You can verify this ability yourself. Hold up both thumbs with their nails facing you. Place them side by side approximately 20 centimeters (about 8 inches) from your eyes. They will look identical in size, as well they should. Next, extend one arm until that thumb is approximately 40 centimeters (about 16 inches) away, twice the distance of the other one. At first glance the two thumbs should continue to appear equivalent in size, even though the image size of the nearer one is now twice that of the farther one. This is what we mean by size constancy.

Now, while maintaining your thumbs at these different distances, move the farther one laterally until it appears just to the side of the nearer one. With one eye closed (to prevent double vision) and your head very steady, carefully compare the apparent size of the two thumbnails. Switching your attention from one to the other reveals that the closer thumbnail does look larger than the farther one. With this exercise you've managed to capture a glimpse of your retinal image. But notice how quickly this glimpse disappears once you open both eyes or move your head.

Bernice Rogowitz (1984) has described another condition where size constancy is defeated. Viewing a natural scene under stroboscopic illumination (such as that experienced at many discos), she noted that objects seemed to expand as she approached them and to shrink as she moved away from them. In the absence of continuous illumination, then, size constancy breaks down dramatically. In a way, stroboscopic illumination is analogous to holding your head very steady with one eye closed; both are highly artificial viewing conditions. One really has to work to override the natural process of size constancy.

At present, it can only be guessed how the visual system actually performs this scaling process of size constancy. Visual neurons, such as those described in Chapter 4, don't exhibit the properties required of such a process. These neurons do encode size information, by virtue of the limited spatial extent of their receptive fields. But this information refers to size on the retina, not the invariant size of the object itself. If at all involved in size perception, the activity of these neurons must somehow be integrated with depth information before size constancy can be realized.

SUMMARY AND PREVIEW

This chapter has examined the cues that the visual system uses to generate the experience of depth. We have emphasized that depth perception occurs automatically, with no conscious deliberation. We have also seen that depth perception influences perceived size, resulting in size constancy as well as certain illusions of size. This connection between illusion and constancy should remind you of a similar connection seen earlier, for lightness perception (Chapter 3). Although we have emphasized distance information in this chapter, the more general contribution made by depth cues should not be overlooked. As David Marr (1982) has pointed out, depth serves to define objects relative to their backgrounds—helping the viewer distinguish those objects and appreciate their shapes. In the next chapter we take up another aspect of vision—movement—that serves the same purpose.

KEY TERMS

absolute distance
accommodation
aerial perspective
Ames room
amodal completion
binocular rivalry
convergence
convergence insufficiency
depth perception
diplopia
disparity-selective cells

egocentric direction
horopter
interposition
linear perspective
motion parallax
neon spreading
oculomotor cues
perceived distance
random-dot stereograms
relative distance
retinal disparity

shading
size constancy
stereoblindness
stereopsis
stereoscope
strabismus
texture gradient
transparency
visual cues

Action and the Perception of Events

The preceding three chapters concentrated on visual experiences in a world of patterns, colors, and depth relationships. Now it's time to bring that world to life by giving objects in it the power to change and the ability to move about. As we have noted, all four of these dimensions of visual experience—pattern, color, depth, and motion—serve a common biological purpose; they all demarcate objects from their backgrounds, making those objects easier to detect and recognize. To see how this applies to motion, imagine walking along in some wooded area. Suddenly a rabbit who's been sitting very still begins to scamper. You realize then how inconspicuous that creature had been before it began to move.

In the example just given, motion helped you detect the presence of some creature, and moreover, it helped you recognize that the creature was a rabbit. Movement, in other words, can provide information about form. This can also be demonstrated in the laboratory, as illustrated in Figure 8.1. A wire hanger has been bent and twisted into a random three-dimensional shape. Using the arrangement shown, the bent wire casts a shadow on a piece of paper. When the wire is motionless, anyone who looks at the shadow will have no idea of the wire's twisted shape. But once the wire begins to move (rotate), its three-dimensional shape becomes obvious immediately (Wallach and O'Connell, 1953). Today this perceptual phenomenon, shape from motion, is studied using more complex, computer-generated displays

(Baker and Braddick, 1982; Siegel and Andersen, 1990).

So, motion serves several different perceptual purposes, including detection, segregation of an object from its background, definition of an object's shape, and guidance of limb and eye motion. For all these functions of motion, the nervous system must extract from the retinal image the spatial displacements of features over time. This requirement makes motion a spatio-temporal event. Moreover, the information associated with movement of objects in the environment must be distinguished from image displacements associated with movements of the head and eyes, not a trivial problem as we shall see. Finally, different aspects of that spatio-temporal information must be transformed in ways dependent on how that information is to be used.

In all its forms, motion is so pivotal to daily life that it is hard to imagine life without the experience of motion. But as a result of damage to the brain, some people are deprived of the ability to see motion. To get some idea of what this would be like, consider the following description of one such person's experiences. Although her visual acuity and form perception were quite normal, she could not see movement:

She had difficulty, for example, in pouring tea or coffee into a cup because the fluid appeared to be frozen, like a glacier. In addition, she could not stop pouring at the right time since she was unable to perceive the movement in the cup (or a pot) when the fluid rose. . . . In a room

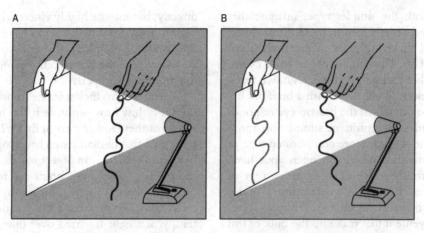

FIGURE 8.1 Movement can provide information about form.

where more than two other people were walking she felt very insecure and unwell, and usually left the room immediately, because "people were suddenly here or there but I have not seen them moving." . . . She could not cross the street because of her inability to judge the speed of a car, but she could identify the car itself without difficulty. "When I'm looking at the car first, it seems far away. But then, when I want to cross the road, suddenly the car is very near." (Zihl, von Cramon, and Mai, 1983, p. 315)

Re-examination years later revealed that her condition had remained essentially unchanged, though she had developed some coping strategies. For example, when listening to someone, she had learned to look away from the speaker's face in order not to be disturbed by the fact that the speaker's mouth never seems to move (Zihl, von Cramon, Mai, and Schmid, 1991).

Obviously, being unable to see motion is frustrating and dangerous. Not only was this woman unable to see the movements of other creatures and objects, she also had difficulty seeing the consequences of her own movements and actions. Her inability to judge when enough tea had been poured is a reminder that perceivers themselves cause many of the changes and movements perceived. Moving about among the world's objects, you see those objects from various perspectives.

Acting on the world's objects can influence how you perceive them. Thus, while your perceptions govern your actions, your actions also influence what you perceive, as Figure 1.1 suggested. We'll discuss the actions that help you explore the world in which you live. Such actions include very large movements of your body as well as very small ones. The large movements allow you to locomote about in the world; the small movements, movements of your eyes, allow you to inspect that world and search out new information. Because these actions are an integral part of visual perception, our discussion of the dynamic perceptual world has to consider what the perceiver does as well as what the perceiver sees.

WHAT IS AN EVENT?

Part of this chapter deals with visual events, so we had better clarify what that term means. An "event" is something that happens in both space and time. Although one can talk about an object solely in terms of space—where it is or what it is—to talk about an event, one needs to consider time. In fact, there are really two kinds of visual events. The simpler type involves only a change in time, not in space; the more complicated type involves changes in both time and space.

Starting with the simpler type, imagine that you've trapped a firefly in your hand. Your closed hand emits a flickering glow as the firefly's tail blinks on and off. This simple type of visual event, involving only a change over time, is known technically as **flicker.** We'll open with a brief discussion of the way in which the human eye responds to flicker and to intermittent stimulation more generally. The second, more complicated type of event is exemplified when you open your hand and see the firefly escape. This common type of event involves change not only in time but also in space. Such events constitute the various forms of visual movement that make up the bulk of this chapter, but first to flicker.

Lights that blink, flicker, or wink are everywhere in industrialized societies. Some of these lights—for example, the flashing lights atop a police vehicle—try to capture attention. Others—for example, the flashing light at a railroad crossing—are designed to warn. For a flashing light to be effective, it must flicker at a rate that can be easily seen. If it flickers too rapidly or too slowly, the flicker will be imperceptible.

Much is known about the **critical flicker frequency (CFF)**—the highest rate of flicker that can be perceived as such (Landis, 1954). When this highest frequency is exceeded, the separate flashes of light blend together to yield the perception of a light that appears to be on continuously. Under the best conditions, the human CFF is around 60 Hz. ("Hz," short for "hertz," is a unit of flicker rate, and is equivalent to 1 per second.) In fact, this is why you cannot see the flicker from a typical fluorescent lamp. Although the lamp actually does flicker on and off at a rate of 120 Hz, you can't see the flicker because its rate exceeds your CFF. However, a bee looking at the same lamp could perceive the 120-Hz flicker, since the bee's CFF is reputed to be around 300 Hz (Lythgoe, 1979).

The CFF depends on many different variables, including the light's intensity and size. In addition, CFF varies with location in the visual field. The rate of flicker of a large stimulus—such as a television set or a bank of fluorescent lights—may be too fast to be seen when you look at the stimulus

directly, but may be highly visible when you look slightly away from it. You may have experienced this annoying peripheral flicker if you've been in a room where the fluorescent ceiling lights were functioning improperly.

Warning lights flicker at rates much lower than the CFF. Just how sensitive is the human visual system at these lower rates of flicker? Recall from Chapter 5 that human vision has an optimal spatial frequency—there is an object size that can be seen most easily. The same holds for temporal frequency—there is a rate of flicker that can be seen most easily. To determine this frequency, the intensity of a light is varied over time, usually in a sinusoidal fashion (see the inset in Figure 8.2). For various frequencies of flicker, the minimum visible fluctuation of light is assessed. At some rates, flicker can be seen even when the light's intensity fluctuates very little. At other rates, flicker can be seen only when the light's intensity fluctuates a large amount. This dependence of flicker perception on rate is shown in Figure 8.2. The vertical axis represents "sensitivity"—how little fluctuation in intensity is needed for flicker to be detected; the horizontal axis represents the rate of flicker. Note two features of the curve. First, the

FIGURE 8.2 Sensitivity to light flickering at different frequencies. The inset shows the sinusoidal variation in luminance over time. High sensitivity means very little fluctuation in intensity is needed to perceive flicker.

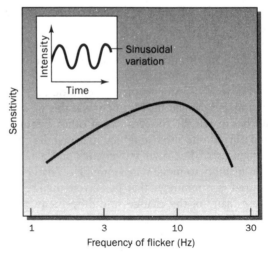

location of the curve's peak indicates that the visual system is most sensitive when the light flickers at around 10 Hz. Second, the highest frequency that the system can detect, the so-called high-frequency cutoff, is the CFF.

Chapter 5 described how separate visual mechanisms process objects of different spatial frequencies. Similarly, separate visual mechanisms process different rates of flicker, as demonstrated by a study of flicker sensitivity in glaucoma patients (Tyler, 1981). The typical patient showed diminished sensitivity to flicker frequencies in the vicinity of 30 Hz. This impairment coexisted with normal sensitivity to other frequencies. For reasons that are not understood, the abnormal pressure within the eyeball reduces the patient's ability to perceive flicker at particular frequencies—implying that glaucoma selectively impairs neural mechanisms that process particular rates of flicker. This impairment for particular temporal frequencies is reminiscent of selective impairment for particular spatial frequencies.

To measure the CFF, it is customary to use a long series of regularly spaced flashes. The close temporal proximity of these flashes makes it hard to distinguish individual flashes—at high rates of presentation, one flash blends into another, destroying their separate identities. Actually, the same sort of temporal "blending" or "destruction" can be experienced with just two successive flashes. This phenomenon is called **visual masking,** because one flash reduces, or masks, the visibility of the other. Any time two stimuli occur close together in time and are near one another in space, there is opportunity for destructive interference between the two (see Fox, 1978). Although masking has been studied in various sensory systems, our concern here is with masking in vision.

VISUAL MASKING

Suppose that you measure a person's threshold for seeing a brief, dim spot of light. The threshold is defined as the minimum amount of light that just permits the test spot to be seen. The threshold is then remeasured while a larger, more intense spot,

the masker, is flashed at the same spatial location as the test spot and following it closely in time. The threshold for seeing the first, small spot is now higher than it was originally—the small spot has to be more intense for it to be seen. This elevated threshold reflects the masking influence of the larger, later stimulus, which has interfered with the perception of the first stimulus. This is known as backward masking, since the second stimulus interferes with the perception of its predecessor. There is an analogous form of masking in which the more powerful masking stimulus is presented before the weaker test stimulus. This kind of masking, as you might expect, is called forward masking.

Over the years, there have been hundreds of studies of visual masking in its various guises (Breitmeyer, 1984). Various motives have driven different researchers; we'll mention three that have impelled much work on masking. These studies assume that the masker, when it is delivered, terminates the extraction of information from the test stimulus. By varying the delay before delivery of the masker, researchers compare the rates at which various forms of visual information are extracted from the test stimulus (Marcel, 1983). Masking also makes it possible to compare the information-processing speeds of various classes of subjects such as the elderly or the very young (Till, 1978). The assumption is that performance on such tasks can eventually be related to the success of perception under more normal, everyday conditions. Finally, masking is often used as an inferential technique for studying neural processes responsive to information in the target and in the mask (Sekuler, 1965; Harvey and Doan, 1990). To the extent that a mask interferes with the visibility of a target, the two must be engaging common neural processes, the reasoning goes.

We'll end this consideration of intermittent stimulation with a warning. In some individuals, seizures can be brought on by exposure to a flickering light. Individuals with this condition, called photoconvulsive epilepsy, should be aware that seizures can be triggered by a strobe light in a disco, a malfunctioning television set, or even the flashing lights of a video game (Glista, Frank, and Tracy, 1983).

BIOLOGICAL MOTION

Though the visual system responds to many different kinds of events, none are more important than the events that distinguish animate from inanimate objects. Imagine walking along the beach and spying what looks like a clear, gooey substance. Something has probably been washed up by the tide, but you can't be sure whether it is still alive. You watch it for a while, waiting for it to move. Finally, you see some movement but not the sort that suggests life. Instead, the gooey substance seems to be simply floating in response to the motions of incoming waves.

This seaside encounter demonstrates a couple of things. First, motion offers powerful clues about an object's biological status, whether something is living or not. The encounter is also a reminder that one kind of motion can be discriminated from another. When a creature's entire body moves en masse, the movement has a different significance than if its parts move in a certain way relative to one another.

Humans regularly watch the motion generated by biological systems. This happens most commonly when we watch another person walk, run, or dance. The motions we see tell us much more than just whether that person is alive or not; the motions may also reveal the person's gender and, perhaps, individual identity. Since this is a particularly important type of event perception, and since it provides some general lessons about motion perception, we'll begin our discussion with biological motion.

RECOGNIZING BIOLOGICAL MOTION

A friend, let's say a female, walks across the room; what is there in her walk that allows you to recognize her just from her gait? Gunnar Johansson, at the University of Uppsala in Sweden, was the first to study this question systematically (1975). Johansson began by determining the minimum information needed to recognize biological motion. Reasoning that the movement of the body's joints might convey particularly important information, Johansson attached one small light bulb to each hip, knee, ankle, shoulder, wrist, and elbow of a person. This person was clothed entirely in black so that looking at the individual in a dark room, you would see only the small set of illuminated spots. Johansson's plan was to eliminate all the familiar, nonmotion cues that might give away the fact that the stimulus was a person.

Figure 8.3 gives some idea of what people saw when Johansson tested them. The figure shows

FIGURE 8.3 Each white dot is a light attached to some part of a person's body. (Drawings adapted from Johansson, 1975.)

A

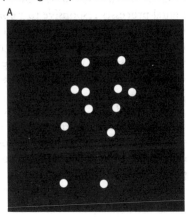

B

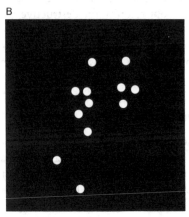

the lights attached to a person who is sitting quite still in a chair. The person in panel A is seated with his feet on the ground; the person in panel B is also seated, but with his legs crossed. There's really not much to give away that it's something alive you're looking at, let alone a person. The lights appear to be a random collection of spots, not unlike a constellation in the sky. Yet, Johansson found that as soon as the person began to move, viewers saw that it was a person. In other demonstrations, Johansson discovered that the same light bulbs were sufficient to reveal when a person was painting, riding a bicycle, or doing push-ups. The overall movements of the lights, and their movements relative to one another, carried this information in a most compelling way.

The following is an even more impressive demonstration of the salience of biological motion. Johansson outfitted two people with light bulbs and had them dance in the dark. Figure 8.4 is a sample of frames taken from a motion picture Johansson made of the two people dancing. Since any single frame contains information only about space and none about time, examination of any one frame gives no clue as to what you're looking at. However, even the briefest section of the film, projected at the proper speed, gives an almost instantaneous impression of two people dancing. It has been found, in addition, that this minimal information enables viewers to identify the gender of someone walking. Viewers can recognize their own gait in such displays, as well as the gait of various friends (Cutting and Proffitt, 1981).

When people do not see Johansson's demonstrations firsthand, but merely read about them, there is a tendency to get the wrong idea. People assume that complex thought processes are required in order to resolve the complex movements of the small lights. But this assumption is wrong. Johansson's studies show that the perception of biological motion occurs automatically; people do not have to puzzle over what they are seeing. The percept is as immediate as it is in viewing any other form of motion. In fact, viewing the moving lights for as little as 200 milliseconds is enough to enable a person to identify familiar biological motion without having been

told what to expect (Johansson, von Hofsten, and Jansson, 1980).

There's other evidence that biological motion perception does not require sophisticated thought processes—even very young infants can discriminate biological from nonbiological motion. Not only can infants tell the two types of motion apart, but they also have a distinct preference for motion that is biological in origin. Robert Fox and Cynthia McDaniel (1982) used a television screen to present two different motion patterns side by side. Infants were propped up in front of the television screen while the biological and nonbiological motions were presented for several seconds. Following Johansson's method, each pattern consisted of several white dots against a dark background. One of the two patterns represented the joints of a human who was running; dots in the other set moved randomly in all directions. An observer sitting near the television screen noted which side of the television screen the infants preferred to look at. By 4 months of age, infants showed a clear preference for biological rather than nonbiological motion.

Fox and McDaniel were concerned that their infants might have been responding not to the biological or nonbiological character of the motion but to how random or constrained the motion was. Since arms and legs usually do not go flying in all directions, biological motion is more constrained than the random motion with which it was paired. So a second experiment was needed to verify that infants had not been responding to differences in the randomness of motion. Fox and McDaniel paired one display in which dots represented a human running in place with another display in which the same running human was presented, but upside down. Again, infants preferred the biological motion—the right-side-up human running. (For a good analytic treatment of other studies of biological motion, particularly ones with infants, see Bertenthal, 1992.)

Studies of infants' responses to biological motion displays do not prove that the ability to recognize biological motion is innate (as Johansson believes); they do however confirm what Johansson's work with brief exposures indicated: rec-

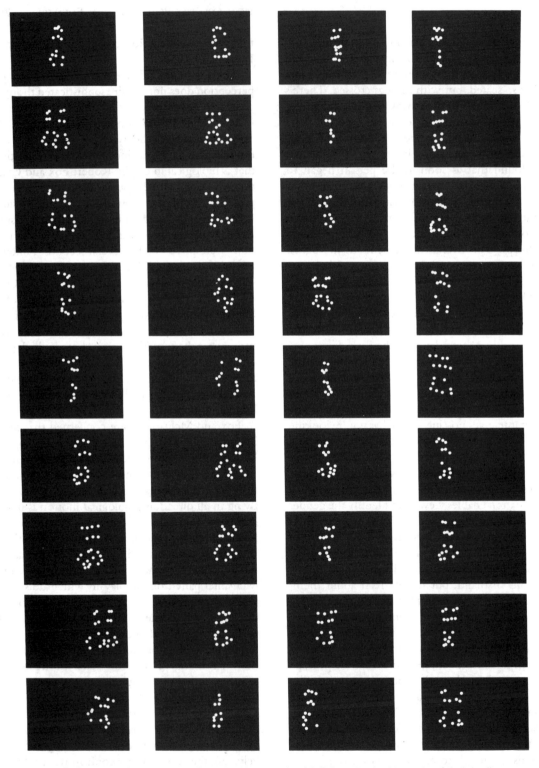

FIGURE 8.4 Frames from a movie of two dancing people with lights attached to parts of their bodies. (Adapted from Johansson, 1975.)

ognition of some forms of biological motion requires little complex intellectual processing. This conclusion is further buttressed by the recent demonstration that cats, too, perceive biological motion in point-light animation sequences (Blake, 1993).

SOMETHING ABOUT THE WAY YOU WALK

Now that you know how easy it is to recognize biological motion, it's natural to wonder about the basis for this ability. What information contained in these displays makes such judgments possible? Although the answers are not known yet, one promising approach to the problem uses computer-controlled displays to isolate particular dynamic (changing) features of the gait. For example, James Cutting (1978), of Cornell University, has used computer displays of moving bright spots to simulate various types of human motion. This sort of research has enabled Cutting to identify characteristic "male" and "female" gaits. To begin, Cutting observed that the typical male adult has broader shoulders than the typical female adult, whereas the female's hips are broader. Because of this difference, the ratio of shoulder width to hip width is about 10 percent greater in males than in females.

But what does this have to do with gait? When you walk, your left leg and right arm swing forward together; then your right leg and left arm follow suit. The result is a kind of oscillating, or shearing, motion. On each step, the body oscillates about a point that is the intersection of two lines: one connecting the left shoulder and right hip, the other connecting the right shoulder and left hip.

Recall, though, that males and females typically have different shoulder and hip widths. Consequently, as males walk, their bodies oscillate about a lower point than do the bodies of females (see Figure 8.5). A computer created a display in which synthetic walkers had centers of movement calculated from the average male body or from the average female body. When viewers saw these displays, they had little trouble identifying the "gender" of the synthetic walker (Cutting, 1978).

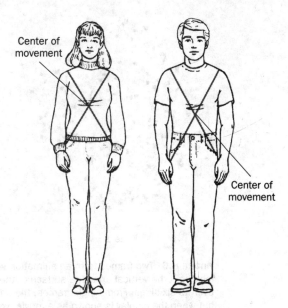

FIGURE 8.5 Males and females have different centers of movement.

These and related studies presumably disclose the stimulus information utilized by the visual system to recognize biological motion (Runeson and Frykholm, 1983).

STRUCTURE FROM MOTION

So far we've considered what happens when people see various forms of biological motion. Of course, nonbiological objects often move too, and the motions of those objects portray valuable information about the three-dimensional shapes of those objects. We are able, in other words, to derive impressions of object structure from motion, an ability called the perception of **structure from motion (SFM).** Earlier in this chapter we mentioned one example of SFM, the bent-wire figure whose shape was readily apparent once it began rotating (Figure 8.1). Another example will amplify the potential importance of SFM as well as illustrate its hallmark characteristics.

Imagine a transparent object such as a glass cube whose surfaces are randomly sprinkled with black texture markings (Figure 8.6). When this

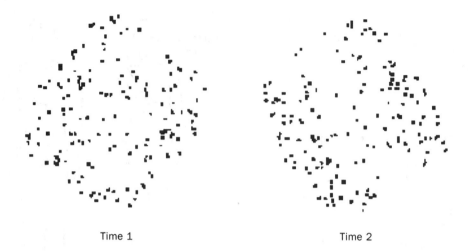

Time 1   Time 2

FIGURE 8.6 Two frames from an animation sequence depicting a transparent cube rotating about the vertical axis. The surface of the cube is textured with dots placed randomly over its six sides. From single frames, the shape and volume of the object are unknown, but when the display is shown as a movie, you would be able to tell the object's structure from its motion.

object is stationary, a person would have great difficulty judging its true shape and volume—the stationary figure looks like a jumble of unconnected dots confined to a rectangular region. But if this object now rotates about any of its axes, its identity as a three-dimensional cube would immediately be seen. The stimulus information specifying its shape and volume comes from the differential motion of the texture markings: dots on a given face of the cube move together coherently in a single direction, with dots on different surfaces moving in different directions. Moreover, dots on the nearest surface will seem to move at a faster speed than those on a farther surface, and this difference in velocity creates the impression of volume. So the key ingredient in creating SFM is the coherent motion of subsets of features, or surface markings. The hallmark characteristics are the impression of depth from this motion ("kinetic depth," as it is sometimes termed) and the perception of object shape and surface layout.

In very recent years, the perception of SFM has been intensively studied, with particular emphasis on the accuracy of shape judgments that use SFM information (Norman and Lappin, 1992), on the stimulus conditions that limit or permit the occurrence of SFM (Todd and Norman, 1991), and on possible neural bases for perceiving SFM (Nawrot and Blake, 1991). For our purposes, it is sufficient to add SFM to the list of sources of information about form and depth.

In the case of biological motion and SFM, we considered the motion from the point of view of a perceiver who was stationary. But when you, as a perceiver, begin to move about, you generate motion on your own retina. This self-produced visual motion helps guide your actions.

THE VISUAL GUIDANCE OF LOCOMOTION

Three centuries ago, the philosopher George Berkeley (1709/1950) had an intriguing idea about vision's main purpose. He wrote that vision was designed to allow animals to "foresee . . . the damage or benefit which is like to ensue, upon the application of their own bodies to this or that body which is at a distance" (p. 39). In other words, he believed that vision keeps creatures out of trouble, which certainly is true. When you move about in the world—walking, running, driving a car, or piloting an airplane—you'd better know *whether* you're going to collide with something, and if so, *when*. This knowledge allows you to change course, thereby avoiding harm. As Berkeley realized, vision guides movement and movement alters vision. Let's consider this interplay between vision and locomotion, starting with the visual information that allows you to steer your movements properly.

FINDING THE RIGHT DIRECTION

Most people get around easily, with a minimum number of collisions, even on sidewalks packed with people. Obviously, then, they exploit some source of information to locomote—keep on course, and, if necessary, change course appropriately. But what exactly is that source of information, and how is it used? As you move about through the world, the image on your retina changes with your movements. To take a simple example, as you move toward some stationary object, the image of that object on your retina expands. Moreover, its *rate* of expansion mirrors the rate of your approach, a point we shall detail later. James Gibson, a leading perceptual theorist, pointed out that this expansion could actually guide complicated and important movements of

the body and head. "To kiss someone," Gibson (1979) instructed, "magnify the face-form, if the facial expression is amiable, so as almost to fill the field of view. It is absolutely essential to keep one's eyes open so as to avoid collision. It is also wise to discriminate those subtle [features] that specify amiability" (p. 233).

Kissing isn't the only activity that produces a flow of visual information. Think about what happens when you walk toward some object such as the door to a building. To appreciate how the retinal image changes in this situation, look at Figure 8.7. Each panel in the figure represents what you might see as you move steadily toward the door. Note particularly how the view changes from one drawing to the next. Though a series of stills cannot fully capture the dynamic character of these changes, there are some important things that can be appreciated. The door you are looking at and walking toward always remains at the center of the field of view. Objects around the door—to its sides, above, and below—shift radially outward, flowing farther and farther into the periphery of the visual field. The center of this flow, known as its focus, allows you to steer yourself toward the door. You will successfully reach the door by keeping the door at the center of the outward flow.

Gibson proposed that the pattern of outward flow could be used to tell where one is headed

FIGURE 8.7 Changes in the field of view as a person approaches a door.

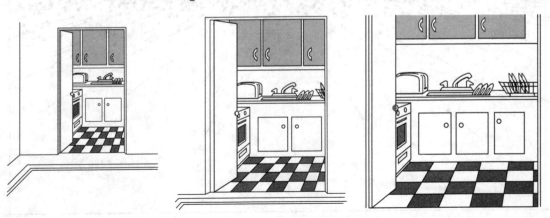

and to steer around obstacles. To test this idea, he filmed the view from the cockpit of an aircraft in flight and found that viewers of this film could identify the direction in which the plane was headed (Gibson, 1947). But in order to guide the high-speed locomotion on the ground, say, of runners or skiers, optical flow information would have to be extremely precise. James Cutting (1986) estimated that various forms of high-speed locomotion would require that forward motion be controlled to an accuracy of about a single part lateral motion for every sixty parts forward motion. This requirement leaves very little margin for error.

There's a more general way to represent the optic flow produced in situations such as the one illustrated in Figure 8.7. Imagine that an observer is looking directly ahead and walking on a perfectly straight course through some environment. At any instant, the optical flow can be portrayed as a velocity field, where the lines signify the instantaneous optical velocity of elements (the dots) in the environment (Figure 8.8). Each line's direction corresponds to the direction of optic flow

at one point in the field; the length of the line corresponds to the instantaneous speed of the optic flow. The single vertical line sticking up from the "horizon" in Figure 8.8 represents the direction in which the observer is headed. So long as the direction of heading and the speed of forward motion were the same, this single diagram would be valid for the optical flow for a walker, a runner, or a driver. Koenderink (1986) gives a detailed mathematical treatment of optic flow.

William Warren, a cognitive scientist at Brown University, examined the accuracy with which observers can use optic-flow information in order to judge the direction in which they're heading. Warren, Morris, and Kalish (1988) created a series of computer-generated "films," each of which consisted of moving dots. A given film of moving dots simulated the optic flow that would be generated on the retina as an individual walked in a particular direction. For each film, the observer had to judge whether he or she appeared to be heading to the left or right of a stationary target located at various positions along the display's simulated horizon. Even with very few dots in

FIGURE 8.8 Instantaneous velocity field produced by an observer moving forward on a straight course parallel to a plane. The single vertical line poking up from the plane indicates the direction in which the observer is moving. Dots represent elements on the surface plane, and line segments indicate the velocity vector associated with each element. Vector orientation signifies the direction of the local optical flow; vector length signifies the speed of the flow. (After Warren, Morris, & Kalish, 1988.)

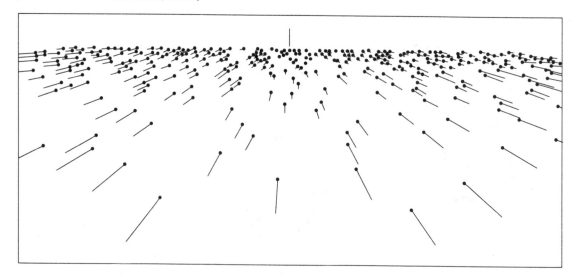

the display, the observers managed to achieve accuracy levels very nearly equal to what Cutting (1986) said would be needed if high-speed locomotion were to be guided by optic flow. In an important follow-up, Warren and his colleagues repeated these measurements with a group of older observers (age range 61 to 78 years) whose vision, despite their age, was quite good. Using displays that simulated speeds of locomotion from a slow walk (1 meter per second) through a fast run (3.8 meters per second), Warren, Blackwell, and Morris (1989) found that at all speeds the older observers were only half as good at judging direction as were young observers tested under the same conditions. Warren and his colleagues speculate that the diminished ability to judge direction of heading could contribute to age-related errors of locomotion and result in an increased incidence of falling accidents.

You've just learned how visual information specifies where you're going. But it's equally important to know when you're going to arrive (or collide). Let's consider the visual information that specifies time of arrival.

JUDGING YOUR TIME OF ARRIVAL

Perhaps you've watched seabirds diving for food. They fly along until a fish is spotted in the water below, then, without warning, they dive into the water at impressive speed. Often they get their fish. The whole process is a marvel to behold, but some species of birds add one additional mystery to their performance: a split second before hitting the water's surface, these birds fold their wings, streamlining their bodies and easing their entry into the water. Watching this performance, you'd think that somehow the bird "knew" exactly when it would hit the water. Though the bird doesn't have sophisticated navigational instruments, it performs this feat with precision and regularity (Lee and Reddish, 1981). Humans perform comparable, albeit less spectacular, feats whenever we walk, run, drive, or catch a ball (Chapman, 1968). Let's analyze the information that enables people to do these things.

Start by considering the information that might be available to a creature who is approaching some stationary object in its environment. Figure 8.7 showed that as you approach an object—a door in that case—the image size of that object expands. If you are walking toward the door at a constant rate, the rate of expansion specifies the time to collision—the moment at which you will reach the door.

Suppose that at time t you're some distance, say D meters, away from the door. You probably recall formulas from physics relating the variables of time, distance, and rate. In those formulas, time is equal to distance divided by rate. So if your rate is R meters per second, and distance is D meters, then time to arrival will be D/R seconds. However, to solve this equation you must have good information about both distance and rate. How does the visual system get such information? It doesn't. Instead, as David Lee (1980) shows, it uses another, dynamic source of information about time to arrival—which makes it unnecessary to know either distance or rate.

Suppose you are 100 meters from a telephone pole when you start walking toward it at a rate of 1 meter per second. Suppose, further, that while walking, you look directly at a knothole on the pole. To simplify calculations, assume the knothole is 1 centimeter in diameter. Using simple trigonometry, we can calculate the size of the image cast by the knothole on your retina. The heavy line in Figure 8.9 portrays the results of this

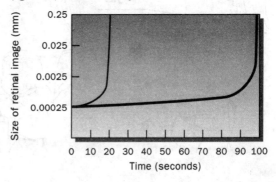

FIGURE 8.9 The retinal image size of an object expands exponentially as you walk (heavy line) or jog (light line) toward that object.

calculation. It will come as no surprise that as you walk steadily toward the pole, the image on your retina expands, nor that because you're traveling at 1 meter per second and must cover a distance of 100 meters, you reach the pole 100 seconds after you began to walk. Note, however, that though you approach the pole at a steady rate, the image does not grow at a steady rate. Instead, its growth accelerates as you approach the pole. Hence, when you're far from the pole, its image grows slowly—signifying that you've got an appreciable time until you hit the pole. As you get very near the pole, however, the image grows rapidly—signifying an imminent collision.

This connection between imminent collision and rapid expansion of the image is not peculiar to the variables in our example; it holds in all situations. To demonstrate, consider the light line in Figure 8.9, which summarizes calculations that would apply if you were jogging toward the telephone pole. Again, your approach begins 100 meters from the telephone pole, but because you are now jogging, not walking, your approach is 5 times faster than before. Since you are now going 5 meters per second, impact should be at 20 seconds—a fact confirmed by the explosion in image size at that time. The connection between imminent impact and growth in retinal image size holds for any distance, rate, or object size. It also holds for any moving creature that has its eyes

open—including the diving birds mentioned earlier. The visual system carries out these complex computations so rapidly that resulting information about rate of expansion can be used to control the braking of an automobile (Lee, 1976), the split-second changes in gait that are needed when running across rough terrain (Warren, Young, and Lee, 1986), or the various movements and adjustments of the hand that are required to catch a ball (Savelsbergh, Whiting, and Bootsma, 1991). Lest you think of this coupling between optical expansion and action as something that is calculated and conscious, it's worth pointing out that people can succeed in these tasks even though they are not aware—or able to articulate—what they're doing (Savelsbergh, Whiting, and Bootsma, 1991).

In fact, animals as dissimilar as fiddler crabs, chicks, and monkeys, as well as human infants, all try to avoid looming patterns created artificially, on television screens (Schiff, 1965). This is true even for newborn infants who have never before encountered a looming stimulus (see Figure 8.10). Apparently, learning plays very little role in this behavior.

Increases in the size of an object's retinal image—expansion—could signal a stationary observer that some object was approaching. Mechanisms that responded to optical expansion could also signal a moving observer that he or she was

FIGURE 8.10 Most animals, including human infants, will try to avoid a looming stimulus, even when that stimulus is portrayed on a television screen.

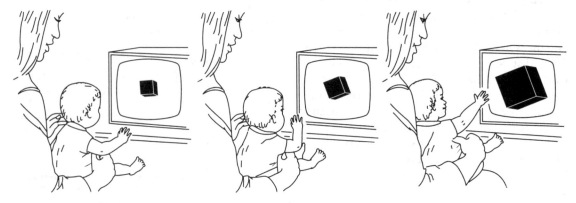

approaching some stationary object. In other words, these mechanisms could help guide locomotion visually. Such mechanisms could also help a pilot control an airplane. Pilots who had particularly sensitive size-change mechanisms should be better able to judge their approach to the runway and should, therefore, execute smoother landings.

This proposal was put to a strong test in studies using U.S. Air Force pilots (Kruk, Regan, Beverly, and Longridge, 1981; Kruk and Regan, 1983). First, a cockpit simulator was used to test the pilots' ability to land an airplane. For each simulated landing, the researchers determined the number of corrective maneuvers a pilot had to make. This provided a quantitative index of the landing's smoothness—the fewer corrections required, the smoother the landing. They then tested the pilots' ability to detect changing size. In this test, the pilot viewed a television display of a square undergoing unpredictable changes in size. The pilot used a "joystick" (like those in arcade and home video games) to compensate for the changing size—movement of the joystick was electronically subtracted from the electrical signal that controlled the square's size. Presumably, someone very sensitive to changing size would quickly spot even the smallest change in size and null that change using the joystick. As these investigators expected, skill in landing a plane was strongly correlated with a pilot's sensitivity to changing size. Keep these results in mind the next time a plane you're on makes an erratic landing: be charitable, and chalk up the rough landing to the pilot's subnormal sensitivity to changing size. In a later section, we describe some properties of these neuronal mechanisms.

LOCOMOTION AND MOVEMENT WITHOUT VISION

Although locomotion and other forms of movement through space tend to be visually guided, there are times when locomotion occurs despite the absence of vision. With eyes closed, you can walk around with fair safety, at least for several seconds. Also, to keep track of some moving object doesn't require keeping your eyes fixed continuously on that object; visually sampling the object's trajectory every half second or so allows fairly accurate tracking (Thomson, 1980). Moreover, if you take a quick look at the objects on your desk, you can then close your eyes and reach fairly accurately for any one of them. You'll be able to bring your hand close to the position you had intended. But small errors will creep in during the final moments of actually trying to grasp the object; here vision seems most important (Goodale, Pelisson, and Prablanc, 1986).

This dissociation between the initial, large movements of the hand and the final, smaller ones shows up dramatically in a neurological condition called **optic ataxia** ("ataxia" designates a disorder of movement). As a result of a suicide attempt, a patient had localized brain lesions (Damasio and Benton, 1979). One affected area, immediately in front of the visual cortex, is thought to integrate visual information about the hands and arms with proprioceptive information about the hands and arms. (**Proprioception** is the sense by which you can feel where your limbs are.) When the patient's eyes were open, she had great difficulty reaching for objects—a cigarette or ashtray might be missed by several inches. Her arm would begin to go in the right direction; but during the final part of the reach, the arm and hand would go astray. She then had to grope about for the object as though she were blind.

Her difficulties with visually guided reaching were not caused by impairment of the sense of touch: with her eyes closed, she had no trouble buttoning or unbuttoning garments, or pointing to some part of her body. The impairments were also not caused by diminished vision. In fact, her visual acuity was quite normal. Moreover, she had no trouble walking with her eyes open. The impairment seemed to be limited to fine hand movements performed under visual guidance. This rare disorder is a reminder of how crucial a role vision normally plays in guiding movements; it is also a reminder that a complete theory of vision must include the action that vision makes possible.

EYE MOVEMENTS: THEIR AIMS AND EFFECTS

There's no doubt that vision helps control your exploration of the world around you. We've already discussed how vision guides one particular form of exploration, locomotion. Now let's turn to visual explorations that are made possible by small, rapid movements of the eye, rather than by larger, slower movements of limbs and the entire body. Eye movement records provide unimpeachable testimony about where someone is looking at any given moment. In fact, instruments are available for tracking the shifts in gaze while someone inspects a visual scene, and from the resulting records it is possible to deduce which aspects of the scene receive closest scrutiny. In one clever application of this technique, Carmody, Kundel, and Toto (1984) monitored the eye movements of radiologists while they scanned x-rays looking for possible tumors. The eye movements actually provided a richer, more comprehensive description of the scanning strategies than did verbal descriptions by the radiologists.

We'll be dealing with two principal kinds of eye movements (Steinman, Kowler, and Collewijn, 1990). To anticipate, we'll briefly describe each type. One type is responsible for shifting your gaze rapidly from one object to another. Such eye movements include the ones you're making right now as you read this book. The other type of eye movement, whose speed may vary from pretty fast to quite slow, allows you to track smoothly a moving target—such as a golf ball that's just been putted toward the hole. We distinguish these two principal types of eye movements because it's likely that each serves a distinct purpose and each depends on somewhat distinct neural circuits in the brain (Steinman, Kowler, and Collewijn, 1990).* We'll also spend some

_____

* The categories of eye movements introduced here have no bearing on the distinction, introduced in Chapter 2, between conjunctive and disjunctive eye movements. That earlier distinction was based exclusively on the direction in which the eyes moved. In fact, one can have rapidly shifting movements that are conjunctive or disjunctive; one can also have slower, smooth movements that are conjunctive or disjunctive.

time on the variety of smooth eye movements that helps your eyes stay fixed on an object even when your head and body move about. You can experience this last type of movement by looking at the number at the top of this page while moving your head slowly back and forth. Anyone who watches your eyes during this maneuver will see them move in their orbits, compensating for the movement of your head.

ACQUIRING THE TARGET

Consider an unpleasant situation that you may have experienced. (We've selected this situation because it is common and also because it involves both types of eye movements just mentioned.) Imagine that while reading, you suddenly spot out of the corner of your eye something scurrying across the floor. Your eyes swing rapidly away from what you've been reading toward the scurrying thing. This kind of high-speed eye movement is designed to shift the image of some interesting object (the scurrying thing) from the periphery of the retina (where resolution is poor) to the fovea (where resolution is good). About one-fifth of a second after spotting the creature, the eyes begin to move. Almost instantly, they reach a very high speed of movement (achieving velocities of almost 20 centimeters per second). Then, usually less than one-tenth of a second after they started to move, the eyes screech to a halt.

When the eyes move about in this way, they do so in abrupt jerks; as a result, eye movements of this type are called **saccades** (from the French verb *saccader,* meaning "to jerk"). The eye does not jerk, or saccade, only when it needs to fixate some object far out in the periphery. Anytime you shift your gaze from one object to another, your eye executes these jerky movements. For example, while you read this page, your eyes are saccading from word to word, four or five times each second. Because you shift your gaze thousands of times each hour, saccades can certainly lay claim to being your most commonly used instrument for visual exploration. Since you need to make so many saccades, it is fortunate that the eye muscles responsible for these saccades never become fatigued (Fuchs and Binder, 1983).

Saccadic Suppression.   There are some peculiar things about saccades, this instrument of visual exploration. For one thing, they are usually invisible to the explorer. Stand in front of a mirror and watch the reflection of your eyes as you make saccades voluntarily; allow your eyes to jump back and forth between two points several inches apart. Though you know that your eyes have moved, you never actually see that movement. This is a puzzle. Furthermore, during the saccade you don't experience blurred vision. Yet if you took a photograph with a camera that moved at the same rate your eyes moved, you'd get a very blurred, low-contrast picture (see Figure 8.11). Why, then, do you not experience impaired vision each time you execute a saccade?

Perhaps the retinal image moves so fast that the motion can't even be perceived. After all, there is a lower threshold, a minimum velocity below which motion cannot be seen (Bonnet, 1982). For example, you cannot actually see the movement of a clock's minute hand even though you know that it's moving. Perhaps, then, there is also an upper threshold, a maximum velocity above which you can't see motion. Several people have suggested that such an upper threshold is responsible for limiting the ability to see the blur and motion accompanying saccades (see Burr and Ross, 1982, for a review).

To test this suggestion, you'd have to move some object at a rate equal to the rate at which the eye would sweep across that object during a saccade. Can an observer see an object moving at this rate? To make sure that motion was being seen, you might ask the observer to identify the direction in which the object moved. It turns out that the ability to see the moving object depends on its size and contrast. Rapidly moving objects of low contrast are impossible to see. So are small objects, regardless of their contrast. However, large, rapidly moving objects can be seen if their contrast is sufficiently great (Burr and Ross, 1982). So rapid movement does not on its own preclude

FIGURE 8.11 Moving a camera while the shutter is open produces a blurred picture.

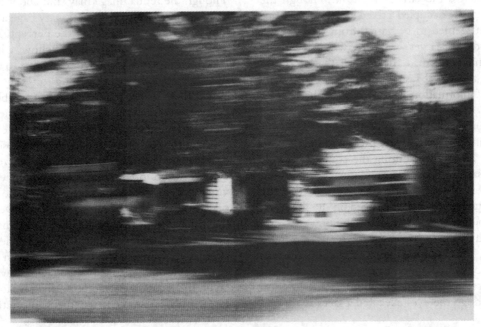

vision. The rapid movement itself is not seen because of visual masking (see discussion earlier in this chapter). Masking is promoted when, immediately before and after each saccade, the eye momentarily fixates. Under normal viewing conditions, these fixations produce a stationary, patterned retinal image with abrupt onset and offset (Dodge, 1900). In the laboratory, these masking effects can be precluded by measuring visibility against a nonpatterned, uniform background. However, even when this step is taken, some saccadic suppression remains. Recent work has identified the culprit.

It's been known for some time that a small, briefly flashed stimulus is harder to see if the observer is at all uncertain about the stimulus' location—even when the stimulus' alternative sites are very close together (Cohn and Lasley, 1974). If during a saccade the visual system does not have an exact, concurrent record of eye position, the observer would be hard-pressed to know precisely what place in space should be attended to. This **stimulus uncertainty,** in turn, would reduce detectability. Greenhouse and Cohn (1991) asked observers to judge the location of a small, very bright target flashed while the observer's eye moved across the target's location. Though the target actually occupied a fixed location, the place where it seemed to be varied from trial to trial; seldom did the target seem to be where it actually was. This confirmed the notion that during a saccade the visual system lacks access to precise reliable information about where the eye is aimed.

Greenhouse and Cohn then measured the detectability of a brief target presented either with the eye held still or during the course of a voluntary saccade. An electronic device monitored the observer's eye position and ensured that the flashed target was always imaged on the fovea. As others before had found, detectability was greatly diminished if the target was presented during a saccade. Then, putting their hypothesis to the test, Greenhouse and Cohn created conditions that would reduce uncertainty about spatial location even though the eyes executed a saccade. In one

experiment, bright, highly visible markers indicated clearly the location where the test target would appear. In another experiment, the test target took the form of an increment to another, bright, easily seen stimulus. In this second experiment, incidentally, the measure was akin to a difference threshold (see Appendix). Both manipulations, which were designed to reduce stimulus uncertainty, greatly improved target detectability, in the latter case, eliminating saccadic suppression altogether.

Perceptual Stability. Greenhouse and Cohn's study revealed that during a saccade the visual system may not have good, current information about direction of gaze. But there is strong evidence that such information is available, just before and immediately after a saccade. Before turning to that evidence, consider why such information would be important. While you're reading this paragraph, each saccade shifts the page's retinal image, sometimes by quite a bit. You can mimic these retinal image shifts by keeping your eyes still (minimizing saccades) while jiggling the page about sharply, to and fro. Though the retina image may shift about in both conditions, saccades with stationary page and jiggling page without saccades, the perceptual consequences are very different. Somehow, when we make saccades, the visual world appears to remain still, despite what's happening on the retina. What, then, is the source of this remarkable perceptual stability? Specifically, how does the visual system monitor the movements of the eyes?

Over the years, researchers have proposed two different mechanisms by which eye movements could be monitored. According to one view, the visual system tracks actual changes in the extraocular muscles; according to an alternative view, the visual system tracks the command signals that go to control the extraocular muscles. (These two alternatives were depicted schematically in Figure 7.3.) The preponderance of behavioral evidence favors the second view; additionally, physiological research has identified neural mechanisms that use the signals sent to the extraoculars to update the brain's representation of visual space (Duhamel, Colby, and Goldberg, 1992). We will not review the literature here, but instead examine several conditions chosen to illustrate some basic principles. These conditions are outlined in Table 8.1.

To make predictions of what ought to be seen in each condition, we'll need some consistent conventions about our descriptions of motions. Our convention assigns a value of $+1$ to leftward motion and a value of -1 to rightward motion. This assignment applies to motions in the external world, to motions of the eyes, and to perceived motion. However, leftward-moving objects produce rightward retinal image motion; for retinal image motion only, we reverse the previous assignments, using -1 for leftward retinal image motion and $+1$ for rightward retinal image motion. To complete the assignments, we denote the absence of motion with a value of 0. Finally, for predictions of the direction in which motion is perceived to go, we assume that perceived direction develops from a comparison between two quantities, the command signals to the extraocular muscles and the accompanying retinal image motion. To derive perceived direction, simply subtract the retinal image motion from the command

signal. In the first two, normal, cases, the observer consciously decides to move the eyes across a stationary visual environment. These being normal conditions, the eyes do as they're bidden, moving left in the first case and right in the second. In each case, subtracting the retinal image motion from the command signal yields 0 (no perceived motion). Now we come to something a bit more interesting. To understand the third condition, close your left eye and push gently and carefully with your finger at the outer edge of your open right eye. You ought to experience, with each displacement of the eyeball, an opposite direction displacement of the world. As the table indicates, this is expected because there is retinal image motion in the absence of command signals to the extraocular muscles. The fourth condition is the most unusual; in it the eyes are paralyzed and, thus, prevented from obeying any command to move. Here, the observer wills a leftward eye movement, but none occurs. Be sure that you work through the details of this condition in order to understand the outcome. Do the same for the last condition as well.

This exercise underscores the rather complicated computations performed by the visual system to achieve perceptual stability as the eyes move about.

TABLE 8.1 Perceptual Consequences of Eye Movements

Conditions of Testing	Command Signals	Eyes Move	Retinal Image Motion	Experience
Normal; stable environment	Left	Left	Right	No motion
Normal; stable environment	Right	Right	Left	No motion
Eye passively displaced left	None	Left	Right	Right
Eyes paralyzed, person *wills* movement left	Left	None	None	Right
Environment translates left	None	None	Right	Environment moves left

The Necessity of Saccades. Besides the quick saccades employed to redirect the focus of gaze, our eyes are constantly executing much smaller saccades even when we're holding our gaze fixed on a given point. These microsaccades, as they're called, are too small to be noticed when you look at someone else's eyes while that person stares in yours, but they can be measured with sensitive monitoring devices. More importantly, these microsaccades are absolutely crucial for vision. To see just how important they are, consider what happens when their contribution is eliminated. This situation can be achieved by means of special optical devices that eliminate all motions of the retinal image. With these **stabilized retinal images,** objects appear to fade and, in some cases, disappear entirely (Pritchard, 1961). Such fading can also be produced by an even more drastic technique—immobilization of the eye by means of a paralyzing drug such as curare (Stevens et al., 1976).

You don't have to paralyze your eyes in order to see some of these visual consequences. Just fixate the small dot in the center of the large fuzzy bar in the photograph in Figure 8.12. If your fixation is very steady, within 10 seconds or so the bar will fade from view. When it does fade, merely shift your gaze slightly to one side and the bar will pop back into view. Once again look at the bar until it fades. Now rather than shifting your gaze, blink your eyes once or twice. This, too, will restore the bar to full visibility. What do

FIGURE 8.12 Fixate the spot in the center of the dark bar and notice how the bar fades from visibility.

these two situations—shifting your gaze and blinking your eyes—have in common? Each of them produces a brief change in retinal stimulation. Such brief changes enhance the visibility of large, low-contrast objects (Robson, 1966). Fortunately, you don't have to shift your gaze or blink your eyes consciously to enjoy this beneficial effect; the normal involuntary movements of the eyes take care of this for you.

* * *

Now that you understand something about saccadic eye movements, including the involuntary microsaccades, we can return once more to the creature we left scurrying across the floor. You visually captured that creature—acquired the target—by making a saccade, but the creature is still moving, so you've now got a different problem: how to keep your eyes on it.

STAYING ON TARGET

Often a saccade brings the image of an object onto the observer's fovea. But if that object happens to be moving, the observer's eyes must track the object in order to keep the image on the fovea. To pursue a moving target, the eyes behave very differently from the way they do when they make a saccade: during pursuit they move smoothly, instead of with abrupt stops and starts. To guide the eyes' pursuit movements, the brain draws on two complementary sources of information. One source comprises sensory information derived from neurons that code direction and speed of moving objects (recall Chapter 4). The other source is the observer's cognitive expectations about object motions that are about to occur (Kowler, 1989). Integrating both sensory signals and cognitive expectations, the brain sends commands to the extraocular muscles for guidance of **pursuit eye movements,** sometimes called **smooth eye movements.**

Unlike jerky saccades, pursuit movements are smooth. Also they are not ballistic; the signals being sent to the extraocular muscles are constantly being updated and revised, thereby altering the speed and direction of the pursuit movements.

Accurate pursuit is important; only if the eye's movements match some object's movement will the image of that object be relatively stationary on the retina—which will have the beneficial consequence of keeping the object sharply imaged on the fovea. If the pursuit is not accurate, the image will be smeared. But how well do pursuit movements actually match the movement of the object the eyes are pursuing? The answer depends on the speed of the moving target that the eyes have to follow (Murphy, 1978). When targets move slowly (less than one-third millimeter on the retina per second), eye movements match target movements almost perfectly. However, at higher target speeds, the eyes have increasing difficulty keeping up with target movement. This difficulty causes the target's image to slip on the retina.

Not everyone appreciates just how difficult it is to pursue a rapidly moving target with the eyes. Take baseball coaches for instance; they're always exhorting batters to keep their eye on the ball, which turns out to be impossible advice (Ripoll and Fleurance, 1988). Baseball, like cricket, tennis, and other sports involving rapidly moving balls, is a game of milliseconds.* A 10-millisecond error in a batter's swing is the difference between a hit over second base and a foul along one of the foul lines (Kirkpatrick, 1963). The pitched ball zooms toward the batter at speeds approaching 50 meters per second (about 100 miles per hour), and as few as 500 milliseconds elapse between the pitcher's release and the ball's crossing the plate. Unfortunately, these conditions actually make it impossible to keep your eye on the ball. Using a realistic batting situation, Bahill and LaRitz (1984) measured the position of the batter's gaze over time. They found that experienced baseball players (including individuals in the major leagues) cannot accurately follow the path of a ball from the pitcher to home plate. Instead, a batter executes a predictive saccadic eye movement a frac-

tion of a second after the ball leaves the pitcher's hand. The predictive saccade aims the batter's eyes where the batter expects the ball will be when it reaches the plate. Contrary to the batter's intuition, then, it is impossible to keep one's eye on the ball throughout its entire travel from pitcher to home plate. Bahill and LaRitz found that really topnotch hitters can pursue the ball for more of its flight before having to resort to the inevitable predictive saccade.

Dynamic Visual Acuity. The eyes' inability to pursue rapidly moving targets helps explain a puzzle. It has been known for quite a while that visual acuity for a moving target gets worse as the target moves faster. (Acuity measured with moving targets is termed **dynamic visual acuity,** to distinguish it from acuity measured with static targets.) Dynamic acuity is quite distinct from static acuity. For example, two people can have identical static acuities, but one person may have dynamic acuity that is 3 or 4 times better than the other person's.

Although all early studies agreed that dynamic acuity is poorer than static acuity, they disagreed about the source of that difference. Some studies suggested that dynamic acuity is poorer simply because the eye (in attempting to pursue a target) is moving and that the eye's movement per se diminishes acuity. According to this view, no matter how well the eyes keep up with the target, dynamic acuity will still be impaired. We know now, however, that dynamic visual acuity is poorer than static not because the eyes move but because the eyes often fail to keep up with the moving target, thus producing retinal image slip. Murphy (1978) found that when the eyes do manage to keep up with the moving target, visual resolution is not impaired at all.

Murphy also found that dynamic visual acuity can be improved by practice. One of his observers showed a substantial improvement in her ability to pursue a moving target. As a consequence, the slippage of her retinal image decreased and her visual resolution improved.

With practice, dynamic acuity improves, more in some observers than it does in others (Ludvigh and Miller, 1958). Since most studies of dynamic

---

* Regan (1992) offers a detailed treatment of visual and cognitive factors in cricket, as well as a brief introduction to the sport itself.

Box 8.1 *Learning to Move Your Eyes*

The ability to move the eyes is one skill that seems to require very little practice—even newborn babies do a pretty good job of it (Wertheimer, 1961). But recent studies suggest that eye movements, like other skills, can improve with practice.

To see an object's details, you must fixate the object. Otherwise, it will not be imaged on that portion of the retina where vision is sharpest. When a bright and clear fixation point is available, a young adult can fixate very well. Over several seconds, the image of a fixated point does move about on the retina, but these movements are extremely small. To what extent is this excellent control of the eyes a learned skill?

To answer this question, Eileen Kowler and Albert Martins (1982) studied eye movements and fixation stability in two cooperative children about 5 years old. In contrast to adults, the children had trouble maintaining steady fixation. During a few seconds of concerted fixation, the children's eyes jumped around, scanning an area 100 times larger than an adult's eyes would.

This relative instability of gaze is not the only characteristic that distinguishes children's eye movements from those of adults—children's pursuit movements are also immature. In fact, extremely young infants can't pursue a moving target smoothly at all. Instead, their eyes try to keep up with the target by means of a series of saccades. Infants don't pursue smoothly in an adult fashion until they get to be 10 to 12 weeks old (Aslin, 1981).

Even after infants acquire the ability to pursue objects smoothly, their pursuit may still lack one important feature—the ability to anticipate. When changes in object movement are predictable, a practiced pursuit system doesn't wait for the change to happen before responding to that change. If the pursuit system did wait, neural and mechanical delays would cause the eye to lag behind the change and thereby lose the object.

It's easy to demonstrate pursuit's knack for

---

acuity have not assessed pursuit eye movements directly, we can only speculate that those who improve in dynamic acuity also improve in the accuracy of their pursuit eye movements. The effects of learning on eye movements are discussed further in Box 8.1.

* * *

Return one more time to the situation where you were sitting and reading when you spotted a creature scurrying across the floor. We've discussed how first you fixate it and then track it visually as the creature scurries across the floor. Now suppose you want to get up and chase it. What new problems would this create for your visual system?

VESTIBULAR EYE MOVEMENTS: A SPECIES OF SMOOTH MOVEMENT

Whenever your head moves, your eyes must make smooth compensatory movements to enable you to maintain the fixation of some object. It's easy to see these compensatory eye movements. While a friend, let's say a male, is standing directly in front of you, have him look at your nose. Now ask your friend to rotate his head back and forth, while keeping his eyes fixed directly on your nose. During the course of all these goings-on, note the position of his eyes. When his head is turned directly toward you, the eyes are centered in their sockets; when his head rotates toward his left, his

anticipating. Tie a key to the end of a piece of string 18 inches (about 45 centimeters) long. While you swing the key back and forth like a pendulum, have a friend follow the key with her eyes. At first, each time the key changes direction, your friend's eyes will lag slightly behind. After a few seconds, though, these pursuit eye movements, anticipating the change in direction, will move in perfect synchrony with the key.

If you were to repeat this experiment with a young child, the result would be different. According to Kowler and Martins (1982), the child's pursuit movements would never anticipate the change in direction; as a result, the image of the moving target would slip off the fovea after each change in direction, requiring one-fifth of a second to catch up again.

No one knows for sure why children's eye movements differ from those of adults. It might be that anticipatory eye movements require maturity at a cognitive level in addition to well-functioning sensory and motor systems. Like other abilities, perhaps the ability to anticipate changes in motion develops only with practice and experience. As Kowler

(1989) noted, control of eye movements "by cognitive expectations allows anticipatory pursuit to deal with abrupt changes in target motion because abrupt changes can often be anticipated correctly by an observer who understands his environment and the significance of the cues it contains" (p. 1056).

It is not known whether individual differences in dynamic acuity are entirely a matter of practice. But whatever their origins, these individual differences can be quite important. For example, Horner (1982) measured dynamic visual acuity in sixty-five college students, some of whom were members of the college baseball team. On average, the baseball players had considerably better dynamic acuity than the rest of the students. In addition, the better hitters among the players had better dynamic acuity. The connection between batting skill and dynamic acuity probably means that better hitters have better pursuit eye movements. We're not saying that with practice anyone could hit as well as Ted Williams; still, it does seem promising to try to improve athletes' pursuit eye movements (see Watts and Bahill, 1990).

eyes rotate rightward; when his head rotates rightward, his eyes compensate by rotating leftward. One can, of course, suppress compensatory eye movements by moving the head and the eyes in the same direction.

When your friend rotated his head, the rotation was sensed by structures within the **vestibule** (a chamber inside the ear). Signals from this vestibular system travel to the brain stem, which ultimately relays them to the extraocular muscles, causing compensatory eye movements (Parker, 1980). These are called **vestibular eye movements** in recognition of the anatomical site at which head movements are analyzed. Like many other functions associated with vision, vestibular

eye movements are so rapid, automatic, and accurate that one virtually never notices them. Not until the vestibular mechanism fails does one become aware of how valuable they are, as the following case illustrates.

Some antibiotics have a particular affinity for the vestibular structures as well as for adjacent portions of the ear. Too heavy a dose of these antibiotics can temporarily destroy certain structures in the vestibular mechanism. A physician described his own experiences after a dose of streptomycin had rendered his vestibular mechanism inoperative. Under these conditions, no eye movements were generated to compensate for the physician's head movements. For example, when he walked about, his eyes jiggled, so that he could not read signs or recognize the faces of his friends. Every head movement, even the very smallest, disturbed his vision. When he sat perfectly still and tried to read, each tiny pulse beat in his head made the letters on the page jump about and blur (Steinman, 1976; see also Walker, 1984).

There's another situation in which vestibular eye movements can spell trouble: when you try on someone else's glasses. When you do, the glasses may cause not only blurred vision but also dizziness and, in extreme cases, nausea. The dizziness is caused by conflict between the vestibular and visual systems. There is an explanation. Suppose you are emmetropic (see Chapter 2) and thus do not need glasses, but you have borrowed some from a friend who has strong glasses. When you put them on, you notice immediately that everything appears blurred. Moreover, when you move your head, the visual world appears to move. This comes about because normal compensatory eye movements produce abnormal amounts of retinal image motion, causing the world to appear to move—a disconcerting and dizzying experience.

The same kind of unpleasant and disorienting experience occurs when you get a new prescription for glasses. For a while, each time you move your head, the resulting vestibular eye movements are inappropriate for your new prescription. This is particularly disconcerting when there is a large change in the prescription, such as when someone has had a cataract operation and must wear very strong lenses. In that circumstance, many people complain about dizziness associated with head movements when first wearing their new glasses. Fortunately, though, the vestibular system is adaptable. Within minutes, the compensatory eye movements change appropriately (Steinman, Cushman, and Martins, 1982; Collewijn, Martins, and Steinman, 1983); the movement of the retinal image is reduced, and the visual world appears stable once again. This adaptation is fortunate because otherwise no one would ever dare to get a new prescription for eyeglasses. Don't think, though, that the capacity for speedy adaptation evolved simply so that you can change your spec-

tacles. Instead, it seems likely that this capacity probably evolved to compensate for growth, degeneration, or disease within the oculomotor system (Collewijn, Martins, and Steinman, 1983).

We've just discussed an unusual interaction between vision and the vestibular system, namely what happens when there's a mismatch between compensatory eye movements and movements of the retinal image. Several other kinds of unusual interactions between vision and the vestibular system are discussed by Dichgans and Brandt (1978). Though many visual-vestibular interactions promote an illusion of self-motion, this illusion can also occur under other conditions, as the following section illustrates.

ILLUSIONS OF SELF-MOTION

You are sitting in a stationary train, next to a window, reading a newspaper. Suddenly another train moves past yours, and while it is passing, you perceive that it's *your* train that's moving. Or you are sitting in the first row of a theater that's showing a movie on a very wide screen. Even though you know better, some of the movements on the screen make you feel that *you* are moving. You feel foolish when you grab the seat to hold yourself down; you don't feel so foolish, though, when you notice that everybody around you has done exactly the same thing.

Illusions of self-motion, like the two just described, have been studied for more than a century, since Ernst Mach did the first work on them in 1875. Though these powerful illusions take many different forms, they usually depend on visual movement in the periphery of an observer's field. Before the invention of trains and widescreen movies, movement of large expanses of the visual field occurred only when the observer moved. When motion occurs in the peripheral field of a stationary observer, the brain mistakenly attributes that visual motion to the self-produced movement of the observer's own body. This misattribution is so compelling that it can knock people out of their chairs or cause them to fall down as they try to compensate for the illusion.

CENTRAL VISION AND PERIPHERAL VISION: TWO VISUAL SYSTEMS?

The center of your visual field, the area imaged on and around the fovea, constitutes a minute portion of what you can see at any one moment; the rest of the field, the periphery, accounts for the vast bulk. Given this fact, it is surprising that most of what is known about visual function concerns the small central portion of the field; very little is known about the outlying territory, except for vague ideas as to its importance. There are many reasons for distinguishing between center and periphery. As you learned in Chapter 3, their acuities differ; but center and periphery also differ in another way: in their responses to motion. As researchers are beginning to appreciate, this latter difference can have important consequences for safety, as we'll now explain.

Over the past hundred years or so, several researchers (for example, Campbell and Maffei, 1981) have reported that the apparent speed of a target changes depending on where in the field it appears. You can try this for yourself. Look directly at the second hand of a clock and note its speed. Now look away from the clock so that the second hand is just barely visible in the periphery of your visual field. The second hand will appear to move more slowly. This means that the periphery and the center of vision give conflicting information about an object's speed. As people drive, both central and peripheral regions are usually being stimulated, and people's judgment of how fast they are traveling is a mixture of information from both regions. However, when visibility is reduced by fog or decreased illumination, the contribution of central vision is reduced and the judgment of speed depends primarily on peripheral vision. Under these conditions, the apparent speed of objects will be underestimated, since objects seen peripherally appear to move more slowly. Consider the impact that fog can have on another form of travel, flying. Under conditions of good visibility, sight of the horizon guides the pilot through complex maneuvers. For example, when the aircraft is being banked for a turn, the image of the horizon moves appropriately. But when flying through dense fog or clouds, the pilot cannot see the horizon; instead he must rely on the plane's instruments and the responses of his own **vestibular** (balance) sense. This inability to see the horizon creates a conflict. When the pilot banks the plane to start a turn, the plane's instruments and the pilot's vestibular sense confirm the maneuver, but the pilot's vision denies it. The pilot's visual world (limited by fog or clouds to the inside of the cockpit) seems unchanged during the maneuver. Every contour in the pilot's visual field—his own knees, the edge of the instrument panel, the cockpit itself—suggests that the plane has not banked. This conflict between vision and vestibular information can so disorient novice pilots that they may assume their instruments are broken. Naturally, this erroneous assumption is extremely dangerous. But the dangerous disorientation can be overcome quite simply. Recent research has developed an unobtrusive artificial horizon that can be presented in the pilot's peripheral field of view. The movements of this artificial horizon, really the image of a small bar of light, mimic the movements of the real, but invisible, horizon outside, making the aircraft easier and safer to fly (Malcolm, 1984).

Box 8.2 describes other ways in which the erroneous perception of motion can cause accidents and suggests ways to prevent them.

FOCAL VISION AND AMBIENT VISION

Herschel Leibowitz has modified the theme of two visual systems, characterizing one as a **focal system** concerned with object identification and discrimination and the other as an **ambient system** concerned with spatial orientation. According to Leibowitz, the focal system utilizes just the information from the center of the retina, whereas the ambient system utilizes information from both the center and the periphery of the retina. He has used this distinction to account for many nighttime automobile accidents (Leibowitz, Post, Brandt, and Dichgans, 1982). Briefly, his argument runs as follows. Driving requires both focal

Box 8.2 *Perceptual Errors Can Cause or Prevent Accidents*

Motion perception can literally be a matter of life or death. It can cause fatal accidents, but it can also prevent them. To document this claim, we'll start with the dark side—collisions at railroad crossings.

According to the Federal Railroad Administration (1992), there are about 5,000 collisions each year between locomotives and other vehicles at railroad crossings in the United States. Most railroad crossings are protected by crossing gates and warning bells; in addition, locomotive engineers must sound a bell or horn as they approach a crossing. Because of these precautions and the ease with which motorists should be able to see these huge and conspicuous locomotives, it's a real puzzle that so many accidents occur. Herschel Leibowitz, of Pennsylvania State University, has come up with some answers to this puzzle. According to him, errors in motion perception are partly to blame (Leibowitz, 1983).

During an accident investigation, Leibowitz rode in the cab of a locomotive that retraced the route on which the accident had occurred. The trip took Leibowitz through an urban area with many gate crossings. He was astonished at the number of motorists who drove around the crossing gates and across the tracks in front of the oncoming train. The train crew, who saw this kind of thing every day, shrugged it off as "typical." Since automobiles don't fare too well in collisions with railroad trains, why do people take such chances?

Leibowitz realized that although the locomotive's bulk made it easy to see, that same bulk would cause its speed to be seriously underestimated. It has long been known that the size of an object and its apparent speed are inversely related. To study this relation, J. F. Brown (1931) asked people to adjust the speed of one square so that it appeared to move at the same speed as another square. When both squares were the same size, observers were very accurate in their adjustments. (Typically a mismatch in speed as small as 10 percent can be easily seen.) However, when the two squares differed in size, the accuracy of the matches was very low. When the squares differed in size, the larger one had to move faster than the small one in order to appear to move at the same rate. As a result, if the two squares moved at the same

and ambient systems. Focal vision allows drivers to read traffic signs, judge distances, and watch out for pedestrians in the roadway; ambient vision allows the driver to orient the car, keeping it safely on the road. With decreasing illumination, such as that encountered at night, the focal system is selectively degraded, as shown by the decline of acuity. But the ambient system is less affected by reduced illumination—the driver can steer the car at even very low light levels. Consider what this means for the driver. Since steering ability is af-fected very little, the driver does not recognize that focal vision is impaired. Therefore, he drives just as fast as he would during the day—a serious error and a potential hazard.

The rationale for this perceptual theory arose from a surprising source—physiological research on hamsters. Gerald Schneider (1969) was interested in the visual functions of two structures in the hamster brain, the visual cortex and the superior colliculus. He lesioned one structure or the other and then examined how the hamster's vi-

speed, the larger one seemed to be moving more slowly than the smaller one.

Leibowitz points out that a comparable phenomenon can be seen at just about any airport. All commercial jets, regardless of size, land at pretty much the same speed. However, the jumbo jets (DC-10s or 747s) appear to land much more slowly than the smaller jets. Leibowitz believes that the same kind of perceptual error causes motorists at railroad crossings to underestimate an oncoming train's speed, and thereby overestimate the time the train will take to reach the crossing.

Let's end on a happier note, the ability of motion perception to prevent accidents. Particularly dangerous spots in any highway system are the intersections called rotaries (roundabouts in the United Kingdom). To navigate safely through a rotary, a driver must slow down. But since motorists often don't slow down enough, many accidents result. Because exhortations and warnings seemed to have little effect, Gordon Denton (1980) took a desperate step. He tricked motorists into believing their cars were traveling faster than they really were. His aim was to frighten motorists into slowing down.

Imagine a road with transverse stripes painted across the pavement. A motorist driving over these stripes will get a sense of how fast the car is traveling by the rate at which it passes the stripes. When they are close together the stripes will be passed at a higher rate, causing the driver to overestimate the car's speed. Denton exploited this phenomenon by having white stripes painted across the roadway near the entrance to a rotary— the stripes nearer the rotary were more closely spaced than those farther back. As a result, motorists approaching the rotary erroneously perceived that they were speeding up. This misperception caused them to slow down. Preliminary tests with this simple and inexpensive scheme indicate that it works: accidents declined at over two-thirds of the rotaries on which stripes had been painted. It's nice to know that illusions of motion perception can save lives as well as take them.

Obviously, there are other causes of accidents under poor visibility, but the differential involvement of the center and periphery is one intriguing possibility. Here we have discussed several connections between safety and peripheral responses to visual movement. These examples don't exhaust the literature on the periphery and motion perception. Finlay (1982) provides a good review of this literature.

---

sion was affected. The effects of cortical lesions seemed to differ from the effects of lesions of the colliculus. In particular, destroying the cortex made it difficult for the hamster to discriminate patterns but did not affect its ability to orient its head and body toward the patterns. Conversely, destroying the colliculus made it difficult for the hamster to orient itself toward the patterns; but if Schneider helped it orient properly, the hamster had little trouble discriminating the patterns. To explain these results, Schneider suggested that many species have not just one but two visual systems. According to this idea, the cortical system helps the animal recognize what object is present, and the collicular system helps the animal locate where that object is. Presumably humans, like hamsters, have both cortical and collicular systems and can draw on both. But when one system is damaged, there may be a selective loss of function. The results of other studies support Schneider's basic idea that one set of visual system structures extracts information about stimulus location and another, different but somewhat overlapping, set of structures extracts the stimulus's other attributes, such as size, texture, color, and motion. In primates, the anatomical substrates of the two subsystems are complex and involve many different structures (Knierim and van Essen, 1992). The distinction between the two visual subsystems has been supported by behavioral and physiological studies of monkeys (Mishkin, Ungerleider, and Macko, 1983; Morel and Bullier, 1990), results with computer networks designed to mimic key aspects of human vision (Otto et al., 1992; Rueckl, Cave, and Kosslyn, 1989), and PET studies of intact human brains (Haxby et al., 1991).

* * *

Think back to that scurrying creature we mentioned earlier. As it darted across the floor, you were able to see not only that it was moving but also the direction in which it moved. When the visual system signals the presence of movement, it also signals what direction that movement takes. Unlike other aspects of motion perception, the neural basis of this aspect of motion perception is fairly well understood. It is to the neural basis of direction perception that we now turn.

THE NEURAL BASIS OF MOTION PERCEPTION

Some cortical cells register direction of motion. They respond vigorously to motion in one "preferred" direction but little, if at all, to motion in the opposite direction (see Figure 4.10). Each **direction-selective cell,** then, prefers its own characteristic direction of motion. As a result, the direction of a moving object can be represented within the nervous system by the responses that object evokes in different cells. Before exploring the perceptual importance of direction-selective cells, we should clarify the origin of direction selectivity itself. How might one build a direction-selective cell?

Although various explanations have been advanced, most are simply variations on a single theme. Werner Reichardt (1961) devised the theme by showing that neurons could be interconnected so as to compare, or correlate, light intensities that strike neighboring retinal regions. (The notion that neurons can perform computations should already be familiar to you from Chapters 2 and 3.) Figure 8.13 schematizes the basic building block of Reichardt's theory. In the

FIGURE 8.13 Schematic drawing of a direction-selective cell responsive to rightward motion (left-hand panel), to leftward motion (middle panel), and to leftward motion faster than that registered by the cell in the middle panel (right-hand panel).

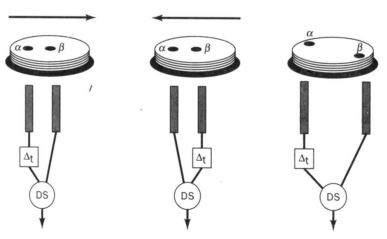

left-hand panel, signals from two regions of the retina (α and β) are collected by neurons (shaded rectangles) and passed along to another neuron, labeled DS (for "directionally selective"). Unit DS takes the inputs and multiplies them together. As a result, DS's response is strongest when its two inputs have the same brightness level and reach DS simultaneously. But note that on its way to DS, the input from region α is delayed by some time, call it Δt. As a result, in order for signals from α and β to arrive simultaneously at DS, the one from α must have a headstart. Putting this another way, we can say that DS responds when the same pattern of light strikes first region α and then, some time, Δt, later, strikes region β. One good stimulus would be an image that moved continuously across the retina from left to right, as represented by the arrow. It's important to realize that this isn't the only stimulus that would work; certain nonmoving stimuli would also be effective in stimulating DS. One example is a stationary light flashed briefly on region α and after Δt, on region β. Later, in the section on apparent motion, you'll see that such nonmoving stimuli do dupe the visual system into treating them as though they had moved.

Returning to Figure 8.13, let's assign the label Δx to the distance separating retinal regions α and β. Defining this distance allows us to be more precise about the moving stimulus that elicits the strongest response from DS. Recall that an optimal stimulus strikes first α and then β, after delay Δt. In order to meet that requirement, the stimulus must move over distance Δx in a time of Δt. As you know, speed is distance divided by time. Therefore the speed of the optimal stimulus is one whose speed is $\Delta x / \Delta t$. Given the proper direction, of course, this speed, which causes an image to fall first in region α and then, Δt later, in region β, will elicit a strong response from DS.

The middle panel of Figure 8.13 illustrates how you might construct a unit that would respond best to retinal image motion in the opposite direction, but with the same speed. Now look at the right-hand panel of Figure 8.13 and try to identify the direction of motion that best stimu-

lates DS. The orientation of the two input areas on the retina, together with the site of the delay, determines the direction to which DS will respond. Note also in the right-hand panel that the two retinal areas α and β are farther apart than were the areas in the other panels. Assuming that Δt, the delay, has not changed, would the optimal stimulus move faster or slower than it did in the cases we considered before? Finally, imagine a whole array of DS units. Suppose that each received signals from retinal regions separated by some distance Δx, and suppose that each preferred some particular delay Δt. If Δx and Δt varied from one DS to another, each DS would be optimally stimulated by a pattern moving in a particular direction and with a particular speed.

We can imagine an array of directionally selective neurons, each "looking for" a particular range of directions of motion within the same small region of space. The direction perceived by the observer could reflect the distribution of activity within the set of direction-selective cells with receptive fields in that part of the visual field. Recall that Chapter 4 proposed a comparable code for visual orientation, and Chapter 5 advanced a similar model for coding spatial frequency.* Here we will explore this hypothesis for perceived direction of motion in greater detail. One technique, **selective adaptation,** has been used to study movement perception both psychophysically and physiologically. Let's see how the two sets of results relate.

MOTION ADAPTATION

Sekuler and Ganz (1963) used selective adaptation to study motion perception behaviorally. Their stimuli were horizontal gratings that moved either upward or downward. An observer viewed an

---

* Analogous models have also been proposed in order to account for another aspect of motion perception—the perception of a target's velocity (Thompson, 1984). The plausibility of such models is enhanced by the discovery that some neurons in the visual cortex of cats and monkeys are tuned to particular ranges of stimulus velocities.

upward-moving grating of high contrast for several minutes. Exposure to this grating produced a twofold increase in the threshold for seeing upward motion. The increase was direction-selective, since the ability to see downward motion was not affected. Sekuler and Ganz proposed that adaptation fatigued cortical cells responsive to the direction of motion seen during adaptation; subsequent physiological experiments confirmed that such an effect does indeed occur in cortical neurons (Hammond, Movat, and Smith, 1985).

Perceptually, prolonged exposure to one direction of motion does more than merely make that direction harder to see. After viewing one direction of motion for several minutes, people experience illusory motion in the opposite direction. This is known as the **motion aftereffect** or sometimes as the **waterfall illusion,** since the illusion is often experienced after looking at a waterfall (Addams, 1834/1964). You may have already experienced this illusion. If you haven't, here is an easy way to generate a strong motion aftereffect. Many television programs have long "crawls"—the steadily moving list of people who were responsible for the show. To read the names, your eyes have to keep up with the crawl. Next time you see a crawl, though, forget about reading the names and just keep your eyes fixed steadily on the center of the screen while the crawl goes by. Then as soon as the crawl is over, you will experience illusory motion in a direction opposite to that of the crawl—this is the motion aftereffect. But how do we explain this illusion within the context of direction-selective neurons? Here's one possibility.

When the visual field is uniformly illuminated and no moving contours are present, all direction-selective cells, regardless of their direction preference, generate approximately equal levels of spontaneous activity. Following prolonged exposure to a particular direction—say, downward—cells preferring downward motion will have virtually no spontaneous activity. This produces a biased distribution of spontaneous activity: cells responsive to downward motion now show little if any spontaneous activity, while cells re-

sponsive to upward motion show a normal level of spontaneous activity. This biased distribution of spontaneous activity produced following adaptation is similar to the activity distribution evoked by actual motion upward—hence the illusory upward motion. In other words, this biased distribution of spontaneous activity could produce the motion aftereffect (Barlow and Hill, 1963; Mather and Moulden, 1980).* Elaborations of this idea have been advanced recently (Hiris and Blake, 1992), still relying on the notion of a biased distribution of activity among direction-selective neurons.

We've just seen one consequence—the motion aftereffect—of a bias in the distribution of responses of direction-selective neurons. Let's examine another perceptual consequence of biased distributions, since it provides additional support for this way of thinking about the perceived direction of motion. If an object's perceived direction of motion does depend on the distribution of activity in direction-selective neurons, it should be possible to alter a moving object's perceived direction by adapting some of those neurons. Levinson and Sekuler (1976) asked observers to judge the direction in which an array of bright dots traveled across a television screen. Prior to adaptation, the judgments were accurate. After adapting for several minutes to dots moving steadily in one direction, the observers again judged the direction in which dots moved. When the dots moved steadily in a direction similar but not identical to the adaptation direction, the observers now made errors of judgment: the direction of motion of the dots always seemed to be shifted away from the adaptation direction. This phenomenon should remind you of the tilt aftereffect demonstrated in Figure 4.19.

---

* The waterfall illusion is not the only case in which stationary objects appear to move. Have you ever noticed how the moon appears to move speedily across the sky as clouds pass in front of it? This is an example of **induced motion**—the real movement of the clouds causes illusory movement of the moon (Duncker, 1929/1938). Unlike the waterfall illusion, induced motion's physiological basis is not known.

NEUROANATOMICAL LOCUS OF DIRECTION-SELECTIVE CELLS

Directionally selective neurons, whose behavior may explain the phenomena just discussed, are found in several different regions of the cerebral cortex. Some researchers argue that an entire pathway (a collection of interconnected cortical regions) is devoted to analyzing various forms of motion information (DeYoe and van Essen, 1988; Wilson, Ferrera, and Yo, 1992). A key stage in this pathway is the medial temporal (MT) region on each side of the brain. Virtually all the neurons in Area MT exhibit strong directional selectivity, which is not surprising since the medial temporal region receives input from directionally selective cells in the visual cortex (recall Chapter 4). However, the directionally selective neurons in the visual cortex respond to local motion within a small patch of the visual field. In contrast, many MT neurons respond strongly to global motion over large regions of the visual field. This suggests that MT neurons perform some complex function, perhaps the integration of several different directions of motion that may be present at the same time (Adelson and Movshon, 1982).

The role of MT neurons in motion perception has been assessed in monkeys, using behavioral techniques that compare psychophysical performance before and after inactivation of Area MT. Injecting a neuronal poison, such as ibotenic acid, into Area MT on the left side of the monkey's brain kills neurons within the injected tissue, creating a localized chemical lesion. Bear in mind that as with other visual regions, MT neurons in the left cerebral hemisphere receive information from the right visual hemifield, while neurons in the right cerebral hemisphere receive information from the left visual hemifield (recall Figure 4.2). These unilateral chemical lesions should hinder motion perception when stimuli are in the right hemifield, but not in the left hemifield.

To test this prediction, Newsome and Paré (1988) created "films" showing many dots that could move in one of two ways, correlated or uncorrelated. With correlated motion, all dots moved in the same direction (either up or down). The two right-hand panels of Figure 8.14 show this arrangement. With uncorrelated motion, each dot could move in any direction and, consequently, appeared to jiggle about randomly, moving like swirling snow. This stimulus is represented in the two left-hand panels of Figure 8.14.

Using a mixture of correlated and uncorrelated motions (such as in the middle panels of Figure 8.14), Newsome and Paré determined how much correlated motion had to be added to an uncorrelated display in order for the monkey to discriminate whether the global motion was upward or downward. Also, by positioning the display in either the right or left hemifield, Newsome and Paré tested the performance of the left (lesioned) and the right (unlesioned) cerebral hemispheres.

Prior to the destruction of MT neurons, the monkey's performance was remarkable: accurate discrimination was possible when as few as 2 to 3 percent of the dots moved in the same direction (either up or down). Performance was equally good in left and right hemifields. After the left hemisphere's medial temporal region had been chemically lesioned, though, things changed. Ability to detect global motion using the lesioned hemisphere decreased by nearly tenfold; ability remained normal in the unlesioned hemisphere. The left hemisphere's deficit, however, affected motion perception only; the monkey's ability to see nonmoving targets, such as stationary gratings, was not changed. Although some deficits in motion perception persisted, the monkey's performance improved significantly over the 3 weeks following the lesion. As Newsome and Paré (1988) point out, "the recovery presumably depends on motion information transmitted via pathways in parallel with those through MT" (p. 2208). Whatever its explanation, the recovery testifies to the brain's amazing plasticity.

Although neurons in Area MT certainly contribute to the perception of motion, one shouldn't get the idea that Area MT is *the* place where motion perception occurs. Actually, various aspects of motion perception depend upon the

Percentage correlation

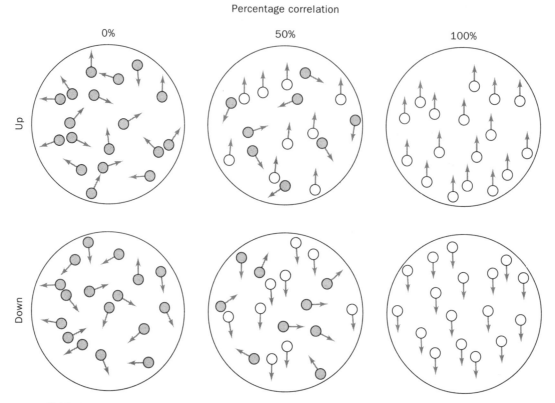

FIGURE 8.14 Schematic representation of a random-dot stimulus that can be used to measure motion thresholds. In each panel, the arrow indicates the direction in which the attached dot moves. In the two left-hand panels, there is 0 percent correlation among the movements of the various dots; they move in every which direction. In the two right-hand panels, movements of all dots are 100 percent correlated, either up (as in the top panel) or down (as in the bottom panel). The middle panels represent an intermediate case: 50 percent of the dots move together, either up (top panel) or down (bottom panel). To make it easier for the reader to distinguish them, dots that move in an uncorrelated fashion are shown in gray; in the actual stimulus, all dots were identical.

neural computations carried out in several different areas of the cortex. Normal motion perception depends on activity distributed over many areas of the brain, each extracting somewhat different information from the retinal image. To emphasize this point, consider the computations carried out in another region of the cortex, Area MST (MST stands for "medial superior temporal," a label that indicates this area lies adjacent to and just above MT, "medial temporal"). Going back to the complex circuit shown in Figure 4.15, you may be able to find MST's two divisions, MSTd and MSTl (for dorsal and lateral, respec-

tively), and confirm that both receive input from MT, among other structures. In a way, MST's view of the world is shaped by MT.

To reinforce the notion that motion perception depends upon computations in multiple areas of the brain, consider the properties of some neurons in MST's dorsal division. Much of our understanding of MST and its contribution to motion perception comes from the work of Keiji Tanaka and his colleagues (Tanaka and Saito, 1989). Tanaka showed that neurons in MSTd have extremely large receptive fields, likely reflecting each neuron's input from many, spatially dispersed neurons in MT. Moreover, MSTd neurons respond most strongly to stimuli that move in a characteristic fashion over large portions of the visual field. These preferred motions are quite different from the translatory motions that V1 and MT neurons prefer. In MSTd, neurons respond strongly to stimulus expansion (or its opposite, contraction) or stimulus rotation. The stimuli preferred by two typical cells are shown schematically in panels A and B of Figure 8.15. The stimuli depicted here are spatially random dots, but strong responses could also be evoked by other stimuli,

so long as they contained appropriate directional vectors. For example, expansion patterns, like those shown in Figure 8.8, would evoke good responses from an MST expansion cell; a rotating spiral or other pattern would evoke good responses from an MST rotation neuron. Additional experiments by Tanaka, Fukada, and Saito (1989) show the likely origin of the stimulus preferences expressed by expansion neurons and rotation neurons. We have schematized these origins in panels C (expansion) and D (rotation) of Figure 8.15. Each MST neuron received input from several

FIGURE 8.15 The two upper panels depict motion vectors associated with expansion (A) and with rotation (B). The two lower panels show possible inputs to a neuron selectively responsive to expansion (C) or to rotation (D).

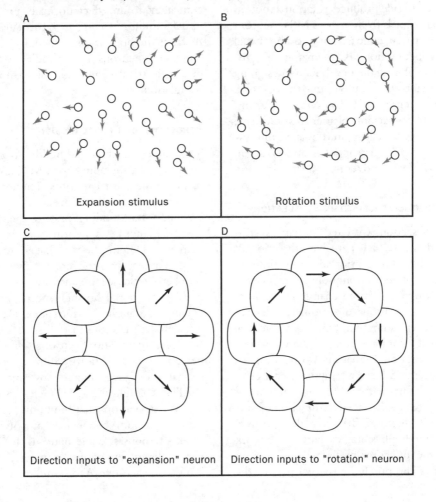

A

Expansion stimulus

B

Rotation stimulus

C

Direction inputs to "expansion" neuron

D

Direction inputs to "rotation" neuron

MT neurons, each of which has its own preference for motion in a particular direction (shown by the arrows). Although the diagrams show eight different input neurons, Tanaka and colleagues indicate that fewer would suffice, so long as their direction preference were appropriate.

What value could these odd neural computations have? Why should the brain bother to register optical expansion or optical rotation? Think back to our earlier discussion of visual guidance of locomotion. There we noted the importance of variables such as optical expansion (looming) and time to collision. In a stable environment, forward locomotion produces expansion of the retinal image; as we saw earlier, the rate of optical expansion carries information about time to collision. In the same environment, twisting your head from side to side produces rotational motion on the retina. Signals from various MST neurons could make crucial contributions to the visual guidance of locomotion. Recognizing this, researchers are exploring the possibility of designing integrated circuits that would mimic the complex computations represented by MST neurons. These MST-like electronic elements would have enormous use, they believe, in robots' vision systems (for example, Hatsopoulos and Warren, 1991; Poggio, Verri, and Torre, 1991).

MOTION PERCEPTION FROM BRAIN STIMULATION

Earlier in this section, we cited human psychophysical studies in which perceived direction of motion was altered by a prior adapting stimulus. The alterations of perception probably reflected a temporary, stimulus-induced change in the normal responses of various directionally selective units. One recent study combined physiological and behavioral techniques to strengthen this view of motion perception. In that study, tiny localized electrical currents induced a temporary change in the responses of particular MT units, and an accompanying change in perceived direction of motion (Salzman, Murasugi, Britten, and Newsome, 1992). The purely physiological part of the work established the direction preferences of various MT neurons. The purely behavioral part of the

work required that the monkeys move their eyes in one direction or another to signal the perceived direction of various random-dot displays. Combining behavior and physiology, perceptual judgments were elicited (1) while electrical stimulation was being applied to particular MT neurons, or (2) without accompanying electrical stimulation.

Electrical stimulation of neurons that share a direction preference biased the monkeys' perceptual judgments of random-dot displays. The result was an increased likelihood that the display would appear to move in the direction preferred by the stimulated neurons. So, for example, direct stimulation of MT neurons that prefer leftward motion made it more likely that the display would appear to move in that direction. Direct stimulation of MT neurons, then, was perceptually equivalent to an effect normally produced by a visual stimulus moving in a particular direction. As far as the brain is concerned, it doesn't matter whether its neurons are responding to this unusual direct electrical stimulation or to normal visual stimulation.

PERCEPTION OF GLOBAL MOTION

The studies just discussed build a strong case that cortical areas, including Area MT, are important in processing visual motion. The excitement of this discovery tends to overshadow one potentially important finding: prior to the chemical lesion, the monkey's performance was truly remarkable. Despite the fact that 97 to 98 percent of the displacements were totally random, the monkey could see the net motion. And when humans are tested on such stimuli, they achieve equally outstanding performance. How does the visual system manage to pull such a weak signal (2 percent correlation) out of so much noise (98 percent noncorrelation)? Some theorists credit special synergistic interactions among neurons (Williams, Phillips, and Sekuler, 1986). The key idea is that neurons that respond to similar directions of motion "cooperate," amplifying one another's responses, while neurons that respond to very different directions "compete," tending to inhibit one another. As a result, the effect of even a small amount of motion in a single direction gets amplified, and the effect of other motions in many different, uncorrelated directions is diminished.

Cooperative-competitive interactions among direction-selective neurons might be important in another well-known perceptual phenomenon. It was long ago recognized that a perception of **global motion**—a general tendency to perceive motion in a given direction—emerges even though many individual motion vectors are random (Koffka, 1935). In other words, nearby elements or features tend to be seen as moving together. This phenomenon, which the Gestaltists called "the law of common fate," is just what one would expect from synergistic interactions among neurons tuned to similar directions (Yuille and Grzywacz, 1988). You can experience "common fate" for yourself when a light breeze blows the leaves of a tree. You can see the tree's net motion (in the direction of the breeze) despite the fact that each leaf also moves on its own. Or, as smoke rises from a chimney, you can see the smoke's net motion despite the random perturbations of its various parts.

Like the Gestalt organizational principles discussed in Chapter 5, the law of common fate may reflect how well our visual systems match the physical properties of the world in which we live. In our world, immediately adjacent regions in the visual field tend to belong to the same object. As a result, there is a correlated tendency for adjacent regions, when they do move, to move in similar directions. In fact, when adjacent regions fail to behave in this way, the visual system treats those adjacent regions as belonging to different objects (recall the discussion of motion parallax in Chapter 7).

MOTION CAPTURE

When we discussed various Gestalt principles in Chapter 5, we noted how they sometimes lead to revealing errors in perception. The same holds for the law of common fate, as the following shows. Ramachandran and Cavanagh (1987) used a computer to create two different random-dot patterns presented in rapid alternation on the computer's display screen. Because the dots in the two were unrelated to one another, this alternation caused the dots to appear to jump about randomly. Ramachandran and Cavanagh then superimposed a low-contrast, moving grating over the noisy display. The grating's motion immediately captured the random jumps of the dots—all the dots now seemed to move along with the grating as though the grating and dots were a single, complex object.

Here's how you can see **motion capture** for yourself. Using a broad-tipped pen, create a grating by drawing a series of parallel lines on a sheet of cellophane or overhead transparency material (a marker such as a fluorescent underliner with transparent ink works best). Then tune a television set to a channel that is not broadcasting; this will create a snowy effect much like the random motions that Ramachandran and Cavanagh's subjects first saw. Place your homemade grating against the television screen and move it smoothly. You'll see that the television's bright spots, which formerly jumped about at random, now follow along quite tamely as the grating is moved.

APPARENT MOTION

Ordinarily, your experience of motion is quite straightforward. You notice a small, timid rabbit standing at one spot nibbling on some weeds. Then, over the next few seconds, the rabbit hops over to another clump of weeds. Without doubt you'll experience the changes in the rabbit's position as movement. But how does your experience arise? Obviously, the image cast on your retina by that rabbit has moved, hence the experience of motion. Conditions such as this one seem to require no explanation—you see motion because there *is* motion. But retinal image motion cannot entirely explain the perception of motion. We've already seen two cases where motion is perceived in the absence of retinal image motion—the motion aftereffect and induced motion (mentioned in a footnote). Now we're about to consider a third, more common case, known as **apparent motion.** This kind of motion has become an important part of our lives. As Stuart Anstis points out,

The flashing lights on a cinema marquee, which seem to move inward toward the lobby and entice us to follow them, are an example of apparent movement. If we go in and watch the movie, we experience two hours of apparent movement: each movie frame projected on the screen is actually stationary whenever the projector is open. If we stay at home and watch TV instead, we are once again experiencing apparent movement. Films and TV, as they exist today, are possible only because of a quirk in our visual systems. (1978, p. 656)

The visual system takes discrete and separate inputs (such as the separate frames of a movie) and knits them into an experience that is smooth and continuous. This is the "quirk" to which Anstis refers. We'll focus on apparent movement now because this quirk provides insights into how the visual system operates under conditions where there is genuine motion of the retinal image. (As we progress through this discussion, keep in mind the scheme, shown in Figure 8.13, by which one can construct direction-selective neurons.)

People have known about apparent motion for quite some time. For example, Sigmund Exner (1888) created brief but intense electrical sparks from two sources. He placed the two sources some distance apart and had observers judge which spark flashed first—the one on the right or the one on the left. When the time delay between sparks was long, the judgment was easy; when the delay was short, the judgment became difficult. Exner found that about one-twenty-fifth of a second had to intervene between the two sparks before their order could be judged accurately. Exner next placed the two sources of sparks very close to each other. With short intervals between the two sparks, people saw apparent motion—a spark moving from one location to the other. Exner then asked people to judge the direction of that apparent motion. Although these people needed delays of one-twenty-fifth of a second to judge the order of sparks that were some distance apart,

they needed less than half that delay to judge the *direction* of movement. This experience of apparent movement could not have been *derived* from judging the sequence of flashes, because the time interval separating the two flashes was too brief to allow for such a judgment. Instead, motion was experienced directly.

Next Exner brought the two sparks so close together that they appeared as a single bright spark. When the twin sparks were flashed one after the other, the observer saw apparent motion even though the sparks were too close together to be resolved. This experience of apparent movement could not have been *derived* from judging the positions of flashes, because the flashes were so close together that they couldn't be distinguished. Again, motion was experienced directly. Apparent motion between points that cannot be resolved spatially has been confirmed by others (Thorson, Lange, and Biederman-Thorson, 1969; Foster, Thorson, McIlwain, and Biederman-Thorson, 1981).

Exner's observations led him to conclude that motion was a primary sensation in its own right, not just an inference derived from comparing temporal order or spatial position. Bearing in mind that apparent motion is not an inference, let's consider the work of Max Wertheimer, the Gestalt psychologist mentioned in Chapter 5.

In one study, Wertheimer (1912/1961) briefly presented two spatially separated vertical lines in succession. What did people *see?* The answer depended on the length of the delay that separated the two presentations. With long delays (greater than one-tenth of a second), one line appeared to succeed the other. In other words, the observer saw one line that came on and went off and then a second line that did the same. With very short delays between presentations (say, one-fortieth of a second or less), the two lines appeared to come on and go off simultaneously. Perceptually there had been only a single presentation. With intermediate delays between presentation of the two lines (say, one-twentieth of a second), a single line appeared to move smoothly from one position to the other. In other words, people saw apparent motion.

To determine whether this apparent motion was retinal or central in origin, Wertheimer arranged conditions so that the first line was seen by one eye and the second line was seen by the other eye. Even under these conditions of interocular stimulation, motion was perceived. This suggests that the neural events giving rise to the perception of motion are central, lying at or beyond the site where information from the eyes has combined. Wertheimer devised a simple but effective demonstration of interocular apparent movement, one that you, too, can try.

Hold a thin book in both hands and lean your forehead against the book's edge, as shown in Figure 8.16. Be sure to place your head so that one eye is on each side of the book. This allows you to use the book as a separator, making it easy to present different objects to the two eyes. Now place your hands on opposite sides of the book with only the index fingers extended upward. Position the left hand so that its index finger can be seen by your left eye, and position your right hand so that its index finger can be seen by your right eye. Don't look directly at your fingers; instead, keep your gaze directed straight ahead at a point several inches beyond the far end of the book. Your fingers should be about 6 inches from your nose. Now comes the hard part. Rhythmically open and close alternate eyes. Though it may take a little practice, at the proper speed of alternation you'll have a strange and amusing experience: your finger will appear to jump back and forth right through the book.

Wertheimer did not know what is known today about cortical function. Thus he mistakenly attributed apparent motion to a short-circuiting of current flow in the brain. Today, apparent motion is more plausibly explained by the responses of direction-selective neurons. As you've already seen, such neurons respond strongly when an object moves through the neuron's receptive field. But many of these neurons can be tricked into responding to an object that doesn't move at all. For example, one neuron may give a vigorous response when a bright bar moves through its receptive field from left to right. The same neuron may give a similar response when a *stationary* bar is briefly flashed, once at the left side of its receptive field and then at the right side. In other words, the neuron's responses to these two very different conditions are virtually identical. If neurons such as this play a role in the perception of motion, these two conditions should be indistinguishable.

THE CORRESPONDENCE PROBLEM IN MOTION PERCEPTION

How does the visual system detect that an object seen at one moment corresponds to the same object seen at another moment? After all, the "finger" example demonstrates that detecting correspondence over time is a prerequisite for motion perception. We can highlight the nature of this prerequisite by comparing retinal images to photographic snapshots of the visual world. Suppose that you have two retinal "snapshots" that were taken a fraction of a second apart. Looking at the two snapshots, how would you determine whether a single object had moved? To accomplish this, you must determine which elements in one snapshot correspond to which elements in the other (this problem is reminiscent of the matching problem in stereopsis, discussed in Chapter 7). Now here's the problem: potentially, any small detail in one of the snapshots *might* correspond to any number of different details in the other. This situation is illustrated by a simple display that has been widely used to study apparent motion (see Figure 8.17). Here, two displays (panel 1 and panel 2) alternate, separated by a brief uniform

FIGURE 8.16 Setup for experiencing apparent motion.

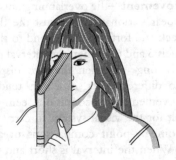

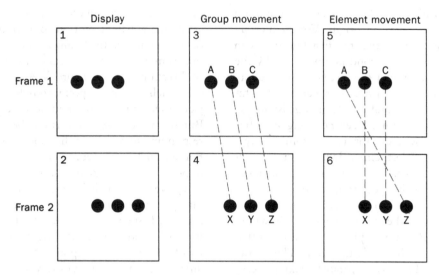

FIGURE 8.17 An illustration of the correspondence problem in motion perception.

field (not shown). Both frames contain a trio of large dots. Note that from frame 1 to frame 2, the trio of dots has been shifted rightward. Before telling you what you would actually see, let's consider the possibilities, bearing in mind that what you'll see depends on the correspondence that vision selects.

Panels 3 through 6 of Figure 8.17 illustrate two possible correspondences. Following the dotted lines from panel 3 to panel 4 shows that your visual system might pair dot A with dot X, dot B with dot Y, and dot C with dot Z. With these correspondences, you would see the entire group of dots moving rightward: A to X, B to Y, and C to Z. Following the dotted lines from panel 5 to panel 6 shows an alternate set of correspondences. Here, your visual system pairs dots B and X, dots C and Y, and dots A and Z. With this set of correspondences, you would see two stationary dots (since B and X occupy the same positions on successive frames, as do C and Y). At the same time, you would see a third dot (A-Z) that moves all the way from the left end of the trio to the right end.

This simple two-frame display is interesting because its ambiguity makes possible two different

percepts, depending on how the correspondence problem is solved. The apparent motion actually seen from such ambiguous displays reveals the rules used by the visual system to establish correspondences. The percept is a choice from among the various sets of correspondences that *might* have been selected.

What, then, do observers actually see when they're shown displays such as that depicted in panels 1 and 2 of Figure 8.17? How does the visual system solve the correspondence problem? The answer is, "It depends" (Pantle and Picciano, 1976; Pantle and Petersik, 1979). Under some conditions, observers see **group movement**—all three dots seem to move en masse (as in panels 3 and 4). Under other conditions, observers see **element movement**—the overlapping dots of each frame appear stationary while just the third dot moves back and forth from one end to the other (as in panels 5 and 6). When the interval between displays is long, or when the two displays are shown to different eyes, observers tend to see group movement. Such conditions seem to make it difficult for the visual system to carry out detailed, point-by-point comparisons of alternate displays. When the interval is short and the two displays are shown to the same eye, observers tend to see element movement. Such conditions facilitate detailed comparisons between displays.

These results demonstrate that vision can be flexible when it has to solve a problem of correspondence. But the world in which we live contains few situations in which correspondences are as ambiguous as those represented in Figure 8.17 or as those that have been generated in other studies (Lappin, Doner, and Kottas, 1979; Ullman, 1979). The number of potential correspondences can be sharply reduced if the visual system takes advantage of regularities in the physical world (Marr, 1982; Ramachandran and Anstis, 1986). After all, the visual system evolved in a world whose objects share particular properties: natural objects don't change color suddenly; natural objects are made of parts that are connected; the surface texture of natural objects tends to be uniform; natural objects, once in motion, tend to stay in motion; and solid objects cannot move through one another. Neurons in the visual system register these and other regularities. In so doing, the visual system is biased against unnatural solutions to the correspondence problem, favoring solutions that are consistent with the properties of real-world objects.

As an example, consider one consistency between apparent motion and the motion of natural objects. Objects in either form of motion seem to obey Newton's first law of motion: once in motion, a body will continue in motion unless acted upon by an external force. In one demonstration of this law, Wertheimer alternated two targets at a rate that he knew would produce apparent motion between them—say, a line at the left and a line at the right. As long as the alternation continued, the line appeared to travel back and forth. Then without warning to the viewer, he occluded one of the lines but kept presenting the remaining line at its appropriate times. Surprisingly, even though only one line was being exposed, it took some time for the apparent motion to cease. For three or four repetitions, the observer continued to see motion. These findings suggest that inertia works not only in the natural world but in the world of apparent motion as well.

Newton's first law of motion applies to all objects in the real world. So perhaps it's not a shock that the visual motion reflects such a general real-world property. But can properties that are far more specific, limited to particular objects, also influence the perception of motion? Maggie Shiffrar, Rutgers University, and Jennifer Freyd, University of Oregon, (1990) proved that the answer is yes. In one of their experiments, two photographs of a human model were alternated in rapid succession. The photographs in each pair were identical except for the position of the model's head or the position of a single limb. One set of photos, for example, showed the hand fully extended and rotated about the wrist in two different positions. To get a sense of this stimulus, extend your right arm fully and directly in front of you; spread the fingers of that hand, palm facing forward. Rotate your wrist so that your fingers point leftward; seen from the front (as in a mirror) that could be one of the pair of photos. To create the second member of the stimulus pair, rotate the wrist as far as it will go in the other direction, without moving your arm (for most people, the fingers will end up pointing downward or nearly so). These stimuli are illustrated in Figure 8.18.

Before reading further, imagine what a person might see when these two views are alternated. In principle, alternation of these two views of the hand, wrist, and arm could produce apparent motion along either of two quite different paths. One path represents a large rotation of the wrist (about 270 degrees); the other path represents a much shorter (about 90 degrees or less) one. These paths differ not only in length but also in biological plausibility; the shorter path requires a rotation that is biologically impossible (unless the wrist were able to rotate through a full 360 degrees). Shiffrar and Freyd found that when the two photos alternated with only a brief time elapsing between them, people saw the shorter (biologically impossible) rotation. This result was not surprising as many previous studies had shown the visual system tends to resolve a choice between two paths in favor of the shorter one. With greater intervals between the photos, though, Shiffrar and Freyd's observers tended to see motion over the

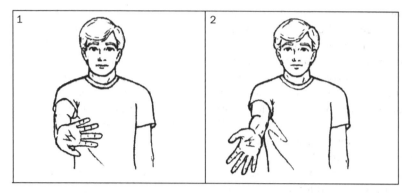

FIGURE 8.18 Drawings based on one set of stimuli used to study biological plausibility's effect on apparent motion (Shiffrar & Freyd, 1990). When the stimuli are presented in alternation, the young man's hand appears to rotate about his wrist, either clockwise or counterclockwise. With a brief interval separating the two stimuli, the hand appears to rotate through a short, but biologically implausible arc; with a greater interval between stimuli, the hand appears to rotate in the opposite direction, over a path that is longer but biologically plausible.

Box 8.3 *Looking One's Age*

Some events happen so slowly that they cannot be perceived while they are happening; you perceive them only later. Despite the leisurely pace of these events, your ability to see them may involve the same processes as those discussed in relation to motion perception. One of these leisurely events is the aging process. Usually, you can judge someone's age merely by looking at that individual. But what stimulus information makes this judgment possible? Some television advertisements claim that the surest signs of age are hand wrinkles that result from washing dishes. Other commercials suggest that grayness of hair is an even surer sign of age. But might there not be some more general visual cue to age?

Examine the accompanying illustration (adapted from Pittenger, Shaw, and Mark, 1979). To create these cartoons of the human head, John Pittenger and Robert Shaw

(1975) began with the head at the right. Next, they produced the remaining heads by transforming the original one according to a formula designed to capture growth's effects on the human head. Going leftward in the row of human heads, you will notice that the heads become younger in appearance. People's judgments of age reflect the information represented in the formula; the perceived relative ages of the faces corresponded closely to the way they had been transformed. Leonard Mark and James Todd (1983) extended this work by applying the same mathematical transformation to a three-dimensional sculpture of a 15-year-old girl's head. They used a computer to carve a new sculpture of the same girl by transforming the original. In its carving, the computer used values that were intended to create a sculpture of the girl at age 6. Mark and Todd took the two sculptures and asked people to judge the ages of

longer, but biologically plausible, path. The visual system, then, can be influenced by the physical plausibility of particular stimulus transformations, provided that there is sufficient time for that influence to be registered.

THE ROLE OF APPARENT MOTION IN ANIMATION

The susceptibility of complex patterns to apparent motion has important commercial applications. About 20 years ago, makers of animated films began to exploit some of apparent movement's quirks (Bregman and Mills, 1982). Before then, animated films (of the Disney style) involved a succession of carefully drawn frames that approximated samples from continuous motion. To create the impression that Donald Duck is walking from one spot to another, an animator would draw and photograph a long series of individual drawings. Each drawing would portray Donald's legs in a position that was just slightly different from that of the preceding drawing. Needless to say, this was an expensive and time-consuming process.

Fred Hanna and William Barbera, creators of Fred Flintstone and other cartoon characters, took a different, more economical approach. To create the impression that Fred Flintstone is walking, they made drawings of Fred's legs in three different positions on pieces of clear plastic. To simulate walking, they photographed the three pieces of plastic alternately in combination with Fred's other parts, which were drawn on separate pieces of plastic. Because his legs can take so few different positions, Fred's gait appears a little jerky. But he does appear to walk. Actually, though, Fred's walk is as illusory as your finger's ability to pass back and forth through a book.

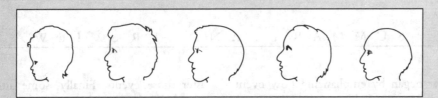

the individuals portrayed. The age judgments averaged 14.5 years for the original and 6.3 years for the derived sculpture. This demonstrates that the formula used to create the cartoon heads also succeeds in capturing whatever information people use when they judge the age of real humans.

In the United States, similar techniques have been harnessed in parents' efforts to find missing children. Technicians can "age" the missing child's face, creating a version that often proves to be a close approximation to the child's current appearance. These fairly simple transformations are related to more complex techniques used in video and film produc-

tion. "Tweening," a technique used in computer-aided animation, allows the animator to draw only two frames, the start and finish, of a character's movement; the computer, using a series of rules, creates all the frames 'tween the two. More spectacular and far more complicated procedures are used in "morphing." Here, one figure is transformed smoothly into a very different figure. In one of its early uses, morphing created the illusion that a pop singer was changing, right before our eyes, into a panther (Sorensen, 1992). Magical? Perhaps, but no more magical than the seemingly routine feats performed by our sensory systems.

For the past several pages we have focused on an error that perception makes. This error—apparent motion—is evoked under artificial conditions, including television and movies. In fact, the conditions that produce apparent motion almost never occur naturally. These artificial conditions stand in sharp contrast to the naturalistic, biological motion discussed at the beginning of this chapter. Some people question the wisdom of using apparent motion to understand a visual system that never saw such motion during the course of its evolution. However, Roger Shepard, of Stanford University, offers some wise counsel about the usefulness of exploiting unnatural conditions in order to study perception:

A recognition of the ecological foundations of perception need not entail experiments that mirror the spatiotemporal properties of the natural environment. [In fact,] the internalized constraints of this system are most clearly revealed when our experimental probings system-atically depart from the patterns to which the system has evolved a complementary fit, for only then does the system lose its "transparency" and so reveal its own inner structure. (1981, p. 311)

Of course, Shepard's plan of attack does not rule out a complementary approach—studying motion perception under more natural conditions (Michaels and Carello, 1981). These two complementary approaches really address different aspects of perception. Studies using artificial or unnatural conditions focus on the mechanisms that underlie motion perception; here the emphasis is on the internal processes within the perceiver. Studies employing more natural or ecologically representative stimuli attempt to identify the stimulus information available in the perceiver's surroundings (see Box 8.3); here the emphasis is on the environment. We believe that a complete understanding of motion perception requires both approaches.

S U M M A R Y　A N D　P R E V I E W

This chapter began by emphasizing how event perception defines visual objects, particularly ones that are alive and move. The chapter went on to discuss how you explore your world by means of visually guided locomotion and by means of eye movements. Next we considered the neural basis of movement perception, noting the good match between the properties of natural events and the properties of neural mechanisms designed to register those events. Finally, some attention was given to an unnatural but common form of motion—apparent motion.

This concludes the four-chapter survey of the visual qualities that enable you to appreciate various biologically important aspects of the world. Next we turn to other senses that also provide vital information about that world. We begin with the ear and hearing.

K E Y　T E R M S

ambient system	dynamic visual acuity	group movement
apparent motion	element movement	induced motion
critical flicker frequency (CFF)	flicker	motion aftereffect
direction-selective cell	focal system	motion capture
	global motion	optic ataxia

proprioception
pursuit eye movements
saccades
selective adaptation
smooth eye movements

stabilized retinal images
stimulus uncertainty
structure from motion
 (SFM)
vestibular

vestibular eye movements
vestibule
visual masking
waterfall illusion

The Ear and Auditory System

C lose your eyes and listen carefully to the sounds around you. Even in the quietest room, it's surprising how much there is to hear. As you listen, try to identify what makes one sound different from another. Undoubtedly, you'll notice that sounds appear to come from sources located at different positions around you. These sources can usually be pinpointed with ease. Notice also how sounds may differ in loudness, ranging from the soft rustle of leaves on a tree to the piercing wail of a siren. Sounds vary in their complexity, too. A birdsong may be composed of just a few notes, or pitches, whereas the traffic on a busy street can generate a cacophony of sound. Besides complexity, sounds can also differ in their cadences, or rhythms. Some sounds have a regularity that makes them recognizable—for example, the sound of footsteps in the hallway. The tempo of those footsteps may even disclose who's coming. In contrast, other sounds, such as the snap of a breaking twig, occur abruptly and without repetition.

So sounds have many features that enable us to identify and locate the objects or people from which they arise. Hearing plays a very important role in defining one's perceptual world. Often, you are able to *hear* things in your environment before you can see them. You rely heavily on hearing when it is dark or when an event occurs out of your field of view. And even when a sound source *is* readily visible, your behavioral reaction to it may depend on the nature of the sound it makes. For example, some grocery shoppers believe that a melon's ripeness can be judged only

from the sound made by thumping it. A similar thumping technique is sometimes used by doctors to check for fluid accumulation within a patient's chest cavity. And hearing provides the basis for many forms of social communication, the most notable being speech. Without the ability to hear voices, an individual must struggle heroically to remain in touch with the flow of social discourse. Perceptual appreciation of the world becomes substantially diminished when hearing is lost, as any deaf person will testify (Noble, 1983).

In this chapter we shall examine the process of hearing, starting with the acoustic energy that carries auditory information, and progressing through what is known about the machinery of hearing. This coverage sets the stage for the next chapter, which considers some of the psychological aspects of hearing, pitch perception, sound localization, and speech perception.

ASPECTS OF SOUND

WHAT IS SOUND?

Sound starts when some mechanical disturbance produces vibrations. These vibrations are transmitted through some medium (usually air) in the form of tiny collisions among the molecules in that medium. If they are sufficiently strong when they arrive at your ears, these vibrations trigger a chain of events culminating in an auditory sensation. All sounds, regardless of their nature, come to you this way. It's odd, but the strains of a symphony and the flush of a toilet share the same physical basis, a series of tiny molecular collisions. To understand this, let's consider sound and its properties in greater detail.

Whenever an object vibrates, or moves back and forth, it causes a disturbance within its surroundings. This disturbance takes the form of waves spreading outward from the source of vibration, and these waves constitute what is known as **acoustic energy.** They travel through the surrounding medium in a manner similar to the ripples produced when a pebble is tossed into a quiet pond (see Figure 9.1). Like ripples on a pond, sound waves must have something to travel through—there can be no sound in empty space or in a perfect vacuum. This was convincingly demonstrated in the seventeenth century by Robert Boyle, a British physicist and chemist. He placed an alarm bell inside a tightly sealed jar and used a vacuum pump to suck all the air out of this jar. When the alarm went off, the bell "rang" but could not be heard. After quickly pumping air back into the jar, Boyle could hear the bell. From this simple experiment, Boyle correctly concluded that air was made up of particles and that sound involved waves of energy traveling *through* these particles. We could liken this energy to the wave of motion produced by toppling a stack of dominoes lined up in a row. In this analogy, the individual dominoes represent individual air molecules; the wave of energy is transmitted by one domino bumping into another—a chain reaction propagated the length of the row of dominoes. For the analogy to be complete, however, each domino would have to return to its upright position after colliding with its neighbor, becoming available for participation in future chain reactions.

FIGURE 9.1 Sound waves resemble the ripples on a pond.

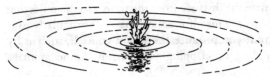

Though one usually thinks of air as the medium for carrying sound, acoustic energy may also be transmitted through other media whose constituent molecules are sufficiently close together to collide with one another when they are set in motion. In fact, the more densely these molecules are packed, the faster sound will travel through them. For instance, at room temperature, airborne sound travels 340 meters per second (or 1,130 feet per second) and slightly less when the air is colder. (The speed of sound is, of course, considerably slower than the speed of light—3,000,000 kilometers per second—which is why we see lightning before we hear the associated thunder.) In the denser medium of water, sound travels about 1,500 meters per second, almost 5 times faster than in air. With this differential in mind, imagine partially submerging your head at one end of a swimming pool so that one ear is under water while the other is above the water's surface in the air. A person at the other end of the pool now snaps her fingers on both hands, one below the water's surface and the other above. The resulting sound will arrive sooner at the ear underwater, probably causing you to hear two clicks. Sound moves even faster through steel, clipping along at over 5,000 meters per second. In general, sound travels more slowly in gases than in liquids, and more slowly in liquids than in solids.

Regardless of the medium through which it is propagated and regardless of the source, sound energy becomes weaker as it travels farther from its source. Yet while it is fading in strength, sound continues to travel at a constant speed, so long as it travels in the same medium. Thus, whether you whisper or shout at a nearby friend, the message will arrive at its destination in the same amount of time, albeit with a different degree of emphasis. This is true for all sound sources—voices, musical notes, and bomb explosions.

As sound waves spread out from their source, they interact with one another as well as with objects in their paths. These interactions can actually be more complex than those involving light. For instance, a solid object casts a visual shadow if exposed to light shining from one direction. But most sounds can be heard with little noticeable change if a relatively small object is situated between the source of a sound and your ears. This happens because sound, unlike light, travels around and sometimes through solid objects. Consequently, it is harder to shut out unwanted sounds than it is bothersome light—pulling a shade, for instance, may eliminate the glare from a nearby streetlamp, but it will not silence the noise of passing traffic.

When sound waves strike a surface, a portion of the acoustic energy bounces off the surface. These reflected sound waves are called **echoes,** and they can be used to compute the distance from a listener to a sound source. Knowing the speed at which sound travels, one can measure the time elapsing between production of a sound and reception of its echo; from this duration it is simple to calculate how far away the reflecting surface is. This is the principle used in sonar, a means for detecting objects underwater.

Echoes actually have a noticeable impact on what we hear. When echoes (reflected sound) collide with other, unreflected sound waves from the same source, these sounds interact by adding or subtracting their component energies. The result of these interactions among sounds can be particularly conspicuous in enclosed spaces such as rooms and auditoriums. Depending on an auditorium's shape and design, for example, there may be some seats where sound is unnaturally loud and other seats where sound is considerably damped. (These seats can actually be quite close to one another within an auditorium.) In an acoustically "good" auditorium, these variations in sound quality are minimal.

As Shankland (1972) documented, it is a real engineering challenge to design and construct auditoriums with superb acoustics. Despite great advances in the science of **acoustics** (the branch of physics concerned with sound), even the most thoughtfully designed structure may, in fact, fail to live up to its billing. The repeated modifications and the eventual complete reconstruction of New York's Avery Fisher Hall demonstrate how sound, particularly reflected sound, has the insidious knack of turning up where it is least expected

while avoiding where it is *supposed* to go (Bliven, 1976).

Not all sound striking a surface is reflected—some acoustic energy is absorbed. The amount of sound absorbed depends on the absorbing material. Smooth plaster, for example, absorbs only 3 percent of the sound striking its surface, reflecting the rest as an echo. This is why your singing voice invariably sounds strongest within the confines of your shower, with its hard-tiled, reflecting walls. Nylon carpet, in comparison, absorbs about 25 percent of incident sound. As you can imagine, a room containing carpet, drapes, and stuffed furniture soaks up a lot of sound energy, thereby providing a rather dead listening environment. For the same reason, the acoustics in a concert hall vary with the season, depending on whether or not the audience is dressed in heavy winter clothing that absorbs sound.

Special rooms called *anechoic chambers* create an environment devoid of echoes. The walls, floor, and ceiling of such rooms are made of porous foam wedges that serve to absorb sound before it can be reflected to your ears. Consequently, you hear only the sounds emitted from the source itself, with no echoes. For instance, when you walk in an anechoic chamber, your footsteps sound quite unnatural, having a muffled, flat quality. This is because you are hearing the sounds of your footsteps unaccompanied by their usual echoes. In general, the dull, muted quality of sounds in an anechoic chamber underscores the contribution of echoes to the normal perception of sound.

Besides contributing to an appreciation of sound, echoes furnish information about objects from which sound is reflected. For one thing, the mere presence of an echo signals that some object besides the sound source must be present in your environment. And as explained earlier, by noting the time elapsing between the production of a sound and hearing its echo, it is possible to estimate the distance from the source to the reflecting object. This information may be particularly useful if you produce the sound yourself, such as by yelling or clapping your hands. Some animals, including bats and porpoises, rely greatly on re-flections of self-produced sound to navigate. While humans don't routinely put echoes to practical use, they can learn to rely on information provided by reflected sound (Griffin, 1959). Sailors claim they can hear echoes from channel-marker buoys located several hundred feet from their boat. It is well documented that blind people can use echolocation to guide their locomotion, and sighted people can learn to utilize this cue, too.

So far we have described the vibratory nature of sound waves and how these waves travel through a medium and may be reflected by surfaces. But to really understand hearing requires understanding the ways in which sound waves differ from one another. This requires a more complete analysis of the physical properties of sound, the topic of the next section.

THE NATURE OF SOUND WAVES

We have characterized sound, or acoustic energy, as a series of collisions caused by molecules bumping into one another. You can neither see these molecular collisions nor feel them, except in un-usual cases of very strong sound waves. To envision the behavior of sound waves, imagine the following setup. Suppose a very thin, lightweight thread is dangled in front of a loudspeaker, with the thread held at one end only, so that it is free to move. Now imagine measuring the amount by which the free end of the thread is deflected as sounds of various sorts are broadcast over the loudspeaker. This setup is depicted in Figure 9.2.

The tiny dots in front of the speaker represent individual air molecules. In the absence of sound energy, air molecules are more or less evenly distributed, as illustrated in panel A. As you may know, a loudspeaker produces sound by moving back and forth, an action that physically jostles air molecules in immediate contact with the speaker cone (the round portion of the unit that actually moves). When the speaker cone moves forward, it produces an increase in air pressure that, if one could see it, involves a bunching up, or compression, of air molecules. This is shown in panel B of Figure 9.2 as a heightened concentration of dots. These compressed air molecules, in turn, collide with their immediate neighbors, thereby projecting the increase in air pressure out from the speaker itself. This miniature "breeze" even-

FIGURE 9.2 Sound waves consist of changes in air pressure.

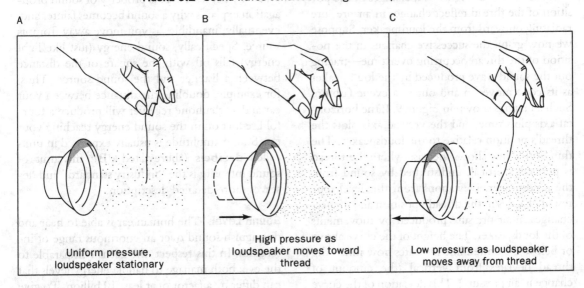

A — Uniform pressure, loudspeaker stationary

B — High pressure as loudspeaker moves toward thread

C — Low pressure as loudspeaker moves away from thread

tually strikes the thin thread, causing it to bend in a direction away from the speaker. In the meantime, the loudspeaker cone has moved steadily back to its initial position. This creates a suction-like action that spreads out, or decompresses, the air molecules, returning them to their initial density (normal air pressure). As shown in panel C, this decompression also travels outward, as air molecules are sucked into the area of decreased pressure; eventually this decompression pulls the thread back to its vertical position. Now suppose the speaker cone continues to move inward, further decreasing air pressure in the immediate vicinity of the cone. This partial vacuum travels outward and eventually sucks the thread in a direction toward the loudspeaker. This bunching up and spreading out of air molecules, caused by mechanical displacement of the speaker, represent waves of high and low pressure. The air molecules themselves each move very little—it is the *wave* of pressure that travels steadily outward from the sound source. You might think back to the ripples on the surface of a pond (Figure 9.1)—the water molecules in the pond, like air molecules, each move only a short distance when disturbed, but by colliding with their neighbors they transmit a wave of motion that can carry over great distances.

As illustrated in Figure 9.2, changes in the position of the thread reflect changes in air pressure radiating outward from the loudspeaker. Suppose we now graph the successive changes in the position of the thread occurring over time—tracing out the sound wave produced by the loudspeaker as its cone moves in and out in a cyclic fashion. Such a graph is shown in Figure 9.3; the horizontal axis plots time, and the vertical axis plots the thread's position relative to the loudspeaker. The thin dotted line shows the case where the thread is perfectly vertical, undisturbed by sound from the loudspeaker. Deviations from this level represent changes in the thread's position and, hence, changes in air pressure produced by movements of the loudspeaker. The height of the curve above or below the dotted line indicates how much the thread deviates from vertical (the amount of change in air pressure). This deviation of the curve

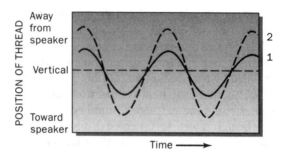

FIGURE 9.3 Change in thread position (representing air pressure) over time.

from the baseline level is known as **amplitude,** and it is determined by the distance over which the speaker moves. When this movement is tiny, the air pressure change is small and the amplitude of the wave is low (the curve labeled "1" in Figure 9.3). As you might guess, small-amplitude pressure waves give rise to weak sounds. But when the loudspeaker's movements are large, the change in air pressure, and hence the wave amplitude, is great (the curve labeled "2"). You would hear this as a loud sound. The peak of this pressure variation curve provides an index of the strength of the sound.

As air pressure changes proceed away from the source, the peak amplitude of the pressure wave gradually decreases. This property of sound propagation explains why a sound becomes fainter and, eventually, inaudible, as you move away from its source. Specifically, sound energy (just like light energy) falls off with the square of the distance between a listener and the sound source. Thus, for example, doubling the distance between your ear and a telephone receiver will produce a four-fold reduction in the sound energy reaching your ear. Sound amplitude is usually expressed in units called **decibels** (abbreviated **dB**); this unit of sound intensity is the "industry standard" and deserves more detailed description.

Sound Level. The human ear is able to hear and distinguish sound over an enormous range of intensities. In this respect, the ear is comparable to the eye: both manage to handle energy levels that can differ by a factor of at least 10 billion. To give you some idea of the energy levels confronted by your ears, take a look at Figure 9.4, a chart listing the values of intensity characteristic of some common sounds. You will notice that these various sound intensities are scaled in units called decibels. This is a *logarithmic* scale with a particular reference level of sound. The logarithmic nature of the scale makes it much easier to show a wide range of values on a single graph. Also, the logarithmic scale specifies sound-level differences in terms of their ratio to one another, not simply in terms of their algebraic difference; this seems to describe more accurately the way one judges intensity differences. Let's consider the definition of a decibel (dB):

$$dB = 20 \log (p1/p0)$$

where *p1* refers to the air pressure amplitude of the sound under consideration and *p0* refers to a standard reference level of air pressure. This reference level is typically set at 20 microPascals (μPa), the microPascal being a measure of pressure. To signify when amplitudes are being given relative to this particular **sound pressure level (SPL),** we'll denote such amplitudes as "dB$_{SPL}$." Sometimes we will use the decibel unit in a different way. Suppose that instead of expressing some sound relative to 20 μPa, we wish to compare the amplitudes of two sounds—say, a sound at 60 dB$_{SPL}$ versus a sound at 35 dB$_{SPL}$. Here we can describe amplitudes relative to each other in terms of dB, omitting the subscript SPL. In this example, we would say that the two sounds differ by 25 dB.

With these definitions in mind, let's consider one of the entries in Figure 9.4. Note that rustling leaves (or a quiet whisper) is 20 dB higher than the 0 dB$_{SPL}$ reference level. This corresponds to a tenfold increase in sound pressure. A loud scream, in contrast, can reach 100 dB$_{SPL}$, which is 100,000 times more intense than the threshold, reference level. Sounds in excess of 130 dB$_{SPL}$ can actually lead to an experience of pain, an adaptive sensation since it causes one reflexively to cover the ears, thereby protecting them from damage. We shall discuss the consequences of exposure to loud noise in the following chapter.

FIGURE 9.4 Sound intensity is expressed in units called decibels.

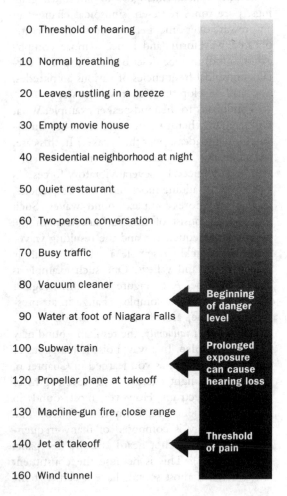

THE DECIBEL SCALE

dB	Sound	
0	Threshold of hearing	
10	Normal breathing	
20	Leaves rustling in a breeze	
30	Empty movie house	
40	Residential neighborhood at night	
50	Quiet restaurant	
60	Two-person conversation	
70	Busy traffic	
80	Vacuum cleaner	
90	Water at foot of Niagara Falls	Beginning of danger level
100	Subway train	Prolonged exposure can cause hearing loss
120	Propeller plane at takeoff	
130	Machine-gun fire, close range	
140	Jet at takeoff	Threshold of pain
160	Wind tunnel	

Sound Frequency. Returning to our loudspeaker example, let's next consider the effect of varying the rate at which the speaker moves back and forth. When the speaker's movements occur slowly over time, the peaks and troughs of the sound wave spread out, as shown in the left-hand portion of Figure 9.5. Rapid movements of the speaker, on the other hand, yield bunched-up peaks and troughs, as shown in the right-hand portion of Figure 9.5. When dealing with steady,

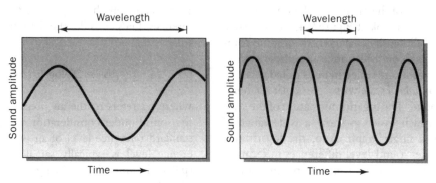

FIGURE 9.5 Rate of change in air pressure corresponds to sound's frequency.

cyclic variations such as those described here, one may specify the *frequency* of the sound. This refers to the number of times per second that air pressure undergoes a complete cycle from, say, high to low and back to high, and the unit used to designate frequency is the **hertz** (abbreviated **Hz**). Thus, for instance, in the case of a 500-Hz sound, a complete cycle of air pressure change (from compression to decompression and back) occurs in 0.002 second, yielding 500 such cycles in 1 second. Think of frequency as the number of cycles of the wave passing a given point in 1 second. You can also consider frequency in terms of the *length* of a single wave; this refers to the distance from a point along one wave (such as its peak) to the corresponding point in the next wave. Considered in this way, a low-frequency sound wave would have a long wavelength, whereas a high-frequency wave would be short in length. Figure 9.6 illustrates the relation between wavelength and frequency. As you can see from this graph, a 400-Hz sound wave is about 3 feet in length, measuring from, say, the peak of one cycle to the peak of the next.

You will probably recognize the waveforms shown in Figure 9.5 as sinusoids, waveforms discussed in Chapter 5 in relation to spatial vision. In the case of vision, recall that complex visual patterns (such as a checkerboard) can be described as the combination of certain spatial frequency components. This is why gratings of various spatial frequencies are so useful in the study of spatial vision. By the same token, complex sounds can

be described as the combination of certain temporal frequencies, or **pure tones** as they are sometimes called. Analogues to sinusoidal gratings, pure tones represent sinusoidal changes in air pressure over time. Let's see how a more complicated waveform (and hence a more complicated sound) may be described as the sum of certain sinusoidal frequencies of various amplitudes. We shall develop this idea in several steps.

Think back to the loudspeaker example: What will happen when two or more tones are simultaneously broadcast over the speaker? In this case, air molecules immediately in front of the cone will be influenced by several vibratory forces. As you continue adding more and more frequencies, you create more complex sound waves. Such waves will consist of the algebraic sum of the component frequencies, and the resulting waveform will quickly resemble a set of irregularly spaced peaks and valleys. One such example is shown in panel A of Figure 9.7. This irregular waveform depicts a complex change in air pressure over time; and if enough components are added together *randomly,* the resultant sound may be heard as **noise.** In a way, noise is analogous to white light, which, as you learned in Chapter 6, itself contains light energy at all wavelengths of the visible spectrum. However, most sounds in the environment are complex—meaning the acoustic energy is composed of many frequencies—but they are not heard as noise (see panel B, Figure 9.7). This is because the constituent frequencies of most sounds have a certain tem-

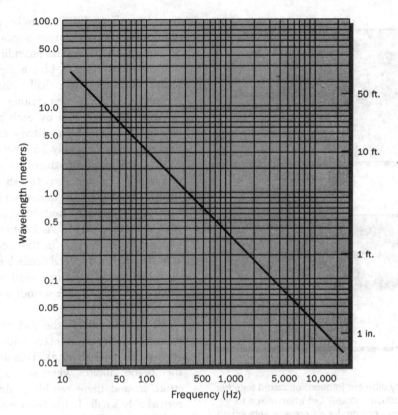

FIGURE 9.6 The relation between wavelength and frequency.

poral structure; unlike the frequencies in noise, they are not added together randomly.

In fact, very seldom does one encounter anything resembling pure tones in the natural environment, which is fortunate. If events and objects in nature were to broadcast their presence using pure tones only, one's ability to identify those objects and events via hearing would be seriously limited—there are not enough discriminable tones to uniquely specify all the recognizable sounds important to us. Because of their virtually unlimited range of unique structure, complex patterns of sound energy provide an enormous vocabulary for conveying biologically and socially relevant information. For instance, your ability to recognize a person's voice over the telephone stems from the unique "signature" provided by the package of frequencies composing that person's voice. Still, it is important to understand that all sounds, regardless of their duration or complexity, can be considered as the sum of many simple frequency components. The auditory system analyzes complex sounds into such simpler components.

THE AUDITORY SYSTEM: THE EAR

The human auditory system consists of the ears, a pair of auditory nerves, and portions of the brain. This section of the chapter is devoted to the ear, which is depicted in Figure 9.8. The top part of the figure shows a cutaway diagram of the right ear, and the bottom part schematically illustrates the operations performed by the three chambers of the ear. In this section, we shall focus on the specifics of these initial stages of auditory processing. As we proceed, the terms appearing in the

A

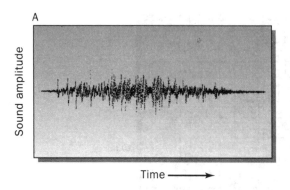

Time ──────▶

B

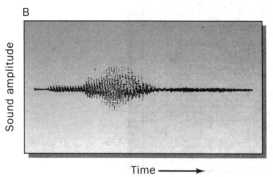

Time ──────▶

FIGURE 9.7 Many different frequencies mixed together randomly can produce "noise," but when mixed together nonrandomly can produce a recognizable sound. These two examples of complex soundwaves would be perceptually quite distinct were you to listen to them.

schematic flow diagram will become clearer; you should mark this page and refer to the diagram from time to time.

THE OUTER EAR

The most conspicuous part of the ear is the **pinna,** that shell-like flap gracing the side of your head. Some animals, such as cats, can rotate the pinnas in order to funnel sound into their ears. Human pinnas, though, are immobile; humans must turn the entire head to orient themselves toward sound. Still, the two pinnas are not useless vestiges; their corrugations act like small reflecting surfaces that modify, or "color," the complexity of sound actually entering the ear (Batteau, 1967). The degree of coloration introduced by the pinnas depends on which direction sound is coming from. Sound originating straight ahead of you

would be affected differently by the pinnas than would sound coming from a source behind you. So these ear flaps, besides providing a convenient support for eyeglasses, play a significant role in sound localization. We shall consider this role in greater detail in the next chapter.

After it is collected by each pinna, sound is channeled down the **auditory canal,** a slightly bent tube approximately 2.5 centimeters long and about 7 millimeters in diameter (the same diameter as that of a pencil, as you should never confirm). Because of its dimensions, the auditory canal has a resonant frequency (see Box 9.1, p. 302) around 3,000 Hz. As a consequence, sounds containing frequencies in this neighborhood are actually amplified several decibels or more (Tonndorf, 1988), which is one reason why human sensitivity to barely audible sounds is best around this frequency.

At the far end of the auditory canal, sound pressure comes in contact with the **eardrum (tympanic membrane).** This thin, oval-shaped membrane vibrates when sound pressure waves strike it, and these resulting vibrations may be remarkably small. It has been estimated (Bekesy and Rosenblith, 1951) that a soft whisper—an intensity of about 2 dB_{SPL}—displaces the eardrum approximately 0.00000001 centimeter, about the width of a single hydrogen molecule! Despite the almost infinitesimal size of this movement, you hear the whisper. This exquisitely sensitive device, the eardrum, is actually quite sturdy; structurally it resembles an umbrella, with a framework of supporting ribs. Even when pierced, the eardrum continues to operate with only a modest reduction in efficiency.

Together, the pinna and auditory canal constitute the *outer ear*. Referring to Figure 9.8, you can see that this portion of the auditory system functions like a directional microphone that picks up sound and modifies it, depending on its frequency content and location in space.

THE MIDDLE EAR

The eardrum forms the outer wall of a small, airfilled chamber called the *middle ear*. In the middle

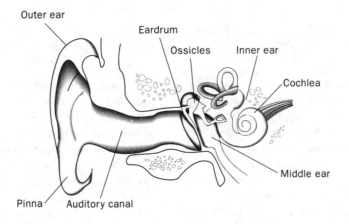

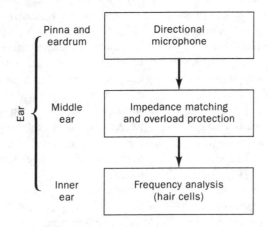

FIGURE 9.8 A schematic representation of the ear and the functions of its constituent parts.

ear, the vibrations impinging on the eardrum are passed along to the **oval window,** which is covered by another membrane, smaller than the eardrum, that forms part of the inner wall of the middle ear. Bridging the small gap between eardrum and oval window are the **ossicles,** the three smallest bones in the human body. Each of the three ossicles is about the size of a single letter on this page; their individual names reflect their shapes (see Figure 9.9). First in this chain, the **hammer** (technically called the **malleus**) is attached at one end to the back side of the eardrum. The other end of the hammer is tightly bound by ligaments to the **anvil,** or **incus,** the midde link in this chain of tiny bones. The anvil, in turn, is

secured to the **stirrup,** or **stapes,** whose footplate is, in turn, anchored against the oval window. Together the three ossicles transfer vibrations from the eardrum to the oval window.

The Role of the Ossicular Bridge. Why did nature build a delicate bridge between these two membranes, eardrum and oval window? Why not have airborne vibrations impact directly on the oval window, doing away with this intermediate chamber, the middle ear? To appreciate the importance of the middle ear and its ossicular bridge, let's consider how things would sound if this chamber and series of tiny bones were eliminated from the ear.

Box 9.1 *Resonant Frequencies: Is It Live or Is It. . . ?*

Perhaps you remember seeing the television commercial where Ella Fitzgerald shatters a crystal wineglass by singing a loud, high note. Or maybe you have felt the window panes in a house rattle following a loud clap of thunder. These are just a couple of illustrations of the ability of sound to produce vibrations in solid objects. Why does this happen?

All objects have a **resonant frequency,** defined as the frequency at which the object vibrates when set into motion. You are probably familiar with the high-pitched ringing sound produced by striking a glass with a spoon. This clear, pure ringing sound corresponds to the resonant frequency of the glass, and it occurs because the molecules of the glass are vibrating back and forth at that frequency. Adding water to the glass causes those molecules to vibrate at a slower rate when you strike the glass with the spoon. The resonant frequency of the glass has been lowered. So long as the amount of water in the glass remains constant, its resonant frequency will stay the same; regardless of how you set up vibrations in the glass, it will produce the same ringing sound. In fact, sound from another source may induce vibrations in the glass, so long as that inducing sound contains energy at the resonant frequency of the glass. For instance, by whistling the right note, you could produce a faint ringing sound from the glass. And if this inducing energy is sufficiently intense (such as a loud, pure note), the vibrations set up in the glass may be sufficiently strong to shatter it.

Presumably this was how the army of priests at Jericho were able to tumble that city's walls, by playing their trumpets in unison! On a less spectacular scale, these induced vibrations, or *resonance,* explain why objects in your room may tremble sometimes when you turn up the volume on your stereo. In general, the resonant frequency of an object depends on the size and rigidity of the object.

We shall be discussing the relation between hearing and the frequency of sound in the next chapter, but at this point it would be helpful for you to have some idea of the subjective experience of different frequencies. Here are a few examples: the tone called *middle C* has a frequency of 261.63 Hz; the faint, high whine produced by a television when the volume control is turned all the way down is 15,750 Hz; and adult human speech consists of frequencies ranging from 200 to 8,000 Hz.

To begin, you need to realize that the inner ear, the chamber located on the other side of the oval window, is filled with fluid; Glen Wever (1978) discusses the evolutionary significance of the fluid-filled inner ear, pointing out that it probably derives from the aquatic environment of the amphibians from which our species' ears evolved. As land dwellers, we hear sounds that are carried to our ears by *airborne* pressure variations. Without the middle ear, these airborne pressure changes would be pushing directly against the oval window and, therefore, against the fluid contained in the inner ear. Because its constituent molecules are more densely packed, the fluid offers more resistance to movement than does air. In other words, more force is required to set up sound waves in water than in air. This explains why when you are under water, you have trouble hearing sounds arising from above the water—about 99 percent of airborne sound is reflected when it strikes the water's surface; only about 1 percent is absorbed by the water (Evans, 1982a).

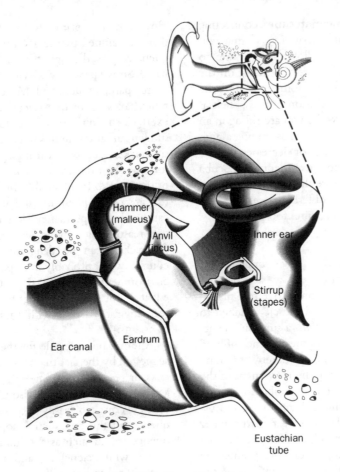

FIGURE 9.9 The middle ear.

This represents almost a 30-dB loss in sound energy. Referring back to the chart in Figure 9.4, you can see that lowering the intensity of sounds by 30 dB would definitely affect your hearing, wiping out altogether some routine sounds (those listed as 30 dB_{SPL} or less in intensity) and reducing the intensity of all others.

So if your ear were to transfer vibrations directly from air to fluid, a great deal of sound energy would be lost. This potential loss in sound energy—or most of it—is avoided within the middle ear, however, because of the difference in surface area between the eardrum and the oval window. The oval window is roughly 20 times smaller in area than the eardrum. Consequently, the force applied on the oval window exerts con-

siderably more pressure than the same amount of force applied to the eardrum. Vibrations from the large area of the eardrum are funneled to the small area of the oval window, effectively amplifying sound energy. This funneling effect recovers about 23 dB of the impedance loss that is caused by the passing of vibrations from air to water. Because it operates to overcome the impedance imposed by the fluid-filled inner ear, the middle ear is sometimes referred to as an impedance matching device.

For this impedance matching system to work efficiently, the average air pressure within the middle ear must equal the atmospheric pressure existing in the outside environment and, hence, within the auditory canal. This equivalence is maintained by the **Eustachian tube***‎ connecting the middle ear and the throat. Every time you swallow, this tube opens, allowing air either to enter or leave the middle ear, depending on the outside air pressure. You can sometimes hear the consequences of this ventilation process, such as when your ears "pop" while you are riding in an elevator, flying in an airplane, or ascending a high mountain. Sudden increases or decreases in outside pressure (such as those experienced by scuba divers) can actually rupture the eardrum; this occurs when the pressure differential on the two sides of the membrane becomes too great.

The Acoustic Reflex. Before we conclude our discussion of this part of the ear, we also need to draw your attention to the protective role played by the *tensor tympani,* a small muscle attached to the eardrum, and the *stapedius,* a tiny muscle attached to the stapes bone. In the presence of loud sound, these muscles contract, thereby stiffening the eardrum and restricting the movement of the ossicles (Møller, 1974). These combined actions, called the **acoustic reflex,** damp the sound vibrations passed from the outer ear to the inner ear; in this respect, the acoustic reflex acts like the damper pedal on a piano, the one that muffles the musical notes by limiting the vibrations of the piano's strings. But why should the ear contain a mechanism to damp sound?

According to one popular theory, the acoustic reflex serves to protect the inner ear from intense stimulation that could otherwise damage the delicate receptor cells within the inner ear (Borg and Counter, 1989). Considering it this way, one can draw an analogy between the acoustic reflex and the pupillary light reflex (the constriction of the pupil in response to light). It is true that the acoustic reflex *does* reduce the intensity of sound transmission by as much as 30 dB (Evans, 1982a).

However, it is primarily low-frequency sounds that are damped by the acoustic reflex; high frequencies pass through the middle ear unattenuated. So as a protective device, the acoustic reflex is only partially successful. Moreover, the acoustic reflex takes about one-twentieth of a second to exert its shielding influence. Consequently, any sudden, intense sound, such as the explosion of a firecracker, can speed through the middle ear before the acoustic reflex can act to damp the force of that sound. Incidentally, abrupt sounds such as this are called *transients,* and if too strong, they can produce a permanent loss in hearing; this is one reason that playing with explosives such as firecrackers can be dangerous. (Explosions, of course, were probably not part of the natural environment in which the human ear evolved; it is not surprising that the acoustic reflex is too sluggish to deal with these kinds of sharp transients.)

Another possible role for the acoustic reflex is suggested by the fact that it occurs whenever one talks or chews something—the same nerves that activate the facial muscles also trigger the acoustic reflex. You can easily experience the consequences of this by listening to a steady low-frequency sound such as the hum of a refrigerator motor while clenching and unclenching your teeth. The sound will seem fainter with teeth clenched, because this engages the acoustic reflex. This general observation has led to the theory that the acoustic reflex reduces the ears' sensitivity to self-produced sounds such as one's own voice. These sounds *do* consist primarily of low frequencies, which as mentioned above are the ones attenuated by the acoustic reflex. We leave it to your reasoning to figure out the advantage of de-emphasizing self-produced sounds.

The functions of the middle ear are summarized in Figure 9.8. Basically, it serves as an impedance matching device and as a circuit overload protector. With these roles established, we are now ready to migrate to the next stage in the auditory system, the inner ear. This is where mechanical vibrations are converted into electrical nerve impulses to be carried to the brain. Within

---

* Named after its discoverer, Bartolomeo Eustachi, a sixteenth-century Italian anatomist (Hawkins, 1988).

the inner ear, the auditory system really gets down to the business of hearing.

THE INNER EAR: THE COCHLEA

The *inner ear* consists of a series of hollow cavities, or labyrinths, carved into the temporal bone of the skull. One set of these cavities, the semicircular canals, is concerned with the maintenance of bodily posture and balance; these are the structures that mediate the vestibular reflexes discussed in Chapter 8. In this chapter, however, our focus will be on the **cochlea** (from the Greek word for "snail"), a coiled, fluid-filled cavity containing the specialized receptors that place us in contact with the sounds in our environment. Vibrations of the oval window produce pressure changes in the fluid within the cochlea. These pressure changes cause movement of the sensitive receptor cells within the cochlea, providing the stimulus for their activity. To understand this process of sensory transduction, we need to examine more closely the structural detail of this tiny, pea-sized organ (a magnified schematic of which is shown in Figure 9.10).

The spiral-shaped cochlea is partitioned into three chambers, which are easier to visualize if

FIGURE 9.10 The cochlea.

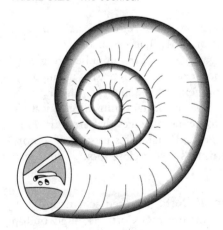

you imagine the cochlea uncoiled, as shown in Figure 9.11. To keep track of its arrangement, we shall refer to the end nearest the middle ear as the *base* and the end normally curled up in the center as the *apex*. The three wedge-shaped chambers of the cochlea each have names: the *vestibular canal,* the *cochlear duct,* and the *tympanic canal*. The vestibular canal and cochlear duct are separated by one membrane, while the tympanic canal and the cochlear duct are separated by another membrane; this latter one is called the **basilar membrane,** and it plays a crucial role in the hearing process. The three chambers run parallel to one another the entire length of the cochlea, except right near the far end, at the apex. There the vestibular canal and the tympanic canal merge at a pinhole-sized passage. Because these two chambers are, in fact, continuous with each other, they contain the same fluid, similar in composition to spinal fluid. The middle chamber, the cochlear duct, contains a fluid that is chemically different from that filling the other two canals. This chemical difference between the two fluids plays a crucial role in the initial stage of hearing. For example, when the two fluids are intermixed (which can occur if the membrane separating them ruptures), hearing is impaired. Besides their apparent role in the hearing process, these fluids also take the place of blood in supplying all the nourishment for cells in the cochlea. Blood vessels, even tiny capillaries, are forbidden within this structure because their pulsations would create violent waves of sound pressure within the closed confines of the cochlea. This arrangement is reminiscent of the eye (Chapter 2), where blood vessels are routed around the fovea to avoid obstructing the image formed on this crucial part of the eye.

Except at two spots where it is covered by elastic material, the walls of the cochlea consist of hard, relatively shockproof bone. At the base of the cochlea, the vestibular canal is covered by the oval window, which, you will recall, is attached to the stapes (stirrup) on the side facing the middle ear. The tympanic canal is likewise covered at the base by the **round window,** another thin membrane that also covers a small opening into the

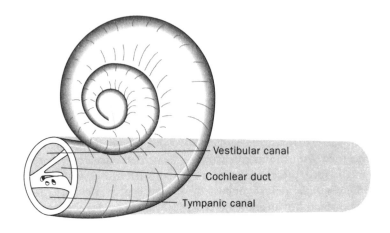

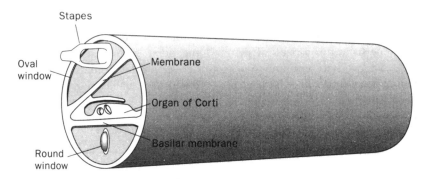

FIGURE 9.11 A section of an uncoiled cochlea.

middle ear. These two elastic surfaces allow pressure to be distributed within the fluid-filled cochlea: when the oval window is pushed inward by the stapes, the round window bulges outward to compensate (see Figure 9.11). This compensation is possible because the two chambers, the vestibular and tympanic canals, are linked. How, though, does the fluid-borne pressure wave generated by the stapes at the oval window give rise to hearing? To answer this question, we must look more closely at the cochlear duct and, in particular, at this complex structure, the **organ of Corti,** situated inside it; the structure is named

after the Italian anatomist Alfonso Corti, who first described it in 1851. The organ of Corti is the receptor organ where neural impulses are generated in response to vibrations passing through the fluid environment of the inner ear. The organ of Corti, in other words, transforms mechanical vibrations into neural messages that are sent on to the brain. To understand this process of sensory transduction, let's take a close look at the organ of Corti.

The Organ of Corti. Pictured schematically in Figure 9.12, the organ of Corti sits snugly on top

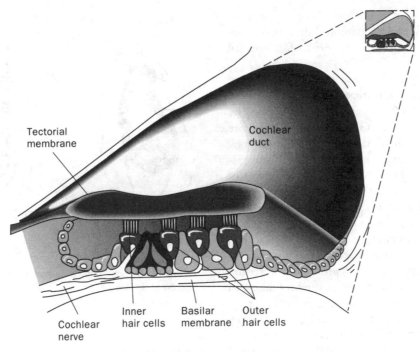

Tectorial
membrane

Cochlear
duct

Cochlear
nerve

Inner
hair cells

Basilar
membrane

Outer
hair cells

FIGURE 9.12 The organ of Corti.

of the basilar membrane (recall that this is the membrane separating the cochlear duct and the tympanic canal), and it runs the full length of the cochlear duct. The following are the major components of the organ of Corti: a layer of supporting cells resting on the basilar membrane, rows of hair cells sticking up from the supporting cells, and an awninglike membrane, the **tectorial membrane,** arching over the hair cells. Note a few things about this arrangement. First, structures called hair cells extend up into the fluid within the cochlear duct; second, the tectorial membrane that arches over the structure contacts the tops of some of these hair cells. Finally, note that because the tectorial membrane is attached at only one end, it can move independently of the basilar membrane. Let's focus more closely on the hair cells, for they hold the key to the transduction of fluid vibrations into nerve impulses.

Hair Cells and Sensory Transduction. The ear is similar to the eye, in that both organs contain two different types of receptor cells. The eye, as you learned, contains rods and cones. These two classes of photoreceptors are different in shape and in retinal distribution, and they are involved in different aspects of visual perception (recall Chapters 2 and 3). The ear's receptors, the **hair cells,** are equally distinctive anatomically and functionally. In all, there are about 15,500 hair cells within a single ear, with this total divisible into two distinct groups. One group, the **inner hair cells (IHCs),** is situated on the basilar membrane close to where the tectorial membrane is attached to the wall of the cochlear duct (see lower right-hand part of Figure 9.12). Numbering about 3,500, these inner hair cells line up in a single row that runs the length of the basilar membrane. The 12,000 or so **outer hair cells (OHCs),** in contrast, line up in anywhere from three to five rows. Let's first look at the anatomical distinctions between the two and then consider their functional differences.

Drawings of an IHC and an OHC are shown in Figure 9.13. Note that each IHC is shaped something like a flask, and each is surrounded by supporting cells. Each OHC, in contrast, is more cylindrical in shape, and each is surrounded by fluid. Both the inner and the outer hair cells terminate in tiny bristles called **cilia.** Figure 9.14 shows a section of the basilar membrane photographed through an electron microscope—in this top-down view, you can actually see the single row of IHCs and multiple rows of OHCs; shown in the right part of the figure are magnified views of each cell type. The most prominent structures visible in these photographs are the brushlike cilia shown sticking up from the tops of the hair cells. Ordinarily these structures would be covered by the overlying tectorial membrane but, to make this photo, the tectorial membrane was lifted away. It used to be thought that cilia from *all* the hair cells actually made contact with the tectorial membrane. Now, however, it is recognized that only cilia from the OHCs actually touch the tec-

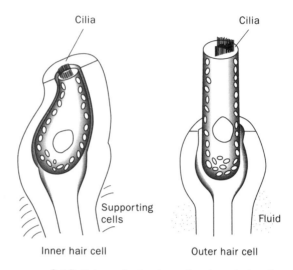

FIGURE 9.13 Schematic drawings of an inner hair cell and an outer hair cell.

torial membrane (Dallos, 1984). Bending of the cilia constitutes *the* crucial early event in the process that leads to hearing, for it is this event which triggers the electrical signals that travel from the ear to the brain. Let's take a look, then, at how

FIGURE 9.14 Electron microscope photographs of the cilia of the multiple rows of outer hair cells and the single row of inner hair cells. The two pictures on the right show a single OHC and IHC in greater magnification. (Photograph courtesy of Dr. David Lim.)

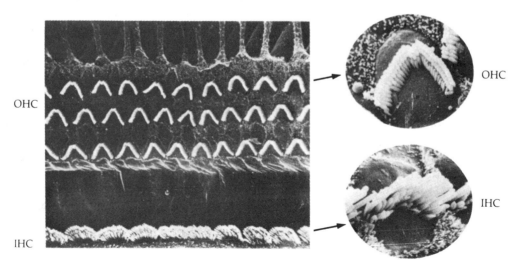

airborne sound ends up producing this crucial event, the bending of the cilia.

As you will recall, airborne vibrations are picked up by the external ear and converted into a mechanical, pistonlike action by the ossicles of the middle ear. Because it is attached to the stapes, the oval window receives these mechanical displacements and passes them in the form of pressure waves into the fluids of the cochlea's vestibular and tympanic canals. As the pressure waves travel through these chambers, they cause waves of displacement along the basilar membrane. The tectorial membrane also moves slightly in response to these pressure waves, but it tends to move in directions that are different from the movement of the basilar membrane. These opposing motions cause the cilia of the hair cells on the basilar membrane to bend, like tiny clumps of seaweed swept back and forth by invisible underwater currents. This bending triggers electrical changes within the hair cells (Russell, 1987). These electrical changes in the hair cell cause it to release a chemical transmitter substance, which is picked up by auditory nerve fibers that make synaptic contact with the hair cells at their base (the portion of the cells at the other end from the cilia). These fibers, in turn, carry electrical impulses from the cochlea to the central nervous system. It is truly remarkable that such microscopic movements of thin membranes, tiny bones, and hairs inaugurate a process—hearing—that can have such an enormous impact on one's feelings and behaviors.

With this sequence of events in mind, let's return for a moment to the two classes of hair cells. As already pointed out, the IHCs and OHCs differ in number (3,500 versus 12,000) and in location along the basilar membrane. In addition, these two classes of hair cells differ in the pattern of their connections to auditory nerve fibers. The more numerous OHCs make sparse contact with the auditory nerve; only about 5 percent of the auditory nerve fibers contact the OHCs. The remaining 95 percent of the fibers contact the IHCs, the smaller of the two cell populations. To draw an analogy, it is as if a telephone company took 50,000 phone lines and divided them up so that 2,500 were devoted to the entire population of Boston while 47,500 were devoted to the much smaller population of neighboring Concord. Why should the more numerous OHCs have so little control over the signals traveling along the auditory nerve? According to recent thinking (Dallos, 1985, 1988, 1992; Shepherd, 1988; Allen and Neely, 1992), the IHCs are the principal actors in the sensory drama that unfolds in the ear, with the OHCs playing an important amplifying role.

Here's how the idea goes. To begin, remember that the cilia of the OHCs are actually attached to the overhanging tectorial membrane. It is now thought that when electric currents are set up in the OHCs, their cilia produce a motor response— they have miniature musclelike elements (actin filaments) that contract and expand the cilia along their longitudinal axes. Suppose that an acoustic disturbance causes maximal vibration at some place along the basilar membrane. As the OHCs at that place ride up and down, their cilia, which are attached to the tectorial membrane, are stretched and relaxed. This sets up an alternating current within the hair cells. The alternating current, in turn, stimulates the OHC cilia to contract and expand, causing them to behave like small motors that pull and push the tectorial membrane. This motorlike action of the OHCs on the tectorial membrane amplifies and concentrates displacement of the basilar membrane created by the back and forth movement of fluid within the cochlea. These amplified movements, in turn, cause the cilia of the IHCs to be displaced by a greater amount than they would have without the extra boost provided by the contractions of the OHC cilia. As a result, the OHCs, despite their minor *direct* contribution to information carried by the auditory nerve, are very important to the hearing process.* It should be noted, by the way, that these amplifying actions must be accomplished at a molecular level; standard mechanical actions such as contraction and elongation of mus-

---

* Acting as amplifiers and tuners, the OHCs primarily modify the mechanical environment of the IHCs; strictly speaking, the IHCs are the only true sensory receptors for hearing. In this sense, the analogy to rod and cone photoreceptors is wrong.

cles could not occur rapidly enough to accomplish the task carried out by the OHCs.

In a later section, we shall learn more about the auditory consequences of this amplification process. But first, there is one important step in this process of sensory transduction that was sidestepped: how do the vibrations traveling within the cochlear fluid affect the basilar membrane? Because the hair cells ride on the basilar membrane, the membrane's reactions to fluid vibrations determine which hair cells are stimulated and, hence, which nerve fibers will be activated. To fill in this missing step, let's turn our attention to the basilar membrane, the thin-walled membrane separating the tympanic canal from the cochlear duct (see Figures 9.11 and 9.12).

The Basilar Membrane. Much of what is known today about the basilar membrane comes from work by Georg von Bekesy, a Hungarian scientist who was awarded the Nobel Prize in 1961 for his research on the ear. To appreciate Bekesy's contributions, you need to be familiar with the two major theories describing the way that pressure waves in the cochlear fluid affect the basilar membrane. Both theories were originally formulated in the nineteenth century, before anyone was able to observe the basilar membrane in action. The opposing theories, called the *frequency theory* and the *place theory,* form the background for Bekesy's important work.

The Frequency Theory. The **frequency theory** proposes that the entire basilar membrane vibrates in synchrony with the pressure changes within the cochlea. According to this idea, the stapes taps out a series of beats on the oval window, and the entire basilar membrane dances along.

Ernest Rutherford, a nineteenth-century English physicist, was the first proponent of the frequency theory. He likened the basilar membrane to the diaphragm inside a telephone receiver. Because it is thin and light, the diaphragm moves back and forth in response to the sound waves of your voice. These movements are converted into electrical current that is carried along a telephone

line; and the current eventually produces the same pattern of movements in the listening diaphragm of another person's telephone receiver, thereby reproducing the sounds of your voice. Rutherford believed that the basilar membrane behaved in a comparable fashion, vibrating as a unit at a frequency that matched the sound stimulus. In turn, this vibration produced in the auditory nerve a train of impulses whose frequency mimicked the frequency with which the entire basilar membrane was vibrating. According to Rutherford's idea, then, a 500-Hz tone would yield 500 nerve impulses per second, while a 1,200-Hz tone would yield 1,200 impulses per second.

Several things are wrong with this theory. For one thing, the basilar membrane is not like a diaphragm in a telephone. The basilar membrane varies in width and in stiffness from one end to the other. As a result, the basilar membrane, unlike a diaphragm, cannot vibrate uniformly over its entire length; a good description of why this is physically impossible is given by Yost and Nielsen (1985). There is another problem, too, with the frequency theory. Single auditory nerve fibers cannot match the performance of a telephone line, because neurons are incapable of firing repetitively at rates beyond 1,000 impulses per second; yet we can hear tones whose frequency greatly exceeds this value. So the neural signal required by Rutherford's theory cannot be realized by individual fibers.

This limitation in firing rate could be surmounted if separate nerve fibers fired not in unison but in a staggered fashion. For instance, two fibers each firing at 1,000 impulses per second in combination could produce 2,000 impulses per second if those impulses were appropriately interleaved (Figure 9.15). This modification of the frequency theory, known as the *volley theory,* was proposed by Wever and Bray (1937), who also described some fascinating findings in support of frequency theory (Box 9.2, p. 312). Also, the volley theory, unlike Rutherford's frequency theory, does not assume that the basilar membrane acts like a telephone diaphragm. It does, however, require that some higher neuron sum the interleaved neural impulses from the fibers responding

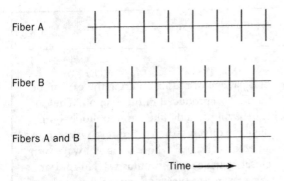

FIGURE 9.15 Two fibers firing regularly but asynchronously.

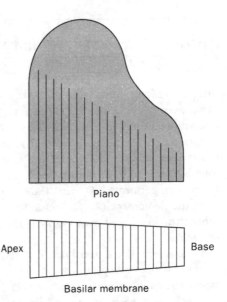

FIGURE 9.16 The basilar membrane's tapered shape resembles the layout of a piano's strings.

near their limits of activity. How this summing neuron could overcome its upper limit of firing rate was never specified by proponents of volley theory. We shall have more to say about the volley theory in our discussion of pitch perception in the next chapter. But let's return now to the basilar membrane and consider the frequency theory's chief opponent, the *place theory*.

The Place Theory. The **place theory** maintains that different frequencies of vibration of the cochlear fluid disturb different regions of the basilar membrane. These different regions of disturbance, in turn, activate different hair cells and hence different auditory nerve fibers. You can see where this theory gets its name—frequency information is encoded according to the location, or *place,* along the basilar membrane disturbed by fluid vibration. The most notable early proponent of the place theory was Helmholtz, whose ideas on color vision we discussed in Chapter 6. Helmholtz's (1877/1954) theory was inspired by the fact that the basilar membrane is narrow at the base of the cochlea and broad at the apex. This layout reminded Helmholtz of the variation in the length of strings of a piano (Figure 9.16)—which led him to propose that the basilar membrane was composed of distinct fibers that individually stretched across its width. Because of the basilar membrane's tapered shape, fibers at one end would be longer than those at the other, just like piano strings. According to Helmholtz, vibrations

within the cochlear fluid would set into motion only those "strings" of the basilar membrane that were tuned to the frequencies at which the fluid vibrated. In other words, fibers of the basilar membrane would vibrate in the same way that piano strings can be induced to vibrate when you sing a loud note. This is the principle of resonance discussed in Box 9.1.

Although based on solid physical principles, Helmholtz's place theory was flawed in several respects. For one thing, subsequent anatomical work showed that the basilar membrane is not composed of separate fibers capable of resonating individually. Rather than a set of piano strings, the basilar membrane looks more like a continuous strip of rubber. Moreover, the basilar membrane is not under tension, like piano strings; it is relatively slack. So the resonance portion of Helmholtz's theory proved incorrect, but his idea that different *places* along the basilar membrane respond to different frequencies *did* survive. In fact, it is this idea that Bekesy's work so elegantly substantiated, and it is to his work that we now turn.

Box 9.2 *A Peculiar Sort of Microphone*

Imagine walking into a radio studio to find a newscaster speaking into the ear of a live cat. Even more astounding, imagine *hearing* the newscaster's voice being broadcast over a loudspeaker in the room! Farfetched as it sounds, this kind of demonstration has actually been performed (Cohen, 1969). Moreover, the demonstration works using animals other than a cat; your own ear would work just fine.

Here is how this unusual sound system works. An electrode placed near the site where the auditory nerve exits the cochlea will pick up an electrical signal arising within the cochlea. This electrical signal results from the high concentration of certain positively charged chemicals within the cochlea's fluid. As the hair cells of the inner ear bend in response to pressure waves within those fluids, the electrical signal changes. When plotted on a graph, this change in electrical potential mirrors the change in the amplitude of the sound wave presented to the ear. For example, playing a 500-Hz pure-tone sound into the ear yields a 500-Hz sinusoidal variation in electrical potential. If this electrically recorded cochlear potential is now fed into an amplifier and then passed to a loudspeaker, you will hear the 500-Hz tone with essentially no distortion: it will be indistinguishable from the original tone played into the ear. In fact, *any* sound stimulus, such as someone's voice

or a passage of music, entering the ear can be faithfully reproduced in this fashion. The ear is behaving exactly like a microphone; both devices convert airborne pressure waves into an electrical signal whose temporal waveform closely parallels the stimulus waveform. For this reason, the electrical potential recorded from the cochlea has been termed the *cochlear microphonic*.

When it was first discovered by Wever and Bray in 1930, the cochlear microphonic was thought to originate from the auditory nerve. This would have meant that the frequency of nerve impulses in the auditory nerve exactly followed the input frequency of sound. If correct, this interpretation would have provided strong support for the frequency theory described in the discussion of the basilar membrane. However, later experiments proved that the cochlear microphonic can be recorded even when the nerve itself is temporarily deadened by an anesthetic. These findings ruled out the auditory nerve as the source of the cochlear microphonic. Current evidence points instead to the outer hair cells as the generator of the cochlear microphonic. This would explain why damage to the outer hair cells diminishes the cochlear microphonic (Davis et al., 1958), whereas damage to the inner hair cells leaves this electrical signal unaffected (Dallos and Cheatham, 1976).

Traveling Waves. Bekesy realized that the essential difference between the place and frequency theories lay in how each thought the basilar membrane vibrated in response to different frequencies. Of course, the simplest way to settle the issue would have been to observe the membrane's

movements, but this was technically difficult in the late 1920s when Bekesy became interested in the problem. Nonetheless, Bekesy knew that the width and thickness of the basilar membrane varied along its length, being wider and thicker at the end near the apex. Armed with these facts, he built a mechanical model of the cochlea, so he could directly observe the behavior of an enlarged replica of the basilar membrane (Bekesy, 1960).

For the tympanic and vestibular canals, he used a brass tube with a small rubber cap stretched over each end; these caps represented the oval and round windows. He cut a tapered slot the length of the entire tube and covered this slot with a rubber "membrane" whose thickness increased as the slot widened; this represented the basilar membrane. For the stapes, he substituted a small mallet placed against the rubber cap on one end of the tube; this mallet was vibrated by a tuning fork. A drawing of Bekesy's large-scale cochlea is shown in Figure 9.17.

To observe the behavior of his mechanical model, Bekesy lightly rested his forearm on the rubber membrane. When a pure tone was produced by striking the tuning fork, Bekesy felt the rubber membrane vibrating against his arm at one particular spot (see panel A of Figure 9.18). By testing with tuning forks that produced different frequencies, he discovered that the location of this tingling spot depended on the frequency with which the tuning fork vibrated the "oval window." With higher frequencies, this tingle occurred near his wrist, a place on the membrane corresponding to the narrow end closest to the stapes. Lower frequencies, in contrast, yielded a tingle nearer his elbow, the region of the membrane corresponding to the wide end near the apex. In panel A of the figure you can see the relation between pure-tone frequency and the point along Bekesy's mechanical model where the frequency yields its peak vibration. Translating Bekesy's results to the actual basilar membrane—a much smaller, coiled structure—yields the scaled diagram in panel B of Figure 9.18. This diagram reveals which point along the basilar membrane vibrates maximally to a particular sound frequency.

Bekesy's ingenious demonstration therefore strongly favored the place theory. In subsequent years, Bekesy went on to confirm this conclusion using other, more precise techniques, including direct visualization of the human basilar membrane under a microscope. He explained the connection between the point of maximum vibration along the basilar membrane and sound frequency in the following way. The fluctuations in fluid pressure produced by the pistonlike movements of the stapes set up a **traveling wave** along the basilar membrane itself. To envision what is meant by a "traveling wave," think what happens when you flick one end of a rope whose other end is tied to, say, a pole. You see a wave of motion traveling the length of the rope. Unlike a rope, though, the basilar membrane varies in thickness and width along its length. If you were to flick the basilar membrane, the resulting wave

FIGURE 9.17 Bekesy's mechanical model of the cochlea.

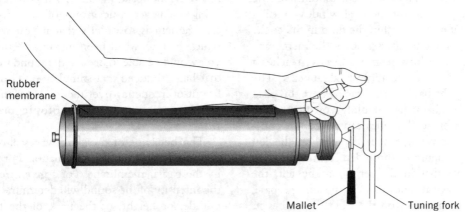

Rubber membrane

Mallet

Tuning fork

A   B

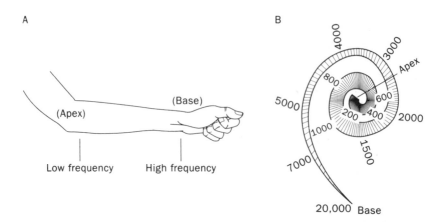

| |
Low frequency   High frequency

20,000 Base

FIGURE 9.18 Summary of the results of Bekesy's experiment.

of motion would actually grow in amplitude as it traveled away from you. But this wave would reach a peak amplitude and then rapidly collapse, never getting to the other end. An example of this kind of traveling wave is illustrated in the drawing at the top of Figure 9.19. In this figure, the basilar membrane is drawn as if uncoiled and viewed from the side. Thus in each panel below the drawing the horizontal axis represents the length of the basilar membrane, with its base at the left and its apex at the right. Each separate panel shows the profile of the basilar membrane at a different instant in time. You might imagine these as successive snapshots of the basilar membrane taken just after you have flicked it as you would a rope. (Flicking it corresponds to the stapes's tapping against the oval window, setting up waves of motion within the fluid in the cochlea.) As the wave progresses down the membrane over time, note how it grows in size, reaches a peak, and then rather abruptly disappears. The place along the basilar membrane where this peak occurs depends on how rapidly you flicked the basilar membrane. This idea can be seen by comparing the traveling waves depicted in the left panel of the figure to those depicted in the right panel. Note that in the series on the left, the traveling wave reaches its peak nearer the base, whereas in the series on the right, it reaches its peak nearer the apex. The waves in the left-hand

series were produced by a high-frequency tone; those in the right-hand series, by a low-frequency tone.

The peak of the traveling wave, you should understand, represents a place where the basilar membrane flexes up and down—which is why Bekesy could feel a tingling spot on his forearm when he tested his mechanical cochlea. This flexion in the actual basilar membrane means that hair cells riding on this portion of the membrane will be displaced further—and their cilia bent more—than elsewhere along the membrane. In turn, these highly bent cilia will activate their associated hair cells. In other words, any frequency of vibration will cause the basilar membrane to flex maximally at one location, thereby maximally stimulating a characteristic group of hair cells. This arrangement is so orderly that if you were told which hair cells had been maximally stimulated, you would be able to deduce the sound frequency that had produced that stimulation. This orderly layout of frequency over the length of the basilar membrane is known as **tonotopic organization.**

The behavior of traveling waves also readily explains how intensity information is registered by the basilar membrane. For a given frequency, the intensity of the sound will determine the amplitude, or height, of the peak of the traveling wave. Increases in the amplitude of these move-

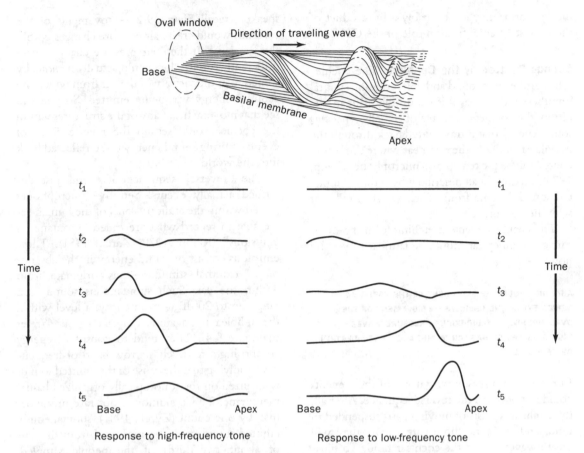

FIGURE 9.19 The top drawing shows a traveling wave deforming the basilar membrane. The set of curves below at the left represents the response of the basilar membrane over time to a high-frequency tone. The curves at the right represent the basilar membrane's response over time to a low-frequency tone.

ments of the basilar membrane will cause the cilia to bend more, leading to greater stimulation of the hair cells, a larger neural response, and ultimately an increase in perceived loudness. Increases in the amplitude of these movements also enlarge the spread of the displaced region along the basilar membrane, which in turn alters the pattern of hair cells stimulated. The perceptual consequences of these changes in the basilar membrane's response to different frequencies and intensities will be discussed in the next chapter.

This gives you a bird's-eye view of the workings of the inner ear. Referring back to Figure 9.8, you can now understand why the inner ear

is characterized as a frequency selective sound transducer. We call it "frequency selective" because, by virtue of its mechanical properties, the inner ear breaks up incoming sound into its component frequencies. In the last section of this chapter we will survey what happens to the signals from the hair cells as they are routed to the brain via the auditory nerve. But before leaving the inner ear, we want to describe one of the cochlea's really unusual properties, its ability to *generate* sounds on its own. These so-called **cochlear emissions** represent one of the most intriguing discoveries about hearing in recent years. While they play no role in your experience of the auditory world, they are probably a by-product of the important amplification role of the OHCs.

Sounds Emitted by the Cochlea. The cochlea is built to receive sound and convert it into neural impulses, and it does this exquisitely. But in addition, the cochlea is capable of actually *generating* sound energy that is transmitted back through the middle ear and into the outer ear where this sound energy can be picked up by a microphone (Kemp, 1979). First we shall describe where these "emitted sounds" come from. Then we shall tell you why they occur.

The chain of events stretching from the outer ear to the inner ear should be familiar to you by now:

AIRBORNE SOUND → MOVEMENT OF THE EARDRUM → MOVEMENT OF THE OSSICLES → MOVEMENT OF THE OVAL WINDOW → FLUID-BORNE PRESSURE WAVES → DISPLACEMENT OF BASILAR MEMBRANE → STIMULATION OF HAIR CELLS

But there is no reason why many of these events could not occur in the reverse sequence. After all, the cochlea consists of moving parts suspended in fluid, and any time those parts move, they will create waves within the cochlear fluid. To illustrate, imagine that you are *inside* the cochlea moving your arms back and forth, splashing about as if you were in a swimming pool. Your movements would disturb the cochlear fluid, setting up waves within it that would spread throughout the volume of the fluid. Because the cochlea (your miniature swimming pool) is a sealed container, these waves will eventually push against the oval window from the inner side. Since the oval window is attached to the stapes, this push would be felt by the stapes and passed in reverse through the other two attached bones in the ossicular chain. The hammer, as a result, would be pushed against the inner side of the eardrum. This pressure would, in turn, cause the eardrum to flex back and forth slightly, displacing air molecules within the auditory canal. The eardrum, in other words, would behave just like the cone on a loud-

speaker (recall Figure 9.2)—movements of the eardrum would create air pressure changes within the ear canal. If these air pressure changes were sufficiently robust, they could actually be *heard* by someone in the vicinity of the ear from which the acoustic energy was being emitted. So you can see that movements of any of the structures within the cochlea could set up the reverse chain of events, causing sound energy to be reflected back into the world.

The "reverse" sequence of events just described actually occurs. Sensitive microphones placed within the auditory canal of the human ear are able to record what are called "spontaneous emissions" (Kemp, 1979; Zurek, 1981). These emissions consist of sound energy in the absence of an external stimulus—they originate from within the ear. Such spontaneous sounds can range up to 20 dB_{SPL} in intensity, a level within the audible range against a quiet background (refer to Figure 9.4). They tend to consist of energy comprising a relatively narrow band of frequencies, implying that the cause of the emitted sounds is localized on the tonotopically organized basilar membrane. This condition is not rare or abnormal; by one count (Zurek, 1981), spontaneously emitted sound could be measured from the ears of about two-thirds of the people sampled, though the measured frequency and intensity level did vary from person to person. These emitted sounds can have bizarre consequences. In some cases, although the emitted sound cannot be heard by the source (the person emitting the sound), it *can* be heard by someone else nearby (McFadden, 1982); these emitted sounds are heard as high-pitched tones. You might try listening for emitted sounds from a friend's ear. In a quiet setting, place your ear close to your friend's and notice whether you hear a steady, faint tone. If you do, have your friend move away from your ear and notice whether you still hear the tone. If the tone persists, it must be originating either from an external source or from within your own ear. But if the tone becomes inaudible when your friend moves, you very likely were hearing an emitted sound from your friend's ear. Incidentally, emitted sounds have been measured from the ears of dogs and cats (McFadden, 1982), so you need not limit your experiment to humans.

Emitted sounds can also be measured immediately following stimulation of the ear by a briefly presented sound such as a click.* Rather than being spontaneous, these sounds emitted in response to clicks are more like echoes in response to the brief acoustic event. But the echo analogy is misleading, for these emitted sounds aren't simply acoustic energy bouncing off the eardrum back to the recording microphone. Instead, they arise from the fluid-filled cochlea. If the real evoking click consists of high-frequency energy, the emitted sound arrives at the microphone earlier than when the evoking click consists of low-frequency energy. Looking back to Figures 9.18 and 9.19, this makes sense, for the region of the basilar membrane registering high-frequency sound is closer to the eardrum and, hence, to the recording microphone.

Most auditory experts now believe these emitted sounds—both emitted and evoked—can be traced to the amplifying actions of the OHCs. Recall that the OHCs behave like tiny motors, amplifying the wave actions in the fluid of the cochlea in response to sound. When that sound is brief—for example, a click—these motorlike actions of the OHCs continue briefly after the offset of the click. They behave, in other words, like tiny post-click tremors, setting up the reverse sequence of events described above. In the case of spontaneously emitted sounds, the amplification process seems to involve self-induced reverberations within the OHCs. Because the middle and inner ears are so delicately designed to amplify and transduce mechanical displacements, it takes very little motion within the cochlea to trigger the chain of events leading to emitted sounds. And the amplification by the OHCs involves molec-

ular movements at least as large as those capable of producing a sensation of hearing. (Recall that motion as small as the diameter of a single hydrogen atom can be heard.) It is ironic that nature has designed an ear so sensitive that it can transmit the effects of the mechanical movements produced by its own parts!†

But if our ears generate sound energy all the time, why don't we hear that sound? For one reason, we are rarely in environments quiet enough for faint sounds to be heard: the normal sounds of the world will "mask" emitted sounds. Moreover, we tend to adapt to a continuous, steady sound, rendering it inaudible. Now despite having said this, there are individuals who *do* experience illusory sounds, meaning that an auditory sensation is experienced in the absence of an external stimulus. This condition is described in the next section.

Tinnitus. It is not uncommon for people to experience a sort of humming or ringing sound coming from within their ears. This condition, termed **tinnitus,** can be very annoying, for even though the ringing is not loud, it is persistent. The incidence of tinnitus is difficult to estimate, for people who do not experience tinnitus may simply have adapted to their self-produced ringing, just as we all adapt to a steady hum from an external source such as a refrigerator motor. Although you should not try this, tinnitus can be temporarily induced by ingestion of a large dose of aspirin (Stypulkowski, 1990). In fact, arthritis patients are sometimes instructed to adjust their dosage of aspirin on the basis of this symptom.

It is natural to guess that tinnitus is attributable to a person's hearing the spontaneously emitted sound from his or her own ear. Although this may be true in a few cases (Wilson and Sutton, 1981), most instances of tinnitus are traceable to neural

---

* The evoking sound has to be brief, so that the recording microphone in the auditory canal can pick up the relatively weak emitted sound against an otherwise quiet background. If the evoking sound remains present, its energy and influence within the cochlea swamp any trace of an emitted sound.

† New hearing tests based on measurement of emitted sounds are being developed (Allen and Neely, 1992); these should be particularly useful for assessing hearing in individuals, such as newborn infants, unable to respond verbally on conventional hearing tests.

degeneration (Tonndorf, 1987; Coles and Hallam, 1987). As a rule, the ringing experienced with tinnitus has a characteristic frequency for any given individual. That frequency, however, typically does *not* correspond to the frequency recorded as spontaneous emission from that individual's ear. Moreover, a large dose of aspirin, which induces tinnitus, can eliminate spontaneous emitted sounds (McFadden, Plattsmier, and Pasanen, 1984). These observations underscore the distinction between emitted sounds and tinnitus.

For a more complete description of the symptoms and incidence of tinnitus, consult Stouffer and Tyler (1990); for a discussion of possible neural bases of tinnitus, see Jastreboff (1990).

THE AUDITORY SYSTEM: THE AUDITORY PATHWAYS

As you have learned, the cochlea converts sound energy (pressure waves) into the only form of information understandable by the brain, neural impulses. This neural information is carried out of the inner ear by the **auditory nerve.** The auditory nerve, in turn, branches into several different pathways that eventually reconverge within the auditory cortex (the region on the side of your brain that would be covered if you put your hand over your ear). These various pathways seem designed to process different aspects of auditory information (Evans, 1974). One pathway contains neurons whose response properties enable them to specify *where* sound is coming from. Another pathway contains neurons that analyze information necessary for identifying *what* the sound is. In other words, the auditory system contains specialized neural analyzers for locating and identifying sound sources within the auditory environment.

Figure 9.20 gives an overview of the pathways originating from the left auditory nerve and the right auditory nerve; the right ear has been omitted for clarity. In the drawing, the dark lines represent pathways from the inner ear, to thalamic nuclei, and on to the brain. At each structure along this route, neurons make synaptic contact

with the next set of neurons in the pathway; the pathways are not a single bundle of fibers passing from ear to cortex. Not shown in the drawing are the neural projections from the brain *back* to the cochlea; these so-called **efferent fibers** make synaptic contact with auditory nerve fibers at the point of innervation of the IHCs; efferent fibers are not distributed to the OHC portion of the cochlea. These efferents, it is thought, modulate auditory nerve fiber activity evoked by IHC stimulation (Dallos, 1981).

We will not trace the flow of information through the maze of pathways depicted in Figure 9.20; interested students may consult the particularly clear description of these pathways given by Hackney (1987). Instead, we'll summarize several aspects of auditory information that the neurons seem to be processing. Our aim is to highlight neural properties that bear on perceptual aspects of hearing to be discussed in the next chapter. This final section of the chapter is divided into three subsections. The first summarizes the properties of neurons composing the auditory nerve. The two remaining subsections focus on the neural analysis of the cues for sound localization (where) and the cues for sound identification (what). In the course of our discussion, you will see a similarity between auditory neural processing and visual neural processing: at successively higher stages, individual neurons become increasingly more discriminating about the sounds that activate them.

THE AUDITORY NERVE

The auditory nerve innervating each of the two ears consists of about 50,000 individual fibers. These are the axons of nerve cells situated in the inner ear. As detailed in an earlier section, about 95 percent of these fibers carry information picked up from just the IHCs (which total only about 3,500), while the remaining 5 percent or so are devoted to input from the OHCs (which total about 12,000). This means, of course, that single IHCs are each innervated by many auditory nerve fibers. The locations at which auditory nerve fibers contact a single IHC are arranged systemati-

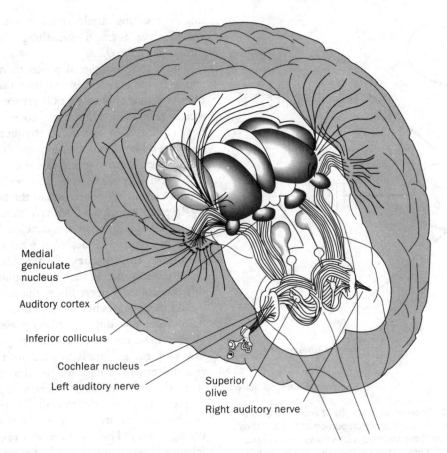

FIGURE 9.20 An overview of the auditory pathways.

cally around the circumference of the hair cell (Liberman, 1982). On the side of the IHC facing the rows of OHCs (refer back to Figure 9.14), contact is made with fibers exhibiting high rates of spontaneous activity; on the opposite side of the IHC are fibers with relatively low spontaneous activity; the remaining locations around an IHC are innervated by fibers with intermediate levels of spontaneous activity. This arrangement is summarized in Figure 9.21. In a moment, we shall return to these three classes of auditory nerve fibers, pointing out another, functionally important distinction among them. But first, let's consider the responses of these fibers to sound stimulation.

By recording the electrical impulses from many individual fibers, physiologists have determined what kinds of sound stimuli must be presented to the ear to activate those fibers. As mentioned in the previous paragraph, fibers of the auditory nerve, like retinal ganglion cells of the eye, are active even when no stimulus is present. Therefore, to register its presence, a sound must alter this spontaneously occurring, random neural chatter. In auditory nerve fibers, sound is registered by a temporary increase in firing rate. However, not just any sound stimulus will do. For any given fiber, there is a limited range of pure-tone frequencies that can evoke a response. Moreover, within this limited range not all frequencies are equally effective. We shall illustrate these observations using the following example.

Suppose we measure the number of impulses

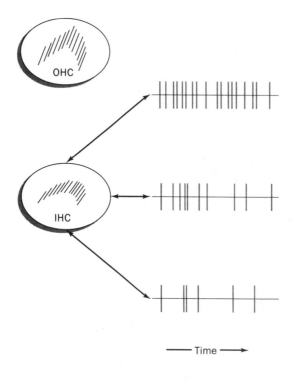

— Time →

Spontaneous neural activity

FIGURE 9.21 Spontaneous activity of auditory nerve fibers varies depending on which portion of the IHC they innervate. The three traces depict spontaneous neural impulses over time: activity in the top trace is ''high''; in the middle trace, ''medium''; and in the lower trace, ''low.''

that pure tones produce in a single auditory nerve fiber. Suppose further that we make such measurements for pure tones of various frequencies (Hz) and intensities (dB). (Keep in mind that a pure tone has a sinusoidal waveform.) For each frequency, we will determine the *minimum* intensity needed to produce a noticeable increase in that fiber's spontaneous level of activity; the resulting intensity value will constitute that fiber's ''threshold'' for detecting that frequency. We refer to this intensity as the threshold because at lower intensities the fiber behaves as if the tone were not presented at all—the fiber is ''deaf'' to all weaker intensities. Such a **threshold intensity** is determined for a number of frequencies. Plot-

ting the resulting thresholds for an individual fiber would yield a graph something like the one shown in Figure 9.22.

There are a couple of points to note in this graph. At the very lowest intensity, this particular fiber responds only to a 5,000-Hz tone (abbreviated 5-kHz). This value, then, constitutes this fiber's preferred, or *characteristic,* frequency. At this quiet sound level, no other tone produces activity in the fiber. But as we increase the sound intensity, previously ineffective frequencies begin to produce measurable increases in the fiber's activity. In other words, the fiber has different intensity thresholds for different frequencies. The entire curve in Figure 9.22 describes what is called the **frequency tuning curve** for that fiber.

When this sort of analysis is applied to many different auditory nerve fibers, the result is a family of tuning curves like those illustrated in Figure 9.23. Note that different fibers possess different characteristic frequencies; some respond best to low frequencies, others to medium frequencies, and still others to high frequencies. As a group, then, the auditory fibers cover a large range of frequencies. Note, too, that all fibers—regardless of characteristic frequency—exhibit asymmetric tuning curves. The loss in neural responsiveness (change in sensitivity) is much sharper at frequencies *higher* than the characteristic frequency. This means, therefore, that small changes in frequency can make big differences in the neural activity of nerve fibers.

The frequency tuning of any auditory nerve fiber depends on the location, along the basilar membrane, of the receptor cells (typically IHCs) from which the fiber collects information. Recall that different sound frequencies produce traveling waves that peak at different places along the basilar membrane. As you might guess, each fiber's characteristic frequency is determined by where along the basilar membrane that fiber makes contact with hair cells. Fibers originating from the apex of the cochlea (the low-frequency region—see Figure 9.18) respond to low frequencies, whereas fibers from the base (the high-frequency region) ''prefer'' higher frequencies.

This idea of representing a stimulus dimension

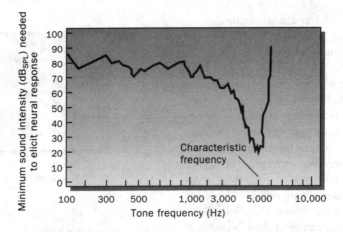

FIGURE 9.22 A graph of the threshold intensities (frequency tuning curve) for a single auditory nerve fiber. (Courtesy of Evan Relkin.)

within an array of tuned neurons should be familiar to you by now. We saw the same principle at work in the visual system: visual cells are tuned for size, orientation, retinal disparity, and so on. In effect, tuned cells make a particular statement about the nature of a stimulus. In the case of the auditory nerve, individual nerve fibers are able to signal the occurrence of a tone whose frequency falls within a limited range of frequencies. Within this range, however, a fiber's activity increases with sound *intensity*, a property we shall discuss shortly. Consequently, within this limited range, the fiber's response is wholly ambiguous: any number of different frequencies could produce the same neural response if their intensities were adjusted properly. So looking just at the firing rate

FIGURE 9.23 Frequency tuning curves for a number of different auditory nerve fibers. (Courtesy of Evan Relkin.)

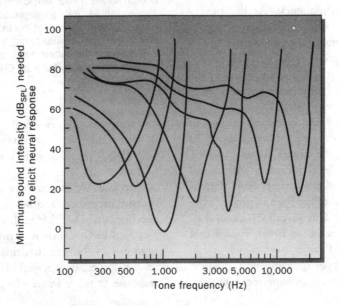

of a particular fiber, we could never be certain which frequency had stimulated it. (This is the same sort of ambiguity problem discussed in Chapters 4, 5, and 6.)

We don't want to give you the impression that auditory fibers respond only to pure tones. In fact, an auditory fiber will respond vigorously to *any* complex sound just so long as that sound contains at least some energy within the frequency range handled by that fiber. For example, the sound produced when you snap your fingers is *broadband*—that is, it contains many different frequencies; so, too, is the static heard when you dial a radio between stations. Either of these broadband sounds would activate a number of frequency-tuned fibers. Any particular fiber, however, would "hear" (respond to) only those frequency components of the complex sound to which it was tuned.

So far our description of auditory fibers has focused on their frequency selectivity, as reflected in their threshold response profile. Before moving to higher levels of auditory processing, let's take a look at two other characteristic features of auditory nerve fiber responses. One feature is the way a fiber responds to sound levels above its threshold. Imagine recording the discharge rate from the fiber whose tuning curve is shown in Figure 9.22. Suppose that we use a 5-kHz tone, that fiber's preferred frequency. As the tuning curve indicates, an intensity of 20 dB$_{SPL}$ will produce a barely discernible elevation in the fiber's activity level—this represents that cell's threshold. Now suppose we plot the discharge level produced by increasingly higher sound intensities of the 5-kHz tone. The result would be a graph like that shown by the solid line in the top portion of Figure 9.24. As you can see, between about 20 dB$_{SPL}$ and 60 dB$_{SPL}$, the fiber's activity steadily grows as the sound level increases. Above 60 dB$_{SPL}$, however, the fiber's activity level flattens out—higher intensities of the tone all produce the same neural response. This so-called *saturation effect,* typical of auditory nerve fibers, means that the fiber has a limited range over which it can signal the intensity level of a given frequency. Hence firing rate provides an *im*perfect represen-

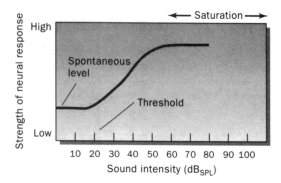

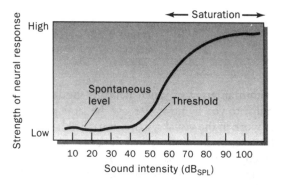

FIGURE 9.24 The neural activity of an auditory nerve fiber increases as the sound level increases, until a saturation point is reached. The graph at the top shows a fiber with high spontaneous activity, low threshold, and low saturation level; the graph at the bottom shows a fiber with low spontaneous activity, high threshold, and high saturation level. The fiber whose activity is shown in the top graph would innervate the IHC on the side facing toward the OHC; the one shown in the bottom would innervate the IHC on the side facing away from the OHC (recall Figure 9.21).

tation of sound level—distinguishable differences in sound intensity (for instance, 80 dB$_{SPL}$ versus 120 dB$_{SPL}$) produce indistinguishable neural responses.

Suppose we repeat these intensity/response measurements on another auditory nerve fiber, also one tuned to 5 kHz. Now we might generate a curve like that shown in the bottom portion of Figure 9.24. Notice that this fiber's spontaneous level is lower, its threshold level is higher, and it responds to more intense levels before saturating.

These two different fibers—sharing a characteristic frequency—correspond to two of the three different innervation patterns described several paragraphs back. (An example of the third fiber type would fall midway between the two shown in Figure 9.24.) Recall that some fibers making synaptic contact with an IHC have low spontaneous activity, others have intermediate spontaneous activity, and still others have high spontaneous activity; and this spontaneous level is closely related to the location around the IHC where the fibers innervate the IHC (recall Figure 9.21). We now see that these three categories of fibers have different thresholds and different saturation intensities. These differences will prove important when we discuss hearing thresholds and loudness perception in the next chapter.

Besides variations in responsiveness with intensity, another significant property of auditory nerve fibers is their response to continuous, prolonged stimulation. When a sound of constant intensity is presented continuously, the level of activity evoked by that sound declines over time; this property is called **adaptation.** As described in Chapter 4, neural adaptation is a common property of sensory neurons. In the case of hearing, this adaptation phenomenon probably has something to do with the gradual reduction in loudness you experience when listening to a steady sound, such as the hum of a refrigerator motor.

This gives an overview of the response properties of auditory nerve fibers, the brain's sole link to the sounds in the environment. The train of neural impulses carried by the auditory nerves from the left and right ears provides the ingredients for all aspects of hearing. Subsequent auditory processing must utilize information contained within these impulses. In the two following sections, you will see how this neural information is utilized for sound localization and for sound identification.

BEYOND THE AUDITORY NERVE: SOUND LOCALIZATION

Having two ears enables you to localize sounds. This section discusses how the processing of in-formation within the auditory system makes such localization possible.

Binaural Neurons. Looking back at Figure 9.20, note that the left auditory nerve projects to the **cochlear nucleus** on the left side of the brain, while the right auditory nerve projects to the cochlear nucleus on the right side of the brain. Thus, at this first stage in the auditory chain, information from the two ears remains segregated. Sound delivered to just the left ear (stimulation that is **monaural,** meaning "one ear") will activate cells in the left cochlear nucleus, but have no effect on those in the right cochlear nucleus. Exactly the opposite is true for monaural stimulation delivered to the right ear. However, at processing stages beyond the cochlear nucleus (superior olive, inferior colliculus, and higher), the auditory system becomes **binaural** ("both ears"), meaning that these higher stages receive neural input from the left ear *and* the right ear. (This property should remind you of the binocular visual cells discussed in Chapters 4 and 7.) Some binaural neurons can be activated by sound presented to either ear, but others are activated by sound presented to one ear but inhibited by sound presented to the other ear. The former category—the pure excitatory neurons—tends to prefer low-frequency sound, whereas the other category—the excitatory/inhibitory neurons—prefers higher frequencies (summarized by Dabak and Johnson, 1992). Some binaural neurons even have a different characteristic frequency for the left versus the right ear (Mendelson, 1992), and they respond to sound sources moving at particular speeds (Ahissar, Bergman, and Vaadia, 1992).

It is now commonly believed that these binaural cells register information about the location of a sound source relative to the head. To understand how these binaural cells work, you first need to be familiar with the two chief cues available for sound localization. In both of these cues, the sounds received by the two ears are compared, which is why the cues are called **binaural cues.** Let's take a moment to discuss them here, to provide some context for understanding the operations of binaural neurons; we'll go into more detail on these cues in the next chapter.

Interaural Time. Imagine keeping your head still and listening to a sound originating from a source located at various positions in front of and to either side of your head. (You might try snapping your fingers while holding your hand at arm's length at various positions around your head.) When the sound source lies straight ahead (a *midline* source), the sound energy reaching your two ears will be identical: the air pressure waves will arrive at the two ears at precisely the same time. Now suppose that a sound source is located to your left, away from the midline. In this case, the sound wave from the lateralized source will arrive at your closer ear, the left one, slightly before reaching your farther ear, the right one. This difference in time of arrival of sound at the two ears is called **interaural time difference,** and it is a potent cue for sound localization.

How might the auditory nervous system register interaural time differences? Do neurons exist that can compute time differences between the two ears? The answer to both questions is yes—neurons at several levels in the auditory pathways are sensitive to small binaural time disparities (Masterton and Imig, 1984; Knudsen, du Lac, and Esterly, 1987). For example, certain cells in the superior olivary nucleus, often called the superior olive (see Figure 9.20), respond maximally when the left ear receives sound slightly before the right ear does, whereas other cells respond best when the right ear receives sound slightly before the left. The interaural time delay that gives the best response varies from cell to cell. But by what means are these interaural delays actually created at the level of binaural cells? The answer, which is elegant yet simple, was proposed decades ago by Jeffress (1948) and more recently substantiated by physiological measurements.

Here's how it seems to work. As you already know, the axon is the neural process carrying impulses from one end of a cell (usually the cell body) to the other (the synaptic zone), where those impulses trigger chemical communication with the next set of neurons in a pathway. Now, it is a fact that a neuron with a short axon conveys impulses to its recepient neurons in a shorter period of time than does a neuron with a longer axon; the impulse travels over a shorter distance and, hence, takes less time. Axon length, in other words, governs the time elapsing between generation of neural impulses and the delivery of the "message" conveyed by those impulses to the next set of neurons. Now imagine a binaural neuron that receives input from two cells whose axons *differ* in length, one axonal path being shorter than the other (see drawing A in Figure 9.25). With this in mind, what will happen if both input neurons are activated at precisely the same time? The input cell with the shorter axon will get its

FIGURE 9.25 Schematic drawings showing how interaural time differences from a lateralized sound source could be registered by a binaural cell receiving inputs from cells whose axons differ in length.

Left ear   Right ear   Left ear   Right ear

Δt   Δt

Binaural neuron   Binaural neuron

A Registers sound to left   B Registers sound to right

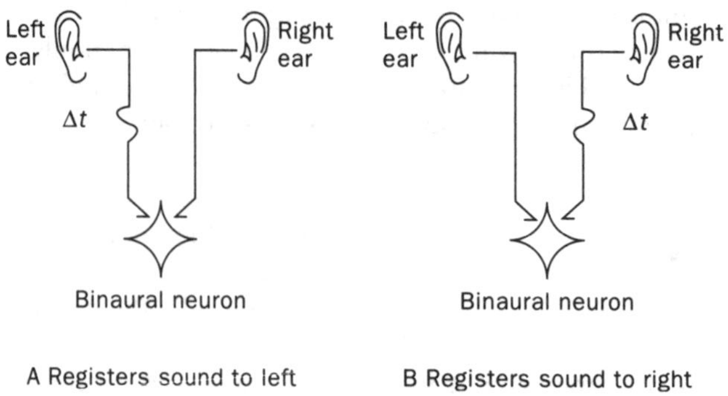

message to the binaural cell sooner than will the input cell with the longer axon, with the disparity in time of arrival at the binaural neuron depending on the magnitude of the difference in axon length between the two input neurons. Given these two input neurons, what would be necessary to ensure that the binaural neuron received *simultaneous* inputs from both? To accomplish this, the input neuron with the longer axon would have to be activated *prior to* activation of the input neuron with the shorter axon; the time disparity between activations would have to match the disparity associated with their conduction times. We could, in other words, compensate for the axon length differences by introducing an appropriate delay between activation of the two input cells. How could we create these differences in activation time? The answer is simple: place the sound source at a location where the interaural time difference creates this exact activation delay. (This scheme, by the way, is similar in purpose but not implementation to the delay line circuit described in Chapter 8 to account for direction-selective motion perception.)

This, then, is the essence of the **delay line** theory proposed by Jeffress (1948). Different binaural neurons receive inputs from pairs of cells, one activated by sound presented to the left ear and the other by sound presented to the right ear. For any given binaural cell, its pair of input cells has a characteristic time delay, governed by the difference in axon length. The binaural neurons respond maximally upon simultaneous stimulation by the input cells, but to achieve this simultaneity, the left- and right-ear input cells must be activated at slightly *different* times. In general, registration of sounds located to the left of the midline would require that the left-ear input cell have the longer axon (to compensate for the left ear's receiving the sound first), as depicted in drawing A in Figure 9.25; sounds located to the right would require the opposite arrangement (drawing B in Figure 9.25). To register particular locations to the left or to the right, the disparity in axonal length could vary among pairs of cells, which means that different binaural neurons would respond best to different interaural time differences.

Actually, there are several means by which impulse conduction delays could be introduced, besides variations in axon length, but the essence of the idea remains the same: binaural neurons with different preferred interaural delays signal different sound locations. Recent physiological work confirms that the auditory system has such a mechanism in place (Carr and Konishi, 1988), and theoretical work has aimed at refining the Jeffress model (Dabak and Johnson, 1992).

Interaural Intensity Differences. There is a second potential source of information specifying sound location: sound energy arriving at the two ears from a single source will be more intense at the ear located nearest the source. This **interaural intensity difference** arises primarily from the "occluding" effect produced by the head. When sound energy passes through a dense barrier—such as your head—some sound energy is usually lost. Thus for a lateralized sound source, a portion of its sound energy will be blocked from reaching the farther ear because the head stands in the way. The head produces what is called a *sound shadow,* a weakening of the intensity of sound at the more distant ear. This binaural difference in sound intensity provides another cue for sound localization. Of course, when the source is located equidistant from the two ears—for instance, straight ahead—the interaural intensity difference will be zero.

The auditory nervous system appears to capitalize on this source of location information, too. Neurons have been discovered that respond best when the two ears receive slightly different intensities, some preferring the stronger intensity in the right ear and others preferring the stronger intensity in the left ear (Wise and Irvine, 1988; Manley, Koppl, and Konishi, 1988). These binaural neurons, incidentally, are found in different neural sites than are those registering interaural time differences (Knudsen and Konishi, 1978). Moreover, binaural cells sensitive to interaural intensity tend to fall into the excitatory/inhibitory category, meaning that the input from one ear is excitatory and the input from the other is inhibitory. In fact, the algebraic subtraction of inhibition from excitation—an operation easily performed by a binaural cell—accounts for a given cell's preferred interaural intensity difference (Manley, Koppl, and Konishi, 1988).

Binaural Cells and Sound Localization. To reiterate: most binaural cells respond best to a sound arising from a particular location. For example, some binaural cells respond best to a source located close to the midline, whereas other cells respond best to sounds arising from various points to one side or the other of the midline. In effect, each binaural cell "listens" for sound within a fairly restricted region of auditory space. This region of space constitutes the cell's receptive field, the area in space where a sound must be located in order to stimulate the cell. As an aggregate, these cells provide a neural map of auditory space (King and Moore, 1991).

There are several reasons for thinking that binaural cells of this sort are involved in sound localization. For one thing, placing an earplug in one ear causes sounds to be mislocalized. Under this condition, sound seems to originate not from the actual location of the source, but from a location displaced toward the unplugged ear. This makes sense. Plugging an ear reduces sound intensity received by that ear. Plugging one ear also produces a shift in the receptive fields of binaural neurons, by an amount and direction predicted from errors in sound localization (Knudsen and Konishi, 1980). This systematic shift in the receptive field locations of binaural neurons reinforces the idea that these neurons encode the location of sound in space.

There is another reason for believing this idea, too. Not all species of mammals possess the kind of binaural neurons just described. In particular, the size of the superior olive varies greatly from one species to another. This structure is one of the brain structures containing binaural neurons. Bruce Masterton tested the abilities of different species to localize sound (Masterton, Thompson, Bechtold, and Robards, 1975). The animals were trained to listen for a short tone that came from one of two loudspeakers, one located to the animal's left and the other located to the animal's

right; the tone informed the animal which way to go, left or right, in order to obtain a drink of water. Masterton found that cats and tree shrews, both of which have sizable superior olives, could perform this task with ease. However, hedgehogs and rats, who have a much smaller superior olive, made numerous errors, indicating an inability to localize sound accurately. Masterton's behavioral study reinforces the idea that binaural neurons of the superior olive are responsible for analyzing interaural cues for sound localization.

This concludes our discussion of how the auditory system processes information about *where* a sound originates. Besides localization, though, sensory systems are designed to detect and identify objects and events. Accordingly, we now consider how the auditory system processes information about the identity of a sound—*what* it is that's being heard.

BEYOND THE AUDITORY NERVE: SOUND IDENTIFICATION

Recall that any fiber in the auditory nerve responds to a limited range of frequencies, a range that defines the fiber's frequency tuning. The responses of such fibers to more complex sounds (such as noise or a vocalization) can be simply predicted from each fiber's tuning curve. Moving from the auditory nerve to more central processing stages (for example, the cochlear nucleus), we find that cells continue to respond to tones of certain frequencies, but the range of frequencies over which any given cell responds becomes narrower. Thus over the first several stages of the auditory system, tuning curves become more selective for frequency. In addition, information destined for the auditory cortex passes through the **medial geniculate nucleus** (see Figure 9.20). This structure, the analogue to the LGN in vision, also receives input from the reticular activating system (recall Chapter 4, page 109). So again, an organism's level of arousal probably modulates auditory sensitivity by means of neural influences occurring within the medial geniculate nucleus.

Within the **auditory cortex,** temporal frequency is organized tonotopically, meaning that the frequency selectivity of neurons changes systematically within this cortical region. There is, in other words, an auditory cortical map that mirrors the tonotopic organization of the basilar membrane; in a sense, this tonotopic frequency map is analogous to the retinotopic map in the visual cortex. Moreover, this auditory map exhibits a form of cortical magnification, since there are more neurons tuned to mid-frequencies than to either higher or lower values; this is the region of the frequency spectrum, incidentally, responsible for carrying information for human speech.

Not all neurons, however, are selective solely for temporal frequency (Moore, 1987). Many neurons in the auditory cortex, rather than being "interested" in the frequency or intensity of sounds, instead respond best to more complicated, biologically significant sounds. We'll give just a few examples. Some cortical neurons fail to respond to any steady tone but do respond vigorously to a tone that changes in frequency. For some of these neurons, the frequency change must be in a particular direction, either up or down. One sound whose frequency goes up is the "Hmmm?" sound you make when you don't understand something (try it). A sound whose frequency goes down is the sound you make when you yawn (try it). In general, frequency changes are responsible for the voice inflections during speech; without these inflections, the voice has a flat, monotone character.

Other cortical neurons respond only to complex "kissing" sounds that resemble the noise often used when calling a dog. In animals that utilize vocalizations to communicate, the auditory cortex contains neurons specifically responsive to individual vocalizations. Such cells often fail to respond to tones, clicks, or noise, and instead can be activated only by a certain "call" that forms part of that animal's natural vocabulary. For instance, in the auditory cortex of the squirrel monkey there are neurons activated exclusively by "cackles," other neurons activated only by "shrieks," and still others activated only by "trills" (Wollberg and Newman, 1972). Each of these natural vocalizations conveys a particular message

within the repertoire of calls made by the squirrel monkey.

Many cortical neurons, then, unlike those at lower levels of the auditory system, respond to more *abstract* features of sound—features that identify the sound source itself, not just the constituent frequencies in that sound. This is why damage to the auditory cortex impairs performance on tasks where an animal must discriminate between complex sounds, but spares performance on tasks involving the detection or discrimination of simple tones.

Insight into cortical processing of auditory information in humans has come from several sources. One is application of the PET technique described in Chapters 1 and 4. (PET, you will recall, pictorially depicts regions of the human brain active during specific tasks.) From the work of Petersen et al. (1988), it is known that listening to words activates regions in the temporal lobe and near the junction of temporal and parietal lobes. There is also evidence that the extent and focus of activity in these areas are modulated by the degree of attention directed to those words (Hari et al., 1989). In the following chapter, we shall describe some evidence suggesting that these regions of the human brain contain neurons selective for certain acoustic cues important for speech recognition.

Studies of brain-damaged patients provide another source of information about the auditory cortex in humans. The clinical literature on brain damage and hearing is too extensive to review here; interested readers should see Tanaka, Kamo, Yoshida, and Yamadori (1991). Suffice it to say that damage to different portions of the auditory pathways can create different kinds of hearing losses, ranging from temporary deficits in the ability to hear tones to permanent inability to recognize otherwise familiar sources from their sounds. There is even an auditory analog to blindsight, the syndrome described in Chapter 4. Tanaka, Kamo, Yoshida, and Yamadori (1991) describe two patients who exhibited seriously impaired hearing from extensive bilateral damage to brain structures in the auditory cortex; the ears and auditory nerves were intact. Despite their

cortical deafness, these patients sometimes behaviorally reacted to a sound—such as a door slamming—while denying any experience of that sound. This suggests that neural pathways subserving auditory reflexes—such as turning the head toward a sound source—are different from those involved in awareness and identification of the source.

This completes our survey of sound, the ear, and the auditory pathways. The stage has been set for consideration of hearing, the next chapter's topic.

S U M M A R Y   A N D   P R E V I E W

This chapter has described the physical events that give rise to the experience of sound. These events are captured by the ears, transformed into neural events by the hair cells, and analyzed by neurons specialized for frequency and sound location. Throughout this chapter we've largely avoided discussing the perceptual consequences of this sequence of events. But now that you know something about the auditory system's machinery, we're ready to consider the accomplishment that this machinery makes possible: hearing.

K E Y   T E R M S

acoustic energy
acoustic reflex
acoustics
adaptation
amplitude
anvil (incus)
auditory canal
auditory cortex
auditory nerve
basilar membrane
binaural
binaural cues
cilia
cochlea
cochlear emissions
cochlear nucleus
cortical deafness
decibels (dB)

delay line
eardrum (tympanic
    membrane)
echoes
efferent fibers
Eustachian tube
frequency theory
frequency tuning curve
hair cells
hammer (malleus)
hertz (Hz)
inner hair cells (IHCs)
interaural intensity
    difference
interaural time difference
medial geniculate nucleus
monaural

noise
organ of Corti
ossicles
outer hair cells (OHCs)
oval window
pinna
place theory
pure tones
resonant frequency
round window
sound pressure level (SPL)
stirrup (stapes)
tectorial membrane
threshold intensity
tinnitus
tonotopic organization
traveling wave

Hearing

Do blind people hear better than sighted individuals? Does exposure to loud music impair one's hearing? How do you manage to ignore the hubbub at a noisy party while at the same time picking out and listening to a familiar voice? These are just a few of the questions we shall consider in this chapter on hearing. Because the properties of the auditory system are crucial to any account of hearing, you'll find that much of the discussion here is grounded in the material presented in the previous chapter.

THE RANGE AND LIMITS OF HEARING

The range of sound frequencies that humans can hear defines the boundaries of auditory perception: outside these boundaries all humans are deaf. The range of audible sound frequencies is analogous to the range of visible spatial frequencies (see Chapter 5). In both instances, the eyes and ears register a fairly wide but definitely limited range of visual and auditory information. Because this range is limited, our perceptual world is limited.

In the case of hearing, the range of audible frequencies is determined by measuring the minimum intensity, or amplitude, necessary to just barely detect tones of various frequencies; these measurements are made in a quiet environment, with no other sounds present. Test tones are typically delivered over earphones or through a loudspeaker. The minimum intensity value is referred to as the **threshold intensity;** values below this threshold intensity cannot be heard, whereas in-

tensities higher than this can be. (The Appendix gives a detailed discussion of techniques for threshold measurements.) Threshold intensity measured for each of a number of tone frequencies can be plotted on a graph like the one in Figure 10.1 Such curves summarize the range of frequencies audible to the human ear.

Curves like this, showing variations in threshold with frequency, are called **audibility functions (AFs).** The analogy between an AF and a contrast sensitivity function for spatial vision should be obvious—both specify threshold performance over a range of frequencies. As the curve in Figure 10.1 indicates, the threshold of hearing varies with the frequency of sound: in the middle frequencies, far less intensity is needed to make a tone audible than in the low and high frequencies. In this figure, intensity values are expressed in terms of decibels (dB_{SPL}), with the value of 0 dB_{SPL} assigned to the weakest intensity that can be heard at any frequency (recall Figure 9.4). In this case, tones in the neighborhood of 2,500 Hz require least intensity to be heard. As a result, their threshold is expressed as 0 dB_{SPL} and all other threshold values are expressed relative to this value. Thus to hear a 200-Hz tone, its intensity must be 40 dB higher than the intensity needed to hear a 2,500-Hz tone.

At its best, the human ear is extraordinarily sensitive: the intensity required to hear a 2,500-Hz tone is hardly any greater than the amplitude of vibrations associated with the random movements of air molecules! At this very low sound level the eardrum moves only about one-billionth

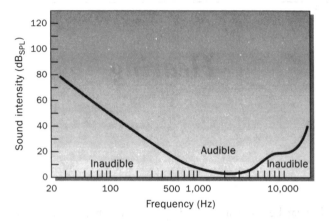

FIGURE 10.1 An ability function (AF) showing the range of tone frequencies audible to a normal young adult.

of a centimeter, a distance less than the diameter of a single hydrogen atom (Bekesy and Rosenblith, 1951). This incredible performance testifies to what a masterpiece of engineering the ears are—all the more remarkable in view of the fact that this very sensitive device is not harmed by sounds several million times more intense. And on top of this, human beings can hear a wide range of frequencies: most people can detect tones as low in frequency as 20 Hz, which is heard as a very low rumble, and young people can detect tones as high in frequency as 20,000 Hz. To get this much performance out of a device so sensitive represents a real design feat.

The performance summarized in Figure 10.1 represents the range of hearing for the normal young adult. This curve is remarkably consistent across individuals, so much so that deviations from this norm usually signify some type of impairment in the peripheral auditory system, either in the ear or in the auditory nerve. Abnormal AFs are *not* commonly associated with disorders of the central auditory nervous system; central neural disorders lead to other kinds of hearing loss, some of which we'll mention later in this chapter. For now, let's consider some of the conditions that can produce abnormal AFs (higher than normal, pure-tone thresholds) and the perceptual consequences of those abnormalities.

HEARING LOSS

Between 17 and 20 million Americans suffer some loss of hearing, making this the most common of all physical disabilities. In its most severe form, impaired hearing means a total loss of sensitivity to sound—complete deafness. People who become completely deaf after years of normal hearing describe the experience as frightening. Since everyday sounds keep one in touch with the environment, loss of hearing isolates the totally deaf person not only from the voices of others but also from the security of life's background hum. As Helen Keller poignantly describes it:

I am just as deaf as I am blind. The problems of deafness are deeper and more complex, if not more important, than those of blindness. Deafness is a much worse misfortune. For it means the loss of the most vital stimulus—the sound of the voice that brings language, sets thoughts astir and keeps us in the intellectual company of man. . . . I have found deafness to be a much greater handicap than blindness (Cited in Ackerman, 1990, p. 191)

In legal terms, a person is said to be "totally deaf" when speech sounds cannot be heard at intensities less than 82 dB$_{SPL}$ (the intensity of ordinary speech is around 60 dB$_{SPL}$). The term "hearing impairment," which can be a far milder condition, refers to any loss in auditory sensitivity relative to the hearing ability of the normal young adult (see AF in Figure 10.1). All hearing difficulties can be divided into two categories: conduction loss and sensory/neural loss. The first category of hearing loss, **conduction loss,** stems from some disorder within the outer ear or the middle ear, those portions of the auditory system involved in mechanically transmitting (conducting) sound energy to the receptors in the inner ear. Hearing disorders originating in these peripheral stages of the auditory system typically involve an overall reduction in sensitivity to sounds of all frequencies. The second category of hearing defect, **sensory/neural loss,** originates within the inner ear or in the auditory portion of the brain; the associated hearing loss may extend over the entire range of audible frequencies or over only a portion of that range. Let's consider some of the more common causes of the two categories of hearing loss, starting with conduction losses.

CONDUCTION HEARING LOSS AND POSSIBLE REMEDIES

Conduction loss can be caused by excessive buildup of ear wax in the canal of the outer ear. Simply cleaning out the plugged-up canal cures the problem. In other cases, however, the problem is more serious. Infection can cause fluid to build up in the middle ear, and if the Eustachian tube (the middle ear's pressure regulator) becomes inflamed, middle-ear pressure can rupture the eardrum. Infection can also spread to the bony chamber housing the middle ear, leading to bone disease that must be treated surgically. With the advent of antibiotics, ear infections can be treated before the symptoms reach these dangerous stages.

There is another type of conduction disorder that affects the middle ear, and this condition is not remedied by drugs. Called **otosclerosis,** this disorder involves the gradual immobilization of the stapes, the last of the tiny middle-ear bones that form the ossicular bridge between the outside

world and the inner ear. Recall that the stapes (stirrup) is the bone actually responsible for transmitting sound vibrations to the oval window, which in turn sets up pressure waves within the cochlear fluids. Hence, when the stapes becomes immobile, the bridge to the inner ear is destroyed. The stapes becomes immobilized by a steady accumulation of a spongy substance near the foot of this bone. This spongy substance eventually hardens, cementing the stapes in a rigid position. No one understands what triggers this disease, but it tends to occur in young adults and more often in females than in males. Fortunately, the disease can be treated. Using a surgical microscope to guide their movements, physicians can remove the immobile stapes and replace it with a plastic substitute. So long as other portions of the ear have not been affected by the disease, this form of surgery can restore hearing to normal levels.

Otosclerosis is a progressive disease that, in time, may spread to the cochlea. In these cases, surgery to replace the stapes cannot restore hearing to normal levels. It is important, therefore, for the physician to know beforehand whether a candidate for stapes surgery also suffers hearing loss due to cochlear pathology. But how can a physician determine functional status when the immobile stapes blocks sound's normal route to the cochlea? The answer is easy—there is an alternate route to the cochlea, through the bones of the skull. You have probably noticed how loud the dentist's drill sounds when it contacts one of your teeth. This is because vibrations from the drill are transmitted from your tooth to your skull. The cochlea, remember, is the coiled cavity formed within the bone of the skull. Thus when vibrations are introduced into the skull, those vibrations reach the cochlea, and if they are sufficiently strong, they set up pressure waves in the cochlear fluids. Those pressure waves behave just like the ones reaching the cochlea through the ear; they set up ripples along the basilar membrane, causing you to experience those bone-transmitted vibrations as sound. This is called hearing by **bone conduction.** Every time you speak, part of what you hear is the sound of your voice transmitted via bone conduction. That's why a tape recording of your voice sounds strange to you but not to others—listening to the recorder, you hear your voice without any contribution from bone conduction.

One wouldn't expect a sound to be as loud when carried via bone conduction as when conveyed through the ear, because this alternate route includes no mechanism like the ossicles for amplifying sound energy. For this reason, pure-tone thresholds measured through the skull of a person with good hearing are roughly 30 dB higher than those measured using tones delivered to the ear. Incidentally, to measure pure-tone thresholds for bone conduction hearing, a tuning fork is set into vibration and placed firmly against the bone just behind the ear. Let's return, then, to the question of whether to operate on a patient with otosclerosis. If that person's bone conduction thresholds are near normal, then the cochlea must be unaffected by the disease, and surgery should be successful in restoring the world of sound to the patient.

Finally, conduction hearing loss can be partially remedied by a hearing aid. Since the loss stems from the damping of sound energy, the hearing aid counters this damping by amplifying sound. Modern hearing aids convert sound into electrical signals, amplifying those signals by up to 60 dB, and then converting the amplified signals back into sound energy. Good hearing aids are designed to amplify mainly those frequencies involved in speech, 200 to 8,000 Hz. Thus other sounds, such as music, may seem distorted—much like nonspeech sounds heard over a telephone. Although not as effective as a modern electronic hearing aid, the simplest, most popular hearing aid is the hand. When the hand is cupped and placed behind the pinna, extra sound waves are funneled into the ear, raising the intensity by as much as 6 dB. Actually, any device or action signaling that an individual is hearing-impaired improves hearing, for other people tend to speak louder if a listener is thought to have impaired hearing. Richard Gregory (1992) suggests that even a string hanging from one's ear serves as an effective hearing aid.

SENSORY/NEURAL LOSS

Anything that deleteriously affects the cochlea (which houses the receptors for hearing) or the auditory nerve will have an impact on hearing. This section outlines several factors that can have such an impact.

Age and Hearing Loss. The most common, perhaps inevitable, cause of hearing loss is age. In industrial societies, people gradually lose sensitivity to high frequencies, a condition known as **presbycusis** (from the Greek *presbys,* meaning "old," and *akousis,* meaning "hearing"), and this selective high-frequency deafness begins at a surprisingly early age. According to one survey (Davis and Silverman, 1960), most people 30 years old are unable to hear frequencies above 15,000 Hz, and by 50 years of age, hearing is impossible beyond 12,000 Hz. By 70 years of age, the cutoff value drops to 6,000 Hz, a value that impinges on the range of normal speech. Moreover, for any given age group, men exhibit a larger degree of hearing loss than do women (Corso, 1981). These figures represent average values and therefore do not invariably apply to all people. Bekesy, whose pioneering work on the cochlea was discussed in Chapter 9, believed that age-related hearing loss resulted from the cochlea's losing its elasticity, thereby diminishing its ability to transmit traveling waves. Contemporary researchers believe that presbycusis results from changes in the vasculature of the cochlea—changes that restrict the blood supply to the delicate neural elements in the inner ear, presumably leading to chronic anemia that starves these elements. Still others feel that cumulative exposure to loud noise may contribute to the steady loss of hearing with age. This noise exposure hypothesis receives some support from cross-cultural studies showing normal hearing in 70-year-old African tribal people living in natural environments unpolluted by noise (Bergman, 1966). Whether their immunity to hearing loss is attributable to their quiet environment, or to other factors such as diet or genetics, remains undetermined. Whatever the cause, those of us living in modern societies better become resigned to a steady loss in hearing with age.

Noise Exposure and Hearing Loss. An unfortunately common cause of hearing loss is exposure to very loud noise; and in most instances, the cause can be traced to damage of the fine receptor structures in the inner ear. For instance, the acoustic energy from explosions—in combat or in industrial accidents—can produce sudden, permanent deafness due to trauma to the organ of Corti. Even the explosion of a single 2-inch firecracker can cause a major loss in hearing (Ward and Glorig, 1961). Comparable hearing losses have been reported in people exposed to the noise of gunfire, such as hunters (Taylor and Williams, 1966), people in the armed forces, and actors in western movies. Included in this last group of hearing-impaired individuals is former United States President Ronald Reagan, whose hearing loss dates back to his days as an actor (Reagan, 1990).

All the cases just mentioned involve sudden explosive noises, but this certainly is not the only type of sound that can damage the inner ear and, hence, cause hearing loss. Sustained loud noises can also lead to permanent hearing loss. Medical authorities point to loud music and headphones as contributors to the high incidence of hearing loss in college students, which by some estimates approaches 60 percent of that age group. In response to these concerns, some manufacturers of headphones now include literature with each set, warning of potential hazards to hearing. One manufacturer has gone so far as to install a warning light on its portable cassette players to indicate when the volume exceeds safe listening levels. The loud, amplified music often encountered at rock concerts and clubs also can cause permanent hearing loss. In one study of this effect (Hanson and Fearn, 1975), pure-tone thresholds were measured in two groups of college students. One group consisted of people who attended at least one rock concert each month, whereas the other group consisted of people who never attended rock concerts. At all frequencies tested, which spanned the range 500 to 8,000 Hz, "attenders"

had higher thresholds—pure tones had to be more intense in order for attenders to hear them. The differences between the groups were small, averaging just a couple of decibels, but they were consistent. The regular attenders, incidentally, were entirely unaware of their deficits, and they had no complaints about their hearing. Besides members of their audiences, pop musicians themselves can develop hearing loss from their chronic exposure to amplified music (Axelsson and Lindgren, 1978).

Chronic noise exposure also represents a serious occupational hazard for individuals who work in such environments as mechanized assembly plants, airports, and construction sites. Chronic exposure to the squeals of farm animals can also damage hearing (Kristensen and Gimsing, 1988). It is well documented that unprotected workers in noisy environments suffer permanent increases in pure-tone thresholds, with the magnitude of the loss related to length of time on the job (Nixon and Glorig, 1961; Taylor, 1965). Moreover, high noise levels in industrial settings are associated with higher accident rates, presumably because noise makes it more difficult to hear warning signals such as whistles or shouts (Wilkins and Acton, 1982). Aware of these deleterious effects of noise (and their likely legal liability in such instances), more industries attempt to shield their workers from harmful noise. This shielding can consist of earplugs (which can reduce noise levels by up to 30 dB) and, wherever possible, sound-attenuating enclosures for workers.

Even people who work and play in everyday environments must tolerate such noises as the roar of a motorcycle or the wail of a siren. On an ordinary day, the sound level on a downtown Chicago street can approach 100 dB$_{SPL}$, and inside a subway tunnel, even this level is exceeded when trains pass through a station. But you don't need to go to a busy city to experience a noisy environment—you can do this in the "quiet" of your own home. Ordinary household appliances can generate surprising levels of noise: a dishwasher can produce 60 dB$_{SPL}$ of sound, a vacuum cleaner 75 dB$_{SPL}$, and an innocent-looking garbage disposal can exceed 100 dB$_{SPL}$ when it is chewing on hard objects such as bones (Stevens and Warshofsky, 1965). While these sound levels won't lead to *permanent* deafness, they are sufficiently loud to elevate your threshold for hearing *temporarily* after cessation of the noise. This transitory reduction in hearing sensitivity following noise exposure is aptly called a **temporary threshold shift.** The phenomenon has been thoroughly studied under laboratory conditions; we'll just mention some of the highlights and implications of that work (summarized by Miller, 1978).

In general, sound levels in excess of 60 dB$_{SPL}$ can produce temporary threshold shifts if the duration of exposure is several hours or longer. The actual threshold shifts can vary from just a few decibels, which for all practical purposes is unnoticeable, to complete deafness. As you might guess, the size of the shift depends on the level and duration of the inducing noise. The length of time it takes for thresholds to return to normal also varies, depending on the strength and duration of noise exposure. Recovery can occur within only a few hours when the noise is modest, but it can take several days following exposure to severe noise. You may have noticed a temporary threshold shift after attending a loud party or a boisterous football game—normally audible sounds such as your own footsteps may temporarily fall below your elevated threshold. For unknown reasons, women seem to exhibit smaller threshold shifts than men when the inducing noise consists of *low* frequencies. Thus after a male and female have been listening to the romantic roar of the ocean for some time, she may be able to hear his passionate whispers, just barely, but he won't be able to make out her whispered replies. However, just the opposite is found when the inducing noise consists of *high* frequencies. Under these conditions, men exhibit smaller threshold shifts than women (Ward, 1966, 1968). So if our hypothetical couple had been listening for some time to the strains of Wagner sung by a lusty soprano, the female of the couple would be at a temporary disadvantage when it came to communicating in whispers.

Drugs and Hearing Loss. Several widely consumed drugs can have deleterious effects on hearing. One is nicotine. Chronic cigarette smokers have higher pure-tone thresholds than nonsmokers of the same age, and this loss is most pronounced at higher frequencies (Zelman, 1973). The loss is probably traceable to poor circulation, since nicotine narrows the ear's blood vessels and makes the ear's blood pressure irregular. These circulatory effects, in turn, reduce the blood supply to the cochlea.

Another common drug that affects hearing is aspirin, which, when taken in large doses, can produce a temporary hearing loss (McCabe and Dey, 1965). A person taking 4 to 8 grams of aspirin per day is likely to experience anywhere from a 10- to a 40-dB shift in pure-tone thresholds, with the loss often more pronounced at higher frequencies. This hearing loss persists as long as aspirin is taken, and normal hearing returns within a day or two after the person ceases to take the aspirin. Since one tablet usually contains one-fourth of a gram of aspirin, hearing won't be affected by taking a couple of aspirin. The aspirin dose that can produce hearing loss (4 to 8 grams) is the typical prescription dose for people with rheumatoid arthritis. The temporary hearing loss induced by aspirin is often accompanied by tinnitus, the high-pitched ringing in the ears we described in the previous chapter. The tinnitus, too, disappears once the consumption of aspirin ceases. It is thought that aspirin has its effect by disabling temporarily the amplification function performed by the OHCs.

Dennis McFadden has found that aspirin makes people more vulnerable to the effects of noise. In a study in 1983, McFadden and Plattsmier exposed paid volunteers to a 2,500-Hz tone for 10 minutes. The tone's intensity was adjusted to yield around a 14-dB threshold shift; the intensity of the tone required to produce such a shift was in the neighborhood of 100 dB$_{SPL}$. Dividing volunteers into two groups, McFadden and Plattsmier then gave them either 1.95 or 3.9 grams of aspirin every day for several days. At the end of this period, volunteers were once again exposed to the loud tone and then retested on their pure-tone thresholds. Some people who were given the higher dosage of aspirin (3.9 grams) now suffered a hearing loss that was almost twice what they had suffered initially. In addition, it took them longer to recover from the noise exposure, although they eventually did. People who were given the smaller dosage (1.95 grams) showed neither of these effects. Results from the study imply that people routinely exposed to loud sounds should restrict their intake of aspirin or, better yet, find a substitute pain reliever. It should be noted that this study and its conclusions speak only to the question of temporary shifts in threshold, not permanent hearing loss.

SOME PERCEPTUAL CONSEQUENCES OF IMPAIRED HEARING

So far we have focused on some of the things that cause pure-tone hearing losses, either temporary or permanent. To appreciate the perceptual consequences of such losses, you need some idea of the frequencies and intensities of sound in your everyday environment. Take, for example, the ringing sound made by a typical telephone, a routine sound we all rely on. Suppose that the acoustic energy associated with the sound lies between 4,000 and 8,000 Hz, and that its sound level is somewhere around 70 dB$_{SPL}$. (The actual distribution of acoustic energy varies from one type of telephone to another.) Suppose also that a person with the abnormal AF shown in Figure 10.2 is expecting a phone call. As you can see, this person suffers about a 50-dB hearing loss in the mid- and upper-frequency range, the region where much of the bell's sound lies. Will this person be able to hear his phone ringing? As mentioned in the previous chapter, sound intensity falls off with the square of the distance between the source and the listener. So in order to hear the phone's ring, the hearing-impaired person must be within about 8 feet of the instrument. Beyond this distance, the sound will be too weak to be heard by his defective ears. This analysis assumes ideal conditions— no distracting noises and no major objects such as

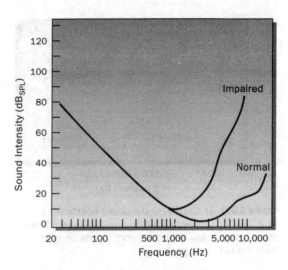

FIGURE 10.2 An AF of an individual with about a 50-dB hearing loss in the middle and upper frequency range.

walls or doors to intercept the phone's acoustic energy before it reaches his ears. Incidentally, people with normal hearing would have no trouble hearing such a bell, even over distances of several hundred feet or through walls and doors.

Let's continue with this example by assuming the hearing-impaired person manages to hear his phone and now answers it. Will he have difficulty understanding the voice on the other end of the line? To find out, we must know something about the frequency content of human speech. Figure 10.3 shows the region of the frequency spectrum responsible for conveying speech sounds; note that acoustic energy in speech spans the range from 200 Hz to about 8,000 Hz. As the diagram shows, vowel sounds consist primarily of low frequencies, whereas consonants cover very nearly the entire range. Of the consonant sounds, the nasal ones (such as "m") are the lowest in frequency and the fricatives (such as "f") are the highest. In terms of their relative intensities, vowel sounds tend to be stronger than consonants, meaning that at normal speaking levels, vowels produce larger variations in sound-wave pressure.

Now, armed with this information, consider

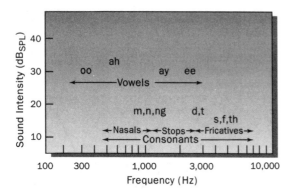

FIGURE 10.3 The region of the sound spectrum responsible for conveying speech sounds. Vowel sounds are primarily of low frequency; consonants cover almost the entire range.

the plight of a hearing-impaired man whose AF is depicted in Figure 10.2. To understand how a telephone conversation will sound to him, let's first examine how the telephone itself alters the frequency composition of the voice it transmits. Modern telephones transmit frequencies only up to about 4,000 Hz, which means that the very highest frequencies contained in normal speech are missing during a phone conversation. Since people are easily able to carry on a phone conversation, these omitted frequencies must be unnecessary for speech comprehension. For our hearing-impaired person, though, more is missing than just these high frequencies—his ears fail to pick up frequencies in speech that are available over the phone. His pattern of hearing loss means that some of the consonants (especially those such as /t/ and /d/) will be heard as mere whispers, if at all. (The slashes, / /, indicate that we are referring to the sounds of these characters, not to their names as letters of the alphabet.) These consonants, in fact, are some of the most important ingredients in speech (Ballantyne, 1977). So a person with an AF of the type shown in Figure 10.2 will have difficulty hearing some of the environment's most important sounds, those of human speech. Simple words such as "time" and "dime" may be mistaken for one another, which in turn may make whole sentences confusing. Clearly, then, a person does not need to be totally deaf in

order to experience the frustrations of unintelligible speech. In a way, the plight of hearing-impaired people is particularly difficult—they hear speech sounds but are confused by the meanings. No wonder some hard-of-hearing people, including the elderly, find it easier simply to withdraw from social encounters.

People with good hearing can gain some understanding of the disturbing consequences of impaired hearing by wearing earplugs for a few hours—those who have done so testify to the psychological importance of nonverbal sounds (Eriksson-Mangold and Erlandsson, 1984). You should try this disquieting exercise yourself; inexpensive earplugs producing a 30-dB reduction in sound level can be purchased at most sports or hardware stores.

THE RANGE OF HEARING IN ANIMALS

The discussion of abnormal hearing illustrates that the AF reveals something important about an individual's perceptual world. The same point can be made by comparing the AFs of different animal species. Look at Figure 10.4. Each horizontal bar shows the range of frequencies audible to a particular species, and as you can see, there is quite a diversity among animals. Many members of the animal kingdom are able to hear sounds outside the limits of the human ear (Fay, 1988). Here's an example: a device called a dog whistle emits frequencies around 14,000 Hz, right at the very limits of the human ear but well within the hearing range of the dog.

One sound that no human will ever hear is the stream of very high frequencies emitted by bats. This acoustic energy bounces off objects in the bat's flight path and then echoes back to the bat. As Figure 10.4 indicates, bats are able to hear these frequencies, and they use them to navigate (Griffin, 1959; Suga, 1990).

So far we have concentrated on normal and abnormal hearing in humans and in animals as specified by pure-tone thresholds measured under quiet conditions. Of course, most of the sounds one usually encounters are loud enough to be easily heard, and they often occur against some

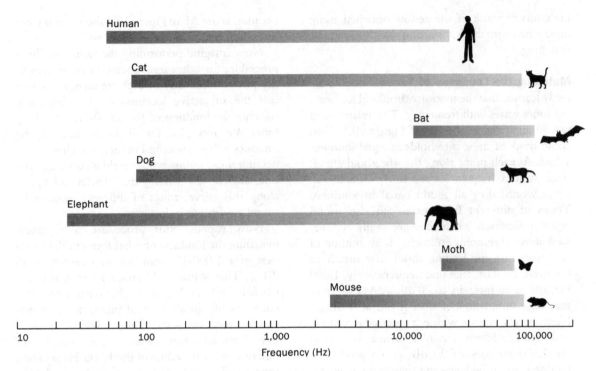

FIGURE 10.4 The range of sound frequencies audible to various species at a fixed intensity of 60 dB$_{SPL}$. (Data for moth from Fullard & Barclay, 1980; data for all other species from Heffner & Heffner, 1985.)

background level of noise. So to understand auditory perception more fully, we need to consider these more common stimulus conditions. We will begin by discussing what determines a sound's loudness, where "loudness" refers to the perceived intensity of that sound. Note that according to this definition, *any* audible sound, whether weak or strong, has some degree of loudness.

LOUDNESS PERCEPTION

MEASURING LOUDNESS

Everyone knows what is meant by **loudness**—one's subjective impression of the intensity of sound. And most people would have no trouble agreeing whether one sound is louder than another, indicating that they all employ the concept of "loudness" in the same way. Yet despite this agreement, there is no way to compare people's impressions of loudness directly—these are subjective experiences that cannot be measured with some instrument. One must rely on language to talk about one's perception of loudness. By the same token, there is no way to determine whether your judgment of a sound's loudness is right or wrong, for there is no right or wrong answer—a sound's loudness *is* whatever you experience. These constraints immediately raise a barrier against attempts to study loudness perception. Fortunately, psychologists have devised several effective procedures for measuring perceived sensory magnitude, including loudness. As applied to hearing, one of these procedures treats the perceiver as a measuring instrument capable of assigning numbers to sounds in proportion to their loudness; this method is generally known as **magnitude estimation.** Another method requires the person to adjust the loudness of one sound until it is equivalent to the loudness of another; this latter method is called **loudness matching.**

Let's survey some of the results obtained using these two methods, starting with loudness matching.

Matching the Loudness of Tones. You've already learned that the intensity threshold for hearing tones varies with frequency. This relationship was summarized in the AF of Figure 10.1. You could think of these thresholds as equal loudness values. At each point along that threshold curve, these various frequencies are *barely* audible—in other words, they all sound equal in loudness. Tones of different frequencies can also sound equal in loudness when they are *clearly* audible, well above threshold. Following is an outline of the procedure for finding tones that match in loudness. To start, take one frequency, say, 1,000 Hz, and set its intensity to 20 dB$_{SPL}$. As expected, that tone sounds louder than it did at 0 dB$_{SPL}$. Next, present a tone whose frequency is 500 Hz and adjust *its* intensity until it sounds as loud as the 1,000-Hz tone of 20 dB$_{SPL}$. To produce a loudness match between the two frequencies requires raising the intensity of the 500-Hz tone to a level *greater* than 20 dB$_{SPL}$. This makes sense

because, as the AF in Figure 10.1 shows, you were less sensitive to 500 Hz to begin with.

Now imagine performing the same matching procedure for other frequencies. In other words, the physical intensity of each frequency is set so that the subjective loudness of that frequency matches the loudness of the 1,000-Hz, 20-dB$_{SPL}$ tone. We now plot, for all the frequencies, the intensity values yielding loudness matches. Connecting those points would yield a curve like the one labeled "20" in Figure 10.5. At all points along this curve, tones of different frequencies sound equivalent in loudness.

Now suppose this procedure is repeated, matching the loudness of other tones to the loudness of a 1,000-Hz tone whose intensity is 40 dB$_{SPL}$. This would yield another curve, the one labeled "40" in Figure 10.5; points along this curve specify another set of intensities at which various frequencies all sound equivalent in loudness. Repeating this maneuver for a number of different intensity values of the 1,000-Hz standard tone would yield a family of curves, each one summarizing the intensity values that make tones of different frequencies sound equal in loudness

FIGURE 10.5 Equal loudness contours.

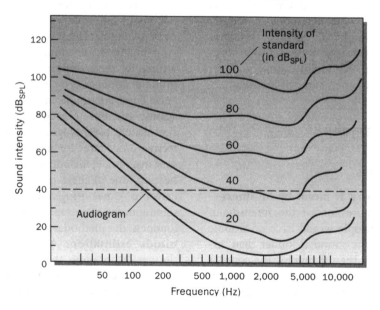

(Fletcher and Munson, 1933). Such curves are appropriately named **equal loudness contours.**

Obviously, the curves in Figure 10.5 are not parallel to one another. This means that loudness does not increase with intensity in the same way for all frequencies. Let's think what this implies. Suppose we draw a horizontal line straight across the graph at the point labeled "40 dB," as shown in Figure 10.5. Note that this line crosses several of the loudness contours. It enables you to compare the perceived loudness of pure tones of different frequencies, all of which have the same intensity—40 dB$_{SPL}$ in this case. Let's make a few of those comparisons.

First, note that a 50-Hz tone would not be audible at 40 dB$_{SPL}$—this intensity level is too weak to be heard at this frequency. At 50 Hz, a tone must be more than 60 dB$_{SPL}$ in order to be heard. At 200 Hz, the tone woud be audible at 40 dB$_{SPL}$, but it would sound considerably weaker than, say, a 1,000-Hz tone at this same intensity. We know this because, for this sound level (40 dB$_{SPL}$), these two frequencies (200 and 1,000 Hz) lie on different equal loudness contours. In fact, to make the two tones sound equally loud, you would need to do one of two things: either turn down the intensity of the 1,000-Hz tone or raise the intensity of the 200-Hz tone. In either case, the curves in Figure 10.5 indicate just how much intensity would have to change in order to produce a loudness match. For instance, the intensity of the 200-Hz tone could be raised to 55 dB$_{SPL}$, thereby placing that tone on the same contour with the 40dB$_{SPL}$, 1,000-Hz tone. See whether you can figure out how much you would have to lower the 1,000-Hz tone in order for it to match the loudness of the 40-dB$_{SPL}$ tone of 200 Hz. These curves indicate that low frequencies tend to sound weaker than higher frequencies of the same intensity. Incidentally, manufacturers of audio equipment know this, and they design their amplifiers to allow listeners to give low frequencies a little extra boost in intensity. Such amplifiers have a "loudness" switch on the front of the unit, to let the listener choose the desired amount of low-frequency boost.

You could compare the perceived loudness of other combinations of frequency and intensity. You would find that in most instances, tones of the same intensity but different frequency do not sound equally loud; to equate them for loudness requires adjusting their intensities appropriately, each to a different level. An exception to this rule occurs at very high intensity levels. As you can see in Figure 10.5, for levels approaching 100 dB$_{SPL}$, the equal loudness contours are relatively flat—indicating that at these high intensities, all frequencies sound more or less the same in loudness. Thinking back to audio amplifiers, you can see that this has an unfortunate consequence: when sound levels are very high, amplifiers adjusted to give a low-frequency boost will now overemphasize low frequencies. This overemphasis can produce what stereo buffs call a "boomy" bass (bass sounds consist predominantly of low frequencies).

So far we have considered how the loudness of one tone compares with the loudness of others. Comparisons of this sort, however, say nothing about the way a sound's loudness depends on intensity. Of course, everyone knows that loudness grows with increasing intensity; but exactly how are loudness and intensity related? For example, does doubling the intensity on your stereo double the loudness of the music you're listening to? In order to answer questions such as this, you need to do more than compare the loudness of one sound with that of another. What you need is some way to measure the actual loudness of individual sounds. This brings us to magnitude estimation, a second method for assessing loudness.

Estimating the Magnitude of Loudness. Magnitude estimation seems deceptively simple: a person is instructed merely to assign numbers to sounds in proportion to their loudness. Thus if one sound seems 3 times louder than another, the louder sound should be assigned a number 3 times larger than the number assigned to the softer sound. The person is free to select any particular numbers, just so long as those numbers faithfully reflect what the person construes as loudness. No upper or lower limits are placed on the range of acceptable numbers, although sometimes the experimenter may arbitrarily assign a given number to one particular sound intensity. For instance, you might be told to let a rating of 100 correspond to the loudness of a 60-dB$_{SPL}$ sound, but from there on your ratings would be entirely up to you.

Given this latitude in assigning numbers to loudness, you might expect the outcome to be a jumble of idiosyncratic numbers, but in fact this does not happen. Although the particular numbers assigned to particular sound levels can vary from person to person, the order and spacing between numbers show a remarkable degree of regularity among individuals. Of course, as sound intensity increases, so does loudness. However, loudness grows more slowly than does intensity. Thus, for instance, doubling sound intensity does *not* double loudness—instead, loudness increases by only about 60 percent. To double the loudness of a sound, its intensity must be approximately tripled (this corresponds to about a 10-dB increase in intensity). This means, for example, that two people singing at the top of their lungs will not sound twice as loud as one of those people singing alone; instead, the duet's singing will sound about 1.6 times louder than a solo. To double the loudness produced by one singer requires adding two additional singers.

So loudness does not grow in a simple, additive fashion, but instead grows multiplicatively (by fractional multiples of intensity). This seems to be true over the entire range of audible sound levels, and it holds for magnitude estimates of loudness obtained from just about everyone. S. S. Stevens (1960), who was among the first to think about loudness in this way, expressed this general finding in mathematical terms: loudness grows in proportion to intensity raised to the power, or exponent, 0.67. In mathematical notation

$$L = k \cdot I^{0.67}$$

where L stands for loudness, I stands for intensity (expressed as sound pressure level), and k is a constant. This general formula is known as the **power law** of loudness growth. Figure 10.6 shows what this relation between intensity and loudness looks

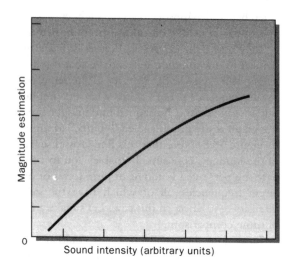

FIGURE 10.6 The growth of loudness plotted on linear axes.

like graphically; plotted on the horizontal axis is the sound level, or intensity, of a pure tone, while plotted on the vertical axis are the numbers (the magnitude estimates of loudness) assigned to those various intensities. Note that in this graph, intensity and loudness are scaled in linear coordinates. Plotted in this way, the resulting "loudness function" appears curved; it is described as negatively accelerating, meaning that loudness grows more slowly than intensity.

Because the relation between intensity and loudness is exponential, replotting the points on logarithmic coordinates should yield a straight line. Taking the logarithm of both sides of the above equation yields

$$\log L = \log k + 0.67(\log I)$$

which is the general form of the equation for a straight line. To show you what this looks like graphically, we have replotted the results from Figure 10.6 in Figure 10.7. Note that both intensity and loudness ratings are now scaled logarithmically. (Recall from the previous chapter that the decibel is a logarithmic unit.) As expected, the exponential curve summarizing the growth of loudness (Figure 10.6) now appears as a straight

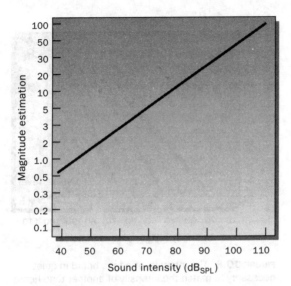

FIGURE 10.7 The growth of loudness plotted on logarithmic axes.

line. The constant *k* specifies where that straight line crosses, or intersects, the vertical axis; the point of intersection depends on the particular set of numbers used by the person to estimate loudness. The exponent, 0.67, specifies the slope (steepness) of the straight line. A slope less than 1.0 means that loudness grows more slowly than intensity, as we described above. The Appendix further discusses magnitude estimation and the power law, including its application to senses other than hearing.

The measurement of loudness is not limited to pure tones. People are also able to rate the loudness of sounds consisting of many frequencies (Zwicker and Scharf, 1965), including noise—which, as you learned in the previous chapter, consists of all audible frequencies. As a rule, the loudness of complex sounds can be predicted by adding up the loudness contributions from the component frequencies, making allowance for the ability of one sound to reduce, or mask, the loudness of others.

Neural Bases of Loudness Perception. Having seen how loudness varies with stimulus intensity, we now examine the neural transformations that

govern that relationship. What happens within the auditory system as the loudness of a sound varies? In other words, what is the neural code for loudness? The most obvious answer is that the discharge rate of auditory neurons increases with sound level, and this constitutes the information for loudness. After all, we did learn in the last chapter that the activity of auditory neurons increases with intensity (recall Figure 9.24). However, although discharge rate is probably involved in the coding of loudness, it alone cannot be the whole explanation. The reason is that auditory nerve fibers increase their firing rate over a limited range of sound intensities; this range typically covers only about 40 dB (Kiang, 1968). Yet one can hear variations in the loudness of sounds over a much larger range, around 120 dB. So one's range of loudness perception exceeds the range that can be coded by individual neurons.

There are two ways the nervous system may overcome the relatively limited range of individual neurons. First, we pointed out in Chapter 9 that different neurons operate over different levels of sound intensity. One set of neurons responds, for instance, to intensity changes within the range from 20 dB_{SPL} to 60 dB_{SPL}, another set to intensity changes from 40 dB_{SPL} to 80 dB_{SPL}, and a third to intensities from 60 dB_{SPL} to 100 dB_{SPL}. As you can see, each *set* covers only a 40-dB range, but as a *population* the neurons would then span an 80-dB range of intensities. Neurons responsive to different intensity ranges would be fairly simple to "construct"—it could be done by adjusting the intensity level where different neurons first start to respond. And as pointed out in Chapter 9, physiological evidence points to the existence of three categories of auditory nerve fibers, distinguished by their different threshold intensities and their different points of contact on the IHCs (see Figure 9.24). For the coding of loudness information, then, one way to overcome the limited range of individual neurons is to design them to operate within different intensity ranges.

There is a second possible way that increasing sound levels may produce greater and greater neural activity, and this has to do with the tuning curves for individual auditory nerve fibers. Recall that single fibers respond to just a limited range of temporal frequencies, with the preferred frequency varying from fiber to fiber (see Figure 9.22). At weak sound levels, the only fibers to respond will be those whose preferred frequencies match the frequencies contained in the sound; fibers preferring other frequencies will be unresponsive at these low sound levels. However, it is possible to recruit some of those fibers into activity by raising the sound level. At such higher levels, the sound (though it does not contain those fibers' preferred frequencies) *will* produce activity in such fibers because their tuning curves do encompass frequencies contained in the sound. We saw a hint of this spread of activity in the previous chapter, where it was noted that more intense sounds caused the traveling wave to spread out over a larger region of the basilar membrane. This is tantamount to recruiting more and more nerve fibers into action at higher and higher sound levels.

At present, evidence is lacking to rule out one or the other of these hypotheses, and there is no reason both mechanisms could not be operative.

Loudness of Tones in Noise. The loudness function shown in Figure 10.7 was for a pure tone heard in an otherwise quiet environment—an atypical situation indeed. More often, one is called on to listen for tones occurring against some background of sound; for practical purposes, we can consider this background sound as *noise.* For instance, imagine listening for the phone to ring while taking a shower; the noise of the water makes the ring harder to hear. Using a matching procedure, it is possible to specify the loudness of a sound occurring within noise (Stevens and Guirao, 1967). Figure 10.8 illustrates the result. These data were obtained by having a listener adjust the intensity of a tone heard in quiet to match the loudness of a tone heard against a background of noise; the different curves represent different levels of noise, ranging from moderate to very loud noise (the "100-dB" noise line). The loudness function gets steeper as the noise level increases, implying that the exponent of the

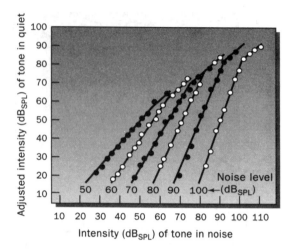

FIGURE 10.8 The intensity of a tone heard in quiet necessary to match the intensity of another tone heard against noise. (Adapted from Stevens & Guirao, 1967.)

power function becomes larger—loudness grows more rapidly when sounds occur within noise. In other words, the loudness of *intense* sounds is less affected by background noise than is the loudness of *weak* sounds.

This effect of noise on loudness has several implications, one bad and the other not so bad. To start with the bad news: weak sounds may be impossible to hear when they occur in noise. This stands to reason; we've all had the experience of being unable to hear a phone conversation when there is lots of static on the line—the noise of the static masks the sounds of the other person's voice. For sounds that are more intense, though, the situation is not so bad. Note that all the lines in Figure 10.8 converge toward the same loudness levels at the top of the graph—intense sounds seem loud regardless of the background noise level. This is actually a fortunate circumstance. If the slope of the loudness function remained the same regardless of background noise level, we'd grossly underestimate the intensity of sounds occurring within noisy settings. For example, the same siren might sound faint under one condition but loud under another. This could be dangerous: imagine hearing an ambulance and trying to judge from the loudness of its siren whether it was still far enough away for you to proceed safely through an intersection. If the loudness of intense sounds were greatly affected by noise, judgment could be fatally flawed depending on the other traffic sounds being heard. So it is adaptive that only weak sounds are significantly affected by background noise.

So far, we've focused on *loudness* of pure tones heard in isolation or in the presence of noise. The next section focuses on a related phenomenon, the *detectability* of pure tones heard against a background of noise; this represents one of the most widely studied problems in hearing.

NOISE MASKING AND CRITICAL BANDS

As mentioned above, background noise can make it more difficult to hear a weak pure tone. Expressed more precisely, the detection threshold for a pure tone is elevated when that tone is presented coincident with noise. This phenomenon is called auditory **masking** (note the analogy to visual masking discussed in Chapter 8); the magnitude of masking is expressed as the difference between masked and unmasked thresholds. The magnitude of masking varies with the noise level, which makes sense intuitively: intense noise yields greater masking (greater threshold elevation) than does moderate noise. But another, equally important determinant of masking effectiveness is the frequency content of the noise relative to the tone. This relation deserves careful analysis, for it reveals important properties of the neural processes underlying hearing.

To explore this point, we need to develop some notations. In what follows, the listener's task will always be the same: to detect a pure tone of a given frequency—call that frequency Hz_t—presented either alone or in the presence of noise. In the last chapter, noise was characterized as a complex of sound composed of energy at many different frequencies. When noise contains energy at all audible frequencies, it is called **broadband noise** and, perceptually, it resembles the sound made by a waterfall. The diagram in the middle panel of Figure 10.9 pictorially represents the energy spectrum of broadband noise, with the area under the rectangle defining the frequencies present in the noise. In the laboratory, unlike in nature, the intensity of broadband noise can be systematically varied, which would correspond to varying the height of the rectangle in the graph. (In fact, energy levels in noise vary randomly within limits from moment to moment; the rectangular shape shown in the drawings is meant to depict the average noise level over time.) In the lab, it is also possible to restrict the range of frequencies contained within the noise by passing the noise through an electronic filter; alternatively, a computer can be used to synthesize noise of specified frequency content. Using either technique, suppose we remove energy from the low-frequency end and from the high-frequency end of the broadband noise spectrum. This form of energy filtering creates what is called **bandpass noise.** Pictorially, this reduces the width of the rectangle (see graphs in the left and right panels of Figure 10.9), and perceptually it makes the noise sound different in quality and reduced in intensity. It is possible to vary systematically the width of bandpass noise while keeping the center of the distribution at the same point along the frequency spectrum; this center point of the noise is called the **center frequency.** Examples of this type of bandpass filtering are shown in the left panel of Figure 10.9. Alternatively, it is possible to keep the width of the noise constant but vary its center frequency, in effect moving the noise package along the horizontal axis. Examples of this type of filtering are shown in the right panel of Figure 10.9.

With these concepts in mind, let's see how the detectability of a pure tone of frequency Hz_t might be affected by various kinds of noise. First, suppose we again measure the threshold for a test tone of Hz_t while varying the bandwidth of the bandpass noise and holding the noise's center frequency constant at the frequency of the test, Hz_t (the manipulation depicted in the left panel of Figure 10.9). The result would look something like the graph in the upper panel of Figure 10.10, which plots threshold elevation against noise bandwidth; the inset serves as a reminder that

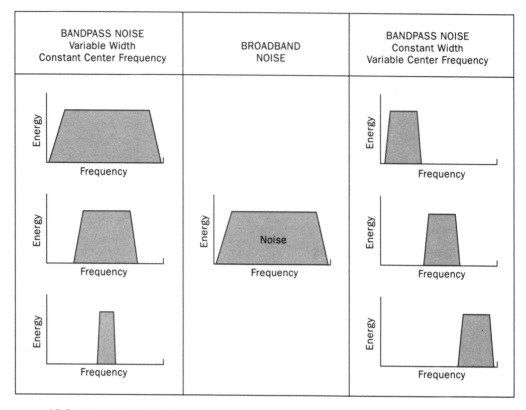

FIGURE 10.9 Schematics of the frequency distribution of acoustic energy content of noise—the shaded area in each drawing represents the presence of energy. The middle panel shows broadband noise—energy covering the entire audible spectrum. The two side panels show noise from which energy at low and high frequencies has been removed. This form of filtering produces what is called bandpass noise. The spectra in the left-hand panel show three examples of bandpass noise whose bandwidth varies and whose center frequency remains constant. The spectra in the right-hand panel show noise whose bandwidth remains constant and whose center frequency varies.

whatever the noise bandwidth, the noise center frequency matched the test-tone frequency Hz_t. The far left-hand value in the graph (inset) represents the threshold measured in the absence of noise—the unmasked threshold. Once noise is introduced, the tone becomes harder to hear, as indicated by the steady increase in threshold. Increasing the bandwidth of the noise produces greater and greater threshold elevation, which makes sense because the tone must be detected in the presence of more and more noise energy. Significantly, though, there is a critical bandwidth beyond which threshold is no further elevated even though additional energy is added to the

noise and even though the noise sounds louder still. This indicates, then, that only a limited portion of the energy in broadband noise acts to mask a tone; this effective portion was termed the **critical band** by Fletcher (1940). Why should noise energy outside the critical band have no influence on the audibility of a tone? What, in other words, is the basis for the critical band?

A clue to the answer appears in Figures 9.22 and 9.23 in the previous chapter; shown there are tuning curves for auditory nerve fibers. One of those curves is reproduced in the lower panel of Figure 10.10, the curve for a fiber whose characteristic frequency (the one to which it is most

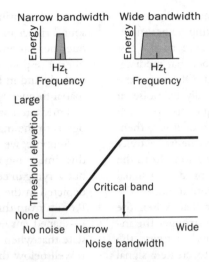

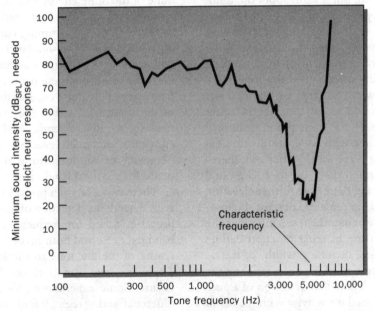

FIGURE 10.10 Upper panel: Hypothetical result from a noise masking experiment. Intensity thresholds for detection of a given pure-tone frequency are plotted as the function of the width of bandpass noise within which the tone must be detected. Threshold increases with noise bandwidth, up to a critical band beyond which threshold remains constant even though noise energy increases. Upper panel inset: Schematics of narrow and wide bandpass noise used in hypothetical experiment; note that noise is centered about H_{zt}. Lower panel: Tuning curve for an auditory nerve fiber maximally responsive to the test frequency used in the masking experiment. The activity level in this fiber will increase as the bandwidth of the noise is increased, as long as the added frequencies fall within the tuning curve of the fiber. Frequencies outside this curve will have no effect on the fiber's activity.

sensitive) corresponds to Hz_t, the test frequency used in the hypothetical masking experiment. This being the fiber most sensitive to the test frequency, it is activity in this fiber that mediates pure-tone detection at threshold. Of course, the fiber will also be activated neurally by noise, if that noise contains energy at frequencies to which the fiber responds. The presence of noise, then, creates a background of elevated neural activity against which the neural activity arising from the tone must be discriminated. To produce a signal discriminable from this background noise, the tone's intensity must be higher than when the background noise is absent. The stronger the influence of the noise on the fiber's activity, the more intense the tone must be to create a signal audible within this noise.

With this in mind, think again about the result depicted in the upper panel of Figure 10.10. Presumably, the magnitude of masking increases with bandwidth because widening the bandpass noise adds more and more frequencies that stimulate the fibers mediating detection of the tone.* Increasing the bandwidth, in other words, increases the fiber's background activity, making it harder to detect the tone. But at some point, additional frequencies associated with wider bandwidths fall outside the tuning curve for the fiber and, therefore, have no further effect on its background activity. At this point, there is no further elevation in threshold; masking remains constant. Following this line of reasoning, then, we infer that the inflexion point in the masking function defines the frequency limits, or tuning width, of the fiber(s) used for detection of the tone. (We use the term "fiber(s)" to denote that detection of a pure tone is probably based on activity within a set of fibers, not a single fiber, all with the same preferred frequency.) Adding more frequencies activates other fibers with different characteristic fre-

quencies, causing the noise to get louder and to sound richer in quality. But those additional frequencies fall outside the critical bandwidth of the fiber(s) responsive to the test. This notion of the critical band in hearing should remind you of the spatial frequency channels described in Chapter 5 and measured using an adaptation procedure analogous to the masking technique described here.

Suppose we repeat the masking experiment, this time using bandpass noise of constant width but varying in center frequency (the manipulation depicted in the right-hand panel of Figure 10.9). Results from this procedure resemble an inverted U-shaped curve. To put it in words, we would state that when the center frequency of the noise is well below the test frequency, the noise is audible but ineffective as a masker; presumably, none of the noise energy stimulates the neuron(s) responsive to the test. Not until the noise begins to encroach upon the tuning curve of the detecting neuron(s) will threshold increase, and masking will grow to a maximum as more and more of the noise stimulates these neuron(s). As the center frequency of the noise exceeds this maximum, less of the noise falls within the critical bandwidth; masking is reduced until, finally, the threshold equals the unmasked level. So varying the center frequency of bandpass noise also generates evidence for a critical band in hearing.

These two examples portray the essence of the critical band: the detection of pure tones by neural processes tuned for frequency. Both employed bandpass noise and both involved varying the intensity of the test tone to measure its threshold. There are many variations on this masking procedure. Some experiments, for instance, employ different filtering regimes for producing the masking noise, such as removing frequencies from the *center* of the noise spectrum, not its extremes, thereby producing a notch in the energy spectrum. In other experiments, the intensity of the noise, not the tone, is varied to find the level that just barely masks a pure tone of fixed intensity. In still other experiments, a brief interval of time is inserted between the onset of the tone and the onset of the masking noise. While the details of the resulting masking curves vary with the partic-

---

* Nerve fibers alone, of course, are not responsible for detection of tones; activity in auditory nerve fibers is passed on to neurons at higher stages in the auditory pathways which participate in hearing. But it is reasonable to consider the effects of noise on auditory nerve fibers, for masking effects arising at this level will be transmitted to higher levels.

ulars of these experiments, the general conclusion remains unchanged: noise is effective as a mask only when it contains frequencies at or near the frequency of the test tone (see Scharf and Buus, 1986, for a thorough review of the auditory masking literature). And in some (but not all) instances, the resulting masking curves—masking strength as the function of the frequency content of the noise—resemble the tuning curves of auditory nerve fibers. For instance, a tone of given frequency is more effectively masked by noise whose frequency composition is a bit lower than the tone compared with noise composed of frequencies higher than the tone. The critical band, in other words, appears more broadly tuned on the low-frequency side. This asymmetry in masking effectiveness dovetails nicely with the asymmetric shape of auditory nerve tuning curves (recall Figures 9.22 and 9.23).

The importance of the critical band cannot be overstated—it plays a pivotal role in theories of tone detection, loudness perception, and pitch discrimination. Critical bands in hearing represent an important, initial stage of auditory processing potentially related to the function of the cochlea and the auditory nerve.

INTENSITY DISCRIMINATION

We turn next to intensity discrimination: the ability to tell whether one sound is louder than another. This sort of judgment can be of practical importance. Imagine, for instance, that your sister is upstairs playing her stereo so loudly that you can't study. You holler up to her, asking her to turn it down a little, and she says she will. Just by listening, how do you tell whether your sister has kept her promise? Of course, you would have no trouble hearing a large drop in intensity, but what if the drop was more subtle? How sharp is your ability to discriminate intensity changes, and what transpires within your auditory system when you make such a discrimination?

In the laboratory, intensity discrimination can be measured by varying the intensity of a tone

very gradually until a person first notices that it has gotten louder or has gotten softer. This minimum necessary change in intensity specifies the person's **discrimination threshold.** Although the actual value of the threshold varies, depending on the details of the experiment, people typically require about a 1- to 2-dB change in intensity to be able to notice any variation in loudness.

A listener probably achieves such keen performance by detecting an increment or decrement in the level of neural activity produced by the tone. In the example above, the most informative neural activity would arise within that subset of neurons maximally responsive to the tone's frequency; for instance, if the tone is 1,000 Hz, the listener should monitor neurons whose center frequency is 1,000 Hz (recall our discussion of the critical band in the previous section). But in real life, most sounds are more complex than the pure tones used in this example. Sometimes a complex set of frequencies changes in intensity in unison, and that change must be heard in the midst of many other frequency components whose intensities are also changing. For example, an alert driver can tell that his truck's engine is malfunctioning when its high-pitched whine becomes louder than the other sounds made by the truck. In effect, he hears a change in the intensity of one set of frequencies (the high-pitched whine) in the midst of other sounds. His task is complicated. When he drives slowly, all the truck's sounds—high-pitched whine included—are weak; when he drives faster, all the sounds are louder. David Green, a hearing researcher at the University of Florida, has offered a compelling explanation of how people detect such intensity changes in the midst of other changeable components.

Green (1982) acknowledges that if a listener has to detect a change in the intensity of only a single tone heard against an unvarying background, the traditional view is correct: only one subset of neurons need be monitored, namely, those tuned to the frequency of the varying intensity tone. But when other frequencies are present and their intensities are also changing from one moment to the next (as in the truck driver's situation), Green believes a more complex process comes into play. This process uses neural information about the *relative* activity across different subsets of neurons. Green calls this process **profile analysis** because the relative neural response to various frequency bands could be represented graphically as a profile. According to Green, in an acoustically rich environment the listener picks up intensity changes by detecting a variation in the profile of activity. (This idea should be familiar to you from our discussions of orientation, spatial frequency, color, and motion perception.) To see where Green's view came from, let's consider two of his experiments.

In one experiment (Green, Kidd, and Picardi, 1983) Green and his colleagues created a complex sound consisting of twenty-one different tones, ranging in frequency from 300 to 3,000 Hz, all played simultaneously. He presented this set of tones twice on each trial. In one presentation, all twenty-one tones were identical in intensity; in the other presentation, the intensity of one tone (1,000 Hz) was slightly greater than the intensity of the other twenty tones. The listener's task was to identify the interval in which the 1,000-Hz tone had been incremented. Green made the task even more difficult by randomizing the *overall* intensity of the package of tones from one presentation to the next. For example, in the first presentation all the tones might be 20 dB$_{SPL}$ in intensity, whereas in the second presentation they might all be 50 dB$_{SPL}$. The exception, of course, was the 1,000-Hz tone, which was slightly more intense than its companions during one of the two presentations. Though the 1,000-Hz tone would be incremented *relative* to the rest, its *absolute* level of intensity would provide no clue whatever to the interval in which it had been incremented. This procedure made it impossible for the listener to base a judgment on the amount of neural activity produced by the 1,000-Hz tone alone; the listener was forced to compare the activity produced by the 1,000-Hz tone with the activity produced by its companions. Using these complex tones, Green determined the minimum increment of the 1,000-Hz tone that could be heard. Despite having to rely on *relative* intensity information alone, listeners were able to detect

remarkably small increments in loudness. In fact, in some instances, the just detectable increment in the complex sound was about as small as that measured for the 1,000-Hz tone on its own.

In the second experiment, Green and his colleagues varied the number of different tones that accompanied the 1,000-Hz tone. Starting with very few companion tones, Green found that adding additional tones actually *improved* a listener's ability to hear small increments in the 1,000-Hz tone. Presumably, the additional tones sharpened the definition of the neural activity profile utilized by the listener. These results and others (Green and Nguyen, 1988) show how useful profile analysis might be in explaining hearing performance in certain real-life situations.

Loudness and intensity discrimination alone seldom allow you to identify a sound source—for that purpose, you also need information about the frequencies composing that sound. This brings us to the topic of pitch perception.

PITCH PERCEPTION

What Is Pitch?

Pitch is a rather difficult term to define, because it—like loudness—is an entirely subjective experience; however, unlike loudness (which can be related systematically to intensity) pitch has no single physical dimension to which it corresponds. Different sorts of sounds—both simple and complex—can have the quality of pitch. Generally speaking, **pitch** refers to that aspect of hearing that allows sounds to be ordered from low to high. A few examples will help, starting with relatively simple tones.

Perhaps you have seen a set of tuning forks—within such a set, individual metal forks vary in size, which means that when struck against a hard surface, the forks vibrate at different frequencies, producing what are called pure tones. The perceptual quality associated with these different frequencies we call "pitch." A tuning fork that vibrates at a low frequency, such as 500 Hz, will sound lower in pitch than a tuning fork that vibrates at a higher frequency, say, 1,000 Hz. Besides tuning forks, a set of crystal glasses filled with different amounts of water will also generate pure tones when struck lightly. In this case, a glass that is filled almost to the top with water will produce a lower-pitched tone than the same-sized glass containing just a little water. Again, these differences in pitch are associated with different frequencies of vibration, as determined by the volume of water filling the glass. Using enough glasses, you can create a sufficient number of different tones to play a tune; in fact, Mozart wrote a concerto for string ensemble and crystal glasses!

The notes played on a musical instrument will also give you some appreciation of the relation between frequency and pitch, even though an instrument's sound is not a genuine pure tone. (We'll tell you why in a moment.) Take, for example, the piano. Each note on a properly tuned piano produces a sound of predominantly one frequency; that frequency is called the **fundamental frequency.** As you probably know, a musical note on the piano is produced when a small hammer strikes a string, causing it to vibrate. Strings differ in length, and the shorter ones vi-

brate more rapidly than the longer ones. Consequently, the shorter strings (which are struck by keys located toward the right-hand end of the keyboard) produce higher-pitched notes than the longer strings (which are struck by keys toward the left-hand end of the keyboard). Figure 10.11 shows the fundamental frequencies associated with the notes on a piano's keyboard. From the low notes at the far left to the high ones at the far right, *frequency* changes in regular steps. So, too, does the *pitch* of the tones—your perception of the musical sounds produced by those keys. Played in sequence from left to right, the notes are heard as the steps on the musical scale. The range of frequencies produced by a piano, 27.5 Hz to 4,186 Hz, is narrower than the total range of frequencies audible to the ear of a young adult (from 20 Hz to 20,000 Hz). Still, the notes on keyboard instruments such as the piano should give you some idea of how pitch changes with frequency, at least for periodic sounds like musical notes. The ability, incidentally, to discriminate tones on the basis of frequency alone appears to be one that improves with practice, and that practice effect can be traced to changes within the auditory cortex, as discussed in Box 10.1.

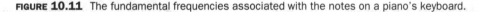

FIGURE 10.11 The fundamental frequencies associated with the notes on a piano's keyboard.

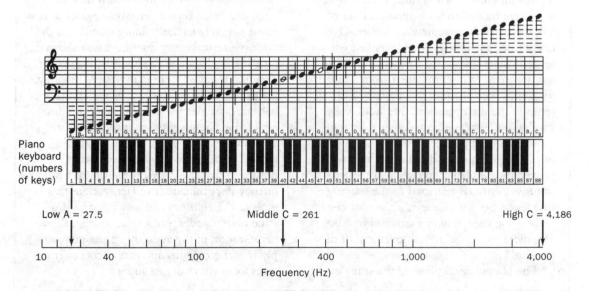

Box 10.1 *Practice Alters the Brain*

As noted in previous chapters, visual abilities improve with practice, and this is true of hearing, too. It is well known, for example, that experience helps people improve their accuracy in tuning musical instruments (Platt and Racine, 1985). We now have a possible idea about the neural concomitant of this practice effect. A recent study of auditory training revealed remarkable plasticity in both frequency discrimination and the trainee's brain. Attempting to train monkeys to make finer discriminations of frequency, Recanzone, Schreiner, and Merzenich (1993) gauged improvement behaviorally and then used physiological techniques to examine possible changes accompanying the improvement. During the behavioral phase of the study, tones were presented as a series of pairs. For most pairs, the tones were of the same frequency. Whenever the tones differed in frequency, the monkey signaled recognition of the difference by lifting its hand from a key. Monkeys were trained to discriminate a standard frequency from one that was slightly different. For example, several monkeys were trained to discriminate a tone of 5,000 Hz from one somewhat higher. Over many trials, the monkeys were trained with several different standard frequencies, learning, for each, to discriminate it from a higher frequency. Performance was described in terms of the discrimination threshold, the smallest difference reliably detected by the monkey (see Appendix). During the course of training, frequency discrimination improved by as much as fivefold. Moreover, improvement was restricted to the training frequency. So, for example, if the monkey were being trained with a standard of 8,000 Hz, there would be no improvement of the threshold at 2,000 Hz.

The physiological phase of the study ex-amined responses of neurons in the monkey's auditory cortex while various tones were being presented to the monkey's ear. In normal, untrained monkeys the auditory cortex contains a frequency map, with neurons tuned to different frequencies occupying different regions of the cortex. In monkeys who had been trained, there were also maps, but Recanzone and his colleagues found the regions of the map devoted to the trained frequencies to be greatly expanded. In fact, the size of these regions correlated strongly with the monkeys' behavioral thresholds: larger areas were associated with lower thresholds for frequency discrimination. This relation between cortical area and perceptual function is reminiscent of cortical magnification (Chapter 4), wherein areas of the retina with greater spatial resolving power are represented over larger areas of the visual cortex. Here, in the auditory system, the amount of cortex devoted to particular frequencies apparently grew as frequency discrimination improved for those frequencies.

Not every monkey in Recanzone's study exhibited cortical changes. Monkeys who listened passively to the training stimuli but did not have to make any discrimination showed little if any change in the auditory cortex. Training requires more than passive listening; the stimuli must be relevant to the animal's behavior, an idea we take up again in Chapter 11. Finally, it's important to appreciate what this study does not tell us. Training-induced changes in the auditory cortex do not mean that the cortex is the site of frequency discrimination. In fact, various structures in the auditory pathway prior to this stage undoubtedly play a role. Indeed, the reorganization of the auditory cortex may simply reflect reorganization that occurs in structures from which it gets input.

Pitch and Frequency Are Not Synonymous. So far we have treated pitch and frequency as though they were two sides of the same coin. In reality, however, the two are dissociable: in some conditions, tones of fixed frequency sound different in pitch. For instance, the loudness of a pure tone influences that tone's pitch. You can experience this yourself by comparing the pitch of a vibrating tuning fork held at arm's length to the pitch of that same tuning fork held close to your ear. Held close to your ear, the tuning fork's note will of course sound louder, but you'll also hear that its pitch changes, too. For instance, a tuning fork vibrating at 300 Hz sounds lower in pitch as intensity increases, even though its frequency remains constant. In contrast, a tuning fork vibrating at 3,000 Hz sounds higher in pitch as intensity increases.

The pitch of a pure tone of fixed frequency may also vary when that tone is heard within a background of noise. In particular, noise composed of frequencies lower than a tone causes the pitch of the tone to appear higher than it does when heard on its own; noise higher in frequency than the tone causes its pitch to sound lower.

One of the most intriguing dissociations between pitch and frequency is the perception of the **missing fundamental.** To explain this phenomenon requires introducing the concept of **harmonics,** which can be accomplished most easily with an example. Any musical note played on an instrument produces not only a fundamental frequency but also a unique set of additional frequency components called harmonics. These harmonics arise because the object producing the sound (a string, a wooden reed, and so forth) has multiple resonant frequencies—recall Box 9.1). To illustrate: Figure 10.12 shows the frequency components produced by a piano when middle C is played. (Each vertical line in the graph means that the instrument is producing sound energy at that frequency; the height of the line indicates the amount of energy, or intensity, present in that frequency.) The fundamental frequency, represented by the bold vertical line, is 261 Hz, and if asked to select a tuning fork whose pitch matched that associated with middle C, you would select one that produced this frequency. But suppose we played a sound containing exactly these same higher harmonics but omitted this fundamental.

FIGURE 10.12 Acoustic energy is produced at multiple, harmonically related frequencies when a given note is played on the piano (or any other musical instrument). This particular set of frequencies is associated with middle C.

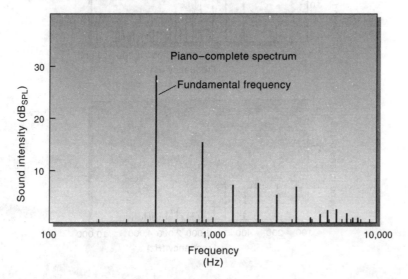

What would be the pitch of this missing fundamental sound? Surprisingly, the pitch remains that associated with middle C, even though there is no acoustic energy at 261 Hz. The demonstration, which works for various sorts of sounds including musical notes and the human voice, represents a dramatic dissociation of pitch from frequency.

The phenomenon of the missing fundamental implies that pitch is determined by the pattern of harmonics associated with a sound, not simply its fundamental frequency. A given type of musical instrument, by the way, generates harmonic patterns that are unique to that instrument. These unique harmonic patterns endow an instrument with its characteristic sound, or **timbre.** The ability to identify various instruments based on sound alone rests on their differences in timbre. For example, look at Figure 10.13 and compare the set of frequency components produced when a guitar and an alto saxophone play the same note—one with a fundamental frequency of 196 Hz. Notice that the two instruments, although producing notes equivalent in pitch, are generating different patterns of harmonics (the vertical lines to the right of the fundamental); these so-called "overtones" enable you to tell the guitar note from the one sounded by the saxophone. Here is another dissociation between frequency and pitch: the two instruments are producing markedly different patterns of frequencies, yet both create the same pitch quality.

The sound quality associated with pure tones and musical notes is often referred to as *tonal pitch.* But the sensation of pitch isn't confined to these so-called periodic sounds composed of energy harmonically placed throughout the frequency spectrum. Complex, aperiodic sounds such as the whine of an engine or a person's voice have a pitchlike quality, which is termed *nontonal pitch.* Even broadband noise can generate a sensation of pitch when its intensity waxes and wanes regularly over time (a form of intensity variation known as

FIGURE 10.13 The various frequency components when a guitar and an alto saxophone play the same note. Here the note has a fundamental frequency of 196 Hz. (Adapted from Olson, 1967.)

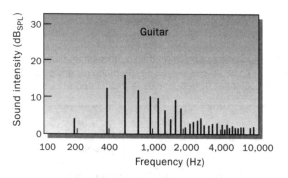

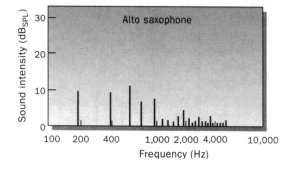

amplitude modulation). Even unmodulated noise alone can produce an illusory perception of pitch. After listening to noise from which a narrow band of frequencies has been removed (noise with a notch in its spectrum), one briefly hears a faint "pitch afterimage" corresponding to the center frequency of the missing noise (Zwicker, 1964). We mention these examples of nontonal pitch and illusory pitch, for they bear on the question of the neural basis of pitch perception, the topic of the next section.

THE NEURAL CORRELATES OF PITCH

What goes on within the auditory system when one perceives a sound as having a particular pitch? To answer this question, think back to the last chapter and the material on the inner ear and the auditory nerve. Recall that the basilar membrane moves up and down in response to sounds impinging on the eardrum, with the crest of this displacement depending on the sound's frequency. This displacement bends the hair cells, and this bending, in turn, triggers neural activity within the portion of the auditory nerve that innervates those hair cells. So what happens when sounds of varying degrees of complexity are heard? Let's start with the simplest situation, listening to a single pure tone.

When the ear is presented with a pure tone, one portion of the basilar membrane will be maximally displaced, a limited set of hair cells will be disturbed, and a subset of auditory nerve fibers will be activated. The frequency of a tone could be registered, therefore, by which set of nerve fibers is currently most active. As you will recall from the last chapter, such a theory is referred to as a *place theory*; it has several things in its favor. First, damage to a limited portion of the basilar membrane causes a loss in the ability to hear certain frequencies. The frequencies affected depend on the region of the membrane damaged, as predicted by the place theory (Crowe, Guild, and Polvost, 1934). Also consistent with the place theory are the results from a study in which an array of small stimulating electrodes was implanted in the auditory nerve of the right ear of a 60-year-

old man who was deaf in that ear because of basilar membrane damage (Simmons et al., 1965). When mild electric current was applied to a single electrode, the man described hearing a single tone; different electrodes evoked tone sensations that differed in pitch. Presumably, different electrodes were contacting different fibers in the auditory nerve. Consequently, the ability of different electrodes to evoke different pitches strengthens the presumed link between activity in individual nerve fibers and pure-tone hearing.

Many aspects of pitch perception, however, cannot be explained by place theory. For instance, frequencies below 1,000 Hz produce a broad pattern of displacement along the basilar membrane. Because of this broad displacement, there is no specific place where the basilar membrane bulges maximally. Yet you have no trouble accurately identifying the pitch of these low-frequency tones. Apparently, pitch perception for pure tones depends on something besides place coding. As an alternative to place, the auditory system could use the firing rate of auditory nerve fibers to register low-frequency information. As you will recall from the previous chapter, this form of neural coding is known as the *frequency theory*. The idea here is that nerve fibers discharge periodically in synchrony with the frequency of the stimulating tone. According to the frequency theory, then, the pitch of a tone corresponds to the periodicity of firing of nerve fibers. And indeed, nerve fibers can fire in synchrony with tones of moderately low frequency (Rose, Brugge, Anderson, and Hind, 1967). Fibers can behave, in other words, like metronomes, generating impulses in time to the frequency of a tone. Thus information about the tone's pitch could be conveyed by the temporal periodicity of fiber activity.

So working in tandem, frequency theory and place theory could account for pitch perception evoked by simple tones of a given frequency. But as stressed in the last section, many aspects of pitch perception defy explanation simply in terms of frequency. Rather than tying pitch perception to maximum activity at a single locus along the basilar membrane, contemporary theories propose that different pitches are associated with unique patterns of activation over the entire basilar membrane (and, by extension, within the ensemble of auditory nerve fibers). (You may recall that this idea of ensemble coding of sensory attributes was introduced in Chapter 4, in regard to visual coding of contour orientation.) Peripheral frequency coding is important in these theories, for it provides the initial decomposition of a complex sound wave into component frequencies; this is the essence of the critical bands discussed earlier. The outputs from these frequency-selective bands, in turn, provide the input signals to a neural process that detects patterns of activity across the frequency spectrum. Different patterns of activity specify pitch. Moreover, removal of one frequency component from a multifrequency sound complex will not destroy the overall pattern—a characteristic pitch can still be heard when a component, even the fundamental, is missing.

Having discussed the possible neural basis of pitch perception, let's now turn to another question about pitch perception, one concerning individual differences in the ability to identify the pitch of a tone.

PERFECT PITCH AND TONE DEAFNESS

Some individuals have what is called **perfect pitch**—an ability enabling them to hum any musical note they're told to or to name any note that is played. Such individuals are encountered in musical circles, although even among musicians the ability is quite rare (Vernon, 1977). One of the most renowned people with perfect pitch was Wolfgang Amadeus Mozart. It was claimed he could tell when the violin he was playing was tuned differently from one he had played the day before, even if those violins were mistuned by no more than "half a quarter of a tone" (Stevens and Warshofsky, 1965). Because it tends to run in families, perfect pitch used to be regarded as genetic in origin (Seashore, 1938). However, this sort of family tendency proves very little, since family members with perfect pitch are very likely to be musicians and would have received lots of exposure to musical notes, the only kind of sound

in nature that allows the development of perfect pitch.

According to one theory, all individuals are born with perfect pitch, but it is trained out of them early in life (Ward, 1970). This unlearning occurs because people are trained to ignore absolute pitch and to attend, instead, to the relations among various pitches. Consider this example: you recognize a familiar melody such as "Pop Goes the Weasel" regardless of the key in which it is played; hence you perceive a melody not as a specific sequence of notes but rather as a particular relation among notes (Pick, 1979). In other words, you attend to pitch relations and not to absolute pitch. While this discourages the retention of any ability for perfect pitch you may have had as a youngster, it enables you to enjoy the same musical melodies played or sung in different keys. In this regard, it is noteworthy that people with perfect pitch frequently complain that it is disquieting to listen to a piece of music played in an unusual key—the piece sounds "wrong" (Terhardt and Ward, 1982). Box 10.2 (pp. 356–357) describes some additional interesting work on melody perception.

Besides perfect pitch, there is a more common ability known as **relative pitch**—people with relative pitch can identify tonal intervals very accurately, although they are not so accurate at naming the particular notes making up that interval. You can think of tonal intervals in terms of the steps of the musical scale. In particular, a tonal interval is defined by the number of steps that separate a pair of notes. For instance, the first two notes of "My Bonnie Lies over the Ocean" define a larger interval than do the first two notes of "Greensleeves." To be able to recognize and label all these various intervals means you have relative pitch. Many musicians have this ability (Siegel and Siegel, 1977).

Our discussion of pitch perception led to the conclusion that a sound source is defined perceptually by the profile of component frequencies that it produces. This sets the stage for our next question: What stimulus properties promote the perceptual grouping of the constituent frequencies of a given sound source? An answer to this question is crucial for understanding how sounds are recognized.

SOUND RECOGNITION: JUDGING *WHAT* THE SOURCE OF A SOUND IS

PERCEPTUAL ORGANIZATION OF THE AUDITORY STREAM

As stressed earlier, the ear ordinarily receives a stream of acoustic energy from a multitude of environmental sources, and the energy from those sources sums to form a single, complex sound arriving at the ear. To appreciate this fact, think about attending a symphony performance. Without effort, you can pick out and listen to the melody line carried by, say, the woodwinds and then easily shift attention to the harmonic strains of the violins. It is possible, in other words, to hear the separate instruments even though their separate voices blend together into one massive acoustic stream arriving at your ears. Or imagine chatting with a friend at a noisy baseball game. The acoustic environment includes applause, music, shouts from popcorn vendors, cheers of neighboring fans and, of personal interest to you, your companion's voice. Amidst the din, you manage to pick out her voice from all the rest.

As these examples dramatize, we do not hear a single cacophony corresponding to the one complex acoustic stream arriving at our ears; rather, we hear individual auditory events perceptually attributable to external sources. Evidently, the auditory system manages to segregate this complex sound field into separate **auditory images,** as they're called. How the ear and brain derive structure from the auditory stream has become a problem of intense interest to those studying hearing and, more generally, perceptual organization (Bregman, 1990; Yost, 1991). From the outset, realize that this problem of auditory grouping has analogs in vision, smell, and taste. In all these modalities, the nervous system must organize complex sensory inputs into separate per-

ceptual events and objects. However, each modality has at its disposal unique stimulus properties that make this process of perceptual organization possible. Early in this century, the Gestalt psychologists investigated organizing principles that promote segregation of a visual scene into distinct objects and events; some of those principles were outlined in Chapter 5. Now, in the last decade or so, scientists interested in hearing have posed a comparable question: What are the properties that promote perceptual grouping in hearing? Some important ones are summarized in the following sections.

Common Spectral Content. Given the existence of neural processes that parse the auditory stream into component frequencies, it is natural to wonder whether frequency content could determine perceptual grouping. Perhaps, the reasoning goes, acoustic energy activating one set of frequency-tuned neurons is attributed to a single sound source, one that is perceptually distinct from the source associated with acoustic energy activating a different set of fibers. Construed in this way, the detectability of a test tone heard against a background of noise is impaired because the tone is perceptually combined with the noise to form a single perceptual event. But when the frequency spectrum of the noise is sufficiently removed from the tone's frequency, the tone stands out as a separate acoustic event and is, therefore, easily detected.

Bregman (1990) describes a simple auditory phenomenon demonstrating grouping by frequency. He created a multitone sequence consisting of three high tones (f1, f2, and f3) and three low tones (f4, f5, and f6) interleaved to form the sequence f1, f4, f2, f5, f3, f6. When this sequence was repeated over and over with the individual tones played in rapid succession, listeners did not hear the high and low tones played in alternation but instead heard two tone streams simultaneously, one the sequence of high-frequency tones and the other the sequence of low-frequency tones. People tended to group the tones, in other words, according to frequency.

Box 10.2 *What Is a Melody?*

You don't have to be a musician to recognize musical melodies; that's an ability that comes naturally to just about everyone. Moreover, musicians or not, most people can recognize a familiar melody when it is played in different keys or on different instruments, or when it is sung by different voices. In these cases, the particular notes differ, but the melody remains the same. Just as different type fonts can be used to print the same sentence, different notes can produce the same melody. The implication is that people hear melodies not as specific sets of notes but as particular relations, or patterns, among those notes (Pick, 1979).

But what aspects of a melody unite musical notes into a pattern? Is it the rise and fall in the pitch of successive notes—the property known technically as **melody contour?** Does it have something to do with the size of the intervals between successive notes? One way to determine what makes a melody is to alter various properties of a familiar melody and see whether that alteration affects the ability to recognize that melody. To give an example, we mentioned that most people can recognize a melody regardless of the key in

which it is played. A study by Dowling and Fujitani (1971) evaluated the effects of some other melodic alterations.

Dowling and Fujitani asked college undergraduates to identify some familiar melodies—"Yankee Doodle," "Oh, Susannah," "Twinkle, Twinkle, Little Star," "Good King Wenceslaus," and "Auld Lang Syne." Each of these tunes was tape-recorded while being performed on the same wind instrument, in the same key, and at the same tempo. When undistorted versions of these tunes were heard, listeners correctly identified the melodies 99 percent of the time—which merely confirms that the melodies were indeed well known. But how did listeners do when these melodies were distorted?

Dowling and Fujitani studied the effects of several different forms of distortion. In one condition, the *absolute* size of the intervals between notes was altered, but the *relative* size of the intervals remained the same. To illustrate, consider the first three notes of a verse from "Oh, Susannah" (see the diagram below). In the unadulterated version, notes 1 and 2 are separated by one whole tone, as are notes 2 and 3. In the first distorted version,

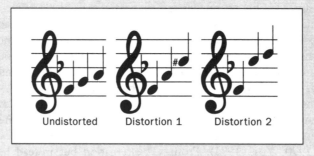

Undistorted   Distortion 1   Distortion 2

notes 1 and 2 are separated by two whole tones, as are notes 2 and 3. Hence in the distorted version, the absolute size of the intervals has been altered but the relative size remains unchanged. Note, too, that the pitch contour remains the same: in both versions, the second note is higher than the first, and the third note is higher than the second. Upon hearing melodies distorted in this way, listeners could correctly identify the tune 66 percent of the time. This decline in performance indicates that absolute interval size (the property distorted in this condition) does contribute to defining a melody. Still, this property isn't absolutely crucial—relative interval size and pitch contour provide enough information for listeners to distinguish one melody from others much of the time.

In a second condition, each melody was distorted even more severely. In this case, only the pitch contour was preserved. With this form of distortion, the sequence of notes moved up and down in pitch in the same manner as it did in the normal version, but the size of the intervals between notes in the distorted version was unrelated to the size of the intervals in the original. An example of this form of distortion, as applied to "Oh, Susannah," appears in the musical staff at the far right (Distortion 2). With such distortion, listeners still managed to identify the melody 59 percent of the time. So pitch contour, all by itself, does provide some information for identifying melodies. In their final condition, Dowling and Fujitani distorted even the pitch contour; the only thing left undistorted was the first note in each measure. With just this scant information to go on, people were not able to recognize the melodies.

In summary, the experiment by Dowling and Fujitani shows that when listeners try to recognize familiar tunes, they make use of several sources of information. These sources include absolute interval size, relative interval size, and pitch contour. Incidentally, most of the participants in Dowling and Fujitani's study had no special musical training. In another study, Dowling (1978) found that musically experienced people were better at perceiving the relative size of intervals than were musically inexperienced individuals. This is not surprising, since relative interval size is a rather subtle structural aspect of any melody. It is the sort of transformation that Bach used in many of his compositions.

There is another salient aspect of melody, and that is its rhythm. To appreciate the salience of a melody's rhythm, have a friend select one of the five tunes mentioned above and then clap out the rhythm of that tune. You'll be surprised how easy it is to identify which of the melodies your friend is clapping. Some of the best examples of rhythm's contribution to a melody come from classical music. One is Franz Liszt's short piece for piano and orchestra, "Totentanz" ("Dance of Death"). It is an amazing example of the musical variety that can be achieved simply by altering the speed and rhythm of one theme. The piece consists of thirty variations on the same theme, the medieval "Dies Irae," and each variation makes its own unique musical statement. An attentive listener should have no trouble hearing the same melody running throughout the piece. Liszt's composition beautifully demonstrates how changes in rhythm alone can influence your perception of a melody.

This grouping of tones according to proximity in frequency is reminiscent of the Gestalt principle of grouping by visual proximity (recall Figure 5.2).

Common spectral content, while effective in some instances, cannot be the entire explanation for auditory grouping. In the natural environment, different sound sources produce frequency spectra with considerable overlap. The spectra associated with two females talking at the same time, for instance, are highly similar. Yet a third person would have no difficulty distinguishing the two speakers on the basis of voice alone. Clearly, information other than spectral content must also be supporting perceptual grouping.

Common Time Course. The energy levels constituting the complex of frequencies associated with a given source fluctuate in synchrony over time: their onsets and offsets correspond, and their modulations in intensity match over time. Consider, for example, your voice, which constitutes a rich package of acoustic frequencies. As you speak, the components in this package of energy rise and fall in unison, and when you're finished, the offsets of the constituent frequencies exactly coincide. In effect, frequency components from the same sound source form a cohesive unit, all members following the same pattern of change. In this respect, the frequency components from a sound source are like sailors in a boat: although the individual sailors differ in size and appearance, all undergo the same up and down motions as the boat rides the waves. This common fate links the individual sailors into a single entity called a "crew." Likewise, common fate could be one way that the auditory system registers which frequencies belong together, meaning that they come from the same source.

Evidently common temporal fate does play a role in perceptual unification, for people have trouble identifying sound sources from recordings heard without temporal modulation (McAdams, 1984). And when one frequency component within a set of frequencies is slightly out of temporal synchrony with the rest, it seems to arise from a separate source (Bregman and Pinker, 1978).

But temporal synchrony alone cannot be sufficient, for we can easily pick out a single individual singing in unison in a quartet even though the temporal modulations of the voices of all four are essentially identical. Moreover, common temporal fate is of limited use in situations where frequency content, not just intensity, varies over time, and one situation where frequencies undergo continuous, often drastic change is music. So, what other source of acoustic information makes it possible to segregate one singer's voice from the rest?

Spectral Harmonics. Another factor influencing whether frequency components seem to originate from a single sound source is the harmonic relations of those components. Frequencies that are multiples of one another are said to be harmonically related. For instance, playing the A string on a violin generates acoustic energy at the frequencies 440, 880, and 1,320 Hz; as you can see, the two higher frequencies are multiples of the fundamental frequency, which means they are harmonically related. And, in general, harmonic tones tend to group together much more readily than do nonharmonic tones (de Boer, 1956). In this regard, it is significant that many relevant sounds in the environment, especially speech and music, are made up of harmonically related frequencies. For example, automobile horns on newer model cars honk at F-sharp and A-sharp, a harmonically related pair that is judged pleasing to the ear (Garfield, 1983).

* * *

In brief, several factors contribute to the perceptual grouping of frequency components into a single, recognizable sound source. We could summarize the operation of these factors by saying that the auditory system picks out patterns among frequency components. These patterns could involve simultaneous changes in the intensities of certain frequency components. Or these patterns could involve a harmonic relation among certain frequency components. In all cases, these patterns unite the constituent frequencies and promote identification of the source.

There is one other rich source of information that promotes perceptual grouping of constituent frequencies into a coherent sound source, and that is information specifying sound location. By tagging "where" in space sound energy arises, it is possible to group frequencies arising from that single location and, thereby, define a single sound source. The next section is devoted to this problem of sound localization.

SOUND LOCALIZATION: JUDGING *WHERE* A SOUND ORIGINATES

Hearing involves more than just recognizing sounds. One also has a sense of the direction from which those sounds are coming. This ability to perceive the location of sounds in space—termed **sound localization**—can be as important as the capacity to identify those sounds. What good is it to recognize the scream of a fire truck's siren if one cannot tell from which direction it is approaching? How frustrating it would be for a parent to hear the frightened cries of a lost child and yet be unable to pinpoint the origins of those cries. Fortunately, hearing does have a distinct spatial quality—sounds always appear to come from somewhere. Moreover, perceiving a sound's location occurs effortlessly and automatically, as common experience tells you. In fact, even newborn infants will turn their eyes toward the source of a sound (Butterworth and Castillo, 1976; Wertheimer, 1961); sound localization is a perceptual ability present from the day of birth. This section discusses the auditory information that endows sounds with this quality of spatial location.*

---

* Spatial location refers to the position of a sound source within an up/down and left/right spatial framework, ignoring the distance of the sound from the listener. Sound intensity provides a potential cue for distance, but people are relatively poor at judging auditory distance unless they are allowed to move toward the sound while listening to it (Ashmead, LeRoy, and Odom, 1990).

From the outset, keep in mind that there is *no* inherent spatial information in the acoustic signals arriving at an ear. In vision, of course, left/right and up/down spatial relations are faithfully retained in the optical image formed on the retina. But in hearing, there is simply nothing contained in the acoustic image that corresponds to these relative locations—spatial coordinates must be computed from available auditory information.

In specifying spatial location of sounds, the terms "azimuth" and "elevation" will sometimes be used (see Figure 10.14). *Azimuth* refers to the horizontal direction of a sound relative to the listener's head; *elevation* refers to the vertical direction of the sound relative to the head. To visualize the meaning of these terms, perform the following simple exercises. Look straight ahead, extend your arm parallel to the ground, and move it from directly in front of you to the side: this action traces an arc corresponding to changes in azimuth. Next, point your arm in a given direction and move it upward: this action traces an arc corresponding to changes in elevation. Any given

FIGURE 10.14 Sound location is specified in terms of azimuth (position along the horizontal plane) and elevation (position along a vertical plane).

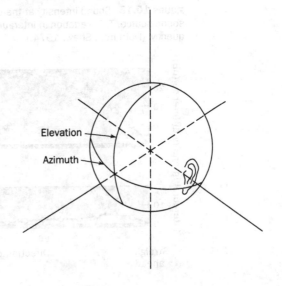

direction in space can be expressed in terms of its azimuth and elevation. As you will learn, these two coordinates seem to be specified by different sources of information.

One thing seems clear: accurate sound localization depends crucially on having two ears. Working together, the ears, like the eyes, enable one to locate objects in three-dimensional space. As any person with unilateral deafness will testify, sound localization using one ear can be difficult.* From the previous chapter, you already have some idea about the information afforded by listening with two ears: sound waves from the same source arriving at the two ears may differ in intensity and in time of arrival, depending on the location of that source relative to the head. The following sections discuss both these sources of binaural information in greater detail and inquire about their effectiveness. We should stress one point. When tested on binaural sound localization tasks, listen-

ers never actually hear differences in intensity between the two ears. Nor can they tell that sound arrives at one ear ahead of the other. Instead, listeners hear a single sound originating from a particular direction relative to straight ahead.

INTERAURAL INTENSITY DIFFERENCES

Figure 10.15 summarizes how **interaural intensity difference (IID)** varies with the azimuth of a sound source. These data were obtained by positioning a sound source at various points around the horizontal plane of an artificial head outfitted with microphones in each "ear" (Shaw, 1974). The vertical axis plots the intensity difference between the sounds arriving at the two ears. The horizontal axis plots the position, or azimuth, of the sound source relative to the straight ahead position. Two curves are shown, one using a 6,000-Hz tone and the other using a 200-Hz tone. Notice that when the high-frequency (6,000 Hz) tone is located to the side of the head, the interaural intensity difference grows to almost 20 dB.

Notice also that for each IID (values on the vertical axis), there are *multiple* distinct locations (on the horizontal axis) where a sound source could produce that intensity difference. Take, for example, sound originating from a location di-

---

* Briefly presented sounds are particularly difficult to localize when using just one ear, but monaural localization performance improves significantly when listening to long, continuous sounds—under these conditions, people are able to turn their heads, which modulates the intensity of the monaural sound and, thus, provides additional information specifying location (Perrott, Ambarsoom, and Tucker, 1987).

FIGURE 10.15 Sound intensity at the two ears varies with the location of the sound source. This variation in interaural intensity difference depends on frequency. (Data from Shaw, 1974.)

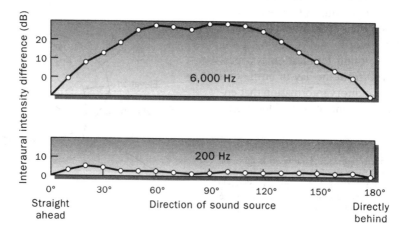

rectly behind the head. As Figure 10.15 shows, this location yields an IID value of zero. Yet the same value—zero—occurs when the sound originates from a location straight in front of the head. Besides this pair of sound source locations, there are other positions where IID provides ambiguous information. Since distinctly different spatial locations can produce the same information about interaural intensity, that ambiguous information could lead to confusions about the location of a sound source. These confusions can in fact occur, but we'll postpone describing why until we have completed our review of the binaural cues for sound localization. For now, let's continue our examination of Figure 10.15.

As the 200-Hz curve indicates, IIDs are much less pronounced when the sound source consists of low frequencies. This means that IID is a less potent cue for low-frequency sounds than it is for high-frequency sounds. There is a simple reason why the intensities of low frequencies are so similar at the two ears. With low-frequency sounds, the wavelength of the sound wave (recall Figure 9.6) is actually longer than the diameter of the head, which is about 20 centimeters. For the sake of comparison, the length between successive peaks of a 900-Hz tone is approximately 40 centimeters, double the head's diameter. The head, in other words, is too small to interfere with propagation of low-frequency sound waves. Because they are unimpeded by the head, these low-frequency waves lose nothing in the way of intensity from one side of the head to the other. High frequencies, however, are more effectively blocked by the head. Their waves are too small to avoid the shadowing effect of the head. Consequently, the head more effectively blocks sound waves of high frequency from reaching the farther ear, thus weakening their intensity at that ear. Because of this physical property of sound, IIDs associated with high-frequency sounds will be larger than those associated with low-frequency sounds; in fact, IID falls to zero at frequencies below 1,000 Hz. Think for a moment what this means for other species whose head sizes differ from ours. In particular, small heads (such as a

mouse's) will generate very little "shadowing" effect, meaning that IIDs will be vanishingly small for frequencies where IIDs are potent for us.

Next let's review the other binaural source of localization information, **interaural time difference (ITD)**.

INTERAURAL TIME DIFFERENCES

Figure 10.16 summarizes how the time of arrival of a sound at the two ears varies with the location of the sound source relative to the head. These measurements were made in much the same way as the ones described above, only using brief clicks as sound stimuli in this case (Shaw, 1974). The horizontal axis again plots the azimuth of the sound source; the vertical axis, the difference in time of arrival of the sound at the two ears. As this graph shows, a sound coming from somewhere off to the side of the head strikes one ear before the other. The largest difference in time of arrival occurs when the sound source is located directly to the side of the head, in which case the ITD is somewhere around 600 to 800 μsec (1 μsec equals one-millionth of a second); the precise value depends on the size of the head. Sounds located just slightly to the left or the right of the straight ahead position produce ITD values as

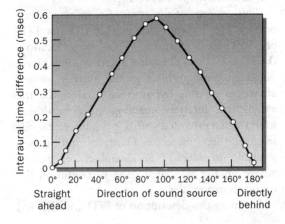

FIGURE 10.16 The time of arrival of sound at the two ears varies with the location of the sound source. (Data from Shaw, 1974.)

small as 10 to 20 µsec. Listeners can discriminate, however, among these slight differences in location, indicating that the auditory system is remarkably sensitive to ITD information.

As with the case of interaural intensity differences, interaural time differences can be potentially ambiguous: the same values of time difference (vertical axis) can be produced by sources in multiple locations (horizontal axis). For instance, a zero interaural time difference could arise from a source located either directly ahead of the listener, directly behind, or anywhere on the median plane connecting these two points.

THE CONE OF CONFUSION

In a moment, we shall look at results from experiments that have examined how well people are able to localize sounds in auditory space. First, however, it will be helpful to point out a fundamental limitation in the information provided by IID and ITD, the two binaural sources of location information. For any given IID or ITD, there is a family of potential spatial locations which could generate that interaural difference. To a first approximation, the surface describing these points of ambiguity (constant IID or constant ITD) corresponds to a cone and, for this reason, the set of ambiguous locations is termed the **cone of confusion** (Woodworth, 1938). You should understand that different values of IID and ITD have different associated cones of confusion; one exemplar is shown in Figure 10.17.

This concept of the cone of confusion is important, for it means that neither IID nor ITD provides *unique* information about sound location. Based on IID or ITD alone, listeners should have difficulty distinguishing sound sources located anywhere on this hypothetical surface. To the extent that listeners unambiguously localize a sound when provided with a given interaural difference, there must be additional information available to specify, or disambiguate, exactly where on the associated cone of confusion the sound source resides.

So given this description of ITD and IID and

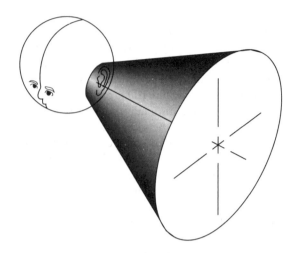

FIGURE 10.17 The cone of confusion, a conical plane defining locations where a sound source would produce the same value of interaural time difference or the same value of interaural intensity difference.

the potential points of confusion, just how well *do* people perform on localization tasks?

THE EFFECTIVENESS OF INTERAURAL TIME AND INTENSITY DIFFERENCES

A classic study of sound localization was performed by Stevens and Newman (1934), and their results highlight several major points about IID and ITD. For their experiment, Stevens and Newman tested a listener seated on the roof of a building. This outdoor setting eliminated sound reflections from walls and ceilings; to minimize disturbance from extraneous sounds, data were collected during the wee hours of the morning. Extending out from the listener's chair was a long metal arm that could rotate around the listener's head in the horizontal plane at ear level; thus they varied azimuth while holding elevation constant. Attached to the end of this mechanical arm was a loudspeaker that could play pure tones of various frequencies. The listener sat blindfolded with his head held very still. He was instructed to point in the direction from which the sound seemed to originate, and the measure of sound localization was accuracy in reporting position. For tones below 1,000 Hz, localization accuracy was high. But for tones between 2,000 and 4,000 Hz, errors became increasingly frequent. At still higher frequencies, performance again improved, eventually becoming as good as it had been with low frequencies. Stevens and Newman took these results as support for the **duplex theory** of sound localization, which says a listener utilizes one source of information (ITD) to localize low-frequency sounds and another source of information (IID) to localize high-frequency sounds. Presumably, the transitions in performance corresponded to shifts in the cue used to make localization judgments. The high error rates at intermediate frequencies indicate that this is a region where neither time nor intensity is particularly effective.

Following the experiment by Stevens and Newman, there have been many other studies of sound localization. Some have used an array of loudspeakers surrounding a listener sitting in an anechoic chamber (Wightman and Kistler, 1980; Oldfield and Parker, 1984a, 1984b). Sound is played from different speakers, and the listener indicates where the sound comes from. In other experiments, listeners have been outfitted with headphones* through which sounds are played (Mills, 1960; Jeffress and Taylor, 1961). In general, the results from all these experiments support the conclusions reached by Stevens and Newman: sound localization depends on interaural time differences at *low* frequencies and on interaural intensity differences at *high* frequencies. In most ordinary listening situations, sounds consist of both high and low frequencies, which means both sources of information, time differences and intensity differences, are available for localizing those sounds. Wightman, Kistler, and Arruda

---

* Headphones have the advantage of allowing the experimenter to vary interaural time and interaural intensity independently, making it possible to examine the effectiveness of the two cues separately. Headphones have the disadvantage of producing a sound sensation localized within the head, not in the external environment. Consequently, headphone studies typically ask listeners to judge the lateralization of sound— whether it comes from the left or from the right of midline.

(1989) believe that ITD dominates in this situation.

SOUND (MIS)LOCALIZATION

People do make errors in sound localization experiments, and those errors tend to be associated with particular positions in auditory space. As you might guess, those positions include the ones where information about interaural time and interaural intensity is ambiguous. Two such positions were mentioned earlier, straight ahead and straight behind. Sounds from either of these positions arrive at the two ears simultaneously and with equivalent intensity. So it is not surprising that sounds arising from these two positions are sometimes mislocalized, especially when the sound consists of a narrow band of frequencies (Butler, 1986); broadband noise yields fewer front/back confusions (Makous and Middlebrooks, 1990) and the presence of sound-reflecting surfaces helps, too (Guski, 1990). Besides directly in front and directly behind, there are many other positions in space where time and intensity cues are also ambiguous; these constitute the cones of confusion described earlier.

Design Features That Minimize Mislocalization Errors. In view of these multiple points of potential confusion, it is surprising that people don't mistake the direction of sounds more often than they do. In fact, there are two reasons why you normally are not confused about the location of sounds. The first reason has to do with *head movements*. In sound localization experiments involving an array of speakers, the listener's head remains in a fixed position. Ordinarily, though, you are free to move your head when listening to a sound, and these head movements can eliminate potential confusion arising from ambiguous localization cues. To illustrate, imagine hearing a sound from a source located directly behind your head. While interaural time and intensity information is momentarily ambiguous, you can eliminate this ambiguity simply by turning your head in either direction. The sound source will no longer be symmetrically located between your two ears, and the available localization information will now specify the sound's location unambiguously. Moving your head changes the pattern of interaural differences associated with a stationary sound source, thereby clearing up any initial confusion about where a sound comes from. Note, however, that head movements are effective in eliminating ambiguity only if the sound is of sufficient duration to allow you to listen to it while turning your head; head movements are too slow to help localize brief sounds, such as the snap of a twig (Pollack and Rose, 1967).

A second factor that minimizes the incidence of localization errors has to do with the *pinnas*. Without them, people have more trouble judging the locations of sound sources (Burger, 1958). You can demonstrate this for yourself by performing the following test. While you are blindfolded, have a friend stand close enough to you that she can snap her fingers at various positions around your head. See how well you can guess where that sound comes from. Now repeat this test while wearing earmuffs or a set of headphones, either of which largely eliminate any contribution from the pinnas. Although still able to hear the sound, you'll find it more difficult to pinpoint exactly where the finger snap originates, especially when that sound originates from either directly in front of you or directly behind you. This simple exercise demonstrates that the pinnas make it easier to locate sound.

But why is that so? It is thought that the pinnas aid localization because sound bounces around in the folds of the pinnas before entering the ear canals; the number and direction of the bounces depends on the direction from which the sound originated. The pinnas, in other words, alter the frequency spectrum of the acoustic signal entering the external canal, imposing a unique "spectral signature" that specifies the direction from which that sound arrived at the ear (Batteau, 1967). The auditory system, in turn, manages to "read" that signature, thereby avoiding any ambiguity about the location of the source of that sound wave.

Pinna cues would be particularly useful for specifying the vertical location of a sound source—its elevation—for binaural cues are plagued by ambiguity in this dimension. And, in fact, listeners are able to determine the elevation of a source with some accuracy. Oldfield and Parker (1986) compared monaural to binaural localization performance for brief bursts of noise positioned at various locations throughout the auditory field. For elevation judgments, the two conditions were very similar, implying that pinna cues (the only source of information available in the monaural condition) specify a source's elevation. For azimuth judgments, however, listeners performed quite well with two ears but woefully when forced to use one ear only. This disparity between monaural and binaural performance implies that IID and ITD are the primary sources of information for judgments of azimuth (but see Butler, Humanski, and Musicant, 1990). Middlebrooks and Green (1991) provide a comprehensive review of the localization literature, especially studies bearing on the question of information supporting judgments of azimuth and elevation.

Because the size and shape of the pinnas vary so much from person to person (see Figure 10.18), this labeled information about a sound's direction should be highly specific to one's own ears. Thus, if you and a friend were to trade pinnas, your ability to localize sound might be impaired. Such an impairment has actually been demonstrated by Fred Wightman and Doris Kistler, now at the University of Wisconsin (Wightman and Kistler, 1989a, b). They placed a tiny microphone inside each ear canal of a person and recorded sounds originating from speakers located at various positions around the person's head. Because of the microphone's position, the sounds it picked up had already been influenced by the person's pinna. Wightman and Kistler also had the person judge the location of the sounds, and as expected, few errors were made except for the ambiguous sound locations we mentioned earlier. Wightman and Kistler collected localization judgments and ear canal recordings from several people. They then played back those recorded sounds over head-

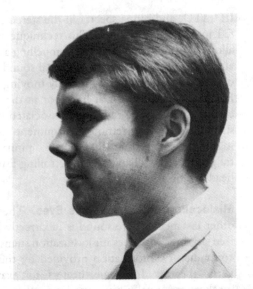
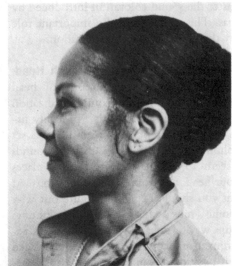
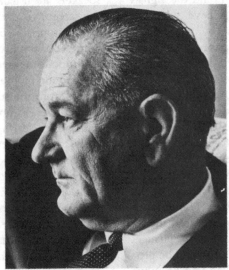

FIGURE 10.18 Pinnas come in all sizes and shapes. (Top, left and right: K. Bendo; bottom: courtesy of the Lyndon Baines Johnson Library.)

phones and had the same people once again make localization judgments. Listening to the sounds that had been recorded through their own ears, people had no trouble accurately localizing sounds. But when listening to sounds that had been recorded through someone else's ears, people were less accurate at localization. By exam-

ining the sound waveform recorded from within the ear canals of these people, Wightman and Kistler could identify the individual differences in those waveforms introduced by each person's pinnas. The individual differences in performance when listening with one's own pinnas or with someone else's imply that the auditory system does register the sound coloration introduced by the pinnas. This underscores the important role played by the pinnas in sound localization.

Mislocalization: Sound Heard Through Headphones. This discussion of the role of head movements and the pinnas in sound localization raises an interesting point. You've probably listened to music in stereophonic sound over a set of headphones. If so, you know that the sounds usually seem to originate from various places *within* your head, not from external locations. At this point you should be able to figure out why stereophonic music heard over headphones sounds the way it does. Typically, music is recorded from an array of many microphones placed at various positions around the musicians. Furthermore, technicians then combine the signals from those microphones to achieve whatever sound balance they desire. So by the time it reaches your ears over the headphones, the sound bears little resemblance to the binaural stimulus you would have heard in person.

Using just two microphones, recordings can be made that mimic what would be heard live; music recorded in this manner and heard over headphones *does* seem to emanate from out in space and not within your head (Koenig, 1950; Belendiuk and Butler, 1978). Even then, however, you must hold your head still for the illusion to be compelling. Here's why. The microphones were stationary at the time the recording was made, so the reproduced sound carries none of the changes in interaural time or intensity that would be produced by head movements. When you do move your head, the brain receives contradictory information: the vestibular system (the one responsible for signaling head orientation) informs your brain of your head movement but the auditory system does not report an associated change in interaural time or intensity. These contradictory messages reduce the otherwise compelling illusion that sounds heard over a headphone appear to come from out in space. Auditory researchers are now trying to devise a computer-controlled headphone system that senses the direction and magnitude of head turns and immediately alters the

IID, ITD, and pinna spectra in the stereo signals fed into the headphones. This technique would allow a computer to generate compelling and realistic acoustic experiences of virtual sound fields over headphones worn by a freely moving head. For example, a listener at home or in the office could experience all the sounds associated with a stroll through some remote environment, including subtle variations in IID, ITD, and pinna spectra produced by changes in the strolling listener's head position.

Mislocalization: Ears Versus Eyes. There are other instances where sound is incorrectly localized. In these instances mislocalization stems from contradictory information provided by the eyes versus the ears. In movie theaters, for example, speakers are usually positioned on either side of the screen, yet we hear the sounds coming from the appropriate sources pictured on the screen. Another example of this kind of mislocalization is ventriloquism—speech is perceived to come from the mouth of the dummy when, of course, it comes from the still mouth of the ventriloquist. Both these examples underscore vision's dominance over hearing when it comes to specifying the location of events (Welch and Warren, 1980).

Probably the most convincing proof of vision's dominance is provided by the *pseudophone*—the odd-looking listening device pictured in Figure 10.19. The pseudophone effectively interchanges input to the two ears, causing the left ear to hear what would normally be heard by the right, and vice versa. What this binaural swap does to sound

FIGURE 10.19 A pseudophone reverses the inputs to the two ears.

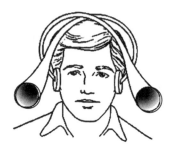

localization depends on whether you listen with eyes open or closed (Young, 1928). Imagine that you are wearing a pseudophone and are sitting between two friends, a male to your left and a female to your right. They are arguing. With your eyes closed, the male's voice will sound as though it were coming from your right and the female's voice from your left. Although wrong, this way of hearing the two voices is not surprising; it is caused by the reversing mechanism of the pseudophone. What is surprising, however, is what you hear with your eyes open. Now the male's voice will seem to originate from your left and the female's voice from your right. While this corresponds to the true seating arrangement, your brain has to *ignore* interaural time and intensity cues to arrive at this perception. Your brain, in other words, believes your eyes, not your ears.

In a way, this bias toward vision makes some sense. For one thing, sounds can bounce off solid surfaces and be reflected to your ears in the form of echoes. Hence the direction from which sound arrives at your ears may not always correspond to the actual location of the sound source. The same is not true of vision—the light reflected from an object travels in a straight line to your eye. Thus the principles of optics ensure that the light arriving at your eyes usually specifies an object's actual location. Physics offers another reason why your brain may trust your eyes more than your ears— sound travels much more slowly than light. Consequently, the sounds from a distant object (such as an airplane in flight) can belie the true position of that object, whereas the light from that object almost never lies. Considered together, these properties of light and sound may have encouraged the brain to rely more on vision for localization. But, as the next section discusses, there may still be an intriguing link between eyes and ears when it comes to localization.

Do the Eyes Determine Sound Localization Accuracy? A variety of animals have been tested on sound localization tasks, and the levels of accuracy vary widely from species to species. Heffner and Heffner (1992) have surveyed the life styles and anatomies of these various species in an attempt to discover what factors seem to govern sound localization ability. Two related factors stood out, both having to do with vision. Species with panoramic vision—eyes located on the sides of the head—exhibit relatively crude acuity for localizing sounds; these species, incidentally, tend to be prey, meaning they are hunted by predators. Species with narrow visual fields—both eyes located in the front of the head—exhibit superior localization acuity; these species are typically predators. Prey species also tend to have regions of maximum acuity* extending over larger portions of the retina than do predatory species (see Figure 10.20). And from Chapter 8 you will remember that one purpose of eye movements is to direct the region of highest acuity to the object of regard. If that region of high acuity is spatially extensive over the retina, the eye movements need not be as precise. Small, concentrated regions of high acuity, in contrast, require the eyes to be very accurately directed at the object of regard.

So what does this have to do with sound localization? We know that sounds can reflexively trigger head movements toward the source (Thurlow and Runge, 1967) and that head movements also serve to direct the eyes to an object of regard. Putting two and two together, Heffner and Heffner (1992) proposed that sound localization operates to guide the eyes to a source of interest. If eye movement accuracy is crucial (as it is with frontally placed eyes with narrow regions of high acuity), sound localization ability must be good also. But if eye movements need not be precise (because the area of maximum acuity is more extensive, as it is in animals with panoramic vision), sounds need not be localized with great accuracy. This putative linkage between eye movements and sound localization is further strengthened by physiological evidence showing that neurons in certain brain structures, including the superior colliculus, may be activated by either

---

* For each species, the region of maximum acuity was determined by assessing retinal ganglion cell density—you may want to look back to Chapter 3 to refresh your memory about the relation between ganglion cell density and acuity.

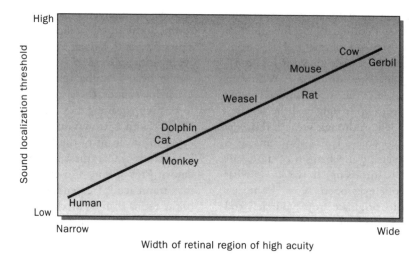

FIGURE 10.20 Graph showing sound localization acuity as the function of the size of the retinal region of high acuity estimated from ganglion cell density. (Adapted from Heffner and Heffner, 1992.)

visual patterns or sounds (see Chapter 4, page 105).

Heffner and Heffner note that this relation applies only to terrestrial animals that don't rely on echo location They conjecture that a major role for hearing is to direct visual attention to sound-producing objects of potential interest within the environment.

THE COCKTAIL PARTY EFFECT: MASKING AND UNMASKING SOUND

Besides sound localization, binaural hearing affords another advantage—listeners are better at picking out one sound from among many in a noisy environment. Because this skill is often required at loud parties, it is aptly called the **cocktail party effect.** In the laboratory, it has been studied using a version of the masking procedure described earlier in this chapter. Using headphones, various levels of noise may be presented to one or both ears, and signals of various intensities may likewise be presented to one or both ears. Moreover, the interval between presentation of the signal and the noise may be varied. As you can imagine from this brief description, these experiments can get rather complicated, as can the

results (see Durlach and Colburn, 1978, for a review of this work). For our purposes of explaining the cocktail party effect, we have summarized the results as follows.

We've already discussed how background noise interferes with the detection of weak sounds, especially when that noise contains strong energy at the same frequencies as the signal. However, even loud noise becomes less effective in masking a sound if the noise comes from a location different from that of the sound. The following observation demonstrates this point. Imagine wearing headphones and having an audible tone delivered to your left ear only. Now suppose noise is also delivered over the headphones to that same ear, with its intensity adjusted so that you are no longer able to hear the tone; the noise, in other words, masks the tone. Finally, suppose the same amount of noise is added to the other ear as well, the one not receiving the tone. Ironically, this additional noise in the other ear actually makes the previously masked tone audible once again. This is called **binaural unmasking.** Besides unmasking the tone, adding noise to the other ear does something else, too—it seems to place that tone and the noise in different locations. With the tone and noise going to the left ear only, both are localized at that ear. But noise introduced to the right ear pairs with the noise already going to the left ear. This now causes the noise to be localized in the center of the head, no longer in the same position as the tone. In other words, when the noise and tone coincide in apparent location, masking is strong; when the two are separated, masking is weak. Binaural unmasking illustrates, then, how localization of sounds can promote perceptual segregation of acoustic events, the idea mentioned earlier in the discussion of auditory perceptual organization. The neural events underlying this unmasking effect are not known, although they most probably have something to do with the neural events involved in sound localization.

Binaural unmasking enables you to focus on one person's voice in the presence of competing conversations elsewhere in a room. However, you are not totally oblivious to those other conversations. If your name happens to be mentioned in one of those conversations, your attention may be drawn to what is being said. This implies that your auditory system continues to analyze unattended sounds. Psychologists interested in selective attention have studied this phenomenon by presenting different, unrelated messages separately to the two ears (Moray, 1959). These experiments typically involve studying a listener's ability to interpret structured verbal messages. Since such tasks probably tap rather refined mental processes, most psychologists would refer to these as cognitive processes, not perceptual ones. In view of this distinction, we shall not discuss the problem of selective attention any further here. Instead, we'll move on to the last topic of this chapter, the perception of speech sounds.

PERCEPTION OF SPEECH SOUNDS

Animals, including people, seem compelled to make sounds, and they will use just about any device at their disposal to do so. Woodpeckers drum their beaks against trees, rattlesnakes shake their tails, gorillas beat their chests, grasshoppers scrape their legs together, and termites grind their mandibles. The variety of resulting sounds is remarkable, ranging from the happy melodies of the robin to the mournful calls of the humpback whale; from the faint, rhythmic ticking of a beetle to the piercing shriek of a baboon. Although some of these biological sounds may just be idle chatter to break the silence, most serve to communicate messages to friends and to foes. Obviously, then, for the sender's messages to be effective, those messages must be received by the other party. In nature, this is one of auditory perception's primary jobs, enabling animals to hear what others have to say.

Of all nature's creatures, humans have developed the largest repertoire of sounds. Human beings can make sounds using various parts of their bodies, including their hands, their feet, and of course their vocal apparatus. Not satisfied with these means, they have also invented devices to assist them in making sounds—including musical instruments, sirens, doorbells, and thousands of other noise makers. But among the many ways that humans have of producing sound, speech is undoubtedly the most important. It used to be commonly believed that the capacity to produce and to perceive speech sounds, more than anything else, set *Homo sapiens* apart from all other creatures. However, as we learn more about the language capabilities of nonhuman species such as the dolphin and the chimpanzee, it becomes necessary to question this belief that speech is the hallmark of the human species. Nonetheless, there is no denying that speech, the vehicle of language, has been immensely valuable in the biological and cultural evolution of the human species.

The study of speech encompasses several disciplines, ranging from neurology to linguistics. Each discipline analyzes speech from a particular perspective. For instance, the neurologist might be interested in the neuromuscular mechanisms responsible for the production of speech—here the emphasis would be on the components of the vocal tract and on the motor areas of the brain that guide the movements of those components. In contrast, a linguist might focus on the structure of grammar—the emphasis here would be less on the hardware of speech and more on the rules governing the formation and interpretation of sentences.

Where does auditory perception fit into this picture? Obviously, to understand a verbal utterance you must be able to hear the associated sounds. So speech perception must take into account the initial stages of hearing, those involved in the reception and processing of sound waves; these are the stages discussed earlier in this chapter and in the previous one. In addition, however, speech perception entails more complex auditory processing. Spoken words are composed of sounds whose acoustic properties are special. In this final section we shall summarize some of the major findings concerning the auditory processing of speech sounds.

THE SOUNDS OF SPEECH

Let's begin by considering the acoustical properties of speech sounds, since these define the relevant information that the auditory system must process in order for speech to be perceived. Speech sounds are produced when air from the lungs is forced through the vocal folds,* a pair of elastic membranes stretched across the upper part of the air passage from the lungs. Air passing through the vocal folds causes them to vibrate, just like the reed on a wind instrument. Male vocal folds are slightly larger than their female counterparts, which means that the male folds vibrate at a somewhat lower frequency than do the female folds. This partially explains why the typical male voice is lower than the typical female voice.

The airborne vibrations produced by the vocal folds, in turn, are modified by changes in the shape of the throat, mouth, lips, and nasal cavity; these components of speech production are intricately innervated by complex sets of muscles that can execute hundreds of articulatory actions per second (Handel, 1989). These actions result in the vowel and consonant sounds that make up speech. Each of these sounds results from a particular po-

sitioning of the elements of the vocal tract. Take a moment to voice slowly several of the vowels and consonants, paying attention to the position of your lips, teeth, tongue, and throat. Notice how these positions differ for various vowels and consonants, which is why they sound different from one another. Not all sound differences are important, though. For example, sound differences associated with regional accents in the United States usually don't prevent people from understanding one another. Sound differences that are important are ones that actually change the meaning of an utterance. Any sound that can produce such a change is called a **phoneme.** Phonemes are considered the distinctive features of speech—together they form the vocabulary of sounds used in a language. When speaking at a normal pace, we produce about 12 phonemes per second, and we are able to comprehend speech at rates up to around 50 phonemes per second (Werker and Tees, 1992). To understand speech perception requires knowing how phonemes are processed by the auditory system. To tackle this problem first requires specifying the acoustical properties of phonemes.

Any phoneme contains acoustic energy at a number of different frequencies. It is impractical, therefore, to define phonemes the way we defined pure tones. Instead, hearing specialists use a more appropriate way to characterize speech sounds; this is called a sound **spectrogram.** A spectrogram is a graph showing the amount of acoustic energy at various frequencies over time. An example is the spectrogram shown in Figure 10.21, which shows a "picture" of the speech energy produced when you utter the word "spike." The vertical axis plots sound frequency and the horizontal axis represents time. Spelled out underneath the horizontal axis is the word "spike," indicating when in time each of its phonemes was uttered. The dark portions of the graph denote the distribution of acoustic energy produced by that utterance; the degree of darkness is proportional to the amount of that energy.

Note that the hiss of the consonant "s" consists of energy distributed over a fairly wide range of frequencies, as indicated by the wide band of

---

* Vocal folds were formerly known as vocal cords.

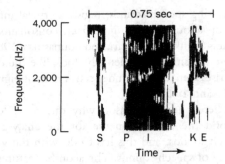

FIGURE 10.21 A sound spectrogram of the utterance "spike."

darkness above that letter. There is a brief period of silence between /s/ and /p/, seen in the spectrogram as an absence of acoustic energy. The vowel "i" consists of several bands of acoustic energy, which in the spectrogram look like a group of worms located above the letter "i." Note that during the course of this utterance, one of these bands of frequencies dips down—this corresponds to the drop in the pitch of your voice when you say the phoneme /i/. (Listen to your voice as you speak this vowel.) In other words, the spectrogram also depicts the intonation of your speech. The spectrogram neatly summarizes the acoustic properties of speech sounds. And as Figure 10.22 illustrates, spectrograms can be created for sentences as well as words. The beauty of the sound spectrogram is that it depicts the entire package of frequencies making up each phoneme

FIGURE 10.22 A sound spectrogram of a sentence. Note the longer time scale in this spectrogram relative to the one in Figure 10.21.

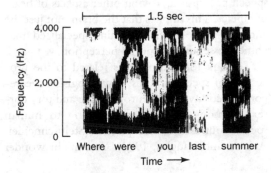

in an utterance, and it shows how those frequencies change over time. The spectrogram visually depicts the transitions and irregularities that characterize different speech sounds. Because an individual's voice reflects the many distinctive features of that person's vocal apparatus and speech intonation, a spectrogram of a voice may be as unique as an individual's fingerprints (Kertsa, 1962). But unlike fingerprints, an individual's spectogram changes with age, coincident with noticeable changes in the sound of the aging person's voice (Liss, Weismer, and Rosenbek, 1990). Incidentally, the spectrographic analysis of sound can also be applied to nonspeech sounds such as the cries made by infants (Green, Jones, and Gustafson, 1987), the vocalizations made by animals (Seyfarth and Cheney, 1984), and the characteristic sounds of the footsteps of males and females (Li, Logan, and Pastore, 1991). It is even possible to create a spectrographic picture of the chilling sound of fingernails scraped over a chalkboard (Halpern, Blake, and Hillenbrand, 1986)!

Armed with this powerful tool for describing the acoustic properties of speech sounds, let's turn to how the auditory system responds to these properties.

THE NEURAL ANALYSIS OF SPEECH SOUNDS

We'll start by thinking about how speech sounds might be represented within the fibers of the auditory nerve which, as you know, respond to narrow ranges of sound frequencies. Each fiber, in other words, "listens" for the presence of particular frequencies in the sound wave arriving at the ear, and different fibers "listen" for different frequencies. With this in mind, look back at the spectrogram shown in Figure 10.21. You could envision points along the axis labeled "Frequency" as representing auditory nerve fibers. Fibers that respond to low frequencies would be situated at the bottom of the axis, whereas fibers that respond to high frequencies would be situated at the top. Thought of in this way, distance along the vertical axis would correspond to distance along the basilar membrane. The horizontal axis would still correspond to time. The changes in the degree of darkness within the spectrogram would now correspond to the amount of neural activity within various nerve fibers.

This way of thinking about nerve fiber activity was introduced by Nelson Kiang (1975), who called the resulting plot of neural activity a **neurogram.** For a given utterance, such as the word "spike," there is a close correspondence between the pattern of acoustic energy in the sound spectrogram and the pattern of neural activity in the neurogram. This correspondence merely confirms that the ear and the auditory nerve perform a frequency analysis on the incoming sound. This cannot be the whole story of speech perception, though. For one thing, there are instances where speech sounds that are perceived as equivalent produce distinctly different sound spectrograms. To give an example, the sound spectrogram representing a particular consonant can vary depending on what vowel happens to follow that consonant. This point is illustrated in Figure 10.23, which shows the spectrographic representations of two utterances, /di/ and /du/. Notice how the transition corresponding to the /d/ sound rises in one case (/du/) but falls in the other (/di/)—yet in both instances, we hear the same /d/ sound. And these variations in the sound spectrogram are registered in the pattern of fiber activity, meaning, for example, that different fibers would be activated by /di/ versus /du/. Yet despite these variations in the pattern of activity, the same consonant is heard. This is because the brain, when

processing speech sounds, registers crucial information about the *transitions* from consonants to vowels (Kaukoranta, Hari, and Lounasmaa, 1988). These transitions, incidentally, look like the dips and rises seen in the sound spectrograms of Figures 10.21 and 10.22.

There's another reason why one must look beyond the auditory nerve for the analysis of speech sounds, and this has to do with the variability of speech sounds. The acoustic features of human speech differ from person to person, which is why it is easy to identify people just by hearing their voices (Itoh and Saito, 1988). Yet despite these individual differences in speech acoustics, we usually have no trouble understanding what people are saying, even when they speak in a whispered voice (Tartter, 1991). This invariance of perception despite variability in the associated stimulus constitutes a form of constancy, similar in principle to size constancy (Chapter 7) and color constancy (Chapter 6) in vision.

So, the brain, in interpreting utterances, uses more than just the specific frequency components making up speech sound. In fact, those concerned with speech perception vigorously debate whether speech perception entails processes fundamentally different from those involved in the analysis of other, nonspeech auditory events (Mattingly and Liberman, 1988). Werker and Tees (1992) summarize this debate, which is presently unresolved. From neurological case studies, it is known that speech perception (Phillips and Farmer, 1990) and voice identification (Lancker, Kreiman, and Cummings, 1989) depend crucially on neural activity in specific areas of the brain—damage to those areas produces selective losses in speech perception, leaving other aspects of hearing intact. This implies that the brain, not just the auditory nerve fibers, contains specialized machinery essential for speech perception.

To look for brain events related to the processing of speech sounds, physiologists have recorded activity from neurons in the auditory cortex of monkeys who are listening to human speech sounds over headphones (Steinschneider, Arezzo, and Vaughn, 1982). You might wonder

FIGURE 10.23 Spectrogram of the utterances /di/ and /du/. (Adapted from Werker and Tees, 1992.)

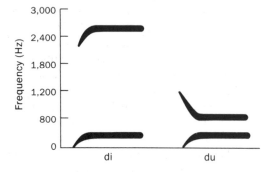

what neural activity in a monkey's brain could tell anyone about perception of human speech sounds. However, these physiologists feel justified in generalizing their results from monkeys to humans because monkeys can discriminate the same speech sounds as humans (Sinnott, Beecher, Moody, and Stebbins, 1976). Without going into details, we can summarize the results as follows. A number of perceptually significant acoustic properties of human speech affect the responses of neurons in the auditory portion of the brain. These properties include (1) the time elapsing between the release of the lips and the start of sound production (the property enabling you to distinguish between such syllables as /pa/ and /ba/); (2) the acoustical context of a sound (such as whether a particular vowel is preceded by one consonant or another); and (3) the rate of frequency changes (an important feature distinguishing certain vowels from one another).

FACTORS INFLUENCING SPEECH PERCEPTION

The Role of Feature Detection in Speech Perception. We've just seen that the auditory system of the monkey contains neurons that respond to perceptually relevant portions of human speech sounds. These neurons are located in a region of the monkey's brain that, when damaged, makes it difficult for the monkey to discriminate human speech sounds (Dewson, Pribram, and Lynch, 1969). Damage to comparable regions of the human brain also produces deficits in speech perception (Marin, 1976). This parallel between monkey and human makes it tempting to believe that the human brain also contains neurons responsive to distinctive features of speech. But how could one go about testing this idea? Think back to Chapter 4, where we described a procedure, selective adaptation, for confirming the existence of visual neurons responsive to lines of different orientations. In that case, staring at lines of one orientation temporarily caused lines of a neighboring orientation to appear tilted away from their orientation. This visual aftereffect presumably re-

sults from the reduced responsiveness of orientation-selective neurons.

The same line of reasoning has been applied in the search for neurons specialized for the analysis of human speech sounds. Peter Eimas and John Corbit (1973) were the first to do this. Using an electronic speech synthesizer, they generated consonant sounds such as /b/, /p/, /t/, and /d/. Included among these consonant sounds were some that were ambiguous, meaning that they might sound like /t/ one time and /d/ the next. These ambiguous sounds, in other words, seemed to lie at the boundary between two unambiguous phonemic categories. Eimas and Corbit had people listen to an unambiguous consonant such as /d/ repeated over and over for several minutes. Following this period of adaptation, people listened to the previously ambiguous consonant, the one that used to sound sometimes like /t/ and other times like /d/. No longer did this consonant sound ambiguous—now it more clearly sounded like /t/ and not like the adapted consonant /d/.

Eimas and Corbit concluded that repeated exposure to one consonant had temporarily fatigued a set of detectors responsive to the distinctive features of that consonant; those feature detectors responsive to other consonants remained at full strength. Thus following adaptation, the ambiguous consonant produced more activity within the set of unadapted feature detectors than within the adapted set. Consequently, listeners heard the consonant sound signaled by the unadapted set of feature detectors. The findings of Eimas and Corbit, along with more recent results using the selective adaptation procedure (Samuel, 1989), point to the existence of neural feature detectors responsive to speech sounds. But this cannot be the entire story of speech perception. As important as they must be for registering the presence of distinctive speech sounds, these feature detectors cannot account for all aspects of speech perception. There are two other important factors that govern how the sounds of speech (the ones signaled by feature detectors) will actually be heard by a listener: the context in which those sounds occur and the perceived boundaries between speech sounds. Let's consider these two factors in turn.

The Role of Context in Speech Perception.

Figure 10.24 illustrates a well-known principle: perception of a stimulus depends on the context in which that stimulus appears. In Figure 10.24, the two center circles are equal in diameter, but one is perceived as larger than the other because of the surrounding dots. The same principle applies in the case of speech perception: how a given speech sound is perceived depends on the context in which it is heard. This context can be defined by any of several sources. One source is the phonetic information occurring closely in time; this influence was illustrated in the /di/ versus /du/ example in Figure 10.23. At a more abstract level, the *topic* of a conversation can itself provide a context for perceiving speech sounds. This form of context is amusingly illustrated by a catchy tune popular during the 1940s. Rendered phonetically, the first several measures go:

Marzi doats n doze edoats n lidul lamzey divey. . . .

Now to those of you who've never heard this song (popularized in the 1940s by Bing Crosby and the Andrews Sisters), this string of "words" may sound like make-believe speech. But in fact the words refer to the eating habits of several familiar hoofed animals. Still puzzled? Try re-

peating the words quickly, paying close attention to the sounds, not the letters. Once you hear the verse as it was meant to be perceived, you'll be able to hear it no other way. Knowing what the song's verses are about will influence what the words sound like to you.

In the case of the nonsense verse, context was provided by the general theme of the song. Speech perception can be influenced by other types of context, too. For instance, the same utterance can sound quite different depending on the *rapidity* with which words preceding that utterance are spoken. To give an example: a syllable may sound like /ba/ when it occurs within the context of a slowly spoken phrase but may sound like /pa/ when occurring within the same phrase rapidly spoken (Summerfield, 1975). The same thing can happen with words in a sentence, as shown by Ladefoged and Broadbent (1957). They tape-recorded multiple versions of the sentence "Please say what this word is," with each version having a characteristic cadence; different versions of the sentence sounded as if they were spoken by different speakers. Listeners heard the different versions of the sentence,* and following each presentation they heard a single word uttered either with the same cadence as the immediately preceding sentence or with one of the other five possible cadences. Listeners simply had to identify the last word. People listening to these recordings frequently misidentified the last word when its cadence differed from that of the preceding phrase. For instance, the same physical utterance was heard as "bit" when preceded by one sentence version and as "bet" when preceded by another. This provides a strong demonstration of context effects in speech perception.

In the examples just cited, the context shaping

FIGURE 10.24 Context influences perception. Are the center dots in these two figures really different sizes, as they appear to be?

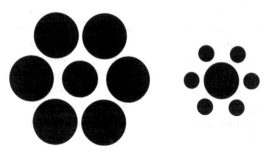

---

* The different versions of the sentence were produced by varying the amount of energy in certain regions of the frequency spectrum; technically speaking, this manipulation alters the formant structure of the speech signal. Perceptually, this manipulation produces utterances that, while readily identifiable as the same sentence, sound as if they were pronounced by different individuals.

the perception of speech sounds was provided by other speech sounds. As the following experiment shows, however, *visual cues* can influence what a verbal utterance sounds like. Harry McGurk and John MacDonald devised a way to put auditory information about a spoken word in conflict with visual information about that word (McGurk and MacDonald, 1976). They had people watch a film of a young woman who was repeating various syllables. In some segments of the film, the audio cue (soundtrack) and the visual cue (lip movement) corresponded to the same syllable, but in other segments the soundtrack for one syllable was dubbed onto the lip movements for another syllable. People reported the syllable accurately when just the sound was heard, and they were able to name the syllable being spoken when just the lip movements were seen with no accompanying sound. (This latter observation merely confirms that people are pretty good at lip reading.) However, people made some very interesting mistakes while watching the dubbed film. One type of mistake involved hearing entirely new syllables, ones corresponding neither to those on the soundtrack nor to those articulated by the speaker's lips. For example, when the syllable /ba/ was dubbed onto lip movements for /ga/, nearly all people reported hearing /da/. In other instances, people heard the syllable formed by the lip movements, not the one actually sounded. Moreover, this strong influence of vision on speech perception is not limited to single syllables. Again using a dubbing procedure, Barbara Dodd (1977) found that people sometimes heard the word "towel" when the sound of a voice saying "tough" was dubbed over the lip movements for "hole." In an interesting twist on this procedure, Green, Kuhl, Meltzoff, and Stevens (1991) generated test sequences in which the gender of the voice heard differed from the gender of the person pictured. Thus, for example, a female voice would utter /ba/ while a male mouthed /ga/. Participants in the experiment readily perceived the incompatibility, but they still heard the phoneme as /da/. In this instance, too, the visual cue influenced the perceived sound but did not dominate.

We can conclude from these dubbing experiments that speech perception depends on more than just the phonetic properties of verbal utterances. In particular, vision provides complementary information about speech. This is fortunate since people often talk to one another in noisy environments where speech sounds may be obscured. Visual information accompanying lip movements can improve speech intelligibility in these situations (Summerfield, 1992). You may be surprised to learn, incidentally, that infants 18 to 20 weeks old can recognize correspondence between auditory and visual components of speech (Kuhl and Meltzoff, 1982). In an experiment to test for this ability, infants viewed a pair of film sequences projected side by side at the same time. Both films depicted a woman's face as she repeated a vowel sound, one vowel for one film and a different vowel for the other. The soundtrack corresponding to one of the two faces was broadcast from a speaker located midway between the two motion pictures. By monitoring the infant's direction of gaze, researchers determined that infants preferred to look at the face whose lip movements matched the sound. This indicates that by 5 months of age infants can detect the correspondence between speech sounds and the lip movements necessary to produce those sounds.

Given vision's influence on speech perception, shouldn't blind people have difficulty in comprehending speech, especially in noisy environments? Paradoxically, just the opposite is true. When asked to discriminate spoken numbers, words, and sentences heard against a background of noise, blind high school students outperformed their sighted classmates (Niemeyer and Starlinger, 1981); this seems to imply that blind individuals hear better than sighted individuals. However, on simpler hearing tests, such as loudness discrimination, the two groups of students were comparable (Starlinger and Niemeyer, 1981). This latter result suggests that the blind students' advantage in speech comprehension reflects superior performance by their brains rather than by their ears or auditory nerves.

The experiments described so far in this section underscore that speech sounds currently cannot be wholly explained by the operation of feature detectors responsive to the acoustic properties of those sounds. Now we shall look at two other important factors that govern how verbal utterances actually sound, namely, the perceived boundaries between words and the intonation, or pitch, of the voice as words are spoken.

The Role of Speech Boundaries and Intonation in Speech Perception. Listening to conversational speech, one usually has no trouble distinguishing words from one another—boundaries seem to exist between words. These boundaries, however, are an illusion. Inspection of a sound spectrogram of a sentence spoken at a normal, conversational speed reveals relatively few identifiable pauses (look back at Figure 10.22). In fact, if one speech sound had to be completed before the next was generated, talking would take forever. So, the boundaries perceived between words have no counterpart in the acoustic signals reaching the ears. Awareness of the paucity of word boundaries occurs when listening to a conversation in an unfamiliar foreign language. In this case, it is difficult to tell where one word ends and another begins—sentences seem to consist of unbroken strings of sounds, with few demarcations to set off one word from the next. Of course, to someone familiar with that language, those individual words are as distinct as the English words you hear during ordinary conversation. What,

then, causes speech sounds to be grouped into separate words?

For one thing, listeners rely on the context of a conversation to help establish those boundaries. An example of this effect of context was provided by the nonsense song introduced earlier—once you discovered what the song was about, the continuous phrase "marzeydoats" sounded instead like "mares eat oats." In the absence of context information, one sometimes errs in establishing boundaries between words, leading to misperceived speech. *New York Times* columnist William Safire (1979) related a particularly amusing instance of misplaced word boundaries. Upon first hearing "the girl with kaleidoscope eyes," a phrase from a Beatles tune, someone thought that the line went "the girl with colitis goes by." Anyone not familiar with the subject of "Lucy in the Sky with Diamonds," the song in which the verse appears, could make such a mistake.

When distinct *pauses* do occur in speech, listeners naturally interpret those pauses as the completion of a clause or of a sentence. These pauses thus serve to inform a listener that it is appropriate to take a turn talking. Pauses, in other words, operate like traffic signals, controlling the flow of a conversation between people. For most individuals, the arrival of an intended pause is signaled by a drop in the pitch of the voice—listen to your voice drop at the end as you speak the sentence "It's ready." Figure 10.25 illustrates this pattern of intonation. A drop in voice pitch signals your listeners that you are through speaking. However, some individuals have a pattern of speaking in

FIGURE 10.25 The continuous line depicts the pattern of intonation as you utter this declarative sentence.

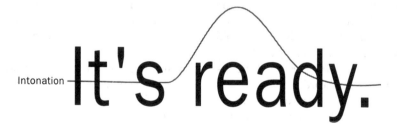

Intonation —It's ready.

which pause signals (drops in voice pitch) occur *before* completion of a sentence. A listener hearing these extraneous pause signals may be confused— the pause signals invite the listener to become the speaker when in fact the other person may not have finished talking.

As you can imagine, people whose speech is punctuated with inappropriate pause signals are inadvertently interrupted quite frequently. One such individual is Margaret Thatcher, the former Prime Minister of Great Britain. A trio of British psychologists, Geoffrey Beattie, Anne Cutler, and Mark Pearson (1982), were intrigued by how often Thatcher seemed to be interrupted during interviews and during debate in Parliament. By analyzing sound transcripts from a television interview with the prime minister, these psychologists discovered that the inflections in Thatcher's speaking voice included frequent drops in voice pitch in the *middle* of her sentences. In other words, Thatcher unwittingly signals listeners that she has finished talking when in fact she has more to say.

Next let's consider the voice intonation accompanying verbalized questions. Listen to the inflection in your voice as you speak the sentence "Is it ready?" Notice how the pitch of your voice rises at the end (see Figure 10.26), in contrast to the falling pitch that characterizes the end of a declarative sentence. Besides signaling the end of a sentence, then, the voice intonation at the end indicates whether that sentence was declarative or interrogative.

Voice intonation, or prosody as it is sometimes called, is also a prime source of information for identifying a speaker on the basis of voice alone. All of us, including newborn infants (DeCasper and Fifer, 1980), are quite good at voice recognition. Evidently the neural machinery responsible for this ability is located in the right hemisphere, for patients with damage to the right parietal cortex (but not the left) exhibit deficits in voice perception, a condition termed **phonagnosia.** This syndrome should not be confused with deficits in speech comprehension, which is typically associated with left hemisphere damage (Evans, 1982b; Corina, Vaid, and Bellugi, 1992). People suffering phonagnosia can understand what is being said but cannot recognize the speaker, even if that speaker is highly familiar (Lancker, Kreiman, and Cummings, 1989).

Voice intonation indicates even more than this. During conversation, one also relies on voice intonation as an index of the speaker's mood. Excitement, whether from enthusiasm or anger, is characterized by marked swings in intonation, whereas calm and boredom are typically signaled by flat, relatively unchanging intonation of the voice. You would be surprised how much information can be conveyed just by humming your sentences—in other words, using only pitch changes to convey a message. Next time you answer the phone, see how long you can carry on a "conversation" using hummed speech. You'll gain an appreciation of intonation's role in speech perception.

FIGURE 10.26 The continuous line depicts the pattern of intonation as you utter this question.

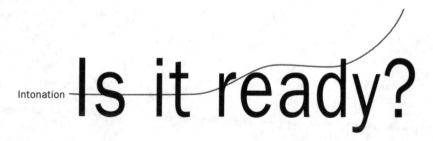

Intonation Is it ready?

S U M M A R Y   A N D   P R E V I E W

These last two chapters have merely scratched the surface of one of perception's most highly developed areas of research, hearing. Acoustics and hearing were among the first fields of study to develop quantitative measures for describing their subject. These developments date back to the early Greeks, who showed experimentally that pitch was related to the length of a vibrating string. Hearing researchers were also among the first to come up with experimental techniques (such as direct scaling) for measuring perceptual reactions to sensory stimulation. These measurements were necessary in order to know what acoustic events actually sound like in terms of loudness, pitch, and so forth. Contemporary research in hearing has made possible a very sophisticated understanding of the initial mechanical and neural events that eventually culminate in auditory perception. Still many of hearing's mysteries remain to be solved, including that very special case of hearing, speech perception.

We are now ready to consider a trio of senses—touch, taste, and smell—that play subtle but important roles in our everyday lives.

K E Y   T E R M S

audibility functions (AFs)
auditory images
bandpass noise
binaural unmasking
bone conduction
broadband noise
center frequency
cocktail party effect
conduction loss
cone of confusion
critical band
discrimination threshold
duplex theory
equal loudness contours
fundamental frequency

harmonics
interaural intensity
    difference (IID)
interaural time difference
    (ITD)
loudness
loudness matching
magnitude estimation
masking
melody contour
missing fundamental
neurogram
otosclerosis
perfect pitch

phonagnosia
phoneme
pitch
power law
presbycusis
profile analysis
relative pitch
sensory/neural loss
sound localization
spectrogram
temporary threshold
    shift
threshold intensity
timbre

Touch

Courtesy of a late-night thunderstorm, your house is plunged into total darkness. As you fumble around the kitchen, you come upon a large bowl filled with fruit. Reaching in, you seize what you hope is an apple. You roll the object around in your hand, exploring various parts with your fingers. You're "looking" at this object with your fingers, searching for information to tell you exactly what it is. Its size, smoothness, and general shape indicate immediately that it's an apple, not a banana or a peach. It takes longer to decide what kind of apple it is. From its firmness and the details of its shape, your fingers tell you it's a ripe Granny Smith.

This hypothetical scenario underscores an important lesson: although we depend heavily on vision to detect and recognize objects, the sense of touch adds a distinctive contribution of its own. Touch helps us identify nearby objects by giving us information about the shape, size, and weight of those objects. Touch also reveals a surface's texture and mechanical consistency, two characteristics that may not be obvious visually. For example, subtle perceptual differences in qualities such as roughness, smoothness, or fuzziness correspond to physical differences in the textures of objects. Similarly, perceptual differences in softness, hardness, and elasticity arise from differences in how readily objects can be compressed. Interestingly, these judgments don't even require direct contact between the hand and the object—many of these tactile qualities can be perceived using a hand-held rod to explore the surfaces of objects (Barac-Cikoja and Turvey, 1991).

To appreciate touch's importance, imagine living in a world devoid of tactile stimulation. Although for most of us the thought is unimaginable, some people do find themselves in such a world. Some patients suffering from multiple sclerosis (a disease affecting the insulating sheath surrounding nerve fiber axons) find it impossible to identify objects by touch; to find their keys in their pocket, for example, they must empty the pocket and inspect its contents visually. Later in the chapter, we'll give other examples of deficiencies in touch perception resulting from brain damage.

But touch does far more than aid object identification; it also plays a major role in development and in social interactions. Dating back to Harlow and Harlow's (1966) classic work with infant monkeys, studies with animals have shown that touch deprivation early in life stunts growth, both physical and social. In rats, for example, the mother's regular grooming of her newborn pups stimulates secretion of growth hormone in the infants; without touch to trigger this secretion, growth is retarded. Touch per se is the key factor here. Secretion of growth hormone in newborn rats is triggered by vigorous, repetitive stroking with a paintbrush (which simulates the normal action of the mother's tongue)—pups receiving this surrogate touch grow at normal rates. Research on premature human infants implies that touch exerts the same therapeutic effect in our species. Diane Ackerman, in her delightful book *The Natural History of the Sciences* (1990), describes case studies in which massaged "preemies" gain weight much faster than do their unmassaged counterparts. In addition, stroked infants seem to be more alert, to be sounder sleepers and, subsequently, to be more advanced cognitively.

Touch makes another important contribution to our lives: it is a universal means of social communication. We shake hands with acquaintances, we embrace close friends and family members, we massage the temples of a distressed companion, we caress the skin of a loved one—all these forms of communication are tactile and all convey specific, unambiguous messages. Some of these touch messages are common to our entire species, no doubt, but others are culturally specific. In Thailand, for example, the top of a girl's head is strictly taboo; to touch the head represents a sexual advance. In many cultures, ours included, touch exchanges between individuals follow unwritten rules of status: the initiator of physical contact is the individual of higher status, and violations of this ritual can be socially awkward. (To confirm this awkwardness, pat the dean of your school on the back the next time you have a chance.)

Despite touch's versatility, this chapter focuses on its ability to provide information about objects and events in the world. In a way, touch can be construed as the most reliable of the sensory modalities. When the senses conflict, touch is usually the ultimate arbiter. Imagine reaching out to grasp an object that you see, only to find nothing there. After the initial astonishment, you'd probably decide that it was your visual system that had been misled—touch, in other words, seems more trustworthy than sight. Or imagine, in the middle of the day, bumping into an object that you could feel but could not see. Again, you'd probably doubt your sense of sight, not your sense of touch. Philosophers such as the eighteenth-century Irish cleric George Berkeley believed that touch provided the basis for calibrating or interpreting the messages of vision. Based on common experience, then, the popular aphorism "seeing is believing" should be rephrased to state "feeling is believing." It is appropriate, though, to say that sometimes we "lose touch with reality."

Touch sensations can arise from stimulation anywhere on the body's surface. Indeed, the skin can be characterized as one large receptor surface for the sense of touch (Sherrick and Cholewiak, 1986).* But most often when you touch an object, your hand is the organ of stimulation. The wonderful and complex abilities of the human hand place it among the most intelligent parts of the body. The skin on the human hand contains thousands of **mechanoreceptors** (receptors sensitive to mechanical pressure or deformation of the skin), as well as a complex set of muscles to guide the fingers as they explore the surface of an object. The mechanoreceptors play a key role in analyzing object detail such as texture; the muscles make their big contribution when grosser features such as size, weight, and shape are being analyzed (Roland and Mortenson, 1987).

But, whether exploring gross details or small details, the hand and the finger pads convey the most useful tactile information about objects. In this respect, the hand is analogous to the eye's fovea, the region of the retina associated with keen visual acuity (Johnson and Lamb, 1981). There is, however, a flaw in this analogy: foveal vision is most acute when the eye is relatively stationary, but touch acuity is best when the fingers move over the object of regard. David Katz (1925), a pioneer of touch research, noted that holding the fingers very still on some surface dulled the ability to sense that surface's spatial features. As Katz noted, moving your fingers across a surface reveals important characteristics about that surface's detailed topography, characteristics that are missed when the fingers are immobile.

It's easy to verify Katz's claim. Think about what happens when you pick up a peach. Upon first grasping it, you can feel the fuzziness of the peach's skin. But if you're now careful not to move your fingers over the surface of the peach, the sensation of fuzziness quickly disappears. Only

---

* Some touchlike sensations originate not from the skin but from inside our bodies. Though such sensations can be important, for instance, in medical diagnosis (Barsky, Goodson, Lane, and Cleary, 1988), we won't cover them here; this chapter, like the rest of the book, focuses on the perception of objects and events in the external world.

by moving your fingers will the true surface quality of the fruit reappear. As you'll learn, this improvement in tactile sensitivity probably reflects the activation of a set of touch receptors that are relatively inactive when stationary fingers make contact with an immobile object.

TOUCH'S DIFFERENT QUALITIES

Touch experiences are triggered by some mechanical disturbance of the skin produced by physical contact with an object. However, the precise nature of that mechanical disturbance varies depending on the physical properties of the object contacted and on the way in which you explore the object tactually. To illustrate what we mean, consider three highly simplified, but representative cases.

First, suppose you're trying to judge the *firmness* of an object by squeezing it with your fingers. Because a hard object won't yield much to the pressure, the skin on your fingertips will be compressed, not the object. A soft object, however, offers less resistance, so the skin will be compressed relatively little. Receptors capable of registering the degree of skin compression could, therefore, furnish information about the firmness of an object.

Next, suppose you're trying to learn something about the *shape* of some small object. Holding it between thumb and forefinger, you roll the object back and forth over your fingertips, looking for telltale clues. If smooth and round like a pea, the object will exert more or less the same forces against your skin at all times. But if it has sharp, irregular edges like a tooth, the object will produce abrupt changes in pressure against your skin. In both cases, moving fingertips have translated the object's shape into a characteristic sequence of skin deformations. Receptors capable of registering the sequence of deformations could provide useful information about the shape and hence identity of the object. Shape information could also come from the changes in the position of your fingers as you explore the surface of any three-dimensional object. Because your finger

movements actually mirror the topography of the object, receptors in the joints of the fingers could signal object shape.

Finally, imagine comparing the *smoothness* of two brands of sheets. As you probably know, rough sheets typically have fewer threads per unit area than do smooth sheets. This means that rough sheets have larger gaps between neighboring threads. These gaps aren't very conspicuous visually, however, so you're better off rubbing your fingers over the two sheets to compare their smoothness. But what actually happens when you make this comparison?

When you rub a finger over a piece of woven fabric such as a bedsheet, the skin's flexibility allows minute sections of skin to be pushed partway into the spaces between the fabric's threads. These small movements of the skin can be thought of as undulations whose frequency mimics the coarseness of the fabric. So touch receptors that register the frequency of skin undulations could provide information about an object's roughness or smoothness.

Here, then, are some distinct perceptual qualities produced by tactile stimulation; each quality corresponds to some physical property of objects. In a moment, we'll see that the skin contains several different types of receptors sensitive to mechanical deformation of the skin. Some of these so-called mechanoreceptors seem well designed to register information about the roughness of a surface, whereas others seem suited for signaling the firmness of an object. But before considering touch receptors and other physiological aspects of touch, let's examine some of touch's capacities.

SENSITIVITY AND ACUITY OF TOUCH

How does one measure touch sensitivity? An old method still in use today was developed by Max von Frey in 1896. Von Frey took hairs of various diameters and lengths and glued each hair to the end of a small stick. Von Frey realized that when the hair was pressed against the skin, it would exert only so much force before bending. Since the force needed to bend a hair depended on its length and diameter, each hair could produce a characteristic maximum pressure and no more. So, for example, a short, thick hair would produce greater pressure than a long, thin hair.

Applying these calibrated hair-probes to several parts of the body, von Frey determined the weakest pressure that could be felt. He discovered that different parts of the body vary dramatically in their tactile sensitivity. For example, the lips and, to a lesser extent, the fingertips are exquisitely sensitive to touch; in contrast, sensitivity is dull on the back and stomach (Geldard, 1972). Interestingly, for any given area of the body, females are generally more sensitive to light touch than are males (Weinstein, 1968). It is also well known that touch sensitivity is dulled when the skin is cooled (Stevens, 1979), in part because the skin (and hence the receptors housed in the skin) is less pliant at colder temperatures.

Besides von Frey hairs, tactile sensitivity can also be measured using a stiff probe that vibrates the skin (Verrillo, 1962; van Doren, Pelli, and Verrillo, 1987). Sensitivity to vibrotactile stimulation is greatest for vibration frequencies around 200 Hz (200 fluctuations in pressure per second). For very low-frequency vibrations (in the range 10 to 30 Hz), sensitivity measured using a large tactile probe is much duller than when measured using a tiny probe (Gescheider, Sklar, van Doren, and Verrillo, 1985). We shall return to this matter of probe size in the section on touch receptors. Regardless of probe size, the region of the body exhibiting the greatest sensitivity to vibration is the palm of the hand, not the fingertips.

Vibrotactile stimulation has some practical uses. For instance, deficits in vibrotactile sensitivity may provide early warning signs of peripheral nerve dysfunction associated with exposure to environmental toxins (Arezzo, Schaumburg, and Petersen, 1983). Vibrotactile stimulation can also be used to present sound information, including speech, to deaf people (Weisenberger and Miller, 1987). Several research groups have developed miniature devices that convert acoustic energy into patterns of vibrotactile stimulation. When such a device is worn on a wristband, different sounds are translated into different patterns of stimulation on the wrist. The vibrotactile stimulation, which is felt as a rapid sequence of taps on the skin, emphasizes the acoustic transients at the onset and offset of a sound. When those sounds are spoken words and sentences, the wearer of the device finds it easier to segment the speech stream, which in turn facilitates lip reading.

It is also possible to measure a different capacity of touch, **touch acuity.** This is conventionally done using the two-point threshold test (see Figure 11.1). To understand this test, imagine using the two points on a drawing compass to stimulate neighboring regions on the skin. How close together can you bring the two points before they meld perceptually into one? This minimum separation is called the *two-point threshold.* Extensive measurements of two-point thresholds have been made over many different places on the body (Weinstein, 1968). When a finger pad is tested, separations as small as 2 millimeters can be reliably discriminated; on the forearm, the just-distinguishable separation is closer to 30 millimeters; and on the back, the minimally discriminable distance grows to 70 millimeters. This form of acuity deteriorates markedly with age (Stevens, 1992).

Places on the body that have very keen touch

FIGURE 11.1 Drawing of apparatus for two-point threshold test. Apparatus is being pressed against extended fingertip.

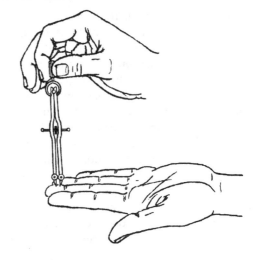

acuity tend also to be places where touch sensitivity is greatest. Those same places also exhibit superior **localization ability:** when a stimulus is applied to the skin within such an area, the location touched can be judged quite accurately. As will become clear in a moment, these acute, highly sensitive areas of the skin contain densely packed mechanoreceptors. Moreover, these supersensitive skin regions enjoy a disproportionately large representation in the cerebral cortex.

LOCALIZATION OF TACTILE STIMULATION

Although touch localization and touch acuity do tend to be linked, they differ in one important way: the ability to discriminate the relative locations of two probes impressed on the skin is considerably better than spatial resolution measured by the two-point technique described above. To explore this performance disparity, Jack Loomis (1981) used tactile probes made from metal sheets with raised dots on them. One type of stimulus, illustrated in panel A of Figure 11.2, used two

FIGURE 11.2 Stimuli used to measure smallest resolvable separation (A) and smallest detectable lateral displacement (B). From left to right in panel A, small raised bumps in each pair grow progressively farther apart. These stimuli can be used to determine the minimum *separation* that the fingertip can just discern. From left to right in panel B, the bump in each pair shifts systematically from the line's left to its right. These stimuli can be used to determine the smallest lateral *displacement*. In an actual experiment, stimuli would be presented randomly rather than in the systematic progressions illustrated here.

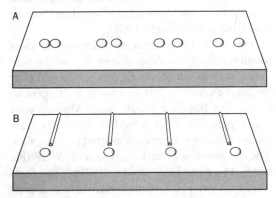

raised dots separated by varying amounts to remeasure spatial resolution. The smallest resolvable separation between two dots was 2.8 millimeters (0.11 inch); dots closer together were indistinguishable from a single dot. In contrast to this poor performance was performance in judging relative position. To measure this, Loomis used a single raised dot presented at various distances either to the left or to the right of a reference line embossed in the metal (see panel B of Figure 11.2). With this stimulus, lateral displacements as small as 0.17 millimeter (0.0067 inch) could be detected. Note that this value is many times smaller than the two-point threshold. To explain the discrepancy between two-point discrimination and discrimination of relative position, Loomis proposed that localization of a point, and hence discrimination of relative position, is governed by the relative responses in an array of receptors. Such a cross-fiber code, as we've seen elsewhere in this book, could represent target location to an accuracy beyond what might be produced by a single receptor operating alone.

In view of the extreme accuracy with which tactile stimulation can be localized, you might expect touch localization also to be very good. Surprisingly, this expectation is very wrong: localization shows large, consistent errors. Two touch researchers, Frank Geldard and Carl Sherrick (1986), explored these mislocalizations using research methods that they likened to a party game. For example, consider a game in which one child lightly touches another child's arm with a pencil. The second child, whose gaze is averted, must indicate exactly where the pencil touched. If you've tried this "game," you know how far off the judgment can be; if you haven't tried it, do. Embarrassingly large errors are the rule as much as the exception.

In a related game, one "writes" on someone's bare back or palm, tracing a letter or word with a finger or the eraser end of a pencil (Heller, 1986). So long as the person can't see the tracing in progress, he or she will find it difficult to tell what's been written. Part of the difficulty comes from mislocalizing various parts of the letter or word. The task can be made even more difficult by frequently lifting the finger or pencil as it writes. These frequent interruptions play on the touch system's tendency to lose track of absolute spatial location.

PERCEPTION OF SURFACE TEXTURE BY TOUCH

Objects often have distinctive texture surfaces that serve as a tactile signature for the object. This texture signature is determined by physical characteristics of the surface. People are quite adept at identifying objects from surface texture alone (recall our hypothetical example of selecting an apple from a bowl of mixed fruit). By using texture information, the sense of touch allows you to make subtle distinctions among objects.

Naturally occurring stimuli, however, don't lend themselves to the systematic study of surface texture. You need an artificial stimulus whose physical properties can be specified quantitatively and varied over a large range. Recall that Chapter 5, on spatial vision, extolled the virtues of one particular type of artificial stimulus, the grating pattern. Gratings have been successfully used in touch research, too. In the case of touch, the gratings are formed by regularly spaced grooves carefully cut into a metal plate or a plastic sheet (see Figure 11.3). A plate containing many grooves per unit area constitutes a high spatial frequency grating; in fact, the grooves can be spaced so close together that the spatial undulations are not even felt, so the surface feels smooth. In a medium spatial frequency tactile grating, the grooves are not so closely spaced; the undulations are more apparent and the surface feels bumpy. Finally, when the spatial frequency is low and each groove is very wide, the undulations again become harder to sense.

So the closeness of spacing of a series of grooves defines the tactile grating's spatial frequency. The depth of the grooves can be varied, too: when the grooves are extremely *shallow,* the surface will tend to feel smoother than when the grooves are deeper. The depth of the grooves in a tactile grating corresponds to the contrast in a visual grating.

Imagine running your fingers across one tactile grating and then another to judge which one is

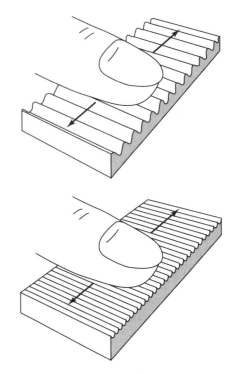

FIGURE 11.3 Drawing of two tactile gratings differing in spatial frequency.

higher in spatial frequency. You'd be able to discriminate between spatial frequencies differing by a little as 3 percent (Lederman and Taylor, 1972). Obviously, then, you could easily tell the difference by touch alone between wide-wale and narrow-wale corduroy fabric. The same stimulus dimension, roughness, also influences affective responses. People tend to find smoothly textured fabrics, such as silk, more pleasant to touch than coarse fabrics, such as burlap (Gwosdow, Steven, Berglund, and Stolwijk, 1986).

The ability to discriminate different degrees of roughness does not depend critically on the particular way in which the fingers are moved over the object's surface, just so long as the fingers do move. But there's a puzzle here. Moving your finger gradually over a surface generates slow modulations in the pressure exerted on your skin, whereas moving your fingers quickly over that same surface produces rapid modulations in pressure. That you perceive the surface as having constant roughness regardless of how you "inspect" it implies that information from touch receptors is referenced to information about the motions of your hand.

With continued use, the fingers develop calluses (thickened keratin layer of the epidermis, the skin's outermost layer). A callus on the fingertip reduces the skin's elasticity and, according to Lederman (1976), should reduce perceived roughness by damping the pressure changes in the skin produced by surface roughness. Lederman asked people how often they used their various fingers to touch objects. She found that the index finger was used most often, the ring finger least often, with the middle finger coming out in the middle. If the degree of callus varies with frequency of finger use, a surface ought to feel least rough with the index finger and most rough with the ring finger. Though it takes carefully controlled experimentation to really verify the prediction, you can check Lederman's conclusion for yourself: one after another, use each of those three fingers to examine the texture of the skin on your cheek. If you're like the participants in Lederman's experiment, your cheek will seem rougher to your ring finger than to your index finger. You can modify the experiment somewhat to confirm also that absolute touch sensitivity is greatest on the tip of your ring finger.

Why should perceived roughness and tactile sensitivity be influenced by the elasticity of the skin on the fingers? We'll postpone answering that question until we get to our discussion of the specialized tactile receptors located just underneath the surface of the skin. Meantime, you now know why safecrackers file their finger pads before going about their business.

READING WITH THE FINGERTIPS

The Braille system consists of sixty-three characters, each made up of closely spaced raised dots. To an inexperienced person, these characters feel like a random collection of bumps. But a person literate in Braille can "read" the characters at 60 to 120 words per minute by moving the fingers over the dots. (Louis Braille, who was blind from childhood, invented this system in the early 1800s, when he was just 16.*) Panel A of Figure 11.4 shows the spatial arrangement of dots used in Braille's system to represent the Roman alphabet's "K," "Q," "A," "P," "O," "D," and "C"; panel B shows the same characters created by raising, or embossing, the letters into the paper. Using the fingers, it's much easier to read text written in **Braille** letters than it is to read text written in embossed (raised) Roman letters. Readers of

---

* Braille's inspiration came from a system that was supposed to allow soldiers to communicate silently and without light on the nighttime battlefield. That system, invented by a French artillery officer, represented various letters by means of twelve raised dots arranged on a grid. This scheme failed because of its complexity; with raised dots in twelve possible positions, it was quite difficult to write the characters, let alone read them (Boorstin, 1985, p. 538).

FIGURE 11.4 Panel A shows the Braille characters for "K," "Q," "A," "P," "O," "D," and "C." Panel B shows the Braille characters as embossed Roman characters. Panel C shows the same Braille characters after blurring. Panel D shows embossed Roman characters (as in panel B) with the same blurring as in panel C. (After Loomis, 1981.)

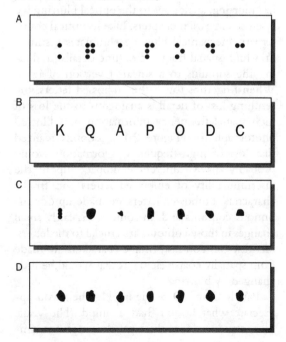

Braille, it turns out, tend to confuse different embossed characters, which slows reading in the same way that a typed page with many typographical errors slows visual reading. This interesting outcome would not have surprised the inventor of the Braille system. When Louis Braille was a student at the Royal Institute for the Young Blind in Paris, the director of the Institute encouraged the sightless students to read from texts written in embossed letters. Louis Braille himself found the embossed alphabet difficult to read, provoking his search for an alternative that did not use alphabet characters (Boorstin, 1985). The widespread use of the Braille system attests to his success.

But why are embossed letters so much harder to read with the fingers than are Braille characters? You might think that with the fingers, continuous lines are harder to follow than raised patterns of dots. But that's not the answer. Instead, as Loomis (1981) showed, the answer lies with the skin's limited ability to pick up fine spatial detail. If you press against the skin with a very thin probe, the probe deforms not just the skin it actually touches, but a fairly wide, neighboring area of skin as well. This spread of effect reflects the mechanical properties of the skin. It can be thought of as mechanical blurring, analogous to the optical blurring we discussed in earlier chapters. Like its optical counterpart, mechanical blurring eliminates a stimulus's high spatial frequencies (fine details), reducing the stimulus to a smeared version of itself. When fingertips touch the embossed letters, the resulting loss of detail is analogous to the loss of high spatial frequency information in a blurred photograph (see Figure 2.11). Loomis realized that loss of high-frequency information would probably have differential impact upon the discriminability of embossed letters and Braille characters. Embossed letters are made up of continuous contours and, in some cases, fairly small changes in those contours are crucial to the letters' identities; in contrast, Braille characters are made from spatially coarse elements that would be little changed by blurring.

Panels C and D of Figure 11.4 help you appreciate what Loomis had in mind. The visual blur introduced into these panels is meant to simulate the mechanical blur produced by the fingertips. Note that blurring leaves the Braille letters fairly distinct (panel C), whereas comparable blur renders many of the embossed letters indistinguishable (panel D). For example, after blurring, the Braille "O" and "D" remain visually distinct, but similar blurring renders the embossed "O" and "D" impossible to distinguish. The low-frequency information available to the skin from different Braille characters is more discriminable than the low-frequency information available from embossed letters. Loomis (1990) has expanded his original insight to create a formal, quantitative model of character recognition and legibility for both tactile and visual characters.

Of course, enlarging the embossed letters would compensate for the limited spatial resolution of the fingers, but this enlargement of letter size would reduce the amount of text that could be imprinted on a page of tactile text, or make it impossible for one letter to fit on a single fingertip. Braille characters represent a good compromise between size and resolution.

Books, particularly textbooks, for visually impaired persons may need to include illustrations, for instance, some drawings or diagrams. Whether the text is in Braille or on audiotape, a computer-controlled stylus embosses the appropriate pattern on stiff paper. The visually impaired person can read the resulting raised material by moving the fingertip over it. One drawback to such material is that it can be difficult to interpret. For instance, common objects presented in the form of raised images are recognized tactually only after great effort and only after considerable time. These same drawings would have been recognized in an instant if they had been presented to the eye.

What causes this divergence between vision and touch? It was probably not a matter of the fingertip's limited spatial resolution. In fact, blurring simple line drawings so as to simulate "blurring" by the fingertips has little effect on visual recognition (Loomis, Klatzky, and Lederman, 1991). The answer probably lies instead in yet another notable disparity between touch and vision.

When we look at a scene or a drawing, the eyes extract visual information simultaneously from a large area. When we use a fingertip to scan an embossed version of the same scene or drawing, at any moment the fingertip gives us information about a very restricted portion of the whole. In order to recognize or appreciate the embossed representation, those small, momentary samples must be somehow pieced together, which would put a huge load on the person's short-term memory.

To decide whether the fingertip's narrow field of view was to blame for the difficulty of deciphering embossed material, Loomis, Klatzky, and Lederman (1991) handicapped vision so that, like tactual input, vision's input would consist of a series of spatially restricted samples. The stimuli, for both vision and touch, were simple line drawings of common objects, for example, a key, a hammer, or a pair of glasses. The subject's task, for either vision or touch, was to identify the object. For tactual recognition, subjects scanned embossed versions of the drawings using either a single fingertip or the tips of two adjacent fingers. For visual recognition, the drawing, presented on a computer display, was first blurred in order to match the finger's low spatial resolution. Additionally, to limit vision's sampling area, only a small section of each drawing was visible at any moment, in the center of the computer screen. The size of this area was adjusted to equalize the sampling areas of vision and touch. Expressed as a proportion of the whole drawing, the visible section's area equaled the fraction of the tactual version that would stimulate either a single fingertip or two fingertips (matching the tactual test conditions). Of course, a moving fingertip does not touch just one single part of the drawing; over time, the fingertip scans many different parts of the drawing. In order to imitate this scanning, during visual testing various parts of the stimulus were made visible. As the subject moved a stylus on the surface of an electronic tablet, the computer sensed the stylus's position and displayed the corresponding section of the drawing that corresponded to that position. For example, moving the stylus to the upper left corner of the tablet caused the upper left corner of the drawing to come into view.

The results were unequivocal. With the larger of the two apertures, visual recognition was vastly superior to tactual recognition. But when vision was limited to sampling the drawings in the smaller bites, analogous to the sampling area of a single finger, visual recognition and tactual recognition were equally poor.

PERCEPTION OF SURFACE TEMPERATURE

Objects often tend to feel warm or cool (Geldard, 1972). When you use your hands to examine a piece of fine furniture, touch receptors register the roughness or smoothness of the wood grain, while temperature receptors respond to the wood's thermal conductivity. "Thermal conductivity" describes the rate at which a surface draws heat away from a hand that's touching the surface. Surfaces such as cement, stainless steel, oak, and maple seem cold to the touch because they have high thermal conductivities; surfaces such as beech wood and various plastics seem warm to the touch because they have low thermal conductivities. This perception of surface temperature of an object has been termed "touch temperature," to distinguish it from the perceived temperature of the ambient environment (Gibson, 1966).

But what determines touch temperature? The temperature of your skin normally falls right around 33°C, with small variations depending on time of day, state of health, and other variables. When you touch an object, the temperature of the area of skin in contact with the object shifts in the direction of the temperature of the object's surface. So when an object feels warm or cool, it is the gradient in temperature between that object and your skin that you perceive, not the actual temperature of the object. This is the basis for a well-known illusion of touch temperature: a surface at room temperature will feel hot to a cool finger but cool to a hot finger. (You can easily experience this illusion by placing one hand in a container of hot water and the other hand in cold water. Now place both hands in the same container of tepid water and note the disparity in perceived temperature between the hands.*) People are actually quite good at detecting even slight deviations from "physiological zero," the temperature described as being neither warm nor cold (Kenshalo, 1972).

The rate of change in skin temperature also is related to the hardness of a surface. For example, metal at room temperature feels cooler than wood at room temperature; this is because a hard surface is a better conductor of heat, including the heat from your skin. Temperature also modifies the perceived weight of an object, as you can experience by performing the following simple experiment. Place a coin on a piece of ice (to cool it) while maintaining a similar coin at room temperature. Now place both coins on the underside of your bare forearm—you should find that the cool coin feels heavier than the neutral coin (Stevens, 1979). This observation suggests that peripheral nerve fibers responsive to pressure are also activated by thermal stimulation.

We won't discuss touch temperature further in this chapter, in part because so little is known about the neural system carrying information about surface temperature.

MENTAL SET AND TACTILE SENSITIVITY

During everyday activities, you sometimes unexpectedly touch—or are touched by—some object. A mosquito lights on your earlobe, a friend taps you on the shoulder, your hand accidentally bumps a glass while reaching for the salt shaker. It's impossible to be certain when or where you're liable to be touched. What are the perceptual consequences of uncertainty about the source and location of tactile stimulation?

This question has been addressed by James Craig (1985), who asked how well people could divide attention among several potential sites of tactile stimulation on the fingers and hand. Stimuli

in Craig's experiment consisted of 108 blunt pins arranged in a rectangular array 6 columns wide by 18 rows high (see Figure 11.5). This array was pressed against the person's finger pad, and each pin could be made to vibrate at 230 Hz. A computer controlled which pins vibrated and which were still. By varying which subset of pins actually vibrated, different spatial patterns of stimulation could be presented to the person's finger. For example, the computer could present tactile patterns that corresponded to different letters of the alphabet.

In one experiment, Craig examined whether uncertainty about location of tactile stimulation influenced a person's ability to identify the pattern of stimulation. With the person's left hand resting on the array of blunt pins, tactile vibrations were delivered simultaneously to both the index finger and the middle finger; on each trial, the index finger received one tactile letter while the middle finger received a different tactile letter. Following each brief presentation, the person had to identify the letter delivered to the particular finger. Craig tested people under two conditions. In one, the

FIGURE 11.5 Two views of Craig's tactile stimulator.

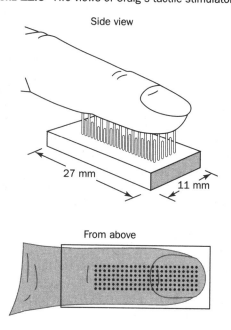

Side view

27 mm

11 mm

From above

---

* This illusion of temperature was first described in the seventeenth century by John Locke (1690/1924). As we noted in Chapter 1, Locke misinterpreted this illusion as proof that the senses were unreliable.

person was instructed before stimulation which finger to pay attention to, whereas in the other, the person was informed only after stimulation. People were much more accurate in identifying the tactile letter when they knew in advance which finger to attend to.

In a second experiment, Craig studied whether people could integrate tactile information from adjacent fingers. On some trials the vibrotactile pattern was presented to a single finger, whereas on other trials the pattern was distributed over two adjacent fingers. Craig predicted that spreading the pattern over two fingers would force a person to shift attention quickly from one finger to another, which would diminish performance. As Craig expected, identification was significantly better when the entire vibrotactile pattern was delivered to one finger. In general, Craig's work shows that uncertainty about the location of tactile stimulation makes it more difficult to identify the stimulus.

At times, uncertainty about touch is more than a mere nuisance; it is a matter of life or death. Each year, 35,000 American women die of breast cancer. Thousands of these deaths could have been prevented if women had simply examined their own breasts for telltale lumps and changes. But it's not enough just to know that you *ought* to do these monthly self-examinations: there are many different ways to tackle a self-examination, and most of them are wrong. Part of the problem seems to be uncertainty about what to "look" for.

Unfortunately, women vary in their native skill at breast self-examination. Physicians, too, vary in the skill with which they examine patients' breasts (Fletcher, O'Malley, and Bunce, 1985). Because perception can often be improved by training, a phenomenon called *perceptual learning,* it is natural to ask what sort of training would improve skill in breast self-examination. Combining basic information about touch sensitivity with an understanding of perceptual learning, some researchers developed a highly successful method for teaching women the right way to conduct a self-examination.

Virtually all studies of perception begin with the proper choice of stimulus. So before they could study breast examination, Bloom and his colleagues (1982) had to develop artificial breasts that would feel natural to the touch. These breast models, made of a silicone material covered with a membrane that mimics the feel of skin, allowed the researchers to study the ease with which simulated tumors (lumps inserted into the model) could be detected. When volunteers palpated the models, detectability improved systematically with lump size, as expected. Practice made it possible to detect smaller lumps. Moreover, the improvement was retained after a layoff of several months. Simply reading about the procedure had no effect: apparently, improvement depends on the actual tactile experience.

In one particularly effective program, the trainee first learns to distinguish between the feel of normal breast tissue and the feel of tissue containing some typical tumors. Trainees are taught to move their finger pads in small circles, first in one spot and then in another, eventually covering the entire breast. Of course, lumps can form anywhere in the breast from just below the skin to quite deep inside. By systematically varying the pressure that they apply, trainees learn to detect relatively superficial lumps (with light pressure) or deeper lumps (with stronger pressure).

Box 11.1 describes other strategies for overcoming the handicap imposed by uncertainty. The effects of certainty show up as changes in brain activity. So, merely anticipating stimulation of a particular finger increases the metabolic activity in the region of the brain that represents that finger (Roland, 1976). Additionally, in at least one area of the brain, the temporal cortex, some cells distinguish clearly between tactile stimuli that are expected and those that are not. These cells respond strongly when the animal's skin is touched unexpectedly but fail to respond to the same touch if the animal has been able to see that touch was impending (Mistlin and Perrett, 1990).

* * *

Having considered some of the psychophysics of touch perception, we're now ready to turn our attention to the neural hardware responsible for registering and processing tactile information.

Box 11.1 *Seeing with the Hands*

Sometimes a person who is both deaf and blind will put his or her hands on a speaker's face. This laying on of hands is part of an effort by the blind and deaf person to understand what is being said. The object is to sense the vibrations produced by the speaker's lips, throat, and jaw. Helen Keller, born deaf and blind, wrote eloquently of all that she could learn from her hands:

By placing my hand on a person's lips and throat, I gain an idea of many specific vibrations, and interpret them: a boy's chuckle, a man's "Whew!" of surprise, the "Hem!" of annoyance or perplexity, the moan of pain, a scream, a whisper, a rasp, a sob, a choke, and a gasp. The utterances of animals, though wordless, are eloquent to me—the cat's purr, its mew, its angry, jerky, scolding spit; the dog's bow-wow of warning or of joyous welcome, its yelp of despair, and its contented snore. (1908, p. 570)

This stratagem allows experienced practitioners to gain remarkably good comprehension of speech, particularly when words are spoken at a moderate tempo. Obviously, when using this technique, the deaf and blind person must divide attention among several sites of stimulation on the hands and fingers.

As described in the text, James Craig has found that dividing attention among different regions of the hand impairs tactile perception. How is it, then, that deaf and blind people pick up the tactile stimulation from speech so well? Just as puzzling, a blind and deaf person will often place a second hand on the speaker's face if he or she is having difficulty understanding what is being said; this maneuver, though seemingly doubling attentional demands, improves comprehension. A clue to this paradoxical observation comes from another of Craig's findings.

Vibrotactile stimulation can be partitioned between pairs of fingers in two different ways. The pattern of tactile stimulation can be divided between two adjacent fingers on the same hand, or the pattern can be divided between one finger on one hand and one finger on the other hand. Surprisingly, Craig has shown that the two-handed condition yields better identification than the one-handed condition. In fact, performance on the two-handed condition is comparable to that measured when the vibrotactile stimulus is delivered to a single finger to which the person is attending.

Why does bilateral stimulation work so effectively? As you will learn shortly, information from the left hand is processed primarily in the right hemisphere of the brain, whereas information from the right hand is processed primarily in the left hemisphere. Craig's paradoxical result may imply that each hemisphere has its own attentional resources and that the deleterious consequence of uncertainty only occurs when a single hemisphere must process multiple tactile inputs.

Here's a brief overview. Mechanical disturbances of the skin are registered by several different kinds of specialized receptors located in various layers of the skin. Afferents from these receptors carry neural impulses evoked by tactile stimulation into the spinal cord, where those impulses are passed to fibers that ascend to the brain. Within the brain, touch information is processed in several specialized cortical regions that contain maps of the surface of the body.

In our discussions of the other senses, we always started with the receptors and progressed to the afferent fibers and finally to the associated sensory areas of the brain. In the case of touch, however, it makes more sense to begin by looking at the nerve fibers that carry touch information to the brain. We'll then backtrack to discuss the receptors that innervate those fibers. We are adopting this approach because the functional roles of touch receptors are easier to appreciate if you first know something about the different classes of afferent nerve fibers associated with touch.

For simplicity, we concentrate on receptors located in—and fibers originating from—the hand. The hand contains just about every type of mechanoreceptor and afferent fiber to be found anywhere on the body's surface. And as we've pointed out, the hand is the principal organ of touch.

PHYSIOLOGY OF TOUCH

TOUCH FIBERS

Information about tactile stimulation of the hand is passed to the spinal cord via two separate nerves, the ulnar nerve and the median nerve. Like all other nerves, these two consist of many *axons,* or *fibers* as they're sometimes called. In the ulnar and median nerves, the axons originate from various regions of the hand. The median nerve, as its name suggests, runs down the middle of the arm, branching out to innervate part of the palm, all the thumb, all the index finger, all the middle finger, and that half of the fourth finger adjacent to the middle finger (Figure 11.6). The ulnar nerve takes its name from the ulna, a large bone in the forearm extending from elbow to wrist on the outside part of the arm. Fibers in the ulnar nerve conduct messages from touch receptors in the rest of the palm, the whole of the little finger, and the adjacent half of the fourth finger.

Each individual fiber signals when a particular region of the skin has been touched. This fact was

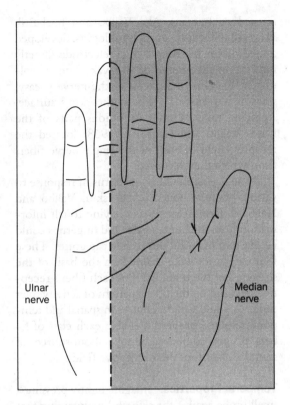

FIGURE 11.6 Innervation pattern of median and ulnar nerves.

established by Edgar Adrian (later Lord Adrian) and Yngve Zotterman (1926), who recorded neural activity from individual fibers while applying tactile stimulation to the skin. The area of skin within which stimuli can influence a fiber's activity constitutes that fiber's *receptive field.* You should see the analogy between a touch fiber's receptive field and a visual neuron's receptive field (the area of the retina within which light affects activity of the neuron).

Following Adrian and Zotterman's classic work, many other physiologists have studied the responses of touch fibers in a variety of species. Of course, when recording neural activity in a nonhuman species, a physiologist doesn't know what kinds of touch sensations are being evoked by the tactile stimuli. This limitation has been overcome in some important experiments performed on humans. Ake Vallbo and Karl-Erik Hagbarth, Swedish neurophysiologists, developed a method for inserting a microelectrode directly into the median nerve of an awake human volunteer. Experimental access to the nerve is easy, since it is relatively close to the skin's surface. Applying touch stimuli to various parts of the hand, Vallbo and Hagbarth (1968) located the receptive field of each of the single nerve fibers from which they recorded.

By analyzing the fibers' patterns of response to various stimuli applied to the skin, Vallbo and Hagbarth found that fibers carrying touch information from the human palm and fingertips could be put into one of four possible categories. These four categories were defined on the basis of the sharpness of the boundaries of each fiber's receptive field and on the fiber's pattern of activity over time. As you'll see, differences in spatial and temporal response properties enable each class of fibers to signal something unique about sources of stimulation within their receptive fields.

Temporal Properties. Imagine lightly pressing a small probe against the skin and maintaining that pressure for a brief time. Recording the activity in many different fibers to this stimulation, Vallbo and Hagbarth discovered two types of fibers. Some fibers responded when the probe was first applied to the skin and continued to respond more or less constantly so long as the pressure was maintained. Fibers of this type are called **slowly adapting (SA) fibers.** Other fibers responded only when the probe was first applied to the skin; these fibers also gave a brief, strong response when the probe was removed. Fibers in this category are called **rapidly adapting (RA) fibers.**

So these first two categories of somatosensory fibers can be distinguished by their responses over time to constant stimulation.

Spatial Properties. Now suppose the probe is used to map a receptive field by stimulating a series of neighboring points on the skin. The spatial layout of the receptive fields reveals that fibers, both SA and RA, come in two types. Fibers of one type, **punctate fibers,** possess small receptive

fields with sharply defined boundaries. Their fields tend to be oval in shape and encompass anywhere from four to ten of the closely spaced ridges that cover the palm and finger pads. Within this small region, sensitivity is approximately uniform.

Fibers of the other type, **diffuse fibers,** have large receptive fields with ill-defined boundaries. Receptive fields of diffuse fibers sometimes cover a whole finger or the greater part of the palm. Because of their large size and blurred boundaries, these diffuse fibers are ill-suited for detailed spatial discrimination.

Four Fiber Groups. Combining the two types of temporal responses with the two types of spatial properties yields four fiber types: SA-diffuse, SA-punctate, RA-diffuse, and RA-punctate. Each of these four types may deliver a distinct message to the central nervous system, since each is best at signaling the presence of a particular kind of tactile stimulation.*

FIBER ACTIVITY AND THE EXPERIENCES OF TOUCH

One approach to functional differences among types of fibers compares responses evoked in each type by stimulation of restricted regions of the skin. Adjusting the temporal pattern of stimulation applied to this single location on an immobile fingertip mimics the effect of moving a fingertip across some pattern, such as an embossed letter. For instance, if a fingertip moved horizontally across the middle of an embossed letter "O," the finger would be stimulated twice, separated by an interval that reflected both the width of the letter and the speed of fingertip movement. In this way,

---

* From various alternatives, we've adopted this set of names for the four fiber groups because they are descriptive and relatively easy for novices to remember. One alternative scheme uses the terms SA-I, SA-II, RA, and PC to stand for what we term SA-punctate, SA-diffuse, RA-punctate, and RA-diffuse, respectively (Johnson and Hsiao, 1992). As you'll see later, the PC system takes its name from Pacinian corpuscle, the receptor from which that system arises.

researchers have recorded afferent fibers' response to various embossed letters, to determine how faithfully the fibers register the spatial details of the letters (Johnson and Hsiao, 1992; Phillips, Johansson, and Johnson, 1992). When stimuli were raised dots consisting of Braille characters, responses within SA-punctate afferents did an excellent job of reproducing the spatial detail of the characters. RA-punctate fibers were a distant second in fidelity of reproduction, with fibers in the other two classes failing almost completely (meaning that their responses to different letters gave no clues as to what the letters were). This suggests strongly that SA-punctate fibers carry the primary information for tactual form and roughness perception.

We could conjecture about the functional significance of different fiber types based on their response properties. But there are two more direct ways to get at this question of functional significance. One is to have a person describe what is felt when a stimulus is applied to the skin during a recording experiment. Keep in mind, of course, that the stimulus used to evoke neural activity in a single fiber actually activates many more fibers than just the one under study—the person's description of that stimulus is not solely attributable to activity in that single fiber (Torebjork, Vallbo, and Ochoa, 1987). The other technique is to stimulate the nerve fiber directly and have the person describe what is felt. Let's consider some results obtained using these two strategies.

NEURAL RESPONSES AND PERCEPTUAL JUDGMENTS EVOKED BY TACTILE STIMULATION

While stimulating a person's hand with weak tactile probes, Johansson and Vallbo (1979) measured the activity in individual fibers and at the same time had the person report whether or not a sensation of touch was felt. When a barely detectable touch probe was applied to the glabrous (smooth, hairless) skin of the hand, RA fibers reliably responded but SA fibers were silent. Activation of SA fibers required a considerably stronger tactile stimulus. So this implies that sensitivity to very light touch is mediated by RA fibers.

Of course, the sense of touch is designed to do more than signal weak, near-threshold tactile stimulation. What kinds of fiber activity are produced by more forceful touch stimulation? Localized indentation of the skin is one common source of stimulation. Such indentation occurs, for example, when you rest a pencil against your chin while thinking. And, of course, applying greater pressure with the pencil produces a stronger sensation of touch on your chin. Suppose that psychophysical and electrophysiological measures are taken while calibrated amounts of pressure are applied to the skin with a tactile probe. The psychophysical measures could be verbal ratings, that is, magnitude estimates (see Chapter 10 and Appendix), and the electrophysiological measures could consist of changes in the activity of touch fibers. When this kind of experiment is done, the SA fibers best mirror the person's verbal ratings: the growth in response with tactical pressure roughly parallels the increase in magnitude estimation ratings made by the person. This finding with humans is reminiscent of earlier work on monkeys by Mountcastle, Talbot, and Kornhuber (1966), who found that SA fibers registered information about touch intensity. We should note, though, that psychophysical and neural responses at the level of nerve fibers are not perfectly correlated, suggesting an important role for subsequent processing (Vallbo and Johansson, 1984).

TOUCH QUALITIES EVOKED BY NERVE STIMULATION

If a given fiber is signaling something fairly specific about a touch sensation, then directly activating that fiber with mild electric current should produce an illusory version of that sensation at a particular location on the skin. (We would term such a sensation "illusory" because there would be no real object on the skin causing that fiber to respond.) The location of the illusory touch would correspond to the location of the stimulated fiber's receptive field, and the quality of the sensation would tell us something about the information signaled by that fiber (Johansson and Vallbo, 1983).

Stimulation of an SA fiber produces a qualitatively different sensation than does stimulation of an RA fiber. When an SA fiber is stimulated electrically, one typically reports a sensation of light, uniform pressure. This can be likened to the pressure of a soft brush held steadily against the skin. When an RA unit is electrically stimulated, the person reports a kind of buzzing or vibration on the skin. You can get some idea of this feeling by rubbing your fingers across the grooves of a long-playing record or the fine mesh of a window screen.

In general, electrical stimulation studies support the idea that SA and RA fibers carry different sorts of information from touch stimuli. There is also evidence that certain types of losses in touch sensitivity resulting from the prolonged operation of vibrating power tools (such as a jackhammer) can be related to damage within particular touch fiber types (Brammer and Verrillo, 1988; Taylor, 1988).

* * *

We are now ready to look more peripherally, at the different types of mechanoreceptors housed in the skin. Each afferent fiber terminates in at least one receptor and carries touch information from that receptor to the central nervous system. Again, remember that the distinguishing characteristics of fiber types reflect structural differences in the receptors that innervate those fibers. The same is true for the other senses. For example, some individual fibers in the auditory nerve respond best to high-frequency acoustic disturbances, whereas other fibers respond best to low-frequency acoustic disturbances. These response differences are not inherent in the fibers themselves; they reflect the different regions of the basilar membrane from which the fibers receive their input. The same principle applies to the touch fibers, which is why it is important to look at the structural details of the mechanoreceptors.

RECEPTORS FOR TOUCH

The smooth, hairless portion of the skin on your hand contains four different types of mechanore-ceptors, together numbering about 17,000 (Johansson and Vallbo, 1983). As mentioned above, each receptor type is associated with nerve fibers that have distinctly different response characteristics: either RA-diffuse, RA-punctate, SA-diffuse, or SA-punctate. The receptors themselves are remarkably diverse in their structure and complexity, and this diversity shapes the functional specificity of different fiber types. Mechanoreceptors are transducers that respond to indentation or pressure on the skin. Some types of receptors are surrounded by a specialized capsule filled with a compressible liquid or gel. The capsule's shape, size, and location determine which kinds of touch stimuli will affect the receptor within that capsule. Consider, for example, a receptor housed within a large, oval-shaped capsule situated in the skin with its long axis parallel to the skin's surface. This capsule's receptor would respond to deformation anywhere within the fairly large area of skin over the capsule. If, however, an oval capsule had its long axis oriented perpendicular to the surface of the skin, tactile stimulation would have to occur within a more circumscribed area to activate the enclosed receptor.

The skin of the fingertips and palm, the touch-sensitive regions emphasized here, contain two types of encapsulated receptors. The two are **Meissner corpuscles** in the upper layer of the skin and the **Pacinian corpuscles** located in the lower layer of the skin. Figure 11.7 depicts these structures and shows their typical locations within the skin. It is believed that the Meissner corpuscle and the Pacinian corpuscle are innervated by RA-type fibers. Also shown in Figure 11.7 are two other, nonencapsulated mechanoreceptors, the **Merkel disks** and the **Ruffini endings.** These two receptor types, which lie at intermediate depths within the skin, are innervated by SA-type fibers. Next, we look more closely at each of these receptor types, starting with the one located most superficially in the skin.

Meissner Corpuscles. Lying just below the surface of the skin, each Meissner corpuscle is tucked into small papillae that line the grooves in the skin of the palm and fingers. The capsule is oriented

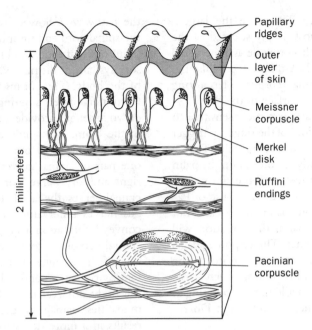

FIGURE 11.7 Cross section through skin of primate finger pad showing location of specialized nerve fiber terminals. (After Darian-Smith, 1985.)

with its long axis perpendicular to the skin's surface. In humans, anywhere from two to six RA-punctate-type nerve fibers enter a single Meissner corpuscle. Because this afferent unit adapts rapidly, it responds best to transient stimulation such as that produced when something rubs against the skin or when the finger is moved over the surface of an object.

The fingertips of young, preteen individuals contain forty to fifty Meissner corpuscles per square millimeter; by age 50, the number of corpuscles has dropped fourfold, to around ten per millimeter. The rate at which corpuscles are lost correlates well with the age-related loss in touch sensitivity for small probes (Thornbury and Mistretta, 1981).

Merkel Disks. Moving just a little deeper into the skin, we next encounter the Merkel disks. This class of mechanoreceptor, usually found in groups of five to ten, is innervated by afferent fibers of the SA-punctate type. It is believed that

these units are active when the skin is stimulated by the steady pressure of a small object.

Ruffini Endings. Ruffini endings lie deeper in the skin and are elongated parallel to the skin's surface. Each individual Ruffini cell is innervated by a single afferent fiber, and neighboring cells may share a single fiber. This convergence of input is analogous to the situation in the eye, where several rod photoreceptors provide input to a single retinal ganglion cell. And as you may remember, spatial convergence operates in the interest of enhanced sensitivity, at the expense of spatial resolution.

The fibers innervating Ruffini endings are of the SA-diffuse type, and it is believed that these neural units provide information about steady pressure on the skin. Because they are also sensitive to stretching of the skin, these SA-diffuse units are active when finger and other joints move, thereby stretching the skin.

Pacinian Corpuscles. These are the largest, least numerous, and most deeply situated of the mechanoreceptors. Each corpuscle is innervated by a single fiber of the RA-diffuse type. Like the Ruffini endings, a Pacinian corpuscle has a long axis that is parallel to the surface of the skin.

Pacinian corpuscles are extremely sensitive to touch. Minute indentations of the fingertip trigger neural impulses in a Pacinian corpuscle. Take a moment to blow as gently as you can on the palm of your hand. The light feeling of the air on your skin most likely originates in the response of Pacinian corpuscles. If you maintain a steady but gentle airflow to your palm, the sensation will diminish or cease altogether. The response adapts rapidly. In the laboratory, investigators isolate the Pacinian corpuscle system by testing touch sensitivity to relatively large tactile probes vibrating at high frequencies (Gescheider, Sklar, van Doren, and Verrillo, 1985).

Because Pacinian corpuscles are located relatively deep in the skin, deformation anywhere within a large area of the skin can affect a single corpuscle, resulting in a spatially diffuse sensitivity. In fact, a single Pacinian corpuscle can have a receptive field as large as several square centimeters. However, these deeply situated receptors provide only crude information about the location of tactile stimulation.

Free Nerve Endings. The skin, both glabrous and hairy, also contains **free nerve endings**—fine, hairlike structures that form a lacey net throughout the layers of the skin. In hairy skin, the free nerve endings wind around the base of hair follicles so that slight bending of a hair will trigger neural impulses in these tactile afferent units. These free nerve endings are also richly distributed throughout mucous regions of the skin, such as that forming the lips and the genital region. They are also found in the cornea of the eye and, as you'll learn in the next chapter, in the nose.

* * *

We've now completed our overview of touch's peripheral sensory hardware and are ready to trace the pathways followed by the touch fibers into the spinal cord and up into the brain. We should point out that touch, unlike any of the other sensory systems, is distributed over the entire surface of the body. This means that many different afferent nerve fibers entering the spinal cord up and down its length provide the input to touch centers in the brain. This multitude of inputs stands in marked contrast to other modalities, where just one pair of cranial nerves (for example, left and right auditory nerves) or at most three pairs of cranial nerves (the facial glossopharyngeal and vagus nerves innervating the tongue and mouth) convey information from peripheral organs to the central nervous system. Consequently, damage to one of the many touch nerves causes a loss of sensitivity that is confined to just that portion of the body innervated by that nerve. With other modalities, damage to the associated nerve fiber results in a more devastating, widespread loss in sensitivity.

ASCENDING PATHWAY FOR TOUCH

Afferent touch fibers enter the dorsal, or back, side of the spinal cord. Inside the spinal cord, these afferent fibers make synaptic contact with two major classes of neurons. One class, called *interneurons,* synapse onto motor neurons, whose axons exit the cord and travel to muscles located in the vicinity of the body where the afferent fibers originated (see panel A of Figure 11.8). This small circuit of afferent/interneuron/motor neurons mediates reflex reactions such as the immediate withdrawal of the hand when it is pricked by a sharp object. The other class of spinal cord neurons that receives inputs about touch travels upward to the brain, carrying input to particular regions in the brain stem. These neurons constitute the so-called *lemniscal pathway;* a second, phylogenetically older pathway, the spinothalamic tract, carries information about pain and temperature. Because of its importance to touch perception, we will concentrate on the lemniscal pathway (*lemniscus* means "band" or "bundle").

As panel B of Figure 11.8 shows, axons in the lemniscal pathway project to nuclei in the brain

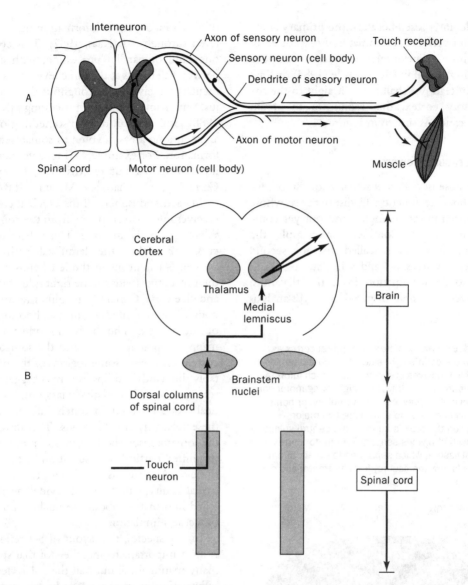

FIGURE 11.8 Panel A is a diagram of the spinal reflex arc mediating response to touch. Panel B is a diagram of the ascending lemniscal somatosensory pathway.

stem. After synapsing, fibers in this pathway cross over the midline, projecting to thalamic nuclei on the opposite side of the brain. At the level of the thalamus, neurons receiving inputs from the superficial and deeper receptors in the skin are segregated. As a result, one set of thalamic neurons responds like the RA-punctate and SA-punctate fibers (the fibers innervating the superficial recep-

tors), whereas another set responds like RA-diffuse and SA-diffuse fibers (the fibers innervating the deeper receptors). Both sets of thalamic neurons send axons to the parietal lobe of the somatosensory cortex, an area of the cerebral cortex largely devoted to sensory analysis of touch information.

We won't go into more detail on the pathways

and nuclei interposed between the primary afferent touch fibers and the somatosensory cortex of the cerebrum. The interested student can read about this material in Mountcastle (1984) or Kaas (1987). Instead, we shall move straight to the somatosensory cortex, that region of the brain whose location is shown in Figure 11.9.

SOMATOSENSORY CORTEX

The somatosensory cortex actually consists of several neighboring, functionally distinct areas whose interconnections are complex and not yet completely understood. Consider, for example, the two major areas, the so-called first and second somatosensory areas, S-I and S-II. Although both receive touch information from the thalamus, S-II also receives input from S-I. So S-II's analysis

of touch incorporates information that's been filtered through S-I (Kaas, 1987). This constitutes one kind of parallel processing, with cross-talk between elements at the same level. This arrangement is widely used throughout the cortex, not just in somatosensory processing (Shepherd, 1988). Still, we can discern something of a hierarchy among areas devoted to somatosensory information. For example, S-II receives much of its input from S-I but returns little, if any (Pons, Garraghty, Friedman, and Mishkin, 1987).

In each hemisphere of the cerebral cortex, S-I receives information arising from the contralateral side of the body and face. This is because of the crossover within the lemniscal pathway (see above). S-I neurons in the left hemisphere have their receptive fields on the right side of the body, and vice versa. Generally, neighboring areas of the body are represented within neighboring regions of the cortex. The body, in other words, is mapped topographically onto the somatosensory cortex. However, some regions of the body, notably the hands and lips, receive exaggerated representation, with a relatively large amount of cortical tissue devoted to touch information from these relatively small regions. This distortion in the somatosensory body map is reminiscent of the magnified cortical representation of the fovea of the eye. And just as the fovea provides detailed spatial acuity, our fingers provide the most detailed information about the quality and location of tactile stimulation.

In any species, the layout of S-I reflects what is most important to members of that species. In many mammals, about half the S-I is devoted to information from the head. In tree shrews and opossums, the nose is emphasized; rats emphasize their whiskers, whereas the brains of squirrels and rabbits are obsessed with the lips. Monkeys and humans emphasize the hand (Kaas, 1987).

The sizes of the receptive fields of neurons in S-I also vary with the fields' locations on the body's surface. As you might guess, cortical neurons activated by stimulation of the fingers or the lips have very small receptive fields compared with neurons devoted to, say, the back (Werner and Whitsel, 1973).

FIGURE 11.9 Drawing of human cerebral cortex as seen from the brain's right side. The somatosensory cortex, which receives and processes touch information, is shown in dark gray; the neighboring motor cortex, shown in light gray, controls voluntary, or nonreflexive, movements. Also shown are two major landmarks on the brain's surface: the central sulcus, a long furrow that divides sensory from motor cortex; and the lateral fissure, which separates the brain's temporal lobe (below the fissure) from its frontal and parietal lobes (above the fissure).

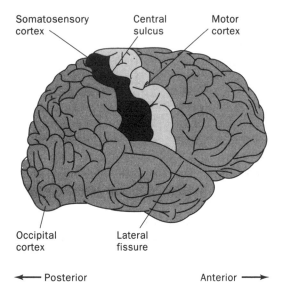

Somatosensory cortex

Central sulcus

Motor cortex

Occipital cortex

Lateral fissure

← Posterior

Anterior →

Early investigators believed that there was just a single map of the body in S-I. We now know, however, that in higher primates the entire region known as S-I contains as many as four separate maps of the body. Each map lies in a strip that runs nearly vertically downward from the top of the brain. The contralateral foot is represented in the upper portion of each map and the head is represented in the lower portion. The details of this layout vary somewhat from species to species and sometimes even between members of the same species (Merzenich et al., 1987). As we'll see later, these differences among individuals in the same species provide important clues about the developmental processes that shape the cortical representations of the body surface.

As just indicated, early investigators underestimated the number of maps in S-I. They also made another error, claiming that the map accurately represented the topography of the body. This map, distorted only to accommodate the exaggerated areas devoted to fingers, lips, and genitals, was usually portrayed as a homunculus, or "little person." Pictures of these bizarre, distorted little people continue to grace various textbooks today. But recent research gives a different picture.

Although neighboring neurons within the somatosensory cortex do tend to represent adjacent areas of the body, overall, the cortical maps only roughly resemble the body's actual topography. As Kaas (1987) notes, a given map may be interrupted at many different locations. Because of these discontinuities, contiguous areas of the body may be represented in noncontiguous parts of the map; also, because of discontinuities in the map, widely separated areas of the body may be represented in neighboring cortical locales. In some cortical maps, for example, neurons representing the hand are sandwiched between neurons representing the back of the head and neurons representing the front of the head.

For historical reasons, the most anterior (forward) of the four strips in S-I is known as Area 3a; the most posterior (rear) strip is known as Area 2, with Areas 3b and 1 lying between. Actually, the four strips, or maps, can be grouped into two sets: neurons in Areas 3b and 1 (the middle strips) respond most vigorously when sites on the skin are touched lightly. They receive inputs, via the thalamus, primarily from the most superficial skin receptors that innervate the RA-punctate and SA-punctate fibers. Neurons in Areas 3a and 2 (the most anterior and most posterior strips) respond poorly, if at all, to light touch on the skin. Instead, they respond strongly either when particular joints are moved—such as the joints of the fingers—or when other structures deep beneath the skin's surface, for example, tendons and muscles, are stimulated. These areas receive inputs, again via the thalamus, primarily from the more deeply situated skin receptors that innervate the RA-diffuse and SA-diffuse fibers.

There's at least a rough correspondence between the receptive field locations of neurons in each strip and the receptive field locations of neurons in adjacent strips. So neurons in Area 3b that represent the skin on a particular fingertip lie near to neurons in Area 3a that represent the tendons and muscles of that same finger.

Turning now briefly to S-II, we find that here also the neurons constitute a map of the body. However, for comparable regions of the body, neurons in S-II have somewhat larger receptive fields than their S-I counterparts. Also, the representations of the hands and lips are less exaggerated in S-II than in S-I.

Compared with the receptive fields of touch fibers, the receptive fields of cortical neurons tend to be more complex. Take two examples of this greater complexity. Certain cortical neurons respond most strongly only when an edge of *particular orientation* lies within the neuron's receptive field. This neuron would respond when the skin pressed against an edge of one orientation but would give little or no response if the skin pressed against an edge of very different orientation. The optimal edge orientation varies from cell to cell. (This may remind you of the orientation-tuned visual cortical neurons described in Chapter 4.) Other neurons, particularly in the posterior strips of S-I, respond most strongly when an object moves *in a particular direction* across the skin. Some neurons give a brisk response when a brush is moved along a finger's long axis or a finger is moved lengthwise across the brush. These same neurons give no response when the brush is moved across the finger or when the finger is moved across the object. Such neurons could provide information during active touch (Warren, Hamalainen, and Gardner, 1986).

SPECULATIONS ABOUT CORTICAL ORGANIZATION

We have stressed the resemblances between the somatosensory cortex's organization and the organization of the visual cortex. Recall that in vision, different subregions, such as V1, V4, and MT, seem to be specialized for processing particular kinds of visual information. Analogously, some regions of the somatosensory cortex handle information from the superficial layers of the skin, while neighboring regions process information from deeper in the skin, as well as from tendons and muscles. What's the purpose, though, of this complex arrangement? What purpose is served by the multiple adjacent maps, such as the maps in Areas 3a and 3b? Although no one can yet say for certain, it may be useful to sketch out some possible answers.

Each individual mechanoreceptor in the skin yields information about just a small portion of the hand. Clearly, then, the appreciation of an object's overall shape, size, and texture requires integration of responses from a large population of receptors (Warren, Hamalainen, and Gardner, 1986). Particularly important may be the integration of information about touch and muscle position. Suppose, for example, with eyes closed, you run the tip of your finger slowly over some grainy wood surface. As the finger moves across the surface, various cortical neurons respond with some frequency of firing. One might imagine that the frequency of the neuron's response reflected, or coded, the surface's grain—the average distance between ridges in the wood's microstructure. In this scheme, a high firing rate might signal that the elements in the wood's grain were quite closely spaced. However, the same neuronal firing rate could have been produced by moving the

fingertip more rapidly across a grain with widely spaced elements. As a result, the neural signal provides ambiguous information about objects and their properties (Darian-Smith, Goodwin, Sugitani, and Heywood, 1984). In order to disambiguate the signal, information about the finger's own movements must enter into the neural equation.

Movement is not the only factor that can introduce ambiguity. Take a nonmoving finger that is pressing against some surface. The receptor response might reflect the depth of the surface's microelements, its scratches, grain, or what have you, but again, the response is ambiguous. Any given response could be produced by a finger that pressed lightly against a deeply structured surface (such as sandpaper with very large grains) or by a finger that pressed more strongly against a finely structured surface (such as sandpaper with very small grains). Again, to disambiguate the receptors' responses, the brain must calibrate the receptor response against the force with which the fingers are pressing.

In both examples, information from touch receptors becomes a useful guide to the properties of object surfaces only when that information is combined with information from receptors deeper in the skin, receptors that signal the state of tendons and muscles. There's good reason, then, for neurons in S-I that signal the responses of superficial mechanoreceptors to adjoin neurons that signal the responses of deeper mechanoreceptors. After all, adjacency could ease the coordination of disambiguating neural computations.

ACTIVE TOUCH: HAPTICS

Usually, when you touch something or someone, you don't simply plop your hand or finger down and leave them still. Instead, you move your fingers about, exploring the object. Think what happens when you grasp and manipulate some delicate object, such as a raw egg. The fingers first move in a coordinated way to form a pouch that fits snugly around the egg, and then, as the egg is lifted or turned, the changing pressure of the fingers on the egg must be regulated carefully.

Feedback from touch receptors controls the fingers' pressure on the egg. Initial contact generates touch signals that guide subsequent finger movements; those finger movements, in turn, generate updated touch signals. You can particularly appreciate the importance of this feedback system when it doesn't work. For instance, when cold has numbed your fingers, it's hard to manipulate delicate objects. This makes complex activities, such as sewing or tying one's shoes, hard to do. Even walking becomes difficult without touch feedback, as you've undoubtedly experienced when your foot has fallen asleep (Sillar and Roberts, 1988).

A foot that's fallen asleep is usually a minor, temporary inconvenience. But when diminished touch results from damage to the brain, its impact can be devastating. In some patients an interruption of the brain's blood supply (a cerebrovascular accident, or stroke) selectively damages the somatosensory cortex, leaving motor function unimpaired. When this selective brain damage diminishes touch feedback from a hand, the patient simply stops using the affected hand for even the most basic everyday activities such as eating or drinking. Ironically, this disuse has further consequences: deterioration of the hand's motor function, which may previously have been spared (Dannenbaum and Dykes, 1988).

For every one of us, finger movements and movements of other parts of the body constitute important actions. Guided by perception, these actions can change the objects being touched and, consequently, can change perception itself, an argument developed by Gibson (1966). The importance of active touch has been confirmed by recent studies of activity in the human brain using neural imaging techniques (Ginsberg et al., 1987).

The hand is an extraordinarily gifted instrument for exploration. When the hand is used to explore an object, information from the skin's touch receptors is actually coordinated or combined with a second kind of information, called **kinesthesis.** Kinesthesis, whose receptors are in the muscles, tendons, and joints, informs us about the movement and position of our limbs. Suppose with eyes closed, you pick up a small, complex object and explore it with your fingers. As fingers encounter various parts of the object, touch receptors signal the properties of those parts. At the same time, kinesthesis provides information about the location of the hand and how the fingers are positioned relative to one another. (This positional information is sometimes referred to as **proprioception.**) As a result, touch information can be related, moment by moment, to the hand and finger positions at which that touch information was acquired. Kinesthesis provides a coordinate system in which various touch experiences can be integrated. An analogy may be helpful. Imagine an unmanned vehicle exploring the surface of another planet. As the vehicle roams about, it sends information back to scientists on earth about the things it encounters. Unless the scientists know the precise location of the vehicle, on a moment-to-moment basis, they will be unable to meld the information they receive into a coherent representation of the planet's surface. Kinesthesis is analogous to information about the changing location of the vehicle. Without kinesthesis, touch receptors in the exploring hand would provide a series of signals about object properties, but those signals could not be translated into a representation of the object being explored—there would be no way to relate touch signals to the position of the hand on the object. Because the coordination of touch and kinesthetic information is so important, a special term, **haptics** (from the Greek "to grasp"), is reserved for sensory information that depends upon both touch and kinesthesis. We say, therefore, that as the hand explores an object, that exploration generates neither touch information nor kinesthetic information alone, but haptic information.

As Gibson (1966) pointed out, our haptic capacities, particularly those of the hand, tend to go unrecognized because they are overshadowed by the hand's extraordinary motor skills and because visual input is usually dominant. But, if visual input is precluded, people are very good indeed at recognizing objects using haptic information alone. For example, Klatzky, Lederman, and Metzger (1985) asked blindfolded subjects to identify 100 different common objects by means of haptic information. Performance was fast and highly accurate.

When people explore objects with their hands, the hand movements are not random, but highly predictable. So, with a small unknown object for example, an observer usually begins the exploration by enclosing the object with the fingers and palm. Lederman and Klatzky (1987) identified several different kinds of stereotyped hand movements, which they termed "exploratory procedures," or EPs. Figure 11.10 depicts the most important of these. Results from a series of related

FIGURE 11.10 Principal exploratory procedures used in haptic examination of objects. Each term in parentheses indicates the stimulus feature most likely to be recognized by the corresponding exploratory procedure. (From Lederman, 1990, as adapted from Lederman & Klatzky, 1987.)

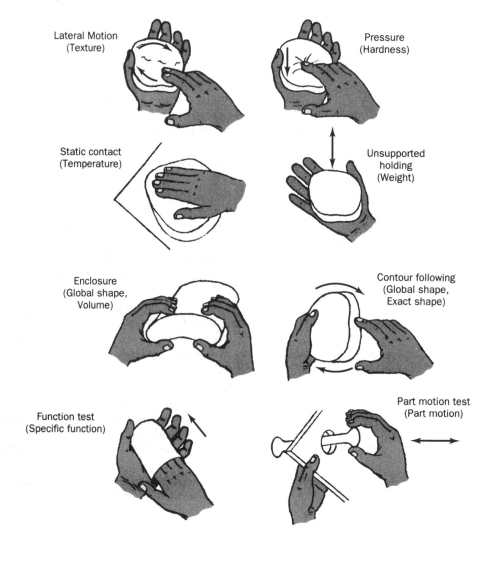

Lateral Motion (Texture)

Pressure (Hardness)

Static contact (Temperature)

Unsupported holding (Weight)

Enclosure (Global shape, Volume)

Contour following (Global shape, Exact shape)

Function test (Specific function)

Part motion test (Part motion)

experiments allowed Lederman and Klatzky (1990) to discover the haptic purposes served by these EPs; here's how they went about it. From earlier work, Lederman and Klatzky knew which stimulus characteristics made it possible for people to discriminate objects haptically. These included texture, temperature, hardness, weight, size, shape, and component motion (movements of an object's parts). Armed with a list of such characteristics, Lederman and Klatzky (1990) began by asking people to imagine handling an object, such as a pencil, and deciding whether this object was a member of some class of objects, say writing implements. For fifty-seven different classes of objects and their members, people identified the haptic properties used to decide about category membership. We'll continue with the pencil example. Observers reported that *shape* was crucial in identifying a pencil as a writing implement; that *texture* allowed them to identify a crayon as a writing implement; and that *size* allowed them to identify a pencil as a used pencil (rather than a new one).

Knowing the characteristic properties for various haptic discriminations, Lederman and Klatzky next tested the role of EPs in extracting those properties. Switching from an imagined discrimination to the real thing, a new group of individuals handled unseen objects one at a time and judged, for each, whether or not it was a member of some class. For example, an observer given a pencil had to state whether it was a writing utensil. On other trials, the person was asked whether the pencil was new or was used. Videotapes revealed that on about 80 percent of all trials, observers began by enclosing the test object with fingers curved and then lifting it (see Figure 11.10). These exploratory procedures provide gross information that was usually insufficient to permit a conclusion. Therefore they were usually followed by one or more other EPs. The selection of a follow-up EP mirrored the property that would be most helpful in deciding category membership. (Recall that this property, for each pair of objects, had been gleaned from the judgments of other people.) For example, if shape were a distinguishing property, people tended to follow the object's contour with their fingers (see Figure 11.10); if texture were most important, people moved their fingers back and forth across the object's surface (see Figure 11.10). Haptic exploration, then, is driven by observers' knowledge of object properties.

From these and related experiments, Lederman and Klatzky (1987) derived two additional characteristics of the EPs: generality and duration. Though each EP was best suited for extracting information about a particular object property, many EPs provided subsidiary information about one or more other properties. This allowed Lederman to rank the EPs on generality of the information, primary and subsidiary, that each gave. Lederman found also that EPs varied dramatically in how long each took to execute. Interestingly, these two measures—generality and duration—tended to be inversely related. One EP, enclosure, offered good generality and rapid execution. Not coincidentally, that one EP typically inaugurated every exploratory sequence in Klatzky and Lederman's experiment.

The analysis of EPs has been extended to children blind from birth (Landau, 1991). In all cases studied, performance by blind children on tasks involving judgments of spatial configurations of objects was similar to that of sighted children tested while blindfolded. We quote the conclusion from this study: "Visual experience is not necessary for the early development of the capacity to explore objects or layouts, the capacity to assemble haptic and kinesthetic information about objects into a unified representation, or the capacity to transform these representations in ways important to mature human spatial cognition" (Landau, 1991, p. 176).

But if vision is not crucial for object representation, what is its role? Outside the laboratory, observers explore and characterize objects in terms of their visual appearance as well as by means of haptic exploration. How is the chore shared between these two sources of information? This question interests not only students of perception but also engineers who must design robots that can operate in distant environments (the moon, for instance) or handle dangerous objects and substances (radioactive material, for example). Suppose the robots have both visual and haptic capacities. Under what conditions should one be used in preference to the other? When do we use one in preference to the other?

Because of the relative speed with which various EPs are executed, haptics is best suited to extract information about properties related to an object's material—its hardness, its temperature, its surface texture—and least well suited as a source about the object's geometric properties—its shape. Lederman, Klatzky, and Pawluk (1993) note that choice of test stimuli can make haptics seem ineffective compared with vision. In particular, imagine having to sort differently shaped three-dimensional objects all made of the same material. Here, compared with vision, haptics would be both slow and inaccurate. Conversely, if the objects were identical in shape but varied only in hardness or in temperature, vision would do poorly compared with haptics. The lesson, then, is that haptics and vision provide complementary sources of information.

Haptics and touch play important roles in another area: both guide skilled motor acts, particularly the grasp and manipulation of objects. Suppose you reach for and pick up a delicate object. Your fingers must exert enough force to hold the object without its slipping but not so much force that the object breaks. The classic demonstration of this trade-off is the robot hand that tries to pick up a raw egg. One approach is to adjust the force of the grip using information from touch receptors in the fingertips. Lederman, Klatzky, and Pawluk (1993) summarize physiological studies that demonstrate the contributions of various touch receptors during different stages of reaching and grasping.

The intimate connection between touch and exploratory motor behavior is mirrored by the proximity of touch areas and motor areas in the cerebral cortex. The area of the brain responsible for activating the muscles of the body, the so-called *motor cortex,* lies immediately adjacent and anterior to the somatosensory cortex. This adjacency simplifies interconnections between these areas and facilitates the coordination of explora-

tory, grasping, and other manipulatory movements needed in active touch.

There is evidence that different regions of the somatosensory cortex control different aspects of active touch. This is most directly shown by temporarily inactivating various localized regions of the somatosensory cortex and measuring the behavioral consequences. In one such study, physiologists at Toho University School of Medicine in Tokyo injected minute amounts of muscimol, a neurotransmitter antagonist, into the finger regions of S-I of the monkey brain (Hikosaka, Tanaka, Sakamoto, and Iwamura, 1985). Before and after various injections, Hikosaka and colleagues tested a monkey's ability to detect and extract small pieces of food embedded in holes in a wooden block (in most tests the monkey's eyes were blindfolded). When the chemical had been injected into Area 3b, the monkey could put its fingers into the hole but seemed unable to detect the presence of food in the hole, even after actually touching the food. This constitutes a sensory deficit. But injections to Area 2 of S-I, presumably a later stage of cortical processing, produced a very different type of deficit.* The monkey's excited behavior showed that the food had been detected, but the animal was unable to move its fingers in the coordinated way needed to extract the food. Other studies, involving permanent lesions to restricted areas of S-I (Randolph and Semmes, 1974) and S-II (Carlson and Burton, 1988), support the idea that these different areas play a crucial role in different aspects of touch.

Touch and motor processes appear to be connected in other ways as well. Some divisions of the somatosensory cortex send signals to more posterior regions of the **parietal cortex,** regions that coordinate touch information with visual information. Such cortical areas participate in the control of eye movements and limb movements. They also make it possible for the animal to orient

---

* We describe Area 2 as "later" than Area 3b because some of Area 2's input comes from Area 3b, although the reverse does not seem to be true.

itself toward important stimuli in the environment (Kaas and Pons, 1988). In humans, a stroke or other damage to these parietal regions produces a remarkable condition called **unilateral neglect.** In this condition, a patient may fail to attend to one side of the body, ignoring it as though it didn't even exist. For example, one patient, as described by the neurologist MacDonald Critchley, reproved his own arm, protesting: "You bloody bastard! It's a lost soul, this bloody thing. It keeps following me around. It gets in my way when I read. I find my hand up by my face, waving about" (Critchley, 1979, p. 118). The ownership of the naughty, wandering arm was denied by the patient despite contrary evidence from the sense of touch.

This condition, in which a person denies ownership of a limb, is the reverse of an equally tragic condition, in which a person claims to have a limb that is objectively not present. In the typical case, long after some body part has been amputated, an amputee experiences what is known as a **phantom limb** (Melzack, 1992). The sense that this phantom is a genuine and integral part of one's body is absolutely compelling. For example, one patient perceived his phantom arm as permanently extended out to the side. This patient, therefore, always walked sideways through any doorway in order to avoid injuring the (nonexistent) limb. Melzack attributes the false sense of limb ownership to responses within the parietal cortex, the same area that is involved in unilateral neglect. But we have ignored the worse aspect of phantom limbs: the excruciating pain that seems to be localized in the limb or in specific parts of the limb. For example, Melzack (1992) mentions that after leg or foot amputation, patients feel that their toes are being "seared by a red-hot poker" (p. 120). Although researchers are actively pursuing a number of leads, there is now no sure way to alleviate such pain.

Often, pain is discussed in relation to touch because the pathways subserving touch can carry information leading to the experience of pain. Moreover, some common forms of pain are generated by strong stimulation of the mechanoreceptors; these experiences can be eliminated by anesthetics that dull the responsiveness of mechanoreceptors or their associated afferent fibers. Although pain, in its many guises, can be both devastating and widespread, we have not devoted a separate section to pain because, unlike seeing, hearing, and touch, it is not a quality that is referred to objects and events in the environment. The phenomenon of phantom limbs demonstrates this fact. Rather, pain is an affective, subjective experience, in the same category as pleasure. Note that we are not saying that pain is unimportant or uninteresting. Pain can be a lifesaving harbinger of impending tissue damage, from either external sources (such as a sharp nail) or internal sources (a swollen appendix). Obviously pain is a powerful motivator, for we try everything possible to avoid or relieve the experience. And pain is certainly grounded in neural activity, for painful stimulation produces widespread activation within the cerebral cortex, as demonstrated by PET activation studies (Talbot et al., 1991). The interested reader can consult Jessell and Kelly (1991) for an up-to-date discussion of pain and contemporary research into this fascinating and frustrating phenomenon.

PLASTICITY IN THE SOMATOSENSORY CORTEX

Earlier, in discussing somatosensory maps, we spoke of species and individual differences in those maps. Recent research demonstrates that throughout life the somatosensory cortex remains malleable, or plastic, and that cortical connections adjust over time to changes in afferent input. This research has intriguing implications for the uniqueness of every human being. But before turning to such implications, we must consider the research itself.

The study of plasticity within the somatosensory cortex was stimulated by Vernon Mountcastle's theory of cortical development (Mountcastle, 1984). Mountcastle depicts the cortex as a dynamic, self-organizing system of interconnected neurons. According to his theory, neurons in a given region of the brain can *potentially* form an

---

Box 11.2 *Illusions of Touch: Keep Your Fingers Crossed*

The oldest known illusion of touch was described by Aristotle more than 2,000 years ago. Suppose that you cross two adjacent fingers and then touch an object, such as a pen, with both crossed fingertips at the same time. It will feel like you're touching two pens, not one. Recently, an Italian psychologist, Fabrizio Benedetti, carried out several ingenious studies of this ancient phenomenon (Benedetti, 1985; 1986). Benedetti started with a puzzle. Suppose, with your fingers *not* crossed and held slightly apart, you touch that same pen with both fingertips. Now, even though two fingertips are being stimulated (as before), you feel only one pen. Why does the illusion not occur in this situation?

Benedetti reasoned from analogy to vision. Under most conditions, when the image of an object stimulates both retinas, we see a single object. This singleness of vision occurs because the two monocular images normally are formed on matching areas of the two eyes. When, however, those images are

formed on nonmatching areas, double vision is experienced—a person sees two objects, not one. Benedetti applied the same reasoning to explain Aristotle's illusion. He hypothesized that we experience perceptual doubling whenever two receptor points (fingertips or retinal loci) not normally stimulated by a single object are stimulated by that object. In the case of touch, if matching sites on adjacent fingers, say, the index and middle fingers, are touched simultaneously, a single object is felt; however, if the same stimulus is somehow applied to nonadjacent fingers, say, the index and fourth fingers, there is an illusory experience of two objects. Note that Benedetti's hypothesis puts visual doubling and touch doubling in a common framework.

Benedetti tested his idea by trying to produce **diplesthesia** (doubled touch) without having to cross the fingers. He used a specially designed clamp to press and hold together volunteers' third and fourth fingers. By changing the amount of pressure on the

---

enormously large number of synapses with other neurons, many more synapses than are *actually* formed. Presumably, afferent fibers coming into the somatosensory cortex from the thalamus compete for contact with—and control over—neurons in the somatosensory cortex. Only a fraction of all possible synapses actually survive this competition. What determines which fibers will win the competition? What controls the selection of particular synapses to be activated from among the horde of potential synapses? In basic terms, the theory claims that the most active inputs win, with less active inputs becoming dormant.

To evaluate Mountcastle's theory, one must study the events that influence the development and maintenance of connections between cortical

neurons and their incoming afferent fibers. This problem has been the focus of research by Michael Merzenich and his colleagues (Merzenich, 1987). Merzenich began by mapping cortical locations that represent touch information from the fingers and hands of adult monkeys. These finger and hand "maps" in the somatosensory cortex turned out to be remarkably plastic, even in adult animals. Though the maps' broad outlines remain fixed, their details can be altered by experience. In one study, Merzenich surgically joined the skin from two adjacent fingers without disturbing the receptors or nerve fibers lying within the skin. This delicate surgical procedure turns previously separate fingers into a single functional unit—anything that happens to one finger also happens to

sides of the fingers, Benedetti was able to displace the fingers' skin by amounts ranging from 3 to 12 millimeters. He then touched the tips of the clamped fingers with either a single sphere or two spheres joined together. The subject reported whether he or she felt one or two objects. Benedetti found that a 4- to 6-millimeter displacement of the skin—without finger crossing—can produce strong illusory doubling of touch sensations.

Extending these observations, Benedetti (1991) used prolonged bandaging to simulate amputation of the middle finger. The bandaged finger was excluded from the hand's exploratory and manipulatory activities; the bandage kept the third finger immobilized. In order to grasp or manipulate an object (say, a pen) the remaining, working fingers had to be used in unusual pairings. For example, people wrote with the pen held between the thumb, index finger, and fourth finger (instead of thumb, index finger, and third finger). These unusual arrangements subjected some pairs of fingers to what was quite rare for them before the amputation: simultaneous

stimulation by a single object. Six months' bandaging brought dramatic changes in diplesthesia. For example, the index and fourth fingers now responded as though they were actually adjacent; simultaneous touch of these new partners no longer produced diplesthesia. One hypothesis, which needs direct testing, is that these perceptual changes reflect some kind of reorganization within the cortical representation of the hand. Such reorganization has been demonstrated by other investigators. Pascual-Leone and Torres (1993) recorded the somatosensory potentials evoked in the human brain by stimulation of the fingers of Braille readers and nonreaders. With Braille readers, who presumably make greater use of their fingertips for fine discriminations, stimulation of the fingertips evoked electrical responses from a larger portion of the cortex than did equivalent stimulation of less-used fingertips. Whatever its physiological underpinnings, though, Benedetti's work throws strong, modern light on Aristotle's intriguing, ancient illusion.

the other. They move as one, and they receive touch information as one.

The procedure had extraordinary consequences. After the newly joined fingers were used for a few weeks, previously sharp boundaries between the maps for the two digits had dissolved, leaving a single cortical representation of the two-finger combination. Moreover, neurons that used to have receptive fields on just one of the digits now had receptive fields extending across both fingers. Next, Merzenich surgically redivided the fingers, restoring them to their normal state. After the fingers were used for a while, the cortical representations of the two fingers again became distinct and separate. The details of the somatosensory map, therefore, are created in response to

experience, and they can be modified by altered sensory input even in adulthood (Wall, 1988). Box 11.2 discusses some behavioral observations on humans that suggest the human brain is capable of analogous remapping.

Up to now we've talked only about cortical reorganization in response to some rearrangement of the fingers, an event that is pretty exotic. Analogous changes in the somatosensory cortex also follow conditions much closer to your own experience. Coordinated behavioral and physiological studies reveal that discrimination of subtle differences in touch stimulation improves dramatically with practice and that this improvement is accompanied by changes in the somatosensory cortex. Recanzone, Jenkins, Hradek, and Merzenich (1992) applied a vibrating stimulator to one spot on a monkey's fingertip. From a series of stimuli, the monkey had to identify the one stimulus that vibrated at a frequency slightly different from the others. Over time, the monkeys were able to make increasingly fine discriminations. Although adjacent, nonpracticed fingers showed some slight improvement as well, the effects on the trained digit were far more impressive, suggesting the practice's effects were localized. Recanzone and colleagues (1992) studied the somatosensory cortex in these same monkeys. Prolonged training produced several changes, including an increase in the area devoted to the trained region of the monkey's finger and a heightened crispness and consistency in responding to stimulus vibration.

This story of cortical plasticity has one other intriguing twist. Changes in organization within the somatosensory cortex induced by training do not occur automatically. If the monkey's finger is stimulated but the animal doesn't have to discriminate one touch stimulus from another, there is very little improvement in performance and correspondingly little change in the somatosensory cortex (Recanzone et al., 1992).* The brain changes only if the monkey pays attention to the stimulated finger. By some means, currently unknown, plasticity of cortical maps is modulated by the behavioral state of an organism.

These laboratory results with monkeys may help shape new therapies for use with humans whose touch sensitivity has been diminished by damage to the somatosensory cortex. Dannenbaum and Dykes (1988) have developed a unique rehabilitation strategy, drawing heavily on Merzenich's work with monkeys. The therapy, which seems quite promising, reeducates one component of touch at a time. To promote reorganization of a damaged somatosensory cortex, Dan-

nenbaum and Dykes encourage the patients to practice skills such as recognizing the presence of rough objects applied to the skin, appreciating the direction in which an object sweeps across the skin, discriminating shapes, and making progressively finer and more accurate localization of touch stimuli. With specific stimulation repeated time and time again, the well-motivated patients who have been studied thus far showed substantial improvement in touch and manipulation of objects.

Whatever their ultimate impact on rehabilitation therapy, Merzenich's findings with monkeys are certainly intriguing. But one must be careful not to misconstrue them. The modifications resulting from altered sensory input occurred within the microstructure of neighboring touch maps; the gross boundaries of the somatosensory area were not affected by experience. It would be wrong to conclude from Merzenich's studies that one area of the brain can take over the function of another. In the *mature* nervous system, the boundaries separating different areas of the brain (for example, somatosensory cortex and motor cortex) become permanently fixed and are not subject to change; only the details of maps within those areas can be reshaped by experience. There is intriguing, preliminary evidence, though, that these boundaries are more flexible in the *immature* nervous system (Kaas, 1991) and that the neuroanatomical and physiological response properties of neurons in various areas can be remarkably reshaped (Schlaggar and O'Leary, 1991; Sur, Garraghty, and Roe, 1988).

Merzenich's studies, together with Mountcastle's theory from which they sprang, carry profound philosophical implications. Human behavior, perception, and personality are all shaped by the billions of connections within the brain. Merzenich has shown some of the influences that can individuate the monkey's brain. Extrapolating from this research on the somatosensory cortex, one suspects that a great many of the neural connections in the monkey's brain reflect what that particular monkey has experienced and paid attention to. It's a small step to the idea that similar influences could also mold the neural connections

---

* The monkeys who did not have to make touch discriminations were actively distracted from attending to what happened on their fingers. These monkeys were serving simultaneously in a second study, on behavioral and physiological effects of practice in making auditory discriminations (Recanzone, Schreiner, and Merzenich, 1993). Those results were described earlier, in Chapter 10.

in human brains. Such influences—your experiences and what you chose to attend to—would make the connections in your brain different from the connections in other human brains. Such differences between brains might explain some of the real differences among people. As you can see, these speculations bear on some truly fundamental issues, including human identity and human diversity. It's exciting even to imagine that in our own lifetimes these basic, long-standing, and perplexing philosophical issues may finally be resolved.

S U M M A R Y   A N D   P R E V I E W

In this chapter we discovered how the sense of touch, working primarily through that remarkable sensory organ the human hand, is capable of fast, highly accurate, and subtle discriminations. We discovered that touch owes part of its success to the information it gets from sets of touch receptors whose different characteristics create diverse and complementary perspectives on the world that lies at our fingertips. An equally important part of its success seems to come, though, from the unique information created by the hand's own skilled and highly purposeful exploration of the world.

The intimate relationships between manual exploration and the resulting sensory response reminded us of the pervasive connections between perception and action. Finally, experiments with controlled, intensive practice dramatized the plasticity of cortical organization and the parallel plasticity of perceptual performance.

We turn in the next chapter to taste and smell, senses that are important not only as channels for information about the world but also as providers of particular delight and pleasure.

K E Y   T E R M S

Braille
diffuse fibers
diplesthesia
free nerve endings
haptics
kinesthesis
localization ability
mechanoreceptors

Meissner corpuscles
Merkel disks
Pacinian corpuscles
parietal cortex
phantom limb
proprioception
punctate fibers

rapidly adapting (RA)
  fibers
Ruffini endings
slowly adapting (SA)
  fibers
touch acuity
unilateral neglect

Smell and Taste

Taste and smell are sometimes called the minor senses, probably out of respect for seeing and hearing. But this designation is arbitrary. Though people do rely heavily on their eyes and ears to guide their everyday activities, the "minor senses" provide crucially important information. The smell of smoke, for instance, can signal a dangerous fire, and the foul taste of spoiled food can prevent ingestion of harmful substances. In fact, many animal species depend almost exclusively on taste and smell to tell them about their world. The mole's very keen sense of smell, to take just one example, allows this animal to live in the dark, safe confines of underground burrows, with virtually no need for eyes. Although humans don't rely as much on taste and smell as do other creatures, we should not underestimate our capacity to use these senses to detect and recognize objects in the environment. In fact, one of the things you are likely to gain from reading this chapter is a healthy respect for your nose and tongue.

As we mentioned above, taste and smell are called the minor senses. They are also sometimes referred to by their technical names, "gustation" (from the Latin *gustare,* meaning "to taste") and "olfaction" (from the Latin *olfacere,* meaning "to smell"). Taste and smell are also sometimes lumped together as the "chemical senses" because the receptors housed in the nose and on the tongue register the presence of chemical substances. In this respect, chemical substances are analogous to light energy that strikes the photo-receptors of the eye. But, as this book has emphasized, you see objects, not light; by the same token, you taste and smell objects and substances, not chemicals. So from the standpoint of an organism concerned with its environment, the term "chemical senses" is a bit misleading. In fact, taste and smell serve precisely the same purposes as vision and hearing; all of them provide behaviorally relevant information about the environment.

Although all the senses work for one common goal, something sets taste and smell apart: the sensations arising from stimulation of the tongue and nose can take on a uniquely pleasurable, sometimes sensual, quality. Sunsets may look beautiful and symphonies may sound enrapturing, but their pleasures are less compelling than the aroma and taste of, say, freshly baked chocolate chip cookies. On the other hand, few sights or sounds are as repulsive as a really putrid smell or foul taste. When there's an annoying song on the radio, you can usually succeed in ignoring it. But try to ignore the stench of a stopped-up toilet. Similarly, just thinking about the taste of some food that made you sick once can nauseate you all over again. Thus in addition to their roles as sources of information, taste and smell wield a powerful emotional impact.

There is a sizable and growing body of data—both perceptual and physiological—concerning taste and smell, and in this chapter we shall discuss some of these findings. (Students interested in a more detailed survey are urged to consult the volume edited by Getchell, Doty, Bartoshuk, and

Snow, 1991.) We shall consider taste and smell separately, although the two are intimately intertwined. Let's begin with smell.

THE SENSE OF SMELL

Smells are with us all the time. From the aroma of your first cup of coffee in the morning to the smell of clean sheets as you doze off at night, you are awash in a sea of odors. Smells enhance the enjoyment of food (which is why appetite decreases when a cold stops up the nose). You can verify this for yourself. Compare the taste of a piece of apple and a piece of raw potato while holding your nose so that you cannot smell them—you'll be astonished to find that on the basis of taste alone, the two are very similar. Odors also influence the ways you spend your money. How often have you passed by a bakery and been enticed in by the smells wafting onto the street? It is said that some bakeries vent their ovens onto the sidewalk, purposely using the aroma of fresh bread to lure customers inside (Winter, 1976). Besides the natural smells of the bakery, some businesses also use artificially created odors to influence people's buying habits. For example, plastic briefcases are impregnated with leather scent to enhance their appeal to prospective buyers, and the market value of a secondhand car increases if it's been sprayed with "new car" smell. Real estate agents like to have a freshly brewed pot of coffee on the stove when a house is being shown, for the aroma is said to convey a sense of "home" to the potential buyer.

Besides the odors of foods, cars, and briefcases, other smells also influence people. TV commercials constantly remind us that we are ourselves an important source of odors and exhort us to buy products that will modify our existing body odors as well as create new ones. In this pursuit, vast amounts of money are spent every year. Such products include deodorants, perfumes, aftershave lotions, mouthwashes, and antiflatulence medications. Nonetheless, every individual continually gives off a unique though invisible cloud of smells.

Your odors constitute a smell signature so distinctive that a trained scent-hound can trace your tracks amid the "noise" of odors from many other people. Only the scents of identical twins seem to confuse good scent-hounds (Kalmus, 1955). But these hounds are not the only creatures that can use scent for tracking. Some humans—the Botocudos of Brazil and members of some aboriginal tribes in the Malay peninsula—can hunt by following their prey's scent (Titchener, 1915). Though few people in industrialized societies perform similar feats, they do have some primitive abilities to use scents for distinguishing people from one another, as the following experiments document.

If you had to judge whether another person was male or female on the basis of smell alone, do you think you could? The answer appears to be yes. Patricia Wallace (1977) tested whether college students could discriminate male from female just by smelling a person's hand. While blindfolded, a student would sniff a hand held one-half inch from the student's nose. The male and female individuals whose hands served as test stimuli had washed thoroughly before the test session and then worn a disposable plastic glove for 15 minutes prior to testing, to promote perspiration. Wallace found that subjects could tell male from female hands, with over 80 percent accuracy. Wallace further found that female sniffers were better at the task than were male sniffers.

In addition to using the smell from sweaty hands, people can also accurately judge gender on the basis of breath odor. Working at the Clinical Smell and Taste Research Center at the University of Pennsylvania, Richard Doty and his colleagues had male and female judges (college students) assess the breath odor of student "donors" who sat on the other side of a partition (Figure 12.1). By inserting their noses into a plastic funnel, the judges were able to smell the breath of the donors, who were exhaling through a glass tube connected to the funnel. Donors had been instructed to refrain from eating spicy food the day before testing and were not permitted to wear any odorous cosmetic products. Most judges scored

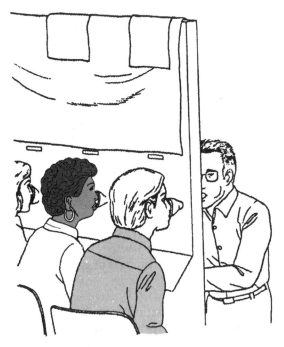

FIGURE 12.1 Setup for measuring gender identification based on breath odor.

better than chance (50 percent) at identifying the sex of the donor, and again female judges outperformed male judges (Doty, Green, Ram, and Yankell, 1982). Doty also had judges rate breath odors for pleasantness and intensity. The breath odors of men were rated on the average as less pleasant and more intense than the breath odors of females. In interpreting their results, Doty and his colleagues noted that fluctuations in reproductive hormones during a female's menstrual cycle cause changes in oral bacteria, which in turn can affect breath odor.

Probably the most remarkable example of acuity for body odor is the case described by William James (1890, vol. 1, pp. 509–510) of a blind woman who worked in the laundry of the Hartford asylum. She would sort the laundry of individual inmates on the basis of smell only, after the clothes had been washed. Less dramatic but impressive nonetheless is the performance of people in the dirty shirt study by Mark Russel, a British psychologist (1976). He had twenty-nine fresh-

men bathe with clear water and then don T-shirts that they wore for the next 24 hours, during which they used no perfume or deodorant. At the end of this period, the T-shirts were collected and individually placed in sealed containers. The same freshmen were now presented with three containers, one with their own shirt, one with the T-shirt worn by an unknown female, and one with the T-shirt worn by an unknown male. Of the twenty-nine people, twenty-two were able to pick out their own T-shirts—a level of performance well above chance. Moreover, twenty-two out of the twenty-nine were also able to identify which of the remaining two T-shirts belonged to a male and which belonged to a female. Male odors were described as "musky," whereas female odors were described as "sweet."

Besides aiding in identification of gender, odors also possess the remarkable ability to call up long-ago memories. A whiff of cedar triggers remembrance of the chest in which your grandmother kept her blankets; scent from a carnation vividly recalls your senior prom; and the smell of clove brings back memories of a dentist's office. Some people have developed a huge repertoire of odor memories and rely on them for their profession. Perfume makers, for example, can discriminate hundreds of aromas, many quite subtle. Astute physicians rely on the nose as a diagnostic tool, using a patient's odors as clues for detecting disease. In fact, any number of disorders have characteristic odors. Here are some examples: typhoid creates a smell like that of freshly baked, brown bread; yellow fever creates a smell like that in a butcher shop; and kidney failure creates a smell of ammonia. (For a complete table of diseases and odors, see Smith, Smith, and Levinson, 1982.)

It is well known that smell plays an enormously important role in the social lives of many animals. Indeed, mammals send and receive at least two dozen different types of odor messages (Doty, 1986), ranging from distress signals to age appraisal. For many animals, mate selection and identification are solely governed by odor. Typically, the females of these species will emit sensuous scents, called **pheromones,** from specialized glands, and these scents can be detected by potential mates. Among such species is the male cabbage moth, an insect whose antennae can sense minute concentrations of the scent released from a sexually receptive female cabbage moth many miles away (Lerner et al., 1990).

The understanding of chemical sex signals has allowed scientists to exploit other species's pheromones. For example, agricultural biologists use pheromones to control some harmful insects. With sex attractants as bait, unsuspecting harmful insects can be lured to their deaths in traps. Pheromones can also be exploited for the eating pleasure of humans. Certain female pigs are trained to hunt truffles, a fungus highly prized by many gourmets. These sows can sniff out truffles buried as much as a meter below ground, and once the truffles are located, the animals root furiously to unearth them. Why do sows expend all that energy, rooting so furiously for a piece of fungus? Truffles contain a chemical with a distinct, musk-like odor that is highly similar to the scent secreted by male pigs during mating behavior. So it appears that the sow's intense interest in truffles is sexually motivated (Claus, Hoppen, and Karg, 1981).

It is natural to wonder whether human sexual behavior is influenced by smell. Is there a pheromone for humans? Certainly the perfume industry would have us believe the answer is yes, but the evidence, while suggestive, is inconclusive. Case studies do disclose that people with serious smell disorders frequently report disinterest in sex (Henkin, 1982), but firm experimental data are lacking. What is clear is that odor signals play a role in the synchronization of menstrual cycles of women living in close contact on a prolonged basis (Graham and McGrew, 1980).

Besides promoting sexual arousal in animals, smells are often employed as defensive weapons. Everyone can testify to the rank odor of a skunk's discharge and can well apppreciate how that odor would ward off enemies (and friends as well). Numerous animal species also employ glandular secretions to mark their territories, often engaging in seemingly bizarre behaviors to ensure that their odor signatures are conspicuous (Macdonald and Brown, 1985). For example, the oribi (a deerlike animal) sticks blades of grass into a gland situated just below its eye, coating the grass with its scent (see Figure 12.2). Odors also guide animals in their search for food, whether it is the bee attracted to the fragrance of flowering plants or the vulture picking up the scent of a dead animal. In fact, the human reliance on eyes and ears to guide vital activities may be fairly unique, since many other animals depend primarily on their noses for such guidance. Indeed, if we were writing this perception book for a nonhuman audience, we'd have to revise it drastically. Instead of emphasizing seeing and hearing, the vast bulk of the book would have to address the most pressing concern of the nonhuman world—the sense of smell.

THE STIMULUS FOR SMELL

Let's start with the basics, asking what physical properties give various substances the power to evoke sensations of odor. As you'll see, the answers are complex. First, to be odorous, a sub-

FIGURE 12.2 Drawing of an oribi coating a blade of grass with scent from its scent gland.

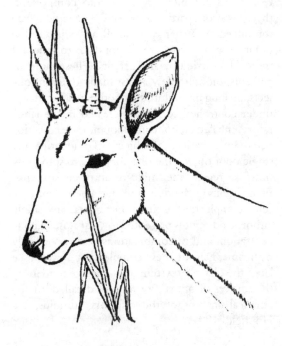

stance must be *volatile*—that is, it must give off vapors (invisible molecules of gas). This requirement has some practical consequences. For example, because heated soup gives off more vapors than cold soup, hot soup smells more inviting. It used to be thought that these volatile molecules had to be airborne to be smelled; according to this view, substances suspended in liquid would be odorless even when they were in direct contact with the sensitive receptors in the nose. Thus if you were to submerge yourself in a pool of perfume, you would smell nothing. Ernst Weber, the nineteenth-century physiologist, actually performed an equivalent experiment: while holding his head upside down, he poured perfume into his nostrils—whereupon he smelled nothing (Boring, 1942). It's now thought, however, that the perfume may have damaged the receptors in Weber's nose, preventing him from smelling anything.

Earlier, in discussing vision and audition, we noted that stimulation reaching the eye or striking the ear usually comprises an aggregate of information from several different objects. We also noted that the perception of distinct visual or auditory objects requires the nervous system to segregate this complex aggregate into components that arose from particular objects. The same is true for olfaction. When you smell an object some distance away, you are responding to odorant molecules carried by air currents. These same air currents, though, blew across many different objects, picking up multitudes of odorants. So except under controlled conditions created in the laboratory, inhaled air contains odorant molecules donated by a variety of objects. To identify any single odor object, the olfactory system somehow must segregate the mixture into constituents. Fluctuations in the direction and speed of air currents complicate the situation further: any single airborne odorant is presented to your nose in concentrations and in combinations that vary greatly over time. Despite these complexities, as we'll see later, the olfactory system does manage to identify the sources of odors. For a more detailed, mathematical analysis of the olfactory stimulus, see Hopfield (1991).

One prerequisite for smell is that the volatile molecules be soluble in fat, because the receptor cells in the nose that capture volatile molecules are surrounded by fatlike materials. When odorous molecules are fat-soluble, they can be absorbed by substances containing fat. This explains why uncovered butter on one shelf of the refrigerator takes on the smell of uncovered tuna fish sitting on another shelf. At the same time, not all volatile and fat-soluble substances are odorous. Additional chemical properties, such as atomic weight, common to all odorous substances, must surely exist (Wright, 1966); identifying these properties remains a challenge. This challenge is closely related to the problem of odor classification, a topic we consider next.

THE CLASSIFICATION OF ODORS

As discussed in Chapter 6, the understanding of color vision was really launched when Newton devised a scheme (the color circle) for describing the relations among different colors. Following Newton's work, there emerged some consensus about the categories of color. It has been widely assumed that odors, too, should fall into distinct categories, comparable in their uniqueness to blue, green, yellow, and red. Knowledge of these odor categories would pave the way for determining the chemical properties shared by members of the various categories. But attempts to identify odor categories have led to much disagreement. We'll consider several of the better-known odor categorization schemes and point out their shortcomings.

The idea of categorizing odors dates back to the ancient Greeks, most notably Aristotle who classified odors as either pungent, succulent, acid, or astringent. Practical concern with odor classification arose in the seventeenth and eighteenth centuries, when it was thought that bad odors were associated with disease and epidemics; by understanding the various "families" of odors, it should be possible to eliminate those that posed danger, or so it was believed (Corbin, 1986).

Probably the best-known system is Hans Henning's (1916) smell prism, a geometric system similar in spirit to Newton's color circle. Henning's geometric model is meant to depict the "principal" odors from which all other odors can be generated. To determine the number of principal odors, Henning used two procedures. First, he instructed people to use verbal labels to describe various scents presented one at a time. Second, he gave people sets of odorous substances and instructed them to line up the substances according to the similarity of their smells (Gamble, 1921). In all, Henning tested well over 400 different odorous substances. Using these sets of judgments, Henning constructed a three-dimensional form—a triangular prism (shown in Figure 12.3)—whose surfaces were meant to reflect people's judgments of odor similarity. Particular odors corresponded to points on the surface of the prism, with nearby points corresponding to odors that were judged similar. Odors were confined to the surfaces and edges of the prism; its interior was considered hollow, meaning that points inside the prism were not used to describe an odor.

Odors near the corners of his prism seemed to Henning to have unique qualities—they could be described using a single verbal label (shown in Figure 12.3). To give you some idea of substances that evoke these six principal odors, we have included in parentheses a substance representative

FIGURE 12.3 Henning's smell prism.

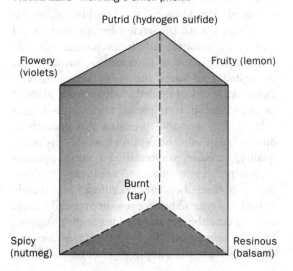

Putrid (hydrogen sulfide)

Flowery (violets)

Fruity (lemon)

Burnt (tar)

Spicy (nutmeg)

Resinous (balsam)

of each. Odors located other than at the corners of the prism (either on an edge or on the plane of one surface) could not be described using a single verbal label. But they could be described by some *combination* of principal qualities represented by the labels at the prism's corners. For example, the smell associated with pine was located along the edge midway between "Fruity" and "Resinous"—implying that the odor of pine possesses both of those qualities. Pine was located where it is on the prism because of its similarity to lemon and balsam. Similarly, the smell of garlic was located on the surface bounded by "Flowery/Fruity/Resinous/Spicy," implying that the odor of garlic possesses all four of those qualities. Again, garlic was placed at that point on the prism because its odor bears at least some similarity to the odors of violet, lemon, balsam, and nutmeg.

Henning's scheme purported to show how odors on the edges or surfaces of the smell prism resemble odors at the prism's corners. This does not mean, however, that a mixture of odors from the corners could produce odors on other parts of the prism. Although it is similar in smell to both balsam and lemon, pine cannot be synthesized by a mixture of those two. In fact, "the resulting odor tends to be a unique percept blend in which both components can be smelled" (Engen, 1982). In this sense, odor shares the analytic character of pitch perception rather than the synthetic character of color perception. For example, if you simultaneously sound a D and an F on the piano, you can hear the separate components in the chord; however, if you mix red and green lights, the result is a synthesis (yellow) in which each component's identity is lost.

Henning's model is appealing for precisely the same reason that Newton's color circle is appealing: both provide a simple, geometrical description of sensory experiences. The accuracy of geometric models is easy to test because they make clear predictions. However, in the case of Henning's smell prism, the predictions have not been confirmed, as William Cain (1978) documents. One major problem is that most people find it impossible to classify odors using just six categories—which implies that Henning may have underestimated the number of principal odors. Critics have also faulted Henning for using a small number of highly trained subjects and for eschewing quantitative analysis of his data. In defense of his procedures, Henning bragged that "the critical introspection of trained psychologists is more valuable than statistics taken on all the students in the University, and the statistical procedure, about which science in America has raved so much, has by no means the precision of a *qualitative* analysis" (Henning, 1916, from a translation by Gamble, 1921).

Following Henning's work, other researchers have also tried to group odors according to qualitative similarities (for example, Crocker and Henderson, 1927). Most of these categorization schemes have started out by identifying a series of semantic descriptors to be used as odor qualities—descriptors such as "sweet," "flowery," "fruity," "burned," and so forth. Whatever odor categories may emerge, therefore, are constrained right from the start; they've got to conform to the specific descriptors chosen by the researcher in the first place. Moreover, there are reasons to question how reliably people can use verbal labels to describe their olfactory sensations (Davis, 1977). The constraints imposed by the descriptors, as well as the difficulty of using any label at all, would distort any classification scheme based on predefined verbal labels.

There is a technique, however, called **multidimensional scaling (MDS),** that sidesteps these problems. This technique was used by Susan Schiffman (1974) to study odor classification. Instead of using descriptor terms for various odors, a person merely compares different odors, numerically rating their similarity to one another. These similarity ratings are then used to place odors within a geometric framework called an odor space. Odors are arranged within the odor space in such a way that the distances separating odors reflect the rated similarity or dissimilarity of those odors. Odors rated as highly similar (such as cinnamon and ginger) would be placed near each other in an odor space, whereas odors judged to be dissimilar (such as vanillin and turpentine) would be located far apart (see the Appendix for

a more detailed description of MDS; Chapter 13 gives another use of this technique). As you can see, the idea of an odor space is reminiscent of Henning's smell prism—both arrange odorous substances in a geometric form based on perceptual similarity. However, the rules for generating an odor space by means of multidimensional scaling differ from those used by Henning. In multidimensional scaling, objective numerical procedures create the geometric arrangement of odors; Henning used his own subjective impressions of data to create his geometric arrangement.

Besides objectivity, the procedures used in multidimensional scaling offer another advantage. The experimenter does not constrain the number of possible dimensions ahead of time; instead, statistical treatment of the similarity ratings determines the number of dimensions needed to place odors in the odor space. (You can think of the dimensions as axes defining the coordinates of a geometrical space, like the Cartesian coordinates used to define the two-dimensional space you're familiar with from plane geometry.)

In using multidimensional scaling, Schiffman found that just two dimensions adequately described the relations among a wide variety of odorous substances. Figure 12.4 replots some of the data from Schiffman's analysis. Look at the various odors in this odor space, and note their relative positions. You'll probably agree that the nearby entries smell more alike than do the widely separated ones. How can the two dimensions that Schiffman's work uncovered be interpreted? To answer this question, Schiffman examined the adjectives people use to describe the various odors she tested. She found that, from left to right in Figure 12.4, odors tended to shade from pleasant (such as vanillin) to unpleasant (such as hydrogen sulfide). It is not too surprising that one strong dimension of odor perception has this "hedonic" quality, for odors so often trigger either approach ("pleasant") or avoidance ("unpleasant"). From top to bottom, however, Schiffman was unable to find any systematic progression in the adjectives used to describe the odors. This finding suggests that this dimension of odor experience does not correlate with any simple psychological dimen-

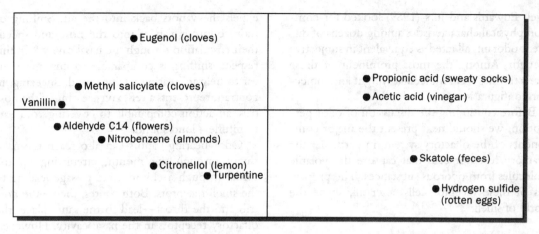

FIGURE 12.4 An odor space, showing the relations among various odors as defined by multidimensional scaling. (Adapted from Schiffman, 1974.)

sion for which there are linguistic descriptors. To what, then, might the ordering in the odor space correspond?

Schiffman (1974) asked whether perceptually similar odors might have some molecular property in common, such as the size or shape of the molecules making up the odorous substances. The discovery of molecular similarities among perceptually comparable odors might furnish important clues about how odorous substances affect receptor cells in the nose. Schiffman considered several molecular characteristics in an attempt to uncover what physical properties, if any, similar smells have in common. Examining the molecular shapes of various substances, she found no relation between the shapes of various compounds and the odors produced by those compounds. This finding, incidentally, contradicts a very popular theory of odor perception. John Amoore (1970), a noted olfactory scientist, proposed that a molecule's shape determines which receptor it is able to stimulate. This theory has been characterized as the lock-and-key model, since the molecule "unlocks" the receptor only if the shape of the molecule matches that of the receptor. According to this theory, molecules that look alike (in terms of the arrangement of their constituent atoms) should also smell alike. However, Schiffman's analysis fails to support this simple idea; she finds

no relation between the shapes of molecules and the similarity of the odors they produce.

Besides molecular shape, Shiffman also examined a number of other chemical characteristics of compounds that smell alike, such as their molecular weight and their solubility in water. However, she found no single characteristic that could explain odor similarity. At the moment, then, the question of the relation between odor quality and molecular structure remains unanswered. Somehow it seems ironic that of all the senses, smell, nature's oldest and most primitive sense, has a stimulus that is one of the most complicated and baffling. This mystery, however, may be close to solution. It is now thought that promising clues concerning the nature and diversity of primary odor qualities may come from studying people with specific losses in odor sensitivity (Wysocki and Beauchamp, 1984). Called **anosmia,** this condition of odor insensitivity may be attributable to genetic deficiencies in the manufacture of olfactory receptor proteins (the importance of which we'll get to in a moment). To the extent that molecular receptor types are related to odor qualities, **specific anosmias** may reveal the diversity of olfactory receptor types.

Besides odor quality—the focus of Henning's model and Schiffman's MDS analysis—odor intensity, too, has been analyzed at the molecular level. Edwards and Jurs (1989) looked for common physical characteristics among dozens of different odorants all rated as equivalent in subjective strength. Among the most prominent of those characteristics were molecular weight and molecular configuration.

Before continuing the discussion of odor perception, we should next present the major components of the olfactory system, in particular the olfactory receptor cells that capture the volatile molecules from odorous substances. The properties of these receptor cells, after all, shape the world of smell.

THE ANATOMY AND PHYSIOLOGY OF SMELL

The stimulus for smell, as noted earlier, consists of airborne molecules, or vapors. The act of inhaling pulls these vapors into the nostrils and then circulates them through the nasal cavity, a hollow region inside the nose where the olfactory (smell) receptors are located (see Figure 12.5). Exhaling

expels the vapors back into the air. Sniffing or more odorous vapors into the nose and speeds their circulation through the nasal cavity.* In this respect, sniffing is comparable to cupping your ear to help in hearing a faint sound. Sneezing, in contrast, represents a reflexive clearing of the nostrils, an action comparable to covering your ears to muffle a loud sound.

Odor-bearing vapors can also reach the nasal cavity through the mouth, circulating up the throat through a chimneylike passage leading to the smell receptors. Both routes, then—the nostrils and the throat—lead to the same place, the olfactory receptors in the nasal cavity. However, vapors from a substance in the mouth may smell

---

* Optimum odor detection occurs when the odorant flows through the nose at a rate of about 30 liters per minute. Interestingly, whenever you try to sniff some odor in your environment, you produce this optimal flow rate without having to think about it (Laing, 1983).

FIGURE 12.5   A cutaway section of a human head, showing the routes taken by air inhaled into the mouth and nasal cavity.

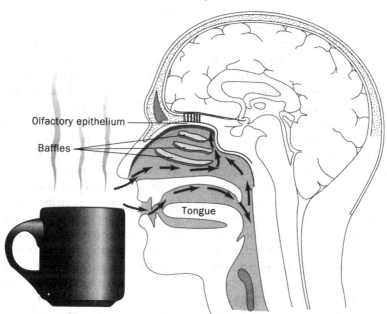

different from the same vapors brought in through the nostrils. This odd disparity is described in Box 12.1 (p. 320).

Most of the air entering the nostrils and mouth flows down the throat to the lungs. However, wisps of air do rise up into the nasal cavity, where they circulate around a series of baffles formed by three bones located in the nasal cavity (see Figure 12.5). As it circulates through this series of baffles, air is warmed and humidified, and debris such as dust is removed by tiny hairs lining the nasal cavity. The entire process has been likened to an air-conditioning system that improves smell acuity (Negus, 1956). As you can imagine, when your nose is congested, the passages of the nasal cavity are narrowed, limiting the amount of odorous vapors that can reach the smell receptors. This is why your sense of smell is dulled when a cold clogs up your nasal cavities. This clogging effect can be chronic in individuals with nasal polyps.

Actually, the two nostrils appear to work in alternating shifts, a phenomenon called the **nasal cycle.** At any given time, the mucous lining in one nostril is more engorged than that of the other nostril, narrowing the nasal passage and offering greater resistance to the inflow of air. This constriction of the nasal passage is under control of the autonomic nervous system and occurs, therefore, unconsciously. You can easily confirm the dominance of one nostril by holding a mirror just under your nose midway between the two nostrils—notice how the two pools of condensation (produced by exhalation) differ in size. Nostril dominance normally switches every 2 to 3 hours (Keuning, 1968), and there is evidence for increased brain activity in the hemisphere contralateral to the dominant nostril (Werntz, Bickford, and Shannahoff-Khalsa, 1987). Some have gone so far as to suggest that people plan their cognitive activities based on which nostril (and, hence, which side of the brain) is currently dominant (Shannahoff-Khalsa, 1986).

So far we've described how vapors are introduced into the nose and how they circulate inside the nasal cavities. Now let's consider how neural elements turn these vapors into the perception of an odor. The receptor cells that register the presence of odorous molecules sit on a patch of tissue called the **olfactory epithelium.** As you can see in Figure 12.5, the olfactory epithelium forms part of the ceiling of the nasal cavity. There are actually two patches of olfactory epithelium, one at the top of each nasal cavity. Each patch of tissue is about the diameter of a dime, but much thinner.

Figure 12.6 shows an enlarged drawing of an olfactory epithelium. Note that the structure labeled **olfactory receptor cell** is embedded in a layer of supporting cells. It is estimated that the

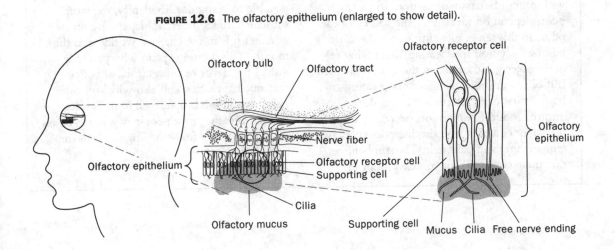

FIGURE 12.6 The olfactory epithelium (enlarged to show detail).

Box 12.1 *Is Olfaction a Dual Sense?*

Have you noticed that some foods smell almost repulsive before you get them into your mouth, but once you start eating them they are enjoyable? Certain strong cheeses, such as Limburger and Roquefort, are good examples of this disparity between odor and flavor. Yet what is referred to as "flavor" is largely the smell associated with the food as it is chewed. This is known from the fact that foods lose their flavor when olfactory cues are eliminated during eating (such as when you have a head cold). How is it, then, that the same food can generate two distinct odor experiences, depending on whether you are sniffing the food or eating it?

Paul Rozin at the University of Pennsylvania, thinks this happens because olfaction is a dual sense—that is, one used to acquire two sets of information: information about objects in the external world and information about objects within the mouth. According to Rozin (1982), these two types of information have different behavioral consequences. Airborne odors arriving through the nostrils can come from a host of objects and events—other people, animals, plants, fire, and so on—only some of which have anything to do with eating. Behavioral reactions to these odors depend on identifying the source of the odor. In this sense, olfaction serves the same interests as vision and hearing, identifying relevant objects and events in the environment. But olfaction's role changes during eating, after food has been selected and introduced into the mouth. Now odors become part of the flavor complex that also includes taste, temperature, and palatability. Rozin believes that these two different contexts (odor in

the mouth versus odor out there) are registered by the olfactory nervous system and give rise to distinctly different perceptual experiences.

Rozin figured that if odor does indeed have different perceptual properties in the mouth versus outside the mouth, people should have trouble recognizing odor through the mouth if their previous experience with the odor was just through the nose. To test this hypothesis, Rozin came up with a set of unfamiliar odors and flavors by mixing together various exotic fruit juices and soups. He then taught blindfolded people to identify these various mixtures on the basis of their odors; each mixture was assigned a number for purposes of identification. Once these individuals had learned to do this, Rozin asked them to identify the same mixtures delivered directly to the mouth through a plastic tube. In this way, any contribution of odor inhaled through the nostrils was eliminated; odor information came entirely from aromas passing up the throat to the olfactory receptors. The results were clear—people made many errors in identifying the mixtures, and they reported that the flavors were impossible to recognize. Evidently, the same substance smells different, depending on whether it is in the external world or in the mouth. This would explain why you may dislike the flavor of things (such as coffee) that smell appealing and also why you can enjoy eating foods that smell foul. Without encouragement, most people would never get around to eating foul-smelling foods in the first place.

human nose contains somewhere between 6 and 10 million olfactory receptor cells. Dogs, in comparison, have about 200 million olfactory receptor cells, which probably accounts for their legendary ability to track the path of a person hours after the individual has trodden that path. Notice also in Figure 12.6 the structure labeled **free nerve ending.** Although these nerve fibers do not themselves give rise to odor sensations, they do significantly influence the perception of odors. We shall consider the role played by these nerve endings shortly, but for now let's continue focusing on the olfactory receptor cells.

There are a couple of things very special about olfactory receptor neurons that set them apart from receptors in the eye and ear. For one, olfactory receptor cells, unlike photoreceptors and hair cells, are genuine neurons, possessing all the paraphernalia of neurons—cell bodies, short dendrites, and long axons. Therefore, olfactory receptor neurons are able to perform two jobs at once: they transduce chemical stimulation into neural impulses, while at the same time carrying those impulses up to the brain along their axons, which make up the **olfactory nerve.** In vision, hearing, and taste, these jobs are assigned to different types of cells. This means, incidentally, that the only neurons in the brain that actually come in contact with the outside world are those located in the nasal cavity.

Even more remarkable, olfactory receptor neurons are constantly dying and being replaced (Graziadei, 1973; Moulton, 1974). Nowhere else in the central nervous system are neurons capable of reproducing. Once in place, neurons elsewhere in the brain are there for life; when those neurons die, the loss is irrevocable. But olfactory cells live for only about 5 to 8 weeks. As a result, the olfactory cells currently at work in your nose have been on the job no more than a few months at most, and already in your lifetime you've gone through hundreds of generations of olfactory receptor neurons. This turnover of neurons is all the more remarkable when you realize that as each new olfactory cell matures, its axon must grow an appreciable distance to reach its target site in the brain. And once there, each axon presumably

must form connections that effectively duplicate those that were undone by the death of its predecessor—otherwise odors would not smell the same from one month to the next. Buck (1992) discusses several possible means by which this amazing developmental feat might be accomplished.

Some people believe that this cyclical turnover of cells may have something important to do with reduced sensitivity to an odor following prolonged exposure to that odor, a phenomenon well documented in the environmental health literature (Ahlstrom et al., 1986). But, in order to appreciate how this might come about, you'll need to know a little more about the structure of the olfactory receptor neurons, in particular the parts that actually extend into the mucous lining of the nose.

From the short, dendritic end of each olfactory receptor cell extends a clump of several **cilia**—thin, hairlike structures suspended in a thin layer of mucus that coats the surface of the nasal cavity. The receptor sites for olfaction are imbedded in the membrane of these cilia; to reach the receptor sites, molecules of odorant must pass from the inhaled air into the mucus layer. In this effort, odorants may have some help from olfactory binding protein (Snyder, Sklar, Hwang, and Pevsner, 1989; Anholt, 1991). Olfactory binding protein, as its name implies, has a chemical affinity for a great many different odorants. It traps and concentrates odorous molecules, ferrying them into the mucus and thence to the receptor sites. This process is illustrated schematically in Figure 12.7. Although some details remain to be nailed down, it's almost certain that the actual receptors are long protein molecules that snake back and forth through the ciliary membrane.* The odor-

---

* Olfactory receptor proteins, of which more than a hundred different varieties have been identified, are members of a large family of receptors, all of which (1) crisscross the membranes of host cells exactly seven times, and (2) employ the same basic mechanisms for initiating signals in those host cells. This superfamily of receptors includes the protein portions of rod and cone pigments, and many chemical receptors in the brain, including those for serotonin and dopamine (Shepherd and Firestein, 1991; Buck 1992).

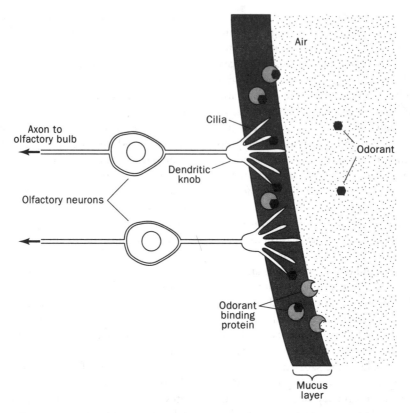

FIGURE 12.7 Odorants received at the olfactory epithelium are picked up by specialized proteins and transported to receptor sites on the cilia. (Adapted from Levitan and Kaczmarek, 1991.)

ant molecules bind to specific sections of the receptor proteins embedded within the ciliary membrane. Binding of the odorant to the receptor triggers a series of molecular events that, in rapid succession, calls into play several different intermediaries located within a cilium (Lindner and Gilman, 1992). The last of the intermediaries is an enzyme that triggers electrical changes in the cell, probably by binding to specific proteins that form the outer membrane of the cilia.

Different olfactory receptor neurons presumably have different receptor proteins, making them differentially responsive to various odorants. Lancet (1986) provides a thorough summary of the evidence favoring the existence of olfactory receptor proteins. According to this protein hy-

pothesis, specific anosmias are attributable to the absence of specific receptor proteins. Temporary anosmia (a temporary, reversible loss in odor sensitivity) would occur whenever the cilia are damaged, as they are by certain toxic chemicals and by some drugs. Once new cilia grow, odor sensitivity returns.

These ideas about odor transduction are controversial, and much remains to be learned about the specifics. For instance, it's not known whether one olfactory receptor neuron houses just a single type of receptor protein or several different proteins. Setting aside these uncertainties about sensory transduction, let's turn to the question of neural coding of odor quality. How are the various qualities of odor represented in the firing patterns of neurons of the olfactory system? What neural responses make it possible for us to distinguish, say, the smell of lemons from that of limes?

Neural Coding of Odor Quality by Olfactory Fibers. You've already learned something about how qualitative (as contrasted with intensive) aspects of a stimulus are represented in other senses. Recall from Chapter 9 that each fiber in the auditory nerve responds to some range of frequencies, giving the strongest response to one particular frequency. Likewise, each fiber in the optic nerve prefers contours of a particular size and, for some, a particular color. Again, the preferred size or color varies from fiber to fiber. In those modalities, then, different subcategories of sensory fibers carry information about different sensory qualities. As a group, olfactory nerve fibers (the axons of the olfactory receptors) do *not* behave in this discriminating, specialized fashion. The vast majority of olfactory nerve fibers respond to a whole host of different odors, some of which bear no qualitative similarity to one another (Kauer, 1991). To be sure, individual fibers don't indiscriminately respond to all possible odors; there must be, and is, some degree of response specificity. But the range of effective odorants is quite large for any given nerve fiber; there is nothing resembling the specialization evident in auditory and visual nerves. Consequently, olfactory fibers individually can signal that some odorous substance is present, but they cannot provide unequivocal information about the identity of that substance. It has been reported that a small fraction of olfactory nerve fibers respond to only a limited set of odorous substances (Gesteland, 1978), but it is arguable whether these few fibers provide sufficient information about the identity of particular odorous substances.

So, the olfactory nerve, by and large, does not treat an odorant as some combination of basic components each separately registered by specialized cells. Nor, for that matter, does there appear to be anything in the olfactory fibers resembling the center/surround antagonism characteristic of visual receptive fields, and there is nothing comparable in the olfactory epithelium to the tonotopic organization of the basilar membrane and the auditory nerve. Simply stated, nature seems to have worked out a unique form of sensory coding within the olfactory system, and to understand more about that code, we must direct our attention to the next couple of stages of processing, the olfactory bulb and the olfactory brain.

The Olfactory Pathways. The previous discussion focused on the olfactory epithelium and the receptor neurons embedded in that tissue. The rest of the olfactory system consists of the **olfactory bulb** (which receives all the input from the olfactory nerve) and the **olfactory brain** (a cluster of neural structures receiving projections from the olfactory bulb). Structurally, the olfactory bulb bears a superficial resemblance to the retina, in that it has several layers of cells laterally interconnected (see Figure 12.8A, p. 424). On the basis of the response properties of neurons in the bulb, however, it is clear that the two structures—retina and olfactory bulb—function quite differently.

For one thing, the incoming axons from the olfactory epithelium activate neurons in the receiving stage of the bulb rather diffusely (those "second-order" neurons receiving this diffuse afferent input are concentrated in clusters called *glomeruli*). There is not, in other words, any kind of topographic, spatial map of the epithelium onto the bulb. There is, though, enormous convergence at this anatomical stage—it is estimated that there are 1,000 receptor cell axons for each second-order neuron in the bulb. Consequently, very weak neural signals, originating in many different olfactory neurons and carried by olfactory nerve fibers, can be summed within the bulb to create reliable responses to minute concentrations of an odorant (Duchamp-Viret, Duchamp, and Vigouroux, 1989).

It is generally believed that odor quality is coded by the spatial *pattern* of neural activity across the entirety of the olfactory bulb (Freeman, 1991; Kauer, 1991)—an idea reminiscent of the explanation of the tilt aftereffect given in Chapter 4. In

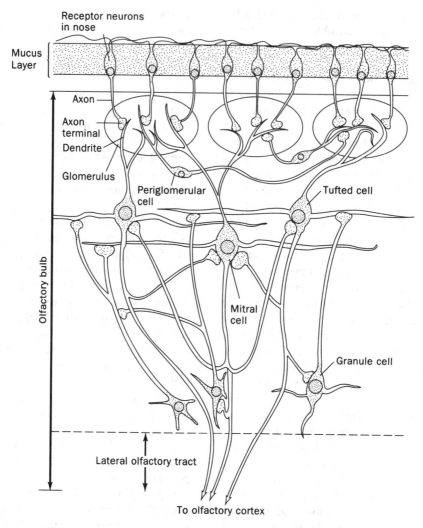

FIGURE 12.8A A schematic drawing of the multiple layers of the olfactory bulb.

this view, virtually all neurons in the bulb contribute to the registration of odor quality; there are no specialized neurons that signal, say, the fragrance of a rose. Support for this view comes from studies in which a map of neural activity was created using the 2-deoxyglucose technique described on page 20 in Chapter 1. (That technique involves the uptake of a radioactively labeled chemical that selectively concentrates in brain regions high in metabolic need.) Different odorants produce characteristic, reliable patterns of meta-

bolic activity within the bulb, but these patterns are rather globally distributed over the structure and are not confined to local clusters of cells (reviewed by Holley, 1991).

Activity of neurons in the olfactory bulb is also shaped by two other important aspects of an odorant. First, neural activity varies throughout the phase of the inhalation cycle, being greatest at the end of each inhalation. And second, neuronal activity in the bulb depends on the level of emotional arousal; if an animal is hungry, thirsty, sex-

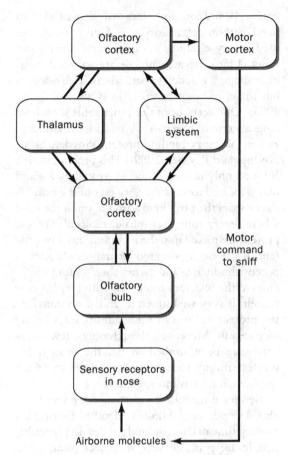

FIGURE 12.8B A flow diagram of the pathway constituting the olfactory system.

by axons from several, morphologically distinct classes of cells within the bulb. Those axons project to the olfactory cortex in the frontal lobe which, in turn, communicates with several other areas of the brain, including subcortical structures in the limbic system (see Figure 12.8B). This latter connection is noteworthy, for the limbic system, which is phylogenetically quite old, is involved in emotional responses. It is thought that the emotion-evoking capacity of odors—and the ability of emotion to affect smell as strongly as it does—arises from two-way links between the olfactory and limbic systems.

Studies of the physiological properties of neurons in the olfactory cortex are few in number. To date, efforts to identify some type of odortopic organization in the cortex (that is, an organized map of different odors represented by different neurons) has failed (Greer, 1991). It is known, though, that people with damage to this region of the brain can have difficulty detecting and/or identifying odors (see review by Richardson and Zucco, 1989), indicating that those regions are critically involved in the processing of olfactory information. As described above, any given type of odorant molecule usually evokes a broadly distributed, characteristic pattern of activity within the olfactory bulb. Of course, the air we ordinarily breathe carries numerous odorous molecules associated with different odor sources. So, the olfactory cortex is receiving from the bulb a complicated pattern of activity associated with this montage of odorant molecules. Researchers are just beginning to grapple with the problem of how the olfactory portions of the brain extract the appropriate invariant response from what must be a fluctuating and unpredictable background of neural responses triggered by the other odorants that are present (Hopfield, 1991).

Neural Representation of Odor Intensity. The previous section focused on odor quality—the difference, for example, between the odor of a banana and the odor of peanut butter. Another dimension of odor perception, of course, is the intensity of a given odor. Odor intensity depends

ually aroused, or fearful, neural responsiveness is enhanced.

If a given odor is indeed represented by a particular global "map" of neural activity within the bulb, we would expect destruction of parts of the bulb to disrupt this map and, hence, impair odor perception. It is remarkable, therefore, that several studies find normal olfactory performance in animals with rather massive lesions of the olfactory bulb (Holley, 1991). Those studies focused mainly on detection and discrimination, not more refined aspects of odor perception such as identification of or memory for odors.

The output from the olfactory bulb is carried

on the concentration of the airborne molecules along with the amount of odorant actually reaching the receptors in the olfactory epithelium. (A given concentration is going to smell weaker when your nose is stuffed up.) Not surprisingly, the nervous system registers information about concentration in the firing rate of neurons responsive to an odor: weak odors elicit fewer neural impulses than strong odors. This property seems to hold at all levels of the olfactory system, from the receptor cells to the cortex. To complicate the picture, though, people can experience changes in the *quality* of an odorant (even chemically pure ones) with changes only in intensity (Gross-Isseroff and Lancet, 1988). So, odor intensity and odor quality are not independent dimensions.

* * *

This overview of the olfactory system sets the stage for considering the perception of odors.

ODOR PERCEPTION

Odor Detection. It is often said that the human sense of smell is rather dull compared with that of other species such as the dog (Moulton, 1976). Although this is true, the human nose is remarkably sensitive nonetheless. For instance, people can detect ethyl mercaptan (a foul-smelling substance) in concentrations as minute as 1 part per 50 billion parts of air. This performance rivals that of the most sensitive laboratory instruments available for measuring tiny concentrations of molecules. Such sensitivity is all the more impressive when you realize that only a small fraction of the odor molecules in this minute concentration actually reaches the olfactory receptors in the top of the nasal cavity. During normal breathing, only about 2 percent of the odorous molecules entering the nostrils actually make it to the receptors; the remaining molecules are absorbed by the lining inside the nose.

Olfactory sensitivity varies greatly from odor to odor. For example, the substance mentioned above, mercaptan, can be detected at a concen-

tration 10 million times less than that needed to smell carbon tetrachloride, a liquid sometimes used in dry-cleaning fluid (Wenger, Jones, and Jones, 1956). Because people are so sensitive to mercaptan, it is added to natural gas, itself odorless but toxic, to warn of gas leaks (Cain and Turk, 1985). One account of this remarkable sensitivity assigns a crucial role to a substance we mentioned earlier, olfactory binding protein (Snyder, Sklar, Hwang, and Pevsner, 1989). This protein, which is found only in nasal tissue, is created by a gland that is located toward the very rear of the nose. A duct carries the protein toward the tip of the nose where, every time you inhale, molecules of the protein are mixed into the incoming air. The protein in the newly inspired air traps molecules of potential odorants and carries these bound molecules to the olfactory receptors. Olfactory binding protein is very well suited to enhance sensitivity: the protein has at least some affinity for virtually all odorants. Moreover, though only a few odorants have been studied so far, the protein has greatest affinity for odorant molecules to which the human nose is most sensitive.

Besides molecular properties, odor sensitivity also depends on a number of other factors, including time of day, age, and gender. In particular, people are generally able to detect weak odors better in the morning than in the evening (Stone and Pryor, 1967); elderly people are less sensitive than young adults (Cain and Gent, 1991; Schiffman, 1983); and females are more sensitive, on average, than males (Koelega and Koster, 1974). Because of these age and gender differences in smell acuity, some people may be put off by body odors that others are not even aware of. Your own experiences in social settings probably confirm this observation. Your experiences may also lead you to believe that your sensitivity to odors increases when you are hungry. But this belief is questionable—some experiments say yes (Schneider and Wolf, 1955); others say no (Furchtgott and Friedman, 1960). Consistent with popular belief, however, smokers are less sensitive to odors than are nonsmokers (Ahlstrom et al., 1987). This dulled odor sensitivity is also found in nonsmokers who live or work with individuals who are heavy smokers (Ahlstrom et al., 1987).

Odor Identification. Having bragged about the sensitivity of the human nose, we must qualify what we mean by "sensitivity." The remarkable performance described above refers to the ability to *detect* the presence of a faint odor, not the ability to *identify* the odor. In fact, at near-threshold concentrations, people can smell an odor but not tell what odor they are smelling. The following experiment illustrates this point (Engen, 1960). When given three empty test tubes and a fourth test tube containing an extremely dilute odor, people can accurately select the tube that "smells different" from the others. But using the same set of stimuli, people make many errors when instructed to pick the test tube that contains some named odor ("pick the tube containing menthol"). So people behave as if they have two thresholds, one for detecting the presence of an odor and a second, higher threshold for identifying what that odor is.

For some odorous substances, part of the identification problem may stem from their bistability: such substances can elicit either of two different qualitative experiences, and these fluctuate over time. (A visual example of bistable perception is the young woman/old lady ambiguous figure shown in Figure 4.23.) For instance, the compound dihydromyrcenol (which is related to turpentine) sometimes has a citruslike odor and other times a woody odor. Lawless, Glatter, and Hohn (1991) were able to bias people's descriptions of this substance by also having the people smell an odorant that was unambiguously woody (for example, pine) or unambiguously citruslike (for example, lemon oil). After smelling citrus, people said the ambiguous compound smelled woody; after smelling the woody odor, the compound smelled like citrus. This shift in perception is not attributable to sensory adaptation, for it did not matter whether the unambiguous stimulus was sniffed before or after sniffing dihydromyrcenol. This context-dependent change in odor identification could be exploited for creative menu planning using dishes with multiple aroma components, such as curried chicken. And when serving wine, it is possible to make a fruity wine such as a German Reisling have either an acidic or a floral bouquet, depending on the accompaniment.

Most odorous substances, though, elicit unique odor qualities regardless of context. Still, individuals differ greatly in their ability to identify odors—to attach a label to the odor of a substance. Odor identification has been measured in two large studies, one a sample of 1,955 people ranging in age from 5 to 99 years (Doty et al., 1984) and the other involving a survey of more than a million readers of a popular magazine (Wysocki, Pierce, and Gilbert, 1991). Conclusions from those two studies were in agreement. Overall, females are significantly better at odor identification than are males, and the best performance is exhibited by individuals ranging in age from mid-twenties to late forties (see Figure 12.9). Some people beyond their sixties show marked impairments in the ability to identify odors, which may explain why elderly people sometimes complain about the blandness of food; after all, smell is an essential component in the enjoyment of food. It should be noted, though, that odor identification performance is much more variable among the elderly: some people in their seventies or older perform as well as middle-aged individuals.

Besides age and gender, there are other important determinants of olfactory performance. Tobacco smoking impairs the ability to identify odors, as the graph in Figure 12.10 documents: the longer the history of smoking, the greater the number of errors on a standardized odor identification test (Frye, Doty, and Schwartz, 1989). Fortunately, cessation of smoking promotes recovery. Ambient air quality, too, affects odor perception. Individuals working in plants manufacturing vaporous chemicals may exhibit long-term impairments in olfactory identification (Schwartz et al., 1989), and people living in cities with poor ambient air quality have difficulty identifying at least some odors compared with matched samples of people from cities with generally better air quality (Wysocki, Pierce, and Gilbert, 1991).

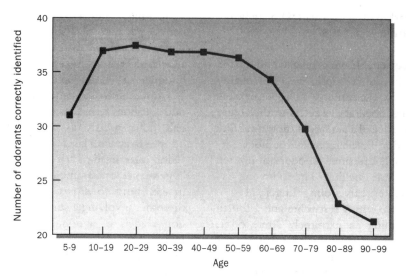

FIGURE 12.9 Ability to identify odors varies with age.

These deficits associated with smoking and with air quality may be related to structural changes at the receptor sites on the olfactory cilia, which become altered with chronic exposure to particular odorants.

Murphy and Cain (1986) have found that blind adults are significantly better at odor identification than comparably aged sighted individuals. Perhaps, then, odor identification should be thought of as a skill that can be sharpened with the enforced practice required without vision. Indeed, even in sighted individuals, practice with feedback improves the ability to identify odors. Desor and Beauchamp (1974) tested people's ability to name

FIGURE 12.10 Ability to identify odors is impaired by cigarette smoking.

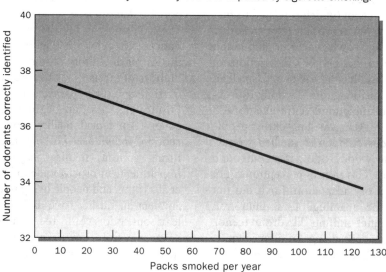

thirty-two common odorous objects contained in individual opaque jars. After sniffing the jar, the person guessed what the object was and rated the familiarity of the odor. Some smells—such as coffee, paint, and banana—were readily identified and were also rated as highly familiar. Other smells—including ham, cigar, and crayon—were incorrectly identified by most people; these odors were also rated as less familiar. Desor and Beauchamp then went through the series again, this time providing people with the correct answer when they made errors. With this practice, everyone was able to learn to name each of the thirty-two odors correctly. Furthermore, the same people were trained on an additional set of thirty-two new odors, and with practice they were able to identify all sixty-four odors with few errors.

Although practice improves odor identification, it does not help everybody to the same degree. For example, practice seems to benefit females more than males, as Figure 12.11 shows. The graph summarizes results from an experiment where Cain (1982) asked male and female college students to identify each of the eighty common odorous stimuli listed in the figure. Each person went through the set of stimuli several times, with feedback provided after every trial. Students of both sexes improved with practice on this task, but the females consistently outperformed the males on just about every odorous stimulus. Each bar in Figure 12.11 summarizes identification performance for a particular stimulus. Stimuli in the upper portion of the figure (for instance, coffee) were readily identified, whereas stimuli toward the lower portion (such as cough syrup) were difficult to identify. Unshaded bars indicate female superiority at identifying that odorant, whereas shaded bars indicate male superiority. The length of the bar denotes the size of the sex difference in

FIGURE 12.11 Odor identification performance for eighty common stimuli, arranged from top to bottom in order of ease of identification. Unshaded bars indicate the superior ability of female subjects to identify a particular stimulus; shaded bars indicate the superior ability of male subjects. (Redrawn with permission from Cain, 1982.)

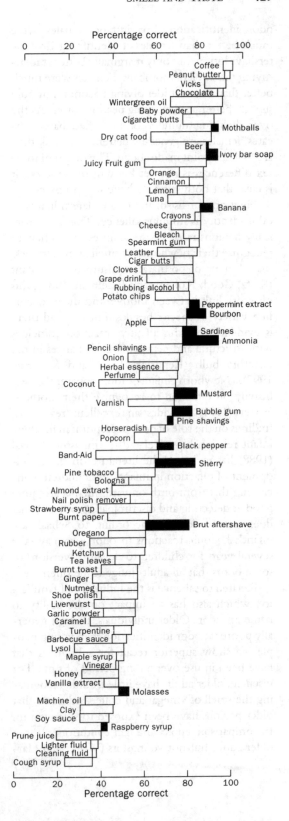

odor identification. For instance, males were much better than females at identifying Brut aftershave lotion, but only marginally better at identifying the smell of mothballs. Females were much better than males at identifying coconut, but only slightly better at identifying peanut butter. As the overwhelming number of unshaded bars indicates, females are generally better at this task than are males, a point made above. The origin of these sex differences is not yet known; nonetheless, it is clear that both sexes do benefit from practice.

Next on our list of important determinants of odor identity is stimulus salience. This is dramatically demonstrated by the abilities of mothers to recognize their newborns by smell alone after less than 1 hour of postnatal exposure to the infant (Kaitz, Good, Rokem, and Eidelman, 1987); this olfactory link between mother and infant occurs in a variety of species besides humans, and there is evidence that this adaptive reaction coincides with structural and neurochemical changes in the olfactory bulb (Kendrick, Levy, and Keverne, 1992). Newborn infants, too, apparently rely heavily on olfaction to recognize their mothers. Porter (1991) provides an excellent review of findings on the role of odor perception in mother-infant relationships. Related to this issue, Schaal (1988) has reviewed the literature on the development of olfaction in infants and children, concluding that from birth onward, infants are quite good at detecting and discriminating odors. What does seem to change, according to Schaal, are infant's hedonic reactions to odors—it may take several years for children to develop aversions to some odors that all adults judge to be offensive.

Related to salience is the influence of familiarity, which also has an impact on the ability to name an odor. Older individuals, though generally poorer at odor identification than young people, *do* show superior recall for substances that have been in use over a long period of time. For instance, older adults have little trouble recognizing the smell of vinegar and coffee, odorants that older persons have been exposed to since youth. In comparison, epoxy and hair conditioner stump older adults but not youngsters (Wood and Har-

kins, 1987). At the other end of the age continuum, newborn infants exposed for about a day to an artificial odorant preferentially orient to that odorant two weeks later when it is paired with a novel one (Davis and Porter, 1991). This olfactory familiarization probably underlies infants' ability to recognize their mothers by smell.

But if experience with odors starts from day one, why are we relatively poor at identifying them, even odors we've experienced over and over? Of course, odors are typically associated with information from other senses, information that unambiguously identifies the source of those odors. For instance, a citruslike aroma is usually accompanied by the sight of a lemon. But in odor identification tasks, people have only the sense of smell to go on, and even healthy, young females may get fewer than half the items correct. Now, the problem isn't one of discrimination: people find it easy to judge correctly whether two odors are "same" versus "different"—the problem involves naming individual odors. In other words, the link between odors and their verbal descriptions is inherently weak (Engen, 1987). This inability to name a familiar odor has been aptly termed the **tip of the nose** phenomenon (Lawless and Engen, 1977)—a variation on the phrase typically used when one blocks on a term or a name. If the problem is indeed one of retrieving odor names from memory, prompting with clues as to an odor's identity should help. And it does. Several researchers (Davis, 1981; Zellner, Bartoli, and Eckard, 1991) have found that merely providing people with a color name related to an odor (such as "yellow" when lemon was being sniffed) is sufficient to trigger correct identification.

Odor Concentrations. Besides having characteristic qualities, odorous substances also vary in the intensity of those qualities. Intensity, as you could guess, depends on the concentration level of odorous molecules. A common misconception about the sense of smell concerns people's alleged poor ability to judge differences in odor concentrations. Until recently, it was generally thought that people require about a 25 percent difference in odor concentration before they can tell that one sample of an odor is stronger than another sample of that same odor. (This implies that a bouquet of five flowers would smell no stronger than a bouquet of four flowers, since they differ by only 20 percent.) Compared with vision and hearing (where difference thresholds are on the order of 10 percent), this represents dull sensitivity indeed. However, William Cain (1977) has shown that this dismal performance does not reflect an inferiority on the part of the olfactory nervous system; instead, the poor performance stems from moment-to-moment variability in the amount of odorous vapor delivered to the olfactory receptor cells. Remember, only a small fraction of these vapors actually reach these cells. Taking account of variability in effective odor concentration, Cain found that concentration differences as small as 7 percent are discriminable. This places the nose in the same league with the eye and the ear as a judge of intensity differences. (Thus if their fragrance was delivered through Cain's apparatus, five flowers *would* smell stronger than four.)

Remember the description of magnitude scaling, in Chapter 10 and in the Appendix, where people assigned numbers to sounds according to their loudness? Comparable scaling measurements have been made of perceived odor intensity. As with loudness, odor intensity grows as a power function of concentration. Although the values vary from odor to odor, many odors give exponents in the neighborhood of 0.6, indicating that perceived odor intensity grows somewhat gradually relative to increasing concentration. For example, doubling odor concentration produces only about a 50 percent increase in perceived intensity, not 100 percent (the value associated with an exponent of 1.0). As a result, a bouquet of ten flowers will not smell twice as strong as a bouquet of five flowers; to smell twice as strong as five flowers, a bouquet would have to consist of seventeen flowers. Intensity ratings can be affected by color. Zellner and Kautz (1990) found that some odorous substances smell stronger when the sniffed liquid substance is colored (for instance,

red, in the case of strawberry). Evidently, simple conditioning cannot explain this finding, since enhanced odor intensity was found even with inappropriate color/odor combinations (for instance, red lemon).

Is discrimination of odor concentration useful? Suppose you walk into your house and smell some foul odor. You can't see where it's coming from, so you have to rely on your sense of smell to guide you to the source. You move around trying to locate where the smell becomes stronger. Since odor concentration varies with distance, this strategy will ultimately bring you to the source.

While tracking the odor, you might also sniff, thereby pulling more of the odorous vapors into your nose. Shouldn't that perceived odor intensity vary depending on the vigor of the sniff? A deep sniff, after all, pulls more odorous vapors into the nose than does a weak, shallow sniff. And since more odorous molecules will be available for stimulating the olfactory receptors, the resulting smell seemingly should be stronger the deeper the sniff. Yet this may not always happen—some investigators have reported that odor intensity remains constant regardless of the vigor of a sniff (Teghtsoonian, Teghtsoonian, Berglund, and Berglund, 1978). This finding is especially surprising since when sniffs are produced artificially, by blowing odorous air into the nose, perceived intensity *does* depend on the rate of air flow (Rehn, 1978). Why would artificial sniffs and natural ones have different effects on perceived odor intensity? After all, with both types of sniffs the flow rate of the odorant varies comparably. According to Teghtsoonian, Teghtsoonian, Berglund, and Berglund (1978), the olfactory system may recognize when the increase in flow rate results from a natural sniff, and it may then calibrate the perception of intensity to take this factor into account. These investigators have dubbed the phenomenon **odor constancy,** since perceived strength of an odor remains constant despite variations in flow rate. You can see the similarity between this phenomenon and shape constancy (Chapter 5), color constancy (Chapter 6), and size constancy (Chapter 7). In all these instances, perception of objects in the world remains constant despite changes in the energy impinging on the receptors. We should note in passing that others have suggested alternative mechanisms by which odor constancy may be achieved (Laing, 1983).

The Common Chemical Sense. While on the subject of odor concentrations, we should note that most odors judged pleasant at moderate concentrations lose some of their attractiveness at high concentrations. This is why a salesclerk in a cosmetics department always urges customers to allow a dab of perfume time to dilute before smelling it. One reason intense odors can be overpowering has to do with the free nerve endings in the olfactory epithelium (a look back at Figure 12.6 will refresh your memory). Those nerve endings are chemical-sensitive cells stimulated by just about any volatile substance of moderately high concentration; they make up what is known as the **common chemical sense.** It is the common chemical sense that is responsible for the *feeling* that accompanies certain "smells"— such as the coolness of menthol or the tingle in your nose when you burp. Even the crisp, invigorating "smell" of fresh mountain air (which itself has no odor) comes from stimulation of the common chemical sense by ozone in the air. In fact, just about any volatile substance can elicit this "feeling" in the nose if the concentration of that substance is high enough. In the case of some substances, stimulation of the common chemical sense produces a burning sensation that causes you reflexively to hold your breath and turn your head away from the source of stimulation. Those of you who have inhaled ammonia fumes know what this feeling is like. Incidentally, cigarette smokers are less sensitive to stimulation of the common chemical sense; for them, the inhaled concentration of an irritating substance must be about 25 percent higher, as compared with nonsmokers, to elicit a reflexive change in breathing pattern (Cometto-Muniz and Cain, 1982). Elderly people, too, show reduced sensitivity to nasal irritants that stimulate the common chemical sense (Stevens and Cain, 1986) and, as you might guess by now, males are less sensitive than females

(Garcia-Medina and Cain, 1982). Some people have totally lost their common chemical sense, from damage to the trigeminal nerve carrying information from the nose's free nerve endings to the brain. In these individuals, harsh chemical substances elicit *no* reaction when inhaled.

The common chemical sense serves as a warning system to signal the presence of potentially irritating substances. However, its operation is not limited to dangerous concentration levels; in fact, even at safe levels of stimulation the common chemical sense influences the perception of odor, as an experiment by Cain and Murphy (1980) demonstrates. In their study, people sniffed amyl butyrate (a fruity-smelling substance) and rated the perceived intensity of the odor. Mixed in with the odorant were various amounts of carbon dioxide. (Carbon dioxide is a gas that does *not* stimulate olfactory receptors but *does* stimulate the free nerve endings in the nose. Hence it has no odor; but because it stimulates the common chemical sense, it elicits a pungent sensation when inhaled.) Cain and Murphy wanted to know whether stimulation of the common chemical sense would influence people's judgments of odor intensity. Some of the results from their experiment are summarized in Figure 12.12; the vertical axis plots the perceived odor intensity of the amyl butyrate

FIGURE 12.12 Stimulation of the common chemical sense (carbon dioxide) affects perceived odor (amyl butyrate).

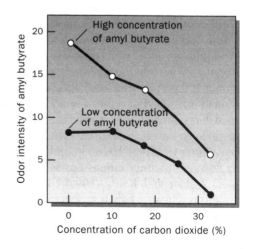

and the horizontal axis shows the concentration of the odorless carbon dioxide. Note that increasing the concentration of carbon dioxide, which itself could not be smelled, reduced the perceived intensity of the amyl butyrate. Even though the actual concentration of amyl butyrate remained constant, its smell changed from pleasant and fruity (at low levels of carbon dioxide) to pungent and irritating (at high levels of carbon dioxide). People also rated how irritating the "smell" seemed. As expected, higher concentrations of the odorless carbon dioxide gas were judged more irritating. However, the pungency of the carbon dioxide was lessened when more amyl butyrate was mixed in with it. We see, then, that the interaction between odor and the common chemical sense works both ways, with each influencing the perception associated with the other. Clearly, the common chemical sense adds an important ingredient to your experience of odorous substances.

Turning back to the topic of odor perception, let's consider "anosmia," a term referring to a loss in the ability to perceive odors.

Disorders of Smell. Deficiencies in hearing and seeing are usually easy to detect because people depend so much on sight and sound to guide their everyday activities. Deficiencies in odor perception, in comparison, can go unnoticed. Though hard to imagine, some individuals are completely unable to distinguish odorless, pure air from strong concentrations of odorous substances. One frequent cause of this "odor blindness," or anosmia, is a blow to the head (Varney, 1988); in such cases, the anosmia often proves to be temporary, suggesting that the olfactory receptors or their axons had been damaged (recall that these neurons can regenerate). Anosmia may also be acquired from inhaling caustic agents such as lead, zinc sulfate, or cocaine. These, too, are believed to injure the olfactory receptors, which is why recovery of smell sensitivity often occurs after ingestion of the caustic agent ceases. Reduced odor sensitivity and identification performance are also observed in patients with Alzheimer's disease (Rezek, 1987). In these patients, impaired odor

perception probably results from degeneration of neurons in the olfactory epithelium (Talamo et al., 1989). Schiffman (1983) reviews the various causes of anosmia.

Sometimes anosmia does not involve a total loss of the sense of smell but is instead specific to particular substances. In these cases, a person shows normal sensitivity to some odors but abnormally poor sensitivity to others. These are the specific anosmias we mentioned earlier, and they are more common than you might think. For example, 3 percent of the U.S. population have trouble smelling the odor of sweat, 12 percent have diminished sensitivity to musky odors, and 47 percent have trouble smelling the odor of urine (Amoore, 1991).

Losing one's sense of smell can have serious consequences. Individuals with acquired anosmia often claim that eating is no longer pleasurable, and these people show a loss of both appetite and weight (Schechter and Henkin, 1974). There is even speculation that anosmia may dull one's sexual drive (Bobrow, Money, and Lewis, 1971). This possibility is not entirely farfetched. As mentioned in the beginning of the chapter, animals rely very heavily on odor to motivate and guide their sexual behavior. And certainly, the large sums of money spent on perfume, not to mention the erotic nature of many perfume commercials, suggest a connection between the nose and sexual behavior.

Before leaving our discussion of disorders of smell, this is a good place to mention **odor hallucinations**—the experiencing of odors for which there is no physical stimulus. Odor hallucinations are sometimes associated with brain tumors (Douek, 1974); they are also a common complaint of people diagnosed as mentally ill (Rubert, Hollender, and Mehrhof, 1961). But don't assume that odor hallucinations necessarily indicate brain damage or mental illness. People sometimes describe sensing strange, metallic odors when they have the flu or other viral diseases (Schiffman, 1983). This effect is thought to result from a virus's having damaged cells in the olfactory epithelium. In any event, you needn't become immediately alarmed when you experience some olfactory hallucination; it is often difficult to distinguish real odors from imaginary ones, since the source of an odor may not be obvious. How many times have you searched your house trying to discover where that "funny smell" was coming from?

Adaptation to Odors. Imagine walking into the lobby of a movie theater and smelling the aroma of fresh popcorn. Driven by this lovely smell, you stand in line to buy some, but by the time you reach the counter, the aroma has faded considerably. This exemplifies how exposure to an odor decreases sensitivity to that odor—a phenomenon called **odor adaptation.** Certain occupations depend crucially on odor adaptation—sewer workers, for instance, can carry out their jobs without being bothered by the stench of their surroundings. Odor adaptation also means that people cease to be aware of their own body odors or of the odors permeating their immediate surroundings. It was Freud (1930/1961) who observed that ". . . in spite of all man's developmental advances, he scarcely finds the smell of his own excreta repulsive, but only that of other people's" (p. 54). Thus, sometimes one must rely on others for information about self-odor, a widely exploited theme in deodorant, mouthwash, and soap commercials.

Odor adaptation has been studied in the laboratory, and the results confirm what experience suggests (see Halpern, 1983). Following even prolonged exposure to an odor, one never *completely* loses the sensitivity to that odor. Instead, its perceived intensity steadily decreases with continued exposure, eventually falling to about 30 percent of its initial level (Cain, 1978). (This is why some people can "tolerate" wearing an overpowering amount of perfume or aftershave—their noses have adapted to the strong fragrance that others wince at.) If an odor's concentration is weak to begin with, it may be impossible to detect that weak odor following adaptation to a strong concentration of the same odor.

Recovery from exposure to an odor takes just a few minutes unless the adaptation odor was

quite strong, in which case an hour or more may be required for complete recovery (Berglund, Berglund, Engen, and Lindvall, 1971). There is also anecdotal evidence for an ultra-long-term adaptation effect, whereby individuals develop a chronic insensitivity to odors common to their work environment. Even when they report to work first thing in the morning, they fail to smell odors that visitors readily sense. The adaptation of these workers carries over from one day to the next. At the same time, these individuals exhibit normal sensitivity for odors not peculiar to their workplace; so they have not completely lost their sense of smell. Moreover, upon returning to work following a short vacation, they are initially able to sense the odors that their colleagues on the job cannot sense; after a few days on the job, however, they again become insensitive to those odors. Gesteland (1986) has speculated that these long-term losses in odor sensitivity may be related to the growth processes in the olfactory receptor cells that we described earlier. Perhaps chronic exposure to a limited set of odors affects receptor cells responsive to that set of odors, and several weeks away from that environment are needed to allow the spoiled cells to be replaced with fresh ones.

This explanation of long-term adaptation probably does not apply, however, to short-term adaptation, where brief exposure to an odor temporarily lessens your sensitivity to it. In this latter case, the process responsible for adaptation probably occurs within the brain, not in the nose. One reason for believing this is that you can adapt one nostril to an odor (keeping the other one closed) and then measure a loss in odor sensitivity using just the unadapted nostril (Zwaardemaker, 1895, cited in Engen, 1982). Since this nostril was closed during adaptation, the olfactory receptors associated with the nostril must have received no stimulation. Nonetheless, your perception of odors introduced into this nostril are still dulled, indicating that the process underlying the loss in sensitivity occurs in the brain, not in the receptor cells. However, the physiology of postreceptor adaptation is poorly understood.

So far we have considered situations where the

perceived strength of an odor is reduced by prior exposure to strong concentrations of that same odor. In some cases, though, a temporary loss in sensitivity to one odor can be produced by exposure to a different odor—a phenomenon called **cross-adaptation.** As you might expect, odors that tend to smell alike (such as nail polish remover and airplane glue) usually show a large degree of cross-adaptation: exposure to one reduces your sensitivity to the other. If you spend several minutes sniffing perfume samples at the cosmetic counter, don't be surprised if the fragrance you're already wearing seems temporarily to have worn off; sniffing perfumes similar to your own has lessened your sensitivity to the one you're wearing. Dissimilar odors, in contrast, do not influence each other nearly so much (Moncrieff, 1956). Thus sniffing perfume samples will not subsequently affect your ability to appreciate the aroma of coffee.

You can experience cross-adaptation by performing the following simple experiment. First, take a sniff of a lemon and get an idea of the intensity of its aroma. Now hold a spoon of peanut butter close to your nose for a minute or so, adapting to its smell. Then quickly take another whiff of the lemon—you will find the lemon's fragrance just as strong as before. Next adapt for a minute to a lime held under your nose, and then again sniff the lemon. This time you will find the lemon's fragrance noticeably weakened. A lesson to learn from this exercise is that your appreciation of food during a multicourse meal depends on the order in which the foods are served. This is particularly true for foods with similar aromas. For instance, cheese with a strong, overpowering smell (such as Roquefort) should not be served before one with a more delicate aroma (such as Gouda).

Initially, it was hoped that cross-adaptation would provide a method of odor classification. Presumably, odors stimulating the same receptors should exhibit maximum cross-adaptation, whereas odors stimulating different receptors should show little or no cross-adaptation. Although this sounds reasonable, the results are confusing. In particular, cross-adaptation is sometimes asymmetrical: adaptation to odor A may strongly influence your perception of odor B but adaptation to odor B may exert hardly any effect on the smell of odor A (Cain and Engen, 1969). This outcome seems to indicate that cross-adaptation is not strictly due to receptor adaptation. Moreover, odors that exhibit marked cross-adaptation sometimes bear no resemblance to each other chemically. Cross-adaptation, like short-term adaptation in general, then, does not appear to result from fatigue of the olfactory receptors.

Odor Mixtures. Besides being subject to cross-adaptation, different odors can affect one another when mixed together in inhaled air. In fact, this occurs quite commonly, as the following examples illustrate. Most meals consist of a bouquet of aromas that when properly mixed can generate a very pleasing experience. Mixing fragrances is the essence of the perfume maker's job; it is also a concern of people who bathe only with a soap that will complement their cologne. Odor mixture also underlies the success of commercial air fresheners sold to cover up house odors. In effect, these products exploit the ability of one odor to mask another by "swamping" the offensive odor with an even stronger pine or floral scent. These products should be distinguished from true deodorizers, which act by actually removing odorous molecules from the air or by preventing the production of odorous molecules in the first place (the mechanism employed in some underarm deodorants).

As indicated before, the nose seems able to sort out and identify the various odors that are in a mixture. This is why you can identify many of the food ingredients that went into some complex dish simply from the smell of that dish. In this sense, the nose's behavior resembles the ear's ability to single out one pitch from a musical chord; the nose does not behave like the eye, which sometimes loses track of the individual hues making up a mixture. However, a person's judgments of an odor mixture cannot be predicted on the basis of the simple addition of the two components. For instance, two different odorants of moderate intensity may not sum to yield an intense mixture; this failure of additivity is termed **mixture suppression,** and its physiological basis is not well understood (Derby, Ache, and Kennel, 1985; Laing, 1988). (For a full discussion of odor mixture, see Engen, 1982.)

Odors and Memory. Even when people cannot identify some odor, they are often able to say with confidence whether or not they have smelled it before—which suggests that odors can reach back into memory (see Box 12.2, pp. 438–439). For Helen Keller, who was blind and deaf from infancy, smell was

a potent wizard that transports us across thousands of miles and all the years we have lived. The odors of fruits waft to me in my southern home, to my childhood frolics in the peach orchard. Other odors, instantaneous and fleeting, cause my heart to dilate joyously or contract with remembered grief. (1908, p. 574)

Odors can be potent reminders of the past—they effortlessly call up memories (Schab, 1991). But can memories call up odors? The answer seems to be no. Most people have great difficulty *imagining* what an odor smells like, even a very familiar one. Can you, for instance, conjure up the smell of a rose? Of course you recognize its fragrance when you actually encounter a rose, but recalling such a smell seems very difficult. Isn't it odd that one can readily hum tunes in one's head, can vividly picture a scene in the mind's eye, but cannot re-create in the mind a remembered smell? Perhaps, during the course of evolution, the sense of smell became fully developed before consciousness came on the scene. And perhaps, as a result, the olfactory system does not have access to the neural machinery needed to imagine odors consciously in the absence of the objects that normally evoke them. But emotional arousal seems quite able to trigger odor memories, probably from the intimate connections between the olfactory system and the limbic system. The so-called "smell of fear" may have neurologic reality. On these spec-

ulative notes we'll end our discussion of smell and move on to its sister sense, taste.

THE SENSE OF TASTE

We say of food, "This tastes good" or "I like the taste of that." But taste determines not only how much we like or dislike some food but also whether we will eat it at all. In effect, the tongue and mouth (assisted by the nose) are designed to ensure that nutritious substances are eaten while noxious ones are not. Living in a civilized environment, one seldom needs to rely on taste to gauge edibility—if the grocer sells it or the restaurant serves it, we assume it must be safe to eat. Taste serves mainly to define our preferences among a large group of commercially available edible foods. Still, taste provides a bounty of perceptual experiences and therefore deserves to be studied.

Technically, the term "taste" is used to refer to sensations caused when various substances dissolved in saliva penetrate the taste buds on the tongue and surfaces of the mouth. If you were to drop a pinch of sugar onto the tip of your tongue, the resulting sensation would constitute what most people call "taste." But when you actually eat something, you learn much more than this about the substances in your mouth—besides taste, you have an immediate appreciation of the food's temperature, texture, and consistency (Gibson, 1966). All these sources of information combine with the substance's taste to form a complex of sensations that is known as **flavor.** Although the remainder of this chapter is concerned with the taste component of flavor, keep in mind that these other sources of information also contribute to one's enjoyment of food.

In our discussion of taste, we shall follow the same general outline used in the section on smell: we'll describe the stimulus for taste, consider the question of taste categories, provide a brief overview of the anatomy and physiology of the gustatory system, and then take up the question of taste sensitivity. Finally, we'll explore the interaction between taste and smell.

THE STIMULUS FOR TASTE

To be tasted, a substance must be *soluble:* it must dissolve upon contact with saliva. This is why you cannot tell the difference between a plastic spoon and a stainless steel spoon simply on the basis of their taste—neither material will dissolve in saliva. Moreover, food seems tasteless when saliva is not present in the mouth, because it represents the vehicle for transporting taste solutions to the receptors within the tongue and mouth. The salivary glands, incidentally, produce in the neighborhood of 25 ounces of fluid in one day, most of it while one eats. Some food substances, particularly those containing citric acid, promote copious salivary secretion, whereas others, including glucose, are less effective. Besides aiding in digestion, saliva contains ingredients that prevent erosion of teeth enamel and eliminate bacteria in the oral cavity. In chemical composition, saliva closely resembles salt water, although the sodium content of saliva varies from one person to the next (Bradley, 1991). It is claimed that you can actually detect this difference in sodium content when you taste someone else's saliva (Bartoshuk, 1980), but we'll leave it to the intellectually curious to confirm this claim.

THE CLASSIFICATION OF TASTES

Nowadays it is widely believed that tastes can be grouped into four distinct categories: sweet, sour, salty, and bitter. However, this particular idea is still controversial. Earlier lists of the basic taste qualities contained more entries. For example, Aristotle believed there were seven basic tastes, the four listed above plus pungent, harsh, and astringent. In the centuries following Aristotle's time, new tastes were added to the list (such as viscous and fatty), whereas others were dropped (Bartoshuk, 1978). It wasn't until the early part of the nineteenth century that the list dwindled to the four categories most people are now familiar with. The person who formalized the four-taste idea is Henning (1916), the same man who was responsible for the odor classification scheme shown in Figure 12.3. Once again, Henning re-lied on geometry to present the relations among the various taste categories. In this case his model, shown in Figure 12.13, took the form of a tetrahedron, with each of the four taste qualities located at one of the four corners.

Henning wanted his geometrical model to emphasize the unity of the four taste qualities; he emphatically rejected the idea that these four taste qualities could be *separately* experienced in any complex mixture of tastes. More recently, however, Donald McBurney (1974) has argued that one *can* pick out and judge the relative contributions of these four primaries, or "basics," as he calls them. He believes this is possible because the tongue analyzes substances into these four distinct categories. Other taste experts disagree with the idea that there are genuinely separate taste qualities. Two of these notable opponents, Susan Schiffman and Robert Erickson (1980), have questioned much of the evidence for the existence of distinct taste primaries. Besides challenging this evidence, Schiffman and Erickson have also performed their own experiments on this topic. Let's consider the results from a couple of their studies.

Schiffman (whose work on odor categories we described earlier) used multidimensional scaling to analyze people's ratings of taste similarity. (Recall that this procedure establishes the number of dimensions required to account for similarity rat-

FIGURE 12.13 Henning's taste tetrahedron.

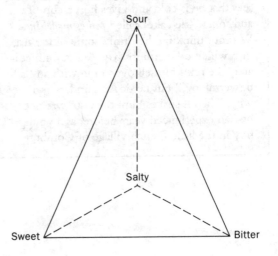

Box 12.2 *Smell, Taste, and Literature*

Languages have limited vocabularies for describing smell and taste experiences. Though it's fairly easy to describe what you see and what you hear, smell and taste are another matter (Bedichek, 1960). This works a special hardship on authors who must communicate their character's smell and taste experiences. Fortunately, good writers rise above the apparent limitations of language. When you read a work in which smell and taste play a key part, you are reminded how important these "inarticulate senses" really are. To illustrate, let's consider some samples of writing in which authors have managed to give these inarticulate senses a voice of their own.

Smell can evoke memories long-buried and obscure; the same thing can happen in the case of taste. Probably the best-known literary description of this phenomenon comes from Marcel Proust's *Swann's Way*. In the book's overture, the narrator muses that it's impossible to recapture one's past merely by trying to think about it. True recapture requires that you reexperience the *sensations* that you felt originally. And he then goes on to provide an eloquent example of this idea. While he is visiting her, the narrator's mother sees that he is cold and gives him a cup of tea and some little cakes called *petites madeleines*. Without thinking, he drinks some of the tea, into which cake crumbs have fallen. Immediately, he finds himself overcome with an "all-powerful joy," but he doesn't understand why. Then it strikes him: the taste was one he had experienced years before, as a young boy in the little French village of Combray.

In that moment all the flowers in our garden and in M. Swann's park, and the water-lilies on the Vivonne and the good folk of the village and their little dwellings and the parish church and the whole of Combray and of its surroundings, taking their proper shapes and growing solid, sprang into being, town and gardens alike, from my cup of tea. (Proust, 1928, p. 58)

Since the next 200 pages of Proust's novel deal with his remembrances of things that happened in Combray, the entire novel actually springs from the taste of those few tea-soaked cake crumbs. What a powerful jolt to the memory!

One lesson from Proust is that any writer who wants to create truly convincing and complete lives cannot ignore smell and taste. James Joyce (1922/1934) understood this as well as any writer of the past 100 years. In his masterpiece, *Ulysses,* Joyce frequently used smells to reach into the minds of various characters. You may know that various episodes in *Ulysses* emphasize different organs of the human body, with the so-called Nausicaa episode highlighting the eye and the nose. This episode takes place just after sunset on a June evening in 1904. Leopold Bloom, the middle-aged Dubliner around whose comings and goings the book revolves, is walking along the beach, trying to clear his head. Bloom finds himself attracted to Gerty MacDowell, a young girl who's sitting on some rocks near the beach. Although they never even speak, Bloom is infatuated. When she leaves, Gerty waves her perfumed handkerchief at Bloom. The scent reaches Bloom, triggering thoughts of Gerty and of his wife, Molly, too:

Wait. Hm. Hm. Yes. That's her perfume. Why she waved her hand. I leave you to think of me when I'm far away on the pillow. What is it? Heliotrope? No, hyacinth? Hm. Roses, I think. She'd like scent of that with a little jessamine mixed. Her high notes and her low notes. At the dance night she met him, dance of the hours. Heat brought it out. She was wearing her black and it had the perfume of the time before . . . Mysterious thing too. Why did I smell it only now? Took its time in coming like herself, slow but sure. Suppose it's ever so many millions of tiny grains blown across . . . Clings to everything she takes off. Vamp of her stockings. Warm shoe. Stays. Drawers: little kick, taking them off. Byby till next time. Also the cat likes to sniff in her shift on the bed. Know her smell in a thousand. Bathwater too. Reminds me of strawberries and cream. (Joyce, 1922/1934, p. 368)

Another great writer with a special appreciation of the chemical senses was Jonathan Swift (1827/1945), the eighteenth-century English satirist. In one of his books, Swift paints a dramatic portrait of adaptation to the smells of a highly unusual environment. In the fourth and final journey related in Gulliver's Travels, Lemuel Gulliver finds himself marooned on an island ruled by the noble Houyhnhnms, a race of intelligent, honest, socially advanced horses. The island is also populated by a nasty, degenerate breed of barbaric humanlike creatures, Yahoos, whom the Houyhnhnms shun and whom Gulliver abhors. After living very happily among the horselike Houyhnhnms for more than 3 years, learning their language and developing great admiration for their culture, Gulliver must leave the island and return to England and the home and family that he had once loved. In Gulliver's words:

As soon as I entered the House, my Wife took me in her Arms, and kissed me, at which having not been used to the Touch of that odious Animal for so many Years, I fell in a Swoon for almost an Hour. At the time I am writing it is Five Years since my last Return to England: During the first Year I could not endure my Wife or Children in my Presence, the very Smell of them was intolerable, much less could I suffer them to eat in the same Room. To this hour they dare not presume to touch my Bread, or drink out of the same Cup, neither was I ever able to let one of them take me by the Hand. The first Money I laid out was to buy two young Stone-Horses which I keep in a good Stable, and next to them the Groom is my greatest Favourite; for I feel my Spirits revived by the Smell he contracts in the Stable. My Horses understand me tolerably well; I converse with them at least four Hours every Day. They are Strangers to Bridle or Saddle, they live in great Amity with me, and Friendship to each other. (Swift, 1726/1890, p. 331)

These literary tidbits give you some idea of how writers of varying backgrounds and literary significance have worked with smell and taste. These samples are a reminder of how impoverished one's own perceptual world would be without these "inarticulate senses."

ings.) Her analysis disclosed that taste judgments could *not* be contained within a "taste space" defined by just four components. (Henning's tetrahedron is one possible taste space utilizing four components.) Schiffman obtained evidence for more than four components even when taste judgments were obtained from anosmic individuals. Because these people could not smell, Schiffman could be certain that the extra dimensions uncovered in her analysis were not the product of olfaction. This led her to conclude that four primaries are inadequate to account for the entire range of taste (Schiffman and Dackis, 1975).

Robert Erickson approached the notion of taste primaries in a different way. He presented people with taste solutions consisting of one or more of the so-called primary tastes and asked those people to judge whether they perceived "one" or "more than one" taste quality. For comparison, Erickson asked for the same judgment about auditory tones presented either alone or in a chord. As expected, a single tone was always judged as one, whereas multiple tones were always judged as more than one. This merely confirms the analytical nature of pitch perception: identification of one tone is possible in the presence of another. The results with the taste solutions were quite different. Solutions composed of a single component were sometimes judged as more than one, whereas multicomponent solutions were sometimes judged as one. Moreover, people were often unable to identify whether a mixture contained a particular component, even when they could reliably identify that component in isolation. For instance, quinine (a bitter-tasting substance) was easily recognized on its own; but when mixed with sucrose (which, of course, is sweet), the quinine in the mixture was unrecognizable. These findings led Erickson to conclude that complex tastes are *not* analyzed into primary components but instead take on their own, unique quality, which may give little hint of their ingredients (Erickson, 1982).

This issue of taste categories is by no means settled (see, for example, McBurney and Gent, 1979). Taste researchers are reluctant to give up the idea of four primaries, for good reasons. In particular, some progress has been made in identifying chemical similarities among substances belonging to the same taste group (Beidler, 1978). Establishing the molecular basis of taste quality is a goal that taste experts have been striving toward for decades. Abandoning the categorization scheme that has guided this search would be a bitter pill to swallow. For the moment we'll set aside the question of primaries and proceed to a less controversial topic, the neural mechanisms of taste perception.

THE ANATOMY AND PHYSIOLOGY OF TASTE

The Taste Receptors. Let's begin by taking a tour of the tongue and the inside of the mouth. The tongue itself consists of muscle covered with mucous membrane. To picture the terrain under study, take a careful look at your tongue in a mirror. Notice that it is covered with little bumps. These bumps are called **papillae** (from the Latin *papula,* meaning "pimple"). When viewed from the side (see Figure 12.14), they resemble regularly spaced columns separated by channels. The walls of the papillae are lined with tiny structures, called **taste buds,** that are shaped like garlic bulbs. These taste buds house the receptor cells responsible for registering the presence of chemical substances. Not all the papillae scattered over your tongue contain taste buds—those in the center of the tongue have none, which is why food confined to this area has no taste. The center of the tongue is analogous to the blind spot in the eye: both are devoid of receptors. There's another parallel. Under normal conditions, you don't notice the blind spot since the brain fills in that gap; similarly, you don't notice the tongue's "blind spot." In fact, taste sensations appear to originate from the mouth's entire surface, including from regions that have no receptors (Todrank and Bartoshuk, 1991). Moreover, when the brain's taste information from an entire side of the tongue is blocked by a virus, there is no subjective change in the daily experience of taste (Pfaffmann and Bartoshuk, 1989, 1990).

Taste buds are not restricted only to the

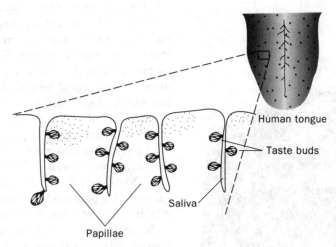

Human tongue

Taste buds

Saliva

Papillae

FIGURE 12.14 A side view of the tongue's papillae.

tongue: taste buds, absent the papillae, are located in the roof of the mouth, inside the cheeks, and in the throat. Some animals have structures similar to taste buds on parts of their bodies other than the tongue and inside of the mouth. Fish, which live in a watery equivalent of saliva, have taste receptors scattered over the surface of their bodies; and some insects have them on their feet, enabling them to taste the surfaces they walk over.

Human papillae that do contain taste buds have anywhere from several hundred buds down to just a single bud (Bradley, 1979), with a grand total of something like 6,000 taste buds distributed throughout the inside of the "average" mouth. We stress average, because the total number of buds varies dramatically among individuals. One count from the tongues of healthy, college volunteers revealed a fourteenfold difference with the sample (Miller and Reedy, 1990). Moreover, the students with taste bud counts toward the top of the distribution rated taste solutions of a given concentration as more intense than did students from the bottom of the distribution of taste bud density.

Developmentally, infants start out life with relatively few taste buds, but during childhood the number steadily increases to the numbers cited above. Around age 40, the trend reverses and the overall number of taste buds declines (Cowart,

1981). This decline in the taste bud population may account for the well-documented loss of taste sensitivity in the elderly (Schiffman, 1983).

Like the olfactory receptors, taste buds are constantly degenerating and being replaced by new ones (Beidler and Smallman, 1965). The life expectancy of an individual taste bud is only about 10 days. Hence throughout your lifetime there is a continuous, rapid turnover within the large population of taste buds. Unlike olfactory cells, however, taste buds are not true neurons, meaning that they do not have axons that project to the brain. In a moment, we'll see how taste information is carried to the brain; for now, though, let's take a closer look at an individual taste bud.

Figure 12.15 (p. 442) illustrates what an individual taste bud looks like under the microscope (buds are too small for the unaided eye to see). Each bud contains an average of fifty individual taste receptor cells, arranged within the bud like the cloves of a garlic. Sprouting out of the end of each taste receptor cell is a slender, threadlike structure called a *microvillus*. A clump of these threads juts into a tiny opening in the wall of the taste bud. It is contact between taste solutions and these microvilli that triggers an electrical potential in the receptor cell. Sensory transduction at these sites involves a cascade of complicated membrane events, some similar to those occurring in olfac-

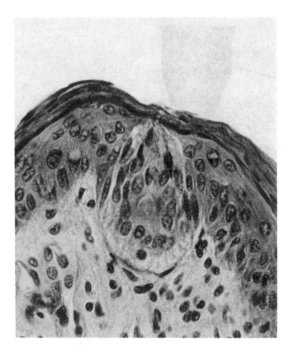

FIGURE 12.15 An individual taste bud. (Photograph courtesy of Dr. Inglis Miller.)

tory transduction (Roper, 1992). Those events differ for the various prototypical taste solutions, and it appears that a single receptor may possess the relevant membrane machinery for several of those solutions. In addition, neighboring taste cells appear to be electrically coupled via intermediary neurons, an arrangement that would promote lateral interactions among receptors. Although the function of these connections is unknown, comparable kinds of circuitry in the retina serve to sharpen differences in activity between neighboring neural elements (Ratliff, 1965). Mucous secretions from supporting cells in the taste buds carry the solution away from the vicinity of the taste bud. This cleaning action is analogous to that described in the case of the olfactory epithelium. But because the tongue's rinsing process is relatively slow, aftertastes can linger after you have swallowed or spit out what was in your mouth.

Back inside a papilla, the taste receptor cells make contact with nerve fibers innervating the tongue. Remember that taste receptors themselves do not have axons to send messages to the brain; like photoreceptors, they must pass their messages on to neurons that in turn carry neural impulses to higher centers. Taste buds in the tongue and mouth are innervated by no less than three distinct cranial nerves, and the same taste bud may be innervated by more than one nerve (Keverne, 1982). We'll not go into which nerves innervate which regions of the tongue and mouth; but keep in mind that taste information arrives at the brain over several different communication lines. Moreover, these communication lines are hooked to a population of receptor cells whose members are constantly dying and being replaced.

So far we've considered the tongue's receptors. Can we relate the responses of specific receptors to specific taste qualities? For decades, textbooks gave the mistaken impression that particular taste sensations were dependent on different regions on the tongue. It was customary to show a "tongue map" with sweet on the tip, salty on the front edges, sour along the edges toward the back of the tongue, and bitter on the midline of the back. But those maps apply only to the ability to identify very weak solutions: different regions of the tongue are differentially sensitive to weak concentrations of the four tastes (Collings, 1974). At higher concentrations any of the four taste sensations can be elicited from any place on the tongue. Moreover, several different distinct taste qualities can be evoked by applying different substances to a single papilla (McCutcheon and Saunders, 1972). So, taste qualities are intermingled over the tongue and cannot be uniquely identified with taste buds at particular locations.

Having looked at the taste receptors, let's now consider how messages generated by those receptors are represented in nerve fibers carrying information from the taste receptors to the brain.

The Taste Pathways. Individual taste fibers exhibit a low, sustained discharge even when no taste substances are on the tongue. When such a substance is introduced, a fiber's activity increases by an amount that depends both on the nature of the substance and on its concentration (Erickson, 1963; Ogawa, Yamashita, and Sato, 1974). With respect to the nature of the substance, most individual fibers respond to several different taste substances—for instance, one particular fiber might respond to both acids and salts.* If individual fibers are indeed not selective for a particular taste, an individual fiber cannot unambiguously specify a certain taste quality. How, then, could the brain know which taste substance was actually present? This question of uniqueness coding in taste is, you will recognize, reminiscent of the same issue in olfaction.

Years ago Carl Pfaffmann (1955) proposed that taste quality is represented in the *pattern* of activity across a population of taste fibers. This **cross-fiber theory** of taste quality has also been championed by Erickson (1968, 1984). Of course, for such a pattern theory to work, taste fibers must respond better to some substances than to others—if they responded to the same extent to *all* taste substances, the cross-fiber pattern of activity would be equivalent for all substances as well. In fact, although most neurons in the taste system are responsive to several taste stimuli, each responds best to a particular taste substance (Frank, 1973). These neurons, in other words, respond selectively to different taste substances. This selective response within a given fiber means that information about taste quality may be coded by the pattern of activity within an ensemble of fibers, as the cross-fiber theory requires (Di Lorenzo, 1989).

Besides differing in quality, the tastes of substances also vary in intensity, depending on the concentration of the substance. Let's consider, then, how taste intensity might be represented within the taste fibers. Most taste experts believe that intensity is signaled by the level of activity within individual fibers, since firing rate increases with the concentration of the stimulating solution. Moreover, if the same solution remains present on the tongue for several seconds, a fiber's activity quickly decreases from the level initially evoked to a somewhat lower one. You might suspect that this drop in neural activity explains why your sense of taste is dulled by repeated sampling of the same food or drink. However, this can't be the entire story, for adaptation of taste sensations may take anywhere from several seconds to a few minutes. Instead of adaptation, the decreased response of taste fibers probably serves a specific function—getting the tongue ready for new tastes. We'll explain why this is important.

Recall that taste judgments allow you to gauge the edibility of food. Taste judgments can be made with astonishing speed: you can identify the taste of what you're eating within the first second of tasting it (Kelling and Halpern, 1987). So after this initial identification, it's less important to continue tasting what you've been tasting than it is to get ready for new tastes. And getting ready for new tastes requires letting the activity in the nerve fibers settle back to a level where they can once again signal the presence of a new substance. Neural adaptation of the kind exhibited by nerve fibers thus makes detection of these changes in taste quality possible (Ludel, 1978). This property of adaptation is particularly important in such sensory modalities as taste, where one fiber may carry information about several different stimulus qualities.

Fibers carrying taste information from the tongue project via several nuclei to two different regions of the brain, with these two regions mediating different aspects of taste perception. One region, the insular cortex, is buried in a region between the temporal and parietal lobes; it is the taste analogue to the visual cortex and the auditory cortex. The conscious experience of tastes presumably arises from activity within this area of the brain, as evidenced by the losses in taste perception occasioned by damage to it (Pritchard, 1991) and by elicitation of taste sensations when it is electrically stimulated in awake humans undergoing brain surgery (Penfield and Faulk, 1955). Still, the percentage of neurons in the insular region responsive to taste stimulation is small; the majority of neurons are activated by chewing or by tactile stimulation of the inside of the mouth.

---

*You should be aware that some people now believe the taste fibers to be more selective than previously thought. If correct, the activity in a single fiber could uniquely specify taste quality (Bartoshuk, 1980).

Nor is there evidence for any sort of topographic arrangement of taste-sensitive neurons by preferred substance (Smith-Swintosky, Plata-Salaman, and Scott, 1991).

The other taste region of the brain constitutes part of the limbic system, whose importance in emotional reactions we mentioned earlier during the discussion of smell. People who have *only* this subcortical pathway intact cannot identify taste substances verbally but still show characteristic facial reactions to sour and bitter solutions. These subcortical taste areas, then, appear to register at least some behaviorally relevant information about taste. It is speculated that this subcortical taste center mediates learned taste aversion, a phenomenon covered later in this chapter.

Finally, keep in mind that taste, besides chemically analyzing substances entering the mouth, must be responsive to the internal, nutritional state of an organism. Selective deprivation from, say, salt leads animals to seek out substances that contain an abundance of that ingredient. It is not surprising, perhaps, to learn that activity levels in gustatory neurons are modulated by appetite (Scott and Plata-Salaman, 1991). The neural pathways mediating this modulation remain unknown.

SENSITIVITY TO TASTE

Detection and Identification. The variation in taste sensitivity across the tongue (Collings, 1974) has already been mentioned. Now we shall consider some other factors that influence the ability to taste substances in weak concentrations. Actually, right at the limit of sensitivity, where the presence of a substance is barely detectable, it is very difficult to identify a taste (McBurney, 1978). Try the following experiment to confirm this point. Fill three identical glasses with equal amounts of water. (The water should be at room temperature.) Place a few grains of sugar in one and a few grains of salt in another and stir both thoroughly. Don't add anything to the water in the third glass. While you keep your eyes closed, have a friend hand you each glass, one at a time.

Take a sip from each and see whether you can pick out the one containing plain water—to do this requires merely *detecting* that the other two contain "something." Next, try to pick the glass containing sugar and the one containing salt. This task requires *identifying* the tastes; if you were sufficiently frugal in the amounts you added to each glass, this task should be difficult, if not impossible. Realizing that you can succeed just by guessing, see how many times you are correct over a series of ten trials. For this demonstration to work, you may need to use less salt than sugar in producing the solutions. The reason is that a salt solution can be detected at one-third the concentration necessary for the detection of sugar, when the solutions are at room temperature.

For most people, the highest sensitivity is to bitter, so if you were to repeat the taste detection test using quinine, you'd have to add just a minute quantity to the water. Some people, however, have difficulty tasting bitter substances. For example, the chemical phenylthiocarbamide (PTC) tastes quite bitter to about two-thirds of all Americans, whereas the remaining one-third are barely able to detect any taste at all from PTC. The same is true for other substances, including 6-*n*-propylthiouracil, known as PROP. In all these substances, atoms of nitrogen, carbon, and sulphur are linked in a particular structure. Studies of families show that sensitivity to the bitterness of PTC or PROP is genetically determined. Individuals to whom PTC doesn't taste bitter ("nontasters," we can call them) have two recessive genes for this trait; those who are sensitive to the bitter ("tasters") have one or two dominant genes for the trait. (Inexpensive paper strips impregnated with PTC are readily available from science supply firms; you might want to purchase some to test yourself and friends.)

Neither PTC nor PROP are commonly found in food, so the inability to taste them is inconsequential. However, Linda Bartoshuk and her colleagues have found that tasters and nontasters also show reliable differences in their judgments of the bitterness of common substances (Miller and Bartoshuk, 1991), including saccharin (an ingredient in many diet sodas) and caffeine (one of the bitter ingredients in coffee). In fact, the caffeine in a typical cup of coffee is not perceived as bitter by nontasters, although it is by tasters (Hall, Bartoshuk, Cain, and Stevens, 1975). This means, then, that a cup of black coffee will taste more bitter to some people than to others. Perhaps individuals who add lots of sugar and cream to their coffee are PTC tasters trying to tone down a degree of bitterness that nontasters never even experience. Again, we are reminded that not all individuals share the same perceptual experiences. Instead, each person lives in a perceptual world that is constrained by the workings of his or her individual sensory nervous system.

In the taste tests suggested above, we specified that the water should be at room temperature because taste sensitivity varies markedly with temperature. Moreover, different taste substances are not equally affected by temperature, as illustrated in Figure 12.16. Note that bitter substances become more difficult to detect at higher temperatures, whereas sensitivity to sweet increases with temperature. Think what this tells you about the effect of temperature on the taste of various foods and drinks. For instance, wine advertisements that urge you to serve their product well chilled may be trying to hide its sweet taste, a common fault with cheap, immature wines. The variations in sensitivity shown in Figure 12.16 also underscore an important rule for cooking: if you season food on the basis of taste, the final seasoning should be done only after the dish has reached serving temperature.

Is there anything to the adage that your ability

FIGURE 12.16 The effect of temperature on taste.

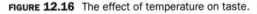
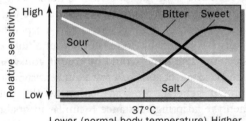

to taste is better when you're hungry? From the results of one study (Moore, Linker, and Purcell, 1965), the answer appears to be no—if by "ability to taste" one means detecting very weak solutions. The study did find, though, that taste sensitivity was better in the afternoon than in the morning, which may explain why people *think* their sense of taste is keener when they're hungry. Another misconception about taste concerns the dulling effects of smoking on a person's sensitivity to taste. Here, too, the evidence is to the contrary—regular smokers are just as good as nonsmokers at correctly identifying taste solutions (McBurney and Moskat, 1975). Why, then, are former smokers always claiming that food tastes better after they have quit? Remember that flavor consists of several mouth-related sensations, taste being just one. Perhaps the reformed smoker's enhanced pleasure from food comes from one of these other sources. For example, smokers are less able to appreciate the pungency of odors (Cometto-Muniz and Cain, 1984), and pungency is a sensation produced by a number of spices used in cooking (Rozin, 1978).

As in the case of odor identification, it has been found that females are better at taste identification than males (Meiselman and Dzendolet, 1967). Though the reasons for female superiority are not yet understood, there seems no doubt that females are better equipped with respect to taste and smell to appreciate food.

Discriminating Taste Intensity. So far we've focused on various aspects of the ability to detect and identify different solutions. Now let's consider how good people are at judging differences in concentration of a single taste substance—another kind of judgment needed in the preparation of food. To get some idea of the difficulty of such judgments, you should try a modification of the taste experiment used to introduce this section. This time fill three large glasses with clear water and place one teaspoon of sugar in the first glass, one and one-quarter teaspoons of sugar in the second, and one and one-half teaspoons of sugar in the third. After stirring, have someone else rearrange the glasses so that you don't know which is which but the other person does. Now try to rank them in order of sugar concentration. This task measures your ability to judge differences in taste concentration.

Although the problem has not been thoroughly studied, available results indicate that people require about 15 to 25 percent difference to be able to judge that one solution is stronger than another (McBurney, 1978). On the basis of these numbers, you should be just barely able to pick out the weakest of the three sugar solutions but will probably be unable to discriminate between the remaining two. The fact that people can discriminate concentration changes in the neighborhood of 15 to 25 percent has implications for cooking: to improve a dish's taste by adding more of some ingredient, add just enough to increase the total amount by about 25 percent each time. This will ensure that you don't suddenly add too much.

Taste Adaptation and Modification. Outside the taste laboratory, people rarely ingest substances in very weak, near threshold concentrations, and moreover, hardly ever are those substances encountered in isolation. When you eat, your palate is typically bathed in a complex of taste substances. So it is of interest to study how the taste of one substance is influenced by the presence of other substances. Such influences can take two forms: (1) the taste of a substance may be weakened by prior exposure to that same substance—the familiar process of **adaptation;** and (2) the taste of a substance may be altered in quality by another substance—a process called **taste modification.**

Let's start with adaptation. You can demonstrate taste adaptation for yourself in the following way. Fill four glasses with equal amounts of water. Now take a freshly sliced lemon and carefully squeeze one drop of juice into one glass, two drops into the second, and the remaining juice into the third (this is the adaptation solution). Thoroughly stir all three solutions. Keep the fourth glass free of lemon—it should contain water only. In this demonstration you should be

aware which glass is which (you may want to number them). Now take a sip of the first solution, the one containing a single drop of lemon juice. You should be able to detect a slightly sour taste (sour is the predominant taste of pure lemon juice), especially in comparison with the neutral taste of water only. Next sip the two-drop solution and compare it with water only. As it is twice as strong, this solution should taste more sour than the one-drop one, and certainly different from water only.

Now adapt your tongue to sour—take enough of the concentrated solution into your mouth to cover your tongue. Don't swallow it; instead, roll it around in your mouth for about 30 seconds, and then spit it out. Now once again sip the two dilute solutions, again comparing them with water only. You should find that the sour taste of both is considerably weaker—perhaps too weak to distinguish from the taste of water only. Wait a few minutes and then repeat this part of the test. You'll find that your sensitivity recovers rather quickly.

This demonstration merely confirms that taste—just like vision, hearing, and smell—shows adaptation. As pointed out in the previous section, this decline in taste sensitivity cannot be caused entirely by the reduced responsiveness of taste fibers; the time course of fiber adaptation is much too short to account for the adaptation of taste sensations. This latter form of adaptation must take place along one of the neural pathways discussed earlier, but exactly where is a mystery (see Gillan, 1984).

Suppose you had adapted to a strong solution of *salt* water and then were tested on the dilute solutions of lemon. Recall that cross-adaptation provides a way to test whether different substances stimulate the same neural elements (look back at page 435 to refresh your memory about the logic of the procedure). You would find that adaptation to salty has essentially no effect on your ability to taste sour. The same would be true if you were to adapt to sweet and then test your sensitivity to sour. In general, cross-adaptation works only when the adapting substance is similar in quality to the test substance (McBurney and Gent, 1979;

Bartoshuk, 1974). Thus you'd find your sensitivity to dilute solutions of lemon temporarily reduced if you were first to eat a sour pickle, since these two share the quality, "sour." The quality "bitter" seems to be an exception to this rule: sensitivity to bitter substances can be reduced by adaptation to a different taste, sour (McBurney, Smith, and Shick, 1972). In all, though, the results from cross-adaptation studies generally point to the existence of distinct taste qualities.

Modification, the second form of taste interaction, occurs when exposure to one substance subsequently alters the taste of another substance. Several of these so-called "taste illusions" have been described by Bartoshuk (1974; Bartoshuk et al., 1969). One that might be familiar to you involves fresh artichokes—after eating this delicacy, people find that other foods and drinks, including plain water, tend to have a sweet taste. (Actually, this is but one example of taste aftereffects involving water; Box 12.3 describes others that you can easily experience.) Another intriguing taste illusion is produced by the leaves of the *Gymnema sylvestre* plant, found in India and Africa. Eating the leaves or drinking tea made from those leaves temporarily abolishes the sweet taste of sugar. In fact, following exposure to *Gymnema sylvestre,* sugar crystals on the tongue are indistinguishable from grains of sand; salt, in contrast, retains its taste—proof that *Gymnema sylvestre* doesn't simply wipe out the entire sense of taste.

Another, equally exotic taste modifier comes from the *Synsepalum dulcificum* bush. Popularly called "miracle fruit," the berries from this bush impart an intensely sweet taste to even the sourest foods, such as lemons. Moreover, this sweetening aftereffect lasts about an hour after eating just a small amount of miracle fruit. This could provide a novel way to reduce your intake of sugar—you could fool your tongue into believing that food was sweet without adding sugar. Although it's not known exactly how miracle fruit works, it is known that it alters the responsiveness of taste fibers (Brouwer et al., 1983). Following exposure of the tongue to miracle fruit's active ingredient, fibers normally responsive to sweet substances but

not to sour ones develop a temporary sensitivity to sour. In other words, these nerve fibers temporarily behave as though sour were sweet. After about an hour, these fibers return to their normal state, once again ignoring sour. Recall that an hour is also about how long the taste illusion persists. Incidentally, the sweet taste caused by miracle fruit can be abruptly abolished by tasting *Gymnema sylvestre,* the leaf that destroys the taste of sugar. Here's an interesting case where one illusion can be used to combat another.

There's one taste modifier that everyone is familiar with: toothpaste. You've probably had the annoying experience of finding that the taste of your morning fruit juice has been ruined because you had just brushed your teeth. This cross-adaptation occurs because toothpaste contains an ingredient that temporarily reduces the sweetness of sugar while making the acid in the juice taste extra sour (Bartoshuk, 1980).

Taste Mixtures. So far our discussion has focused on altering one taste by exposure to another. Next, let's consider what happens when two or more taste substances are mixed together (which occurs routinely whenever one cooks). Everyone knows that it's possible to tone down the taste of one substance by adding another—this is one reason why people add sugar to coffee, to mask its bitter taste. This reduction of one taste sensation by another is called **taste suppression,** and it seems to be a general property of taste mixtures (Bartoshuk, 1975; Gillan, 1982). But what do taste mixtures actually taste like? Is taste analogous to color vision, where two component hues (for instance red and green) can create an entirely new hue (yellow)? Or is taste more like hearing, where two tones played together still maintain their individuality?

The answer to this interesting and important question is not clear. McBurney (1978) maintains that new qualities are not produced by the mixture of taste components. According to this view, lemon juice with sugar added may taste both sour and sweet; but it won't taste salty or anything else new. This outcome is reminiscent of the situation

Box 12.3 *The Taste of Water: An Aftereffect*

You would probably agree that water doesn't seem to have any particular taste, aside from the faint mineral taste found in tap water. Yet by adapting your tongue to different substances, you can make water take on various distinct tastes. This phenomenon—"water taste"—is somewhat similar to the negative color afterimages described in Chapter 6. In the case of water, however, the taste aftereffect is not organized in an opponent fashion. This will become apparent when you perform the following experiment.

Obtain a bottle of distilled water for this experiment, for distilled water has no mineral taste whatsoever (you should confirm this for yourself). Pour a glass full of distilled water—this will be the test stimulus. Next, fill three other glasses with water (the tap variety will do) and add a teaspoon of salt to one, a teaspoon of lemon juice to the second, and a teaspoon of sugar to the third—these are the adaptation stimuli. Be sure each is well stirred. Begin by taking a sip of the distilled water, just to remind yourself what "no taste" tastes like.

Now take a mouthful of the salty solution and roll it around in your mouth for about 30 seconds. At the end of this adaptation period, spit out the salty water and take a sip of the distilled water. The previously tasteless liquid will now have a noticeable sour or bitter taste. Once this aftertaste has worn off, such that distilled water again has no taste, adapt to the sour (lemon) solution for 30 seconds. Now you will find that the same distilled water tastes faintly sweet. After this taste aftereffect has worn off, adapt to the sweet solution. This time distilled water will take on a sour taste.

Can you see the similarity between this taste aftereffect and the negative color afterimages you experienced when you looked at Color Plate 10? In the case of color, a white surface took on the hue that was dependent on the adaptation color. In the case of taste, the distilled water plays the same role as the white surface—both represent a neutral stimulus that becomes temporarily "shaded" by adaptation. There is, however, a real difference between colored afterimages and water taste aftereffects. With color, adaptation obeys an opponent rule: adapting to red makes white look green, whereas adapting to green makes white look red; blue and yellow are comparably related. With taste, adaptation is not reciprocal: adaptation to salty makes water taste sour, but adaptation to sour makes water taste sweet, not salty. Similar nonreciprocal aftereffects are found in the case of bitter (which you can most easily produce using unsweetened quinine water). Bitter makes distilled water taste sweet, but as you experienced, adapting to sweet makes distilled water taste sour, not bitter. All this implies that taste does not involve opponent process mechanisms such as those implicated in color vision (McBurney, Smith, and Shick, 1972). It also implies that the taste of water must be changing all the time during the course of a meal, since you are constantly adapting your tongue to different taste substances. Even the salt in your own saliva can act as a mild adaptation stimulus. Because you've adapted to your own saliva, when you sip distilled water it may appear to have a slightly sour taste.

in hearing, not color vision. Schiffman and Erickson (1980), however, report that sometimes a mixture will produce an unexpected taste, one not usually associated with the taste of any of the components. Such a result would be in line with the behavior of color vision, not hearing.

How does one unravel these seemingly contradictory observations? Part of the problem stems from the inherently subjective nature of these perceptual judgments. In effect, people must "introspect" on their taste sensations, decomposing the mixture into constituents. (To see how difficult this is, try analyzing the tastes evoked by each dish in your next meal.) Introspection, however, is not a simple task, and it is subject to all sorts of extraneous influences, such as the instructions given to people. As an alternative, people could be asked to "construct" a taste mixture that matches the taste(s) of a solution mixed by the experimenter. Such an experiment would be analogous to the metameric color-matching experiments described in Chapter 6. However, to perform such a taste-matching experiment requires having some idea of what components should be provided for the mixture. And this brings us back to the question raised at the outset—the question as to the existence of basic taste qualities. At present, this question represents the fundamental issue in taste research, and until it is resolved, we'll have to be content enjoying what we eat without knowing exactly what we are tasting.

TASTE PREFERENCES

Liking and disliking are not usually thought of as natural properties of sensory stimulation. There seems to be nothing inherently sad about the color blue, for example. Taste may be an exception, however. People can reliably rate various tastes along a dimension of "pleasant/unpleasant," and one person's ratings are very likely to agree with another's. Bitter is usually judged "unpleasant," whereas sweet, at least in low concentrations, is rated "pleasant." Such judgments are called **taste hedonics** ("hedonic" is derived from the Greek

word meaning "pleasure"). Some taste experts believe that these hedonic qualities stem from biological factors governing food selection. Organisms ranging from insects to primates, humans included, crave sweet substances. This may be adaptive, since sugars are easily detected nutrients common in plants (Ramirez, 1990). Bitter is typically associated with toxic substances, which would explain why nearly all animals show an aversion to bitter substances. In fact, some plants and animals have capitalized on this universal aversion by evolving a bitter-tasting skin themselves, a characteristic that wards off potential predators (Gittleman and Harvey, 1980).

Earlier we mentioned that sensitivity to certain bitter substances, including PROP and PTC, varies with one's genetic makeup. This genetic heterogeneity produces a corresponding heterogeneity in preferences for particular foods. Generally, tasters are more finicky in their food preferences, expressing dislike for a greater number of foods (Fischer, Griffin, England, and Carn, 1961; Glanville and Kaplan, 1965). Anliker, Bartoshuk, Ferris, and Hooks (1991) summarize this body of work, noting that adults with normal bitter sensitivity tend to avoid certain strong-tasting foods, including sauerkraut, turnips, spinach, and strong cheese. Anliker and her colleagues also extended these observations to the preferences of tasters and nontasters among young children, aged 5 to 7 years. Although food preferences are governed by many factors, including social, moral, and cultural ones (Rozin, 1990), genetic differences in taste sensitivity have a clear influence as well.

With the mention of social and cultural influences on food preference, we should note that a natural aversion to bitter can be overcome, as evidenced by the almost universal enjoyment of such substances as beer, coffee, and quinine water. And just as natural aversions can be conquered, unnatural ones can be *acquired* (Garcia and Koelling, 1966; Garb and Stunkard, 1974). Extreme nausea following ingestion of some food is a sure bet to cause an animal to reject that food the next time it is available. This phenomenon, called **con-**

ditioned taste aversion, is an extremely potent method for discouraging predators from disturbing farm animals such as chickens and sheep. One meal of sheep meat laced with lithium chloride (a chemical that induces violent nausea) will dissuade a coyote from going near the source of that meat in the future. By the same token, one night of heavy indulgence in whiskey is enough to discourage a person from ordering whiskey sours in the near future.

Although sweet tastes are usually thought of as pleasant, extremely sweet food or drink can be unpleasant. Howard Moskowitz has studied how hedonic ratings vary with the concentration of various substances. He finds that for sweet substances, pleasantness increases with concentration up to a point, after which the substance becomes more and more unpleasant. This transition point Moskowitz (1978) calls the *bliss point*—the concentration yielding the highest hedonic rating. As you might expect, young children have a higher bliss point than do adults, which explains why advertisements for highly sweetened breakfast cereals are aimed primarily at the Saturday morning television audience. Contrary to expectation, however, some obese individuals actually have a lower bliss point than do people of normal weight (Grinker and Hirsch, 1972), although this finding does not hold for all sweet substances (Drewnowski, Grinker, and Hirsch, 1982).

Besides concentration, a food's color can also influence how much people like its taste. One clever study (Duncker, 1939) had people rate the taste of white chocolate and brown chocolate, and they did this while either blindfolded or not. With their eyes open, people judged the white chocolate as weak in taste, whereas the blindfolded group liked it just as much as the brown chocolate. The same pattern of results has been found for fruit-flavored beverages and cake (DuBose, Cardello, and Maller, 1980). The food industry, aware of the influence of color on taste perception, often adds color to products. Margarine, for instance, is naturally very pale but is dyed yellow to mimic the color of real butter. Likewise, orange food coloring is added to many orange juice prod-

ucts, and this strategy improves the flavor scores of these products (see Pangborn, 1960). To convince yourself of the potent effect color has on taste perception, just add green food coloring to milk and see how it tastes.

Related to the issue of taste preference is **sensory-specific satiety,** the reduction in the pleasurable sensory quality of a particular food as it is being eaten (Rolls, 1986). Suppose a moderately hungry person rates the pleasantness of the taste, smell, and texture of some food. Now, following this initial rating, imagine the individual gets a meal that includes the previously rated food, and immediately following the meal the person again rates the food's pleasantness. The postmeal ratings will be lower than the premeal ratings, even though the food itself has not had time to be digested. Evidently it is the sensory quality of the food itself, not its nutritional consequences, that produces the reduced hedonic response to the food. Moreover, this satiety effect is specific to the food items consumed during the meal—foods that were not eaten do not lower their pleasantness (Ross, Van Duijvenvoorde, and Rolls, 1984). The specificity of satiety means that relatively more food may be eaten during a meal that consists of many different foods served over several courses. Understanding sensory-specific satiety may shed light on eating disorders such as bulimia (Drewnoski, Bellisle, Aimez, and Remy, 1987), the condition where an individual engages in an eating binge followed by fasting or self-induced vomiting. Rodin, Bartoshuk, Peterson, and Schank (1990) have found that bulimic patients continued to rate sweet substances as pleasant even after ingesting a healthy dose of glucose dissolved in water; nonbulimics, in contrast, found the sweet substance less pleasant after ingestion of glucose. Rodin and her colleagues speculate that bulimics may engage in food binges because they fail to experience a reduction in its pleasantness during the course of eating.

The general topic of taste preferences is a fascinating one; there is much interesting material that cannot be presented here for lack of space. Those interested in that topic should consult Rozin's (1979) comprehensive chapter; in addition, there are several informative articles on cross-cultural studies of taste perception and preference (Johns and Keen, 1985; Bertino and Chan, 1986).

THE INTERACTION BETWEEN TASTE AND SMELL

Several times in this chapter we have stressed the role played by odor in what we usually think of as taste. Holding your nostrils closed while you eat dramatically demonstrates this role. One study (Mozel et al., 1969) found that the ability to identify food substances is severely hampered when odor perception is eliminated. In this study, twenty-one familiar substances were individually liquified in a blender and dropped onto a person's tongue from an eye-dropper; the person's task was to name the food. The results are summarized in Figure 12.17, which shows the percentages of people tested who could identify each of the twenty-one substances. The shaded bars give the results when the odor of the solution could be smelled; the unshaded bars give the results when odors were blocked from reaching the olfactory epithelium. Obviously, smell improved performance greatly. In fact, for several very familiar substances, including coffee, garlic, and chocolate, correct identification was impossible without smell.

There is something paradoxical about odor's contribution to taste: when odor is added to a substance that is being tasted, people do not report that its smell has increased in strength, they say instead that its *taste* has increased (Murphy, Cain, and Bartoshuk, 1977). Demonstrate this for yourself—begin eating with your nostrils held closed; then release them. Opening your nostrils means that odor will be added, but instead of experiencing this addition as smell, you will find that it is taste that has become stronger. In other words, taste and smell blend into a single experience, and this combined experience is typically referred to as "taste." One of the skills that "taste" experts

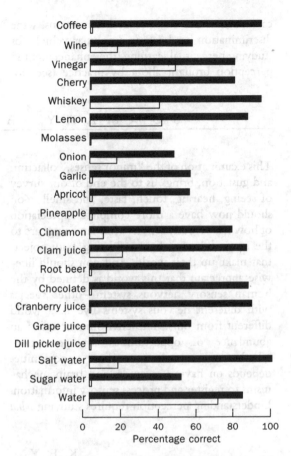

FIGURE 12.17 The percentages of subjects who could identify a substance dropped onto their tongues when they could smell the solution (shaded bars) and when they were prevented from smelling the solution (unshaded bars). (Adapted from Mozel et al., 1969.)

develop is the knack of attending to the odors of the food or drink they are sampling. If you've ever watched a serious wine taster at work, you know what we mean. First of all, wine tasters prefer to evaluate wine when it is close to room temperature, so that the odorous vapors are more abundant. To further promote the release of vapors, a taster will swirl the liquid around in the glass and will then deeply inhale the vapors with the nose placed right at the mouth of the glass. This odor information alone is often sufficient to identify the particular wine being sampled. Because wines vary along several dimensions, wine discrimination has become a popular vehicle for studying perceptual learning, the enhancement in perception brought about by practice (see, for example, Owen and Machamer, 1979). In fact, entire books have been written on the sensory evaluation of wine (Kramer, 1989).

S U M M A R Y   A N D   P R E V I E W

This examination of the "minor senses," olfaction and gustation, brings us to the end of our survey of seeing, hearing, touch, taste, and smell. You should now have a more complete appreciation of how marvelously sensitive human beings are to the noisy, odorous, light-reflecting, tasty objects that make up their world. And you should likewise appreciate that this world is defined by the human sensory nervous system—other species with different nervous systems live in a world different from ours. The environment offers an abundance of opportunities for perception; whether one capitalizes on those opportunities depends on having receptors and brain mechanisms to register and process sensory information. Understanding perception requires studying *what*

there is to be perceived (the environment as a source of stimulation) and *how* the process is implemented (the mechanisms of perception).

As stressed throughout these chapters, perception serves to guide thought and action. This means, therefore, that your perceptions of the world can be influenced by what you intend to do or what you are thinking. You've seen in this chapter and others that the evidence from your senses is often supplemented by evidence from other sources, including what you have learned about the world during previous encounters with it. In the final chapter, then, we shall consider the role of knowledge in perception and the role of perception in such complex activities as reading.

K E Y   T E R M S

adaptation
anosmia
cilia
common chemical sense
conditioned taste aversion
cross–adaptation
cross–fiber theory
flavor
free nerve ending
mixture suppression

multidimensional scaling (MDS)
nasal cycle
odor adaptation
odor constancy
odor hallucinations
olfactory brain
olfactory bulb
olfactory epithelium
olfactory nerve

olfactory receptor cell
papillae
pheromones
sensory-specific satiety
specific anosmias
taste buds
taste hedonics
taste modification
taste suppression
tip of the nose

Knowledge and Perception

ristotle had insightful things to say about many different subjects, including perception:

Under the influence of strong feeling we are easily deceived regarding our sensations . . . for example the coward under the influence of fear and the lover under that of love have such illusions that the former owing to a trifling resemblance thinks he sees an enemy, the latter his beloved . . . men sick of a fever sometimes think they see animals on the walls owing to some slight resemblance in the figures drawn there . . . in cases where the patient is not very sick, he is still conscious of the deceptions, but where his condition is more aggravated, he even rushes upon these animals. (Aristotle, Parva Naturalia, quoted in Davidoff, 1975, pp. 195– 196)

Aristotle's observations capture an idea of fundamental importance: though perception begins with the responses of the sense organs, it draws also on the perceiver's knowledge of the world. In order to appreciate the sum and substance of Aristotle's observations, it's best to put them into a context that connects them to discussions earlier in the book.

KNOWLEDGE'S MODES OF INFLUENCE

Previous chapters emphasized the patterns of stimulation generated by the environment in which we live and the responses of our sense organs and brain to those patterns of stimulation.

We focused on the contribution to perception of information from receptors. This view is schematized in panel A of Figure 13.1. Note that although the three panels in Figure 13.1 use vision as their example, a similar analysis can also be made for other senses.

Panel A outlines a truncated but familiar scheme: the visual system, particularly various cortical structures, extracts information about stimulus features, stimulus location, and spatial arrangement. This scheme represents what is called a **bottom-up** model of perception. In it, essential information flows from early, peripheral levels (the receptors) upward to higher levels (the brain). The neural operations engaged in these early stages of processing are said to be "data-driven," meaning that physical aspects of the stimulus (for instance, its intensity) determine the patterns of activity generated. Thus far, knowledge has yet to make an appearance.

Knowledge's influences on perception can be characterized as **top-down,** in contrast to those sensory influences dubbed bottom-up. Though top-down influences could take many different forms, they generally seem to work in one of four ways. A very brief introductory preview of the four may help when they reappear throughout the rest of the chapter. Here, then, are knowledge's four modes of influence on perception.

1. **Knowledge enables categorization.** Knowledge, particularly as a record of previous sensory data, permits objects and events to be related to what we've ex-

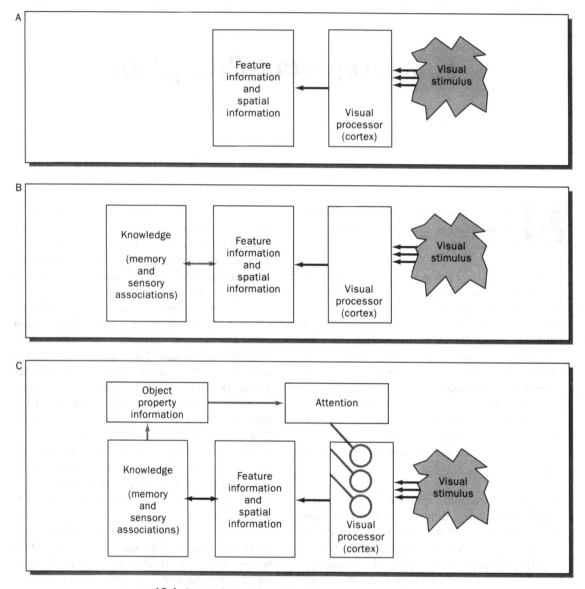

FIGURE 13.1 Interactions among knowledge, attention, and perception.

perienced before and, therefore, to be categorized. One special category, "object experienced previously," constitutes recognition. Without the ability to identify and recognize, perception's usefulness is tremendously diminished.

2. **Knowledge controls attention.** Knowl-

edge steers the selective process known as attention; as you'll see, attention does its work by amplifying the effectiveness of some stimuli and, perhaps, by diminishing the effectiveness of others.

3. **Knowledge guides acquisition of sensory data.** Top-down influences guide the

acquisition of sensory input, including supplementary input. For example, upon hearing the song of a wood thrush, you are better able to canvas the trees' branches for the source of this lovely sound. The first event guides subsequent perceptual activity.

4. **Knowledge supplies context for sensory data.** Top-down influences—knowledge—can add to or supplement sensory input, by providing a context in which that input is interpreted; the interpretation thus can vary depending on the context. This is what Aristotle had in mind when he cited the misperceptions of cowards and lovers (see above). William James helped us appreciate how supplementation might operate: "The natural way of conceiving all this is under the symbolic form of a brain-cell played upon from two directions. Whilst the object excites it from without, other brain-cells, or perhaps spiritual forces, arouse it from within." (1890, vol. 1, p. 441)

This four-part scheme simplifies a very complex domain. Like any simplification, though, this one has limitations. For one thing, the first of these four modes of influence is conceptually different from the others. In particular, the first item represents a use made of residue from *previous* sensory input; the last three items represent specific routes by which knowledge acts on *current* sensory input. Additionally, the four modes of influence cannot always be separated cleanly from one another: there are times when two, or even more, operate simultaneously. Still, it will be helpful to keep the four-part scheme in mind as you read this chapter.

However knowledge influences perception, rarely are we aware of that influence and then only when knowledge leads us seriously astray. Generally, knowledge's influence is unrecognized albeit highly beneficial. Consider this illustration. The knowledge that a visitor is coming sensitizes you to sounds that closely resemble knocking at your door. This makes the knock, when it does occur, easier to hear in the midst of some background noise. But since perception is colored by expectations, perception will be in error whenever those expectations are wrong. No one, no matter how scrupulous, is immune from such influences. For example, the greatest astronomers of the late nineteenth century mistook various geographical features on Mars' surface for rectilinear canals (Sheehan, 1988). Interestingly, once the first of these astronomers reported the canals, virtually all astronomers subsequently saw these markings as canals.

Expectations about more mundane matters can also dominate perception. William James spoke to this in comments on the price we pay for heightened sensitivity:

When watching for the distant clock to strike, our mind is so filled with its image that every moment we think we hear the longed-for or dreaded sound. So of an awaited footstep. Every stir in the wood is for the hunter his game; for the fugitive his pursuers. Every bonnet in the street is momentarily taken by the lover to enshroud the head of his idol. (1890, vol. 1, p. 442)

No one can deny how common—and powerful—such phenomena are. Ordinarily, knowledge is subsidiary to sensory data, but under some conditions, sensory data drop to a supporting role while knowledge takes center stage. Then, knowledge overrides what your senses may be signaling. As you might imagine, knowledge is most likely to overpower sensory information when, for one reason or other, the sensory information is weak, ambiguous, unclear, or in the extreme, absent. But even when sensory information is strong, unambiguous, and clear, knowledge still has an impact.

IDENTIFICATION AND RECOGNITION

As we've noted, the capacity to identify or recognize objects and events is crucial for normal perception. Without that capacity, people cannot effectively use what they see, hear, smell, taste, or touch to guide their behavior. In this section, we'll first give a rough sketch of how identification works and then discuss what happens when it fails.

Consider the middle panel in Figure 13.1. Here we've elaborated on panel A by taking account of knowledge. The two-way arrow in panel B signifies that information about the features and spatial layout of an object is compared with records of the properties of objects experienced on prior occasions; this exemplifies the first mode of knowledge listed above. When we identify an object, we say that it is a member of some class, for example, the class "purple finch" or the class "Mozart string quartet." Classifying the stimulus requires that some correlation be made between (1) the sensory evidence produced by the current object, and (2) stored evidence generated during prior occurrences of that object or similar objects.

The nature of the correlation is currently under intense study, with the debate converging on two issues: the character and cortical distribution of the stored information, and the nature of the process that uses the stored information. For example, although panel B represents knowledge as lying within a single compartment, it may be that records of diverse attributes are actually stored in separate, but intercommunicating, regions of the brain (Damasio, 1989). The first of these issues, the representation question, is discussed at various places in the text, including in this chapter. The second issue, which is beyond the scope of this text, focuses on the neural computations that implement the correlation. One promising approach implements the correlation by means of a hierarchical network of simple elements whose interactions are governed by one or another set of mathematical rules. (Bechtel and Abrahamsen, 1991, provide a good, accessible introduction to this approach.)

TEMPORARY FAILURES OF CATEGORIZATION

When sensory data are impoverished, the correlation process may be stymied, rendering categorization impossible. Imagine you are walking along a country road. It is very foggy and the light has begun to fail. Down the road appear some blurry shapes moving about, but you can't tell exactly what they are. These remote, blurry objects fail to produce a clear, strong match to the stored records corresponding to the representation of any one object. You may not be certain of what you're seeing because the input matches, though only imperfectly, the representations left by several different sorts of objects.

If forced to identify the object, you ought to respond with the single stored representation that best matches the input. This representation would be the best among a series of not-so-great bets. Your identification might be correct, but since the match was equivocal, it could also be wrong. If accuracy is paramount, you're better off getting additional sensory input before making your response. Later we'll consider how knowledge guides the acquisition of that additional input.

Like anything else, the process of correlation—and its result, identification—can and does go astray. Most often "astray" means that you mistake one stimulus for another. As an example, take the confession of the distinguished Scots philosopher Thomas Reid. While he lay in bed, Reid mistook his own heartbeat for a knock at the door. This happened not once, but several times within a short time. At each "knock," Reid got out of bed to open the door for a nonexistent visitor (1813/1970, p. 53). So intelligence, which Reid had in abundance, confers no immunity against misjudgment.

Though Reid's problem with misrecognition may have been aggravating, it was only temporary. Imagine what it would be like if recognition were permanently disrupted. In the extreme, suppose that it were no longer possible to compare sensory information against records of prior experiences. You might still be able to perceive but would not be able to recognize or know *what* you'd perceived or whether you'd encountered the object before. You could see your family and friends but not know who they were or, perhaps, that you'd ever seen them before. To reinforce the importance of recognition, consider one unusual condition that leads to the paradoxical condition of perception without recognition.

PROSOPAGNOSIA: A PERMANENT FAILURE OF CATEGORIZATION

A neurological disorder, as you have learned, can severely disrupt one function but leave others intact. In some cases, the disruption spares a sensory system, say vision, but prevents the perceiver from making sense of what is perceived. Known generically as **agnosias** (from the Greek, meaning "without knowledge"), these disorders take many different forms, depending on the neural structures damaged (Farah, 1992). To appreciate what perception without knowledge must be like, consider one particularly interesting type of agnosia, known as **prosopagnosia.** In this condition, a patient can see and describe another person's face but cannot recognize whose face it is, even if the person is a close relative (Sacks, 1985). We'll discuss this relatively rare condition in some detail, because prosopagnosia illuminates some key theoretical and methodological ideas.

The following case involves a fairly typical patient who has cerebral lesions of uncertain origin:

When her husband or mother visited her, she failed to recognize them immediately, and only when a conversation was begun did she identify her visitors. When she was shown photographs of her two older children of preschool age, she failed to identify them; when she was told that these were indeed her children, she remarked that "they don't look like they should." Her failure in facial recognition extended to public personalities such as television stars. When watching television, she was unable to identify performers who were well-known to her until they spoke or sang. (Benton, 1980, p. 178)

Most patients diagnosed as prosopagnosic, when looking at a set of pictures of different faces, can distinguish one face from another (meaning they can judge whether one is different from the other); they can also categorize the faces by gender (Tranel, Damasio, and Damasio, 1988). They can even say when two photographs are actually of the same face viewed from different perspectives (Sergent and Poncet, 1990). Despite all these abilities, though, they cannot *recognize* faces, including photographs or mirror images of their own face.

The deficit goes beyond not being able to put a name to a face, or being able to relate pertinent information about the face's owner. Faces that should be well known to the patient fail to evoke even a glimmer of familiarity. The condition is so hard to comprehend that

those who have never seen a prosopagnosic patient may be tempted to dismiss the phenomenon as the result of psychiatric illness or dementia. These interpretations are not credible considering that these patients show no evidence of language impairment, have intact cognitive skills and do not have psychiatric symptomatology before or after the onset of prosopagnosia. (Damasio, 1985, p. 133)

This fascinating, sad condition might tempt us to conclude that these patients have suffered brain damage to a region responsible for "face identification." However, the history of neurological research teaches us to be very cautious about interpreting behavioral observations on any patient whose cerebral cortex has been damaged—it can be very tricky to make comparisons among individual patients. Subtle differences in the cortical areas affected can produce dramatic differences in the ensuing behavioral deficits. Patients diagnosed as prosopagnosic are no exception to this rule. For example, most prosopagnosics have associated deficits that are ignored. Damasio, Damasio, and van Hoesen (1982) point out that the distress of not being able to recognize faces of relatives and friends is so devastating that other types of recognition losses are likely to be overlooked. Damasio, Damasio, and van Hoesen describe patients who are unable to recognize other familiar things besides faces. For instance, they tell of an avid bird watcher who knew a bird when he saw one but could no longer identify the species to which individual birds belonged, and a farmer who, though knowing a cow when he saw one, had lost the ability to recognize individual members of his own herd. Thus, patients can show losses in recognition of stimuli other than faces. One of Damasio and colleagues' more bizarre cases was a patient who could not recognize her own car in a parking lot. She had to check the license plate numbers on every car until she found her own car's license number; the appearance of the car was of no help. Thus instead of a loss restricted to recognition of faces, prosopagnosia may involve a more general impairment of the ability to recognize specific, individual members of classes of complex objects.*

Recently Justine Sergent of the Montreal Neurological Institute demonstrated that prosopagnosia can result from defects at different levels of the face-recognition process (Sergent and Poncet, 1990). You may recall from Chapter 12 that by applying multidimensional scaling to the judged similarity of stimuli, it is possible to learn what stimulus information is crucial in similarity judgments (see also the Appendix). Using this technique, Sergent showed prosopagnosic patients eight different faces, two at a time. After each pair, a patient rated how similar the faces seemed to one another. Multidimensional scaling revealed that Sergent's patients operated quite differently. One patient's scaling results were much like the results from normals: facial similarity was judged on the basis of overall similarity of the face's configuration, integrating various facial features into a comprehensive gestalt (Sergent and Poncet, 1990). The other patient, in contrast, manifested what appeared to be a perceptual coding defect. Multidimensional scaling disclosed that this patient compared faces on the basis of the face's separate components taken singly, without real integration into an overall gestalt (Sergent and Villemure, 1989). As a result, Sergent urged a distinction between prosopagnosics who have a defect of perceptual coding and prosopagnosics whose perceptual coding is normal but who do have a defect involving activation of pertinent memories.

Consider those prosopagnosics who have normal or near normal perceptual coding (Damasio, 1985). In these patients, face recognition probably fails because of inability to mobilize pertinent stored information about the face's owner. Assume, though, that the inaccessible memories are present nonetheless in some form. Perhaps their presence could be tapped by probes that bypass conscious recognition. After all, many of our memories have effects that don't reach consciousness (for example, Schacter, 1989). Investigators have used various probes to explore the existence, in some prosopagnosics, of inaccessible memories. In one approach, the skin resistance of prosopagnosics was monitored while they were shown photos of familiar and unfamiliar faces. (Skin resistance reflects the activation level of the body's autonomic nervous system.) Despite the demonstrated absence of conscious recognition, seeing the faces of relatives and friends generated stronger changes in skin resistance than those evoked by nonfamiliar faces (Bauer, 1984; Tranel and Damasio, 1985). Sergent and Poncet (1990) strengthened this point with a number of other probes of prosopagnosics' implicit memory for faces. Together, these probes reveal that in prosopagnosics whose perceptual processing is intact, some part of the brain does register the stimulus, though this registration never reaches awareness.

The foregoing discussion of deficits in face recognition has skirted a key question: What region(s) of the brain participate in face recognition? One recent study set out to answer this question while avoiding the difficulties of making inferences from cases of brain injury (Sergent, Ohta, and MacDonald, 1992). Sergent and her colleagues used brain imaging techniques to study face and object recognition in normal people, not patients. Positron emission tomography (PET; see Chapter 1) measured the spatial distribution of brain activity while an individual engaged in various visual tasks including (1) categorizing objects as living or natural versus nonliving or manmade; and (2) categorizing well-known faces as belonging to actors or nonactors. These two tasks constitute "object identification" and "face identification," respectively. By comparing brain activity

---

* Results like these may tell us how the normal brain organizes knowledge, including knowledge about the representation of objects and their properties. One theory inspired by such evidence (Damasio, 1989) postulates that an object's many different features are separately represented in distributed fashion across various specialized areas of the brain, an idea raised in Chapter 4.

produced by different tasks, Sergent was able to distinguish those brain areas specifically involved in face identification.*

Brain regions associated with face identification were mainly located forward of regions that were active during gender identification or object identification; in addition, virtually all the regions specific to face identification were located within the lower portion of the cerebral cortex, in the area of the temporal lobe. In addition, during face identification, several regions in the right hemisphere showed greater activity than their left hemisphere counterparts. This result harmonizes with clinical observations: when prosopagnosia is found in a patient with unilateral brain damage, the damage is almost always to the right hemisphere.

Another of Sergent's results may explain a baffling aspect of prosopagnosia: the loss of ability to recognize a person as a *particular* person (for example, as one's daughter) but the retention of ability to categorize individuals or objects into classes (for example, as males versus females, or knives versus spoons). Remember that face identification—but not identification of objects—activated regions of the cortex that lay toward the front of the brain. Included among these are regions within the temporal lobe. Sergent conjectures that recognition of a particular person requires the activation of biographical memories that are housed in the temporal lobe. Of course, biographical information is not needed for functions that are spared; we don't need such information to identify a face as belonging to a male or to identify some creature as a fish. Though much work remains to be done before we fully understand identification and recognition, studies like those of Sergent and her colleagues do represent an important beginning. One thing is clear,

though: categorization is a complex process involving multiple stages of processing, any one of which may be disrupted by damage to the brain.

In this next section, we turn to the second mode of influence of knowledge on perception—knowledge's ability to steer the process called attention.

ATTENTION: INFLUENCE AND ORIGIN

William James realized very clearly the central place occupied by **attention** in human experience.

Millions of items of the outward order are present to my senses which never properly enter into my experience. Why? Because they have no interest for me. My experience is what I agree to attend to. Only those items which I notice shape my mind—without selective interests, experience is an utter chaos. Interest alone gives accent and emphasis, light and shade, background and foreground—intelligible perspective, in a word. (1890, p. 381)

What is this phenomenon that James places so near the center of our individuality? Whatever it may be, we owe a debt of gratitude to attention: at a party, we can choose to listen to one person speaking amidst other voices; looking through a phone book, we can scrutinize a long, unorganized list of names looking for one name in particular; trying to identify some wonderful scent, we can take several quick sniffs to determine what we're smelling. All these are the sort of active assertions of which James spoke; they demonstrate that, with the aid of that mysterious process, attention, we really do control our own perceptions. But what guides attention? What knowledge about an object of interest allows you to scrutinize the visual sense for that object? Attentional scrutiny can be metaphorically represented as a magnifying glass that concentrates information-processing resources to particular stimuli at particular locations. That scrutiny constitutes one form of attention and is schematized in panel C

---

* To make a comparison, researchers subtract one set of PET data from another. This approach, which is used in many PET studies, places a premium on the experimenter's choice of appropriate subtrahend (control condition). Sergent, Ohta, and MacDonald (1992) discuss this theoretical issue and several others related to the interpretation of PET data.

of Figure 13.1. The trio of magnifying glasses signifies that attention to particular features or stimulus properties is controlled by various forms of knowledge.

CUES DIRECT ATTENTION: BEHAVIORAL RESEARCH

Various experimental strategies are available for examination of attention and a perceiver's control over attention. One favorite strategy exploits the fact that cues, when delivered in a timely fashion, encourage heightened selectivity and improve perceptual function. In audition, for example, a tone is easier to hear if just prior to the tone's onset the listener is cued about its frequency. If, however, the listener is misled about the tone's frequency (for example, told that it will be a high-frequency tone, when it's actually low), attention is misdirected, and the sound is less audible (Johnson and Hafter, 1980; Scharf et al., 1987).

Cues work much the same way in vision. In one study, Ball and Sekuler (1981) determined the ease with which people detected very dim dots that moved across a video screen. From trial to trial, the dots' direction of motion changed unpredictably. In addition, during half the trials, no dots at all were presented; the viewer saw just a blank screen (see panels A and B in Figure 13.2). The dots could be made so dim that a viewer had great difficulty telling whether or not any dots were present. Ball and Sekuler measured the intensity threshold for detecting the dots under various conditions. Thresholds were initially determined simply by randomizing from trial to trial the direction in which the dots moved. Thresholds were then measured with an explicit cue that reduced the viewer's uncertainty about direction of motion. As illustrated in Figure 13.2, this directional cue was a short line flashed very briefly at different times relative to the presentation of the dots. The orientation of the line indicated the direction in which the dots, if present at all, might move (recall that on half the trials, no dots at all were presented).

Ball and Sekuler made several noteworthy dis-

FIGURE 13.2 On any trial, Ball and Sekuler presented either dim dots (A) that could move in any direction or no dots (B). Panels C, D, and E represent the sequence of events for different trials. The viewer first saw a blank screen. Then a cue (short white line) appeared, followed some time later by moving dots. The orientation of the short lines in panels C and E signifies upward motion; the orientation of the line in panel D signifies downward motion. The interval between cue and motion varied—the intervals represented in panels C and D are longer than the one represented in panel E.

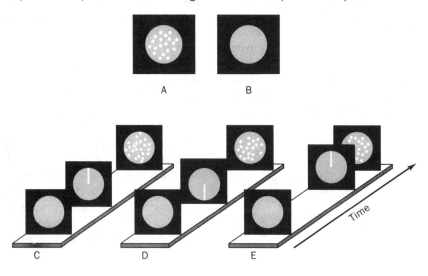

coveries. First, when the orientation of the line corresponded exactly to the dots' direction of motion, the dots were easier to see (threshold was low). Second, the cue was not helpful unless it preceded the dots by about a half-second or so, confirming that attention required some time to operate. Third, if the cue's orientation did not match the dots' direction precisely, but only approximated it, the cue could still lower the detection threshold, but not as much as when it was precisely accurate. Generally, the greater the discrepancy between the cue's orientation and the dots' direction of motion, the more difficult it was to see the moving dots. As in audition, a cue that misdirected an observer's attention to the wrong direction was worse than no cue at all.

CUES DIRECT ATTENTION:
PHYSIOLOGICAL RESEARCH

Physiological counterparts of these psychological studies have helped us understand the mechanisms of attention. Here's one example. Haenny, Maunsell, and Schiller (1988) measured the level of neural activity of single neurons in the visual cortex of monkeys while the animals were engaged in a behavioral task. The neurons studied were in a higher cortical area—known as V4— that receives information already processed by several other areas of the brain (DeYoe and van Essen, 1988). First, consider the experiment's behavioral aspect. The monkey initiated each trial by pressing and holding a lever. This action brought on the presentation of the "cue" for that trial—a grating whose orientation varied randomly from trial to trial. After this grating cue had disappeared, the monkey was then shown a series of gratings in rapid succession, each differing in orientation. The monkey's task was to release the lever when it saw a grating whose orientation matched that of the previously seen cue grating. Over trials, the experimenters varied the number of gratings presented before the matching orientation appeared, thus preventing the animal from simply counting presentations before releasing the lever. The animal was rewarded with a drink of juice following each correct response.

The cue in Haenny, Maunsell, and Schiller's experiment temporarily made one particular orientation very important to the monkey. Physiologically, the boost in importance potentiated cells tuned to that orientation, causing a larger than normal response when their optimum orientation was actually presented. If the grating's orientation had not been cued, a neuron tuned to that orientation gave only its normal response. Intriguing demonstrations of this sort have been offered by other researchers as well (Moran and Desimone, 1985; Spitzer, Desimone, and Moran, 1988).

The experiment just described conclusively demonstrates that attention can modulate the level of activity in brain cells. But what are the neural pathways by which cues affect neurons in, say, Area V4? The research in the next several paragraphs provides some clues. To begin, we must realize that attention is not just a single monolithic process, but arises from a set of separate but interdependent processes, each responsible for a component of attention (Posner, 1992). This realization grew out of three parallel strands of research: single cell recordings from the brains of alert, behaving animals (like the experiment described above), PET studies of humans engaged in various attention-demanding tasks, and work with patients who have suffered localized damage to the brain. Many details of attention's neural bases are yet to be worked out; moreover, the particular structures and circuits involved in mediating attention vary from one attentional task to another. For these reasons, we can't present a comprehensive treatment of attention's neurology. Instead, we describe a neural system that mediates one component of attention. The discussion draws on a sample of experimental results from a particularly exciting and rich study (Corbetta et al., 1991). These results provide an excellent framework for understanding the ensuing discussion of other work on the interplay between attention and perception.

NEURAL CIRCUITS OF ATTENTION

The examples of attention given above underscore that perceptual selectivity is one of attention's essential hallmarks. To investigate the mechanisms of this selectivity, Corbetta and colleagues coordinated measurements of psychophysical performance with measurements of brain activity. Different psychophysical tasks demanded varying degrees of perceptual selectivity. Concomitant records of brain activity, cortical and subcortical, were made with PET, the metabolic labeling technique described earlier.

Observers had to recognize subtle differences between two brief, sequentially presented displays on a computer monitor. Each display consisted of 30 rectangles that moved together across the monitor. The rectangles, which were distributed randomly, were identical in shape and color, and all moved at the same speed. On some trials one or more properties changed slightly from the first to the second display. In particular, the rectangles could change slightly in their elongation; their color might change slightly; and/or their speed of movement might increase somewhat. On other trials, the first and second displays were identical in all respects.

In the "selective-attention" condition, observers knew ahead of time the one feature that might change. In the "divided-attention" condition, observers had no information about which feature might change and so had to monitor all three features simultaneously. Note that the characteristics of the display were identical in the selective-attention and divided-attention conditions; only the observer's mental set changed.

The psychophysical results were as expected: when observers attended to one predefined feature, they spotted the change more easily. The PET measurements revealed that attention to any particular feature activated a characteristic region or regions within the extrastriate visual cortex. These regions correspond to ones that have special responsibility for processing information about the feature that activated it here (see Chapter 4, 6, and 8). This result suggests that attention may be able to drive changes in the responses of neurons within the brain's specialist areas, a point we discuss below. But what inaugurates these changes in visual areas?

Selective attention consistently activated one set of nonvisual areas of the brain, chief among which was a subcortical structure, the **pulvinar,** which is the largest nucleus of the thalamus (see Chapter 4). The pulvinar occupies much of the posterior region of the thalamus and receives inputs from many different cortical and subcortical structures. Among its cortical inputs are ones from the temporal, parietal, and occipital lobes. The pulvinar sends signals back to these same structures. This feedback arrangement puts the pulvinar in position to amplify or to inhibit the normal, stimulus-driven responses of neurons in visual areas (and probably areas devoted to other senses).

Lesion studies and observations with PET established the pulvinar's crucial role in various forms of attention. In particular, the pulvinar directs visual attention to give heightened scrutiny to some particular location or object (Petersen, Robinson, and Morris, 1987) and to filter out irrelevant information such as visual clutter (LaBerge and Buchsbaum, 1990; LaBerge, Carter, and Brown, 1992). Corbetta and his colleagues (1991) added a demonstration that the pulvinar controls feature-specific amplification of neuronal responses within various specialists visual cortical areas. This influence by the pulvinar may also explain some of the cuing effects mentioned earlier (for example, Ball and Sekuler, 1981) as well as physiological demonstrations of attention like those of Haenny, Maunsell, and Schiller (1988).

EXPLOITING INTRINSIC CUES

Earlier, we mentioned that cues presented prior to the onset of a stimulus can guide attention and thereby sharpen perception of that stimulus. We have just identified one neural circuit—centered around the pulvinar—that evidently participates in those effects. In the case discussed, the cue was distinct and apart from the stimulus that had to be detected. Sometimes, however, helpful cues are intrinsic to the stimulus itself. Suppose, for example, a stranger begins talking but you can't understand a thing he is saying. Suddenly you realize that he's speaking English, only with a strong Eastern European accent. Realizing that you are hearing accented English helps you understand what's being said. In other words, exposure to a brief sample of speech makes you a more capable listener. This exemplifies the third mode of knowledge's influence, its ability to guide acquisition and processing of subsequent sensory data.

Such effects occur just as readily with language in written form, as the following example illustrates. When you receive a letter from a friend whose handwriting is particularly hard to read, the letter may first seem difficult to decipher; but after a while you learn the "code," making the scrawl easier to read. This common experience has also been studied systematically. In one study (Corcoran and Rouse, 1970) observers were asked to identify words briefly flashed one at a time. Each word was either typewritten or handwritten. When successive words were all typewritten, observers were quite accurate in identifying the words. Likewise, observers were accurate when one word after another was handwritten. However, when handwritten and typewritten words were randomly intermixed, identification was much poorer. A computer metaphor can be used to explain this result: different perceptual strategies, or "subroutines," are used to analyze typewritten material versus handwritten material. Having to select the appropriate subroutine takes some time. Thus if the subroutine is not already in place, the observer must devote some fraction of the word's brief presentation to selecting a subroutine; less time is left for actually analyzing the word, leading to slower identification. Selection of the proper subroutine requires information about the kind of materials requiring analysis—handwritten or typewritten. The process of selecting the proper subroutine represents a top-down process.

It's easiest to study the effects of intrinsic cues if perception is somehow degraded. For example, when a stimulus cannot be seen or heard clearly and instantly, one can see how the perceiver uses intrinsic cues to guide the extraction of additional information from the stimulus. Jerome Bruner and Mary Potter (1964) took this approach in a study of visual recognition. To impede immediate perception, Bruner and Potter created ambiguous stimuli by blurring a series of slides (see Figure 13.3). Their slides depicted various scenes and objects, such as a dog standing on some grass, a traffic intersection seen in aerial view, and a fire hydrant. For each slide, Bruner and Potter slowly reduced its blur, gradually bringing it into sharper focus. Starting when the slide was extremely blurred, people kept writing down what they saw. When the slide was badly out of focus, people's descriptions were usually inaccurate; for example, a pile of earth might be mistaken for a dish of chocolate ice cream. Not surprisingly, as the slide's focus improved, so did people's accuracy.

Bruner and Potter found that when the initial degree of blur was great, observers often failed to recognize what they were looking at until the image was almost perfectly focused. However, when the initial degree of blur was not so great, observers tended to recognize what they were looking at even when it was noticeably blurred. Why should early exposure to a high degree of blur retard later recognition of a picture? One possible explanation became clear when people expressed their thoughts aloud while looking at the pictures. No matter how blurred the picture, people had an interpretation of what some of its parts might be, and this interpretation influenced their perception of the rest of the picture (the fourth of the four top-down influences listed at the beginning of the chapter). When the picture was extremely blurred, visual information that might contradict that interpretation did not become available for quite a while. Consequently, someone initially seeing a highly blurred picture may become locked into a wrong interpretation. In this case, the top-down influence retarded correct perception.

The ability to capitalize on top-down information varies among people. Potter (1966) showed this by repeating the original experiment but testing observers ranging in age from 4 years to 19 years. For any given age, some observers tended to be rapid recognizers whereas others tended to be slow; as shown in Figure 13.4, however, younger observers took about 50 percent longer to recognize the picture than did older observers. Besides differing in speed of recogni-

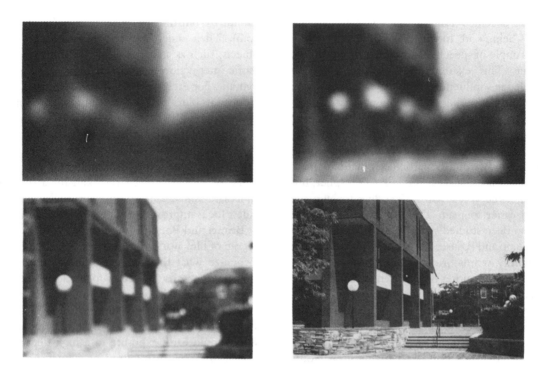

FIGURE 13.3 These four progressively blurred photographs show the same scene. Note that your ability to recognize the contents of the scene is impaired by blur. (Glyn Cloyd.)

tion, young and old observers seemed to arrive at solutions in different ways. The older observers' descriptions formed a coherent series, with a guess at one moment evolving into another, related guess the next moment. In contrast, younger observers' descriptions consisted of a parade of unconnected guesses, often focusing on a single small detail, rather than on the entire scene. This difference between older and younger individuals suggests that experience may be necessary before top-down information becomes maximally effective.

Potter's study underscores individual differences in the speed with which information is extracted from photographs. The x-ray, or radiograph, constitutes a class of photographs for which speed and accuracy of interpretation can be a matter of life and death. Because correct interpretation of an x-ray image may take several seconds, it's a natural theater within which to study the use of intrinsic cues. Such images, of course, are among medicine's most important diagnostic tools. Besides being used to detect breaks in bones, radiographs are used to visualize tumors, benign and malignant. The interpretation of an x-ray requires not only good vision but also considerable practice. A skilled x-ray interpreter works with amazing speed and accuracy, though a significant number of abnormalities get overlooked. To explain these oversights, Harold Kundel, a radiologist, and Calvin Nodine, a psychologist, recorded the eye movements of interpreters who were reading x-rays (Kundel and Nodine, 1983). Because the eye's visual acuity is not uniform over the entire retina, the interpreter must successively fixate different regions of the x-ray.

To guide fixation, the interpreter draws upon several forms of knowledge (Carmody, Nodine, and Kundel, 1980). From the outset, that person usually knows what anatomical structure (for example, the chest) is depicted in the x-ray. This initial knowledge establishes expectations about

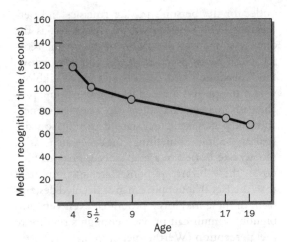

FIGURE 13.4 Median time for recognition of pictures as blur was reduced. (Adapted from Potter, 1966.)

the structure's normal appearance, drawing on memory of previous x-rays. The x-ray interpreter is guided by knowledge that particular parts of that structure are most likely to be abnormal. These parts should be scrutinized first and most carefully. Kundel and Nodine found that when interpreters were instructed where to look, a glance as brief as one-third of a second was sufficient for detection of the abnormality.

Still, on occasion, the interpreter fixated the correct spot but failed to detect the abnormality. You might say that the interpreter was looking at the right place but not attending to the right thing. To perform optimally, the interpreter should know where to look and what to look for.

INTRINSIC CUES CAN DISTORT PERCEPTION

Information that's derived from the stimulus itself can help guide the extraction of additional information. But what happens when that initial information is misleading? Here, the ambiguity of some event or object can also lead the top-down process astray, thereby impairing perception. Just as visual perception can be misled when a person is looking at a blurred picture, auditory perception can be misled by vague, muffled sounds, as the following experiment shows.

B. F. Skinner (1957) had people listen to a tape

recording of low-intensity speech sounds heard against a background of noise. Skinner describes the sound as resembling fragments of "natural speech heard through a wall" (p. 260). Listening to these sounds, some listeners heard a different message with each repetition. The following is one set of responses (successive responses are separated by slashes):

Do not do that / spell the party / have you pummeled him / how do you do / good-night / you know a part / cracker / have you anything / two four one eight / call station / sour pickles / calm down / keep out of it / hobo / do it again / you are mine / I knew her /. (Skinner, 1957, p. 261)

Using a tape recorder and a clean handkerchief, you can repeat Skinner's study. With the handkerchief covering your mouth so as to muffle your voice, tape-record yourself as you read in a monotone three- or four-word fragments from this book. Record a dozen fragments, letting several seconds of silence separate successive fragments. Now have someone listen to the recording played at low volume. During each pause, have the person say what is heard. Repeating this with a number of different people, you'll be surprised at the variety of interpretations you get out of the same fragment. Evidently, people attempt to impose structure on ambiguous sounds, and the structure will vary from one person to the next. But, again, note that the imposed structure is constrained by the physical attributes of the ambiguous stimulus. For example, the people you test will never report the muffled recording as someone singing a song.

This tendency to impose structure on impoverished speech sounds is even more dramatically illustrated by the so-called **phonemic restoration effect.** Richard Warren tape-recorded spoken sentences and then carefully excised one brief speech sound from each, replacing it with a nonspeech sound, such as a cough. Listeners claimed to hear not only the cough but also the excised sound (Warren, 1970; see also Samuel, 1983). In a similar vein, George Miller (1962) presented various words to listeners and asked them to identify what they heard. To make the task difficult, the words were presented in the midst of noise (such as the sound made by static on the radio). Miller presented the words either in random order or in a sentence. He found that in a sentence, the words were much easier to identify. To illustrate, suppose listeners heard the words "who," "some," "red," and "socks." Suppose further that another word ("bought") was presented between "who" and "some," but the listener heard only the first consonant of that word, /b/. Because the words formed a sentence, information from the other words made it easier to identify the incomplete word (Lindsay and Norman, 1977, pp. 276–277). In other words, knowledge of the structure of the English language (top) helped listeners know what to expect and how best to interpret what they were hearing (bottom).

AMBIGUOUS AND IMPOVERISHED STIMULI

It's commonly thought that a person's interpretation of ambiguous sensory messages reveals something about that person's motivation and interests. The Viennese psychiatrist Sigmund Freud discussed this idea in his book *The Psychopathology of Everyday Life* (Freud, 1910/1938). Although most of the errors Freud dealt with were errors of speech or memory, he did consider some to be perceptual errors. Take two examples. Freud described one woman who was so anxious about having children that she often mistook the word "stock" for the word "stork"—presumably reflecting her unconscious preoccupation with the arrival of a child. The second example pertained to Freud himself. An avid collector of antiques, Freud confessed that he saw the word "antiquities" on every shop sign that bore any resemblance to that word. So despite his sophisticated knowledge of unconscious influences on the mind, even Sigmund Freud was apparently not immune to top-down influences.

Rorschach Test. Some psychopathologists have exploited ambiguous stimuli to aid them in personality assessment. So-called projective tests are types of psychological tests that use ambiguous pictures and designs that presumably provide an outlet for the person's private fantasies and perceptions. The best-known projective test is the one developed in the 1920s by Hermann Rorschach, a Swiss psychiatrist. As you may know, the **Rorschach test** consists of a set of inkblots, which the person is asked to describe. Some psychiatrists believe that they can draw inferences about a person's mental state if that person describes seeing something bizarre—such as a bloody axe buried in a man's head. For our purposes, these bizarre responses are less important than the fact that people can give detailed descriptions of these inkblots—proof that even very ambiguous stimuli can provide enough structure to fuel perception (Wertheimer, 1957).

The Autokinetic Effect. A stimulus even more ambiguous than an inkblot—namely, a single point of light in a dark room—can be used as a projective test. Imagine sitting in a dark room looking at a small, stationary spot of light, such as the glow from a cigarette. Under these conditions, the spot of light will appear to drift about (Matin and MacKinnon, 1964). This illusory motion is called the **autokinetic effect** ("autokinetic" means "self-moving"), and some people believe that it results from involuntary drifting movements of the eye. Certain drugs, such as marijuana or alcohol, increase the autokinetic effect (Sharma and Moskowitz, 1972), perhaps because these drugs increase the eye's tendency to drift.

Rechtschaffen and Mednick (1955) exploited the autokinetic effect as a projective test. Observers sat in a totally dark room, about 2.5 meters from a very small, stationary light. They were *told* that the experiment would test their ability to see the words that would be written by the movements of the small light. Though the light never actually moved, the autokinetic effect did produce considerable illusory movement. Every one of the nine observers reported that the light had written at least two words, and one observer reported seeing forty-three words. Some of the words were innocuous (such as "the" or "and"); others were highly personal. In fact, after "reading" the words, one observer became very upset and demanded to know where Rechtschaffen and Mednick had gotten all that information about him. We don't mean to encourage prying into other people's business, but you may wish to try this fascinating projective test on your friends. They may find it hard to believe that the light didn't really "write" all that stuff about them.

Autokinetic "writing" demonstrates how important suggestion can be when perceiving impoverished stimuli. Seeing words is not an inevitable consequence of autokinetic motion. In fact, most people simply see random motions, not words. Rechtschaffen and Mednick's viewers were different though, because they had been told to expect the light to write something. When they experienced illusory motion, the viewers naturally tried to decipher what the light was writing. Under the same circumstances, suggestion could just as well have caused viewers to interpret what they were seeing as outline drawings or the messages on traffic signs.

Reversible or Ambiguous Figures. The power of an unambiguous stimulus to bias the perception of an ambiguous one has been vividly demonstrated with varying versions of the ambiguous figure, a version of which appeared in Chapter 4 (Figure 4.23). Recall that the figure could be seen either as a young woman facing away from the viewer or as an old hag facing toward the viewer.

That figure is reproduced here as the middle panel of Figure 13.5. On the left is a version of the drawing that makes it more clearly depict a young woman; on the right is a version that makes it more clearly depict an old woman.

It has been found that when observers are shown only the ambiguous drawing (middle panel), the majority initially see an old woman (Leeper, 1935). However, this tendency can be altered by having the observer look first at one of the less ambiguous versions of the drawing. When people are first shown the left panel of Figure 13.5 and then the middle panel, virtually all of them initially see the middle panel (the ambiguous drawing) as depicting a young woman. Conversely, when people are first shown the right panel of Figure 13.5 and then the middle panel, virtually all of them then see the ambiguous drawing as depicting an old woman. In other words, exposure to either unambiguous drawing can "prime" the subsequent perception of the ambiguous drawing. Incidentally, this priming effect requires visual experience; it cannot be produced by *verbal* descriptions that emphasize either the young woman or the old woman (Leeper, 1935).

Paranoia. The preceding sections showed how, when stimuli are ambiguous or impoverished, the resulting perceptions reveal much about the per-

FIGURE 13.5 Three versions of young woman/old woman figure—an example of the way priming biases perception.

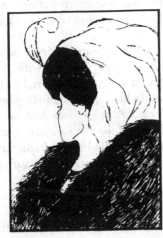 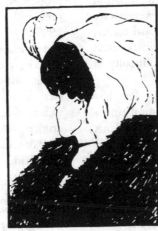 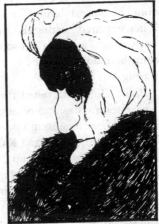

ceiver's own state or motives. Sometimes, however, the stimulus contains a good deal of structure, but some defect in the perceiver degrades the stimulus, introducing ambiguity. For example, an uncorrected myopic eye forces the rest of the visual system to work with a blurred, ill-defined image—a condition resembling the one represented in the top two panels of Figure 13.3. Similarly, a defective ear forces the rest of the auditory system to work with muffled input—a condition resembling that in the Skinner experiment described earlier. Moreover, impaired vision or hearing resulting from defects in the sensory organ can lead to serious psychological disturbance as the following example demonstrates.

Paranoia is a mental disorder characterized by delusions of persecution. Although the idea is controversial, some psychiatrists have attributed paranoia to hearing impairment, since these two conditions are sometimes associated (Zimbardo, Andersen, and Kabat, 1981). It is certainly easy to understand why paranoia and hearing loss might be causally linked. People can gradually develop a hearing loss without being aware of it. Suppose that such a person is surrounded by people who are talking to one another at a normal conversational level. The hearing-impaired person will have difficulty understanding what the others are saying and may conclude that they are whispering to keep her from hearing. If she asks them why they are whispering, they deny that they are. After a while, all the "secretive" discussions may be construed as part of a plot. Note that the situation would be quite different if the person were aware of her impaired hearing. So the irrational condition termed "paranoia" in some cases may result from the rational impulse to explain difficulty in hearing.

Philip Zimbardo tested this possible link between hearing loss and paranoia by simulating a temporary hearing loss in a dozen college students (Zimbardo, Andersen, and Kabat, 1981). He did this by hypnotizing a group of students and implanting the posthypnotic suggestion that they were partially deaf. After coming out of hypnosis, half of the students were told that they would be temporarily losing some of their hearing; the other

half were not told this. A well-rehearsed conversation was then carried on in the presence of each "hearing-impaired" student. This conversation included laughter and grimaces designed to pique the interest of the "hearing-impaired" listener.

Within 24 hours, those individuals who were unaware of their hearing impairment developed significant paranoid tendencies in their thinking, emotional responses, and social behavior. In contrast, individuals who were aware of their hearing loss showed no such tendency. Incidentally, Zimbardo does not claim that all paranoid delusions spring from an unrecognized loss of hearing. However, his research supports the possibility that paranoid tendencies in some middle-aged and older people may develop out of the gradual hearing impairment that often accompanies aging (recall Chapter 10).

FAMILIARITY AND PERCEPTION

An experienced bird watcher can distinguish among hundreds of bird species that to most people look the same. Simply being exposed to a variety of interesting stimuli can sharpen one's capacity to discriminate among them: familiarity can sharpen perception. Previous chapters chronicled demonstrations of this fact, in many cases linking the demonstrations to physiological changes (see particularly Chapters 9 and 11). **Perceptual differentiation** is an umbrella term for the process that makes it possible to discriminate properties, patterns, and distinctive features that previously had been indiscriminable (Gibson, 1969).

For example a novice wine drinker may order "white wine" and be quite content with just about any wine (so long as its color is right). In fact, the novice would have difficulty telling one variety from another. A more seasoned wine drinker, however, would specify a particular variety of white wine and would know whether the wine had a taste that was unusual for that variety (see Owen and Machamer, 1979).

Humans, incidentally, are not the only creatures whose perceptions become differentiated with appropriate training. Recall the preferential looking procedure described in Chapters 5, 6, and 8. There we noted that human infants prefer to look at novel stimuli and tend to ignore stimuli that they have seen many times before. Monkeys exhibit the same behavior. Nicholas Humphrey (1974) took advantage of this ability to determine what animals would be classed as similar by monkeys and what animals would not. When shown a series of pictures of other monkeys, a monkey looked at each picture as though it were novel and interesting. This lack of habituation implies that the monkey distinguished among members of its own species. However, monkeys lumped together members of other species. Once a monkey had initially seen a picture of some domestic animal (such as a pig), the monkey quickly lost interest not only in other pigs but also in other four-legged species as well (such as cows).

However, several months' exposure to pictures of various animals changed the situation drastically. Following such exposure, the monkeys distinguished not only one species from another but also members of a given species one from another. Humphrey (1974) concludes that in some circumstances "insensitivity to visual detail seems to be simply a consequence of visual inexperience" (p. 114). The aphorism claims that "familiarity breeds contempt"; but in Humphrey's study, "familiarity bred perceptual differentiation."

Krueger (1975) reviewed the many other ways in which familiarity affects perception. Although the existence of such effects is beyond question, there are a number of unsettled issues concerning the exact way in which such effects come about. For instance, does familiarity actually alter what you see, or does familiarity alter your ability to use what you've seen? Also, what part is played by practice-related physiological changes that we described in several earlier chapters?

* * *

Thus far our examination of knowledge and perception has been limited to relatively simple stimuli and tasks. How well, though, do the same principles apply to stimuli and tasks that are more representative of everyday activities? To find out, we'll consider two prototypical perceptual tasks.

The first task is the perception of complex visual stimuli, in particular, natural scenes; the other is reading, a demanding and sophisticated task. In both instances, we'll see how context affects perception, the fourth mode of influence listed at the beginning of the chapter.

HOW CONTEXT AFFECTS PERCEPTION

NATURAL SCENES

Irving Biederman measured the time required for an individual to extract visual information from photographs of various indoor and outdoor scenes (Biederman, Rabinowitz, Glass, and Stacy, 1974). The photographs of scenes were presented for varying durations, followed by a masking stimulus that erased any afterimage of that pictorial information. Observers were queried about the general nature of the scene as well as about the presence of particular objects in that scene.

Even when photographs were presented for as little as one-tenth of a second, observers could describe the overall nature of the scene and identify nearly half of the objects contained in the scene. How can so much information be extracted from such a complex stimulus in so short a time? For one thing, real-world scenes are full of redundancies. Consequently, seeing any one object provides a clue about what else is present, particularly in nearby locations. To see how important these redundancies really are, Biederman created real-world scenes in which the natural redundancies were reduced. Biederman began with photographs depicting various scenes, such as streets, kitchens, and desktops. Each photograph was then cut into six rectangular pieces, and the pieces were then randomly reassembled, as shown in the two pictures in Figure 13.6.

Biederman's observers had difficulty describing these random scenes, and they also had difficulty identifying objects contained in them. Though the process of scrambling merely rearranged objects without splitting any of them, disrupting their normal relations nonetheless made the individual objects more difficult to see. Evidently,

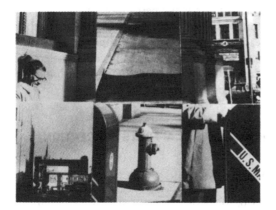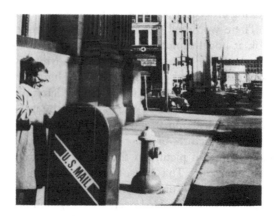

FIGURE 13.6 Scrambled and unscrambled scenes. (From Biederman, Glass, & Stacey, 1973.)

observers use the normal relations among objects to speed perception of a scene and its components. These normal relations, in other words, provided a context that influenced perception.

Point of View. We've just seen that object recognition is enhanced when objects appear in their normal relation to one another. This means that people have expectancies about the appearance of scenes as a whole. Moreover, people seem to have strong expectancies about individual objects, and these expectancies are reflected in the mental representations they have of particular objects (Humphreys and Quinlen, 1987). Stephen Palmer studied these representations by showing people pictures of various common objects, such as chairs, houses, grand pianos, teapots, and horses (Palmer, Rosch, and Chase, 1981). Each object was photographed from twelve different perspectives, including front, side, back, and top. A set of perspectives for one object is shown in Figure 13.7. For each object, Palmer found the perspective that was rated most typical for that object. Figure 13.8 shows the most typical perspective for each of the objects studied.

Palmer then determined whether objects were most easily recognized when seen from their most typical perspective. When observers had to name the objects portrayed in various photographs, they took much less time when the perspective was typical than when it was not. Perhaps pictures of

an object taken from atypical perspectives are less easily recognized because observers do not anticipate seeing the object from those perspectives. Though this seems quite plausible, there is a simple alternative. Perhaps an atypical perspective conceals some visual information that is crucial for easy recognition. Two lessons from Palmer's study help us choose between these alternatives.

First, if the perspective is sufficiently unusual, even a familiar object will be hard to recognize. (This would be the case for the photograph at the bottom right of Figure 13.7.) Second, over a large range of different perspectives, an object is still relatively easy to recognize, even from a perspective probably never taken before. (This would be the case for the top right photograph in Figure 13.7.) These findings are consistent with a provocative new theory of object and scene recognition. This ingenious and highly speculative theory, devised by Biederman (1987, 1990), provides one particular viewpoint on difficult issues in object and scene recognition. You should understand, though, that the theory has yet to undergo extensive behavioral testing.

According to Biederman's theory, when we try to recognize a visible object, the visual system first creates a rough classification of the object on the basis of three-dimensional shape. This rough classification puts objects into categories such as "chair" or "mushroom" or "cup." Note that this classification does not put objects into finer cate-

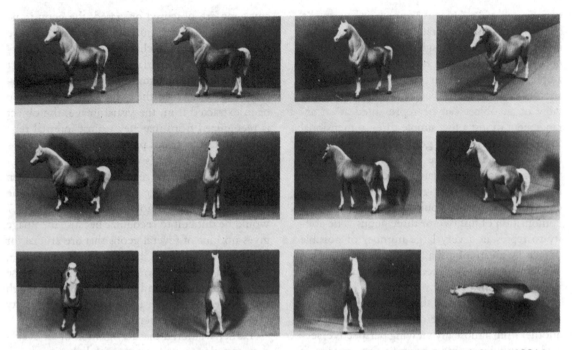

FIGURE 13.7 A single object seen from twelve different perspectives. (From Palmer, Rosch, & Chase, 1981.)

FIGURE 13.8 Twelve objects, each seen from its most typical perspective. (From Palmer, Rosch, and Chase, 1981.)

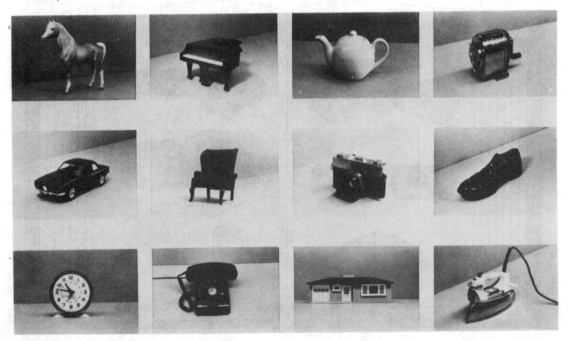

gories, such as "a Queen Anne chair" versus "a chair of the arts and crafts style." Because the initial classification is rough, details that would be needed for more subtle discriminations (for example, to distinguish one type of mushroom from another) are not used. Biederman argues that any view of an object can be represented as an arrangement of just a few simple three-dimensional forms called **geons** (for **geo**metrical ico**ns**). The left-hand panel of Figure 13.9 shows five of the two dozen geons postulated by the theory. The right-hand panel of the figure illustrates how several common objects could be represented by a combination of just two or three geons. The ability to represent a very large number of possible objects by means of just a few components makes Biederman's approach economical from a computational point of view.

Biederman's geons all share two essential properties. First, they can be distinguished from one another from almost any viewing perspective; second, even when some randomly chosen parts of

any geon are obscured or erased, the geon is almost always still recognizable. As a result of these properties, neither a change in an object's perspective nor some partial occlusion of the object ought to disrupt recognition of the object's component geons. Once the appropriate geons have been extracted from the visual image, the object is recognized from matches against internal representations of various previously seen objects.

Among the theory's virtues is its ability to explain the difficulty of recognizing an object seen in a highly unusual perspective. The horse in the lowest right-hand photograph in Figure 13.7 would be difficult to recognize because the image gives no hint of several geons that are crucial for defining the category "horse." At the same time, we would have little trouble recognizing the horse in the upper right-hand photo because, although the perspective is odd, the image makes it pretty easy to extract the crucial geons.

Earlier we noted that recognition of an everyday, complex scene happens with lightning speed.

FIGURE 13.9 Biederman's geons and simple objects created therefrom. (From Biederman, 1990.)

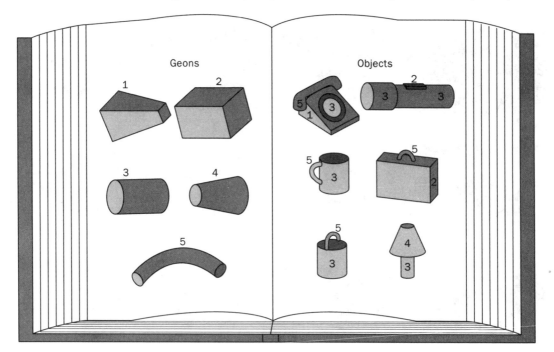

Biederman (1990) suggests that geons might even explain the ease with which natural scenes can be recognized, at least roughly (for example, as "city street" or "office"). For instance, buildings and roadways in a city street scene could be adequately represented as geons or as clusters of geons.

A main theme of this chapter is knowledge's influence on perception. It's noteworthy, then, that Biederman's theory can accommodate top-down influences on object or scene recognition. If some geon is difficult to extract (because, for instance, the visual image is dim or because crucial parts of objects happen to be occluded), an internal model or expectation could guide the extraction of additional image features that would define the geon's identity.

* * *

This section has emphasized how visual information is extracted from natural scenes and artificial displays. The nature of the extraction process varies with the viewer's goals and with the character of the scene or display. When information is to be extracted from displays of visible language, the extraction process is called reading. But the term "reading" is not restricted to what you do with words printed on a page; the same term can be used to describe what you do when you examine a map, study someone's facial expression, or interpret a musical score. The parallels between reading and other forms of sophisticated visual exploration are not accidental, since reading may have evolved out of those other visual skills. After all, long before members of our species had to cope with visible language, they were using their eyes and brains to wring information out of their visual world.

PERCEPTUAL ASPECTS OF READING

As you read this sentence, your eye movements and fixations control the rate at which you take in information from the printed page. Ordinarily, you vary the movements of your eyes to match your comprehension of what you're reading. Thus it's possible to learn a lot about reading by studying readers' eye movements and fixations.

Exactly what do your eyes do when you read? Recall from Chapter 8 that the eyes jump, or saccade, whenever one's gaze shifts from one object to another, and that the eyes are relatively still between saccades. As just noted, reading words is much like reading a map or reading someone's face. All these varieties of reading require a mix of saccades and fixations. The number of saccades and the duration of fixations depend on a reader's skill and on the difficulty of the text (Rayner, 1978). We'll confine the discussion to the behavior of a skilled reader (such as yourself) who is reading moderately difficult material (such as this text).

As you read a single line of this paragraph, your eyes make about five saccades. Between saccades, your eyes fixate every word except the smallest ones (such as "the"), which are usually skipped (Rayner, 1978). On average, a fixation lasts one-quarter of a second, although fixations can range from as little as one-tenth of a second to more than half a second. The actual duration of fixation increases when the word is uncommon, complicated, or unexpected. In addition, the distance traveled by a saccade can vary from just two letters to as many as eighteen letters. Finally, the direction of saccades also varies. About 90 percent of the time, a saccade moves your gaze rightward, to a word you haven't already looked at. Occasionally, though, you make a leftward, or regressive, saccade to recheck a word you've already read and perhaps misinterpreted. Of course, you also make a large leftward saccade at the end of each line.

To understand how you acquire information while reading, we need to consider two questions. First, how fast is the textual information taken in while you're reading? And second, what accounts for the variability among saccades while you're reading? As you know, the eyes move very fast during a saccade, so most processing of visual information must occur during the fixations between saccades. But the entire duration of any fixation cannot be devoted exclusively to text processing, since the visual system has more to do than this. Decisions have to be made about where to move the eyes next, and those decisions must be relayed to the saccadic control system. What part of a fixation, then, is devoted to analyzing the fixated word and what part to programming the next saccade?

Keith Rayner answered this question by using a computer to present text on a television screen (Rayner et al., 1981). While a person read the text, the person's eye movements were registered by the computer, which in turn used that information to modify what appeared on the television screen. In particular, whenever the reader's eyes fixated a portion of the text, a masking stimulus covered the letters in that portion. This scheme is depicted in Figure 13.10. When the mask came on immediately after the eyes began fixating (a condition that resembles trying to read without a fovea), reading was difficult. But when the mask was delayed by as little as one-twentieth of a second, people had little trouble reading the text. This shows that only a small fraction of the entire fixation duration is required to encode the text. Incidentally, if this seems like a very short time to do so much, recall from Biederman's study that a person gets the gist of a complex scene in a comparably short time. Rayner's results suggest that the bulk of a fixation period is spent programming the next saccade. Recognizing this, other researchers (Biederman et al., 1981) have suggested that reading would be considerably faster if the visual system were relieved of this programming chore. In fact, this has been accomplished by using a computer that presents words one after another,

all in the same spatial position (Sperling, Budiansky, Spivak, and Johnson, 1971). With this mode of presentation, an observer needs to fixate just one position, eliminating any time spent on saccadic programming.

These findings make it clear that people can process text very rapidly during reading. But what exactly are they processing? While reading this page, you probably have a sense that each line (or perhaps even the entire paragraph) is focused sharply. But this must be an illusion, since only the very center of your retina allows good acuity. For example, without use of the foveas, one observer in Rayner's studies (McConkie and Rayner, 1975; Rayner and Bertera, 1979) misread the sentence "The pretty bracelet attracted much attention" as "The priest brought much ammunition." Such errors are not surprising, since these people were reading with retinal regions that could specify only the overall length and shape of words but could not clearly identify each letter.

When the foveas are available, though, how many letters does a person see clearly at any one moment? To answer this question, one could determine how reading is affected when the number of letters displayed at any moment is reduced. So long as the number of letters being displayed exceeds the number being used by the reader, reading speed should be unaffected. To produce this situation, Rayner programmed the computer to reveal only that portion of the text on which the person fixated, masking all other portions with

FIGURE 13.10 Setup used by Rayner and colleagues (1981) for studying the ability to read without central vision.

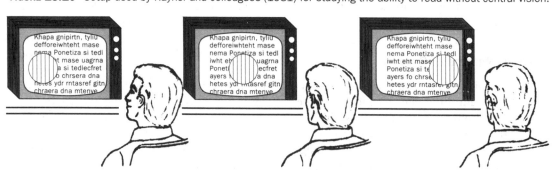

small "x"s. Thus as the person's eyes moved, new letters were constantly being revealed. This procedure, illustrated in Figure 13.11, gave people the impression that they were reading through a "window" that moved along in synchrony with their eyes.

When the window was extremely narrow (so that people saw just one letter at a time), they could read correctly about 90 percent of the words. Needless to say, though, reading under these conditions was slowed. As the window widened to include seven or nine letters, entire words could be read at once, enabling error-free performance. However, reading was still slower than normal. Reading did not even reach normal speed until the window was wide enough to reveal about four words. Presumably, readers use words to the right of fixation to guide decisions about the next saccade. Though only dimly perceived, these words furnish a preview of what will be encountered on the next fixation (Rayner and Pollatsek, 1987).

You can prove to yourself how important peripheral vision is in reading. Take a 5″ × 8″ file card and cut a rectangular "window" in it one-half inch wide and one-quarter inch high. Orient the card so that the window's larger dimension is vertical, then place the card over some pages in this book. When the window is properly aligned on the page, you will be able to see just about one word at a time through the window. Move the card along the line of text as you try to read.

After you've practiced a while, have a friend measure how long it takes you to read a passage of text 100 words long. Now, using new text, repeat this test with a window large enough to expose four words at a time. Comparing your reading speeds with the two windows, you'll discover that peripheral vision does indeed play an important part in reading.

Marcel Just and Patricia Carpenter (1980) identified the major processes involved in reading. This effort is summarized in the flow chart shown in Figure 13.12. Note that a number of the processes represented are top-down ones of the kind mentioned earlier in this chapter. For example, the right-hand box, "Long-term memory," includes rules about letter shape (orthography), the normal structures used in writing (discourse structure), and background information for what is being read (episodic knowledge). As each new word or short phrase is encountered, these top-down processes guide the reader (see Hirsch, 1988).

If you are reading an ordinary novel, these top-down influences can be enormously helpful in processing the text. Here's a simple example. After reading "John hit the nail with a," there is little uncertainty about the next word, making it easier for you to process "hammer." However, certain books minimize the usefulness of top-down influences, forcing you to deal with each word, one at a time. The following brief passage from James Joyce's *Finnegans Wake* illustrates what

FIGURE 13.11 Setup used by Rayner and colleagues (1981) for studying the ability to read with only central vision.

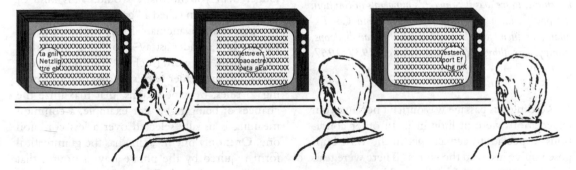

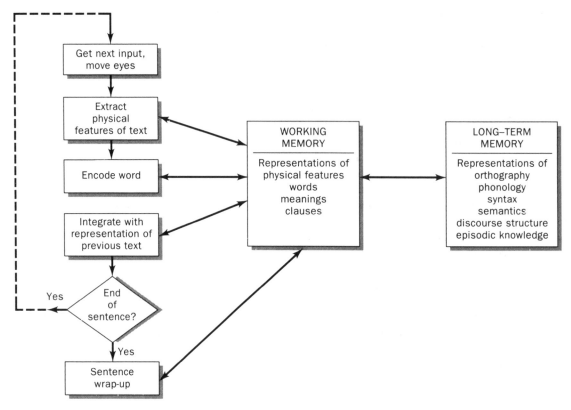

FIGURE 13.12 Schematic diagram of the major processes involved in reading comprehension. (Adapted from Just & Carpenter, 1980.)

we have in mind. First read it silently. Then read it aloud, listening carefully to yourself.

She thawght a knogg came to the dowanstairs dour at that howr to peirce the yare and dowandshe went, schritt be schratt, to see was it Schweep's mingerals or Shuhorn the posth with a tillycramp for Hemself and Co, Esquara, or them four hoarsemen on their apolkaloops, Norreys, Soothbys, Yates and Welks. (1939/1967, p. 480)

Reading this passage was difficult because your expectations were of little help. In other conditions, expectations actually get in the way. Suppose you've just read the words "There were tears in her brown. . . ." Usually you'd interpret the

word "tears" as referring to liquid produced by the lacrimal gland, rather than as referring to a rip in something. This interpretation leads you to expect the next word to be "eyes." So on encountering the word "dress," you fixate that word longer than you normally would. This kind of sentence has been called a "garden path" sentence (Carpenter and Daneman, 1981) because its early part leads the reader astray—down the proverbial garden path. If a word (such as "tears") has several meanings, the reader selects among them according to rules, or expectations, that maximize the chances of being right. For example, a common meaning is usually selected over a less common one. Or if only one meaning has the grammatical form required by the phrase (say, a noun), that meaning is selected. Presumably the errors revealed by garden path sentences reflect these normally helpful selection factors.

Word Superiority. In written English, the letter "u" is redundant after a "q." Once you have seen the "q," you know what follows. But information may be redundant even if it is not as perfectly predictable as the "u" after a "q." In fact, there are varying degrees of redundancy, and methods have been developed to quantify them and their effects on perception (Garner, 1962).

To learn what sorts of redundancy sensory information contains, consider the sense of sight. You use your eyes to view objects or collections of objects. Like the objects themselves, such collections can be natural, such as a flock of birds, or artificial, such as a group of buildings. Whether natural or artificial, the objects are seldom randomly arranged; instead, they occur in predictable arrangements. For instance, suppose that someone is looking out the window at some object you cannot see. As soon as she tells you that the object has leaves, you know that it probably also has branches and a trunk. You make this educated guess because certain objects tend to occur together; the information concerning the leaves

provided a context for your guess. As the following study shows, perception can capitalize on these context effects provided by regularities.

More than 100 years ago, James McKeen Cattell described a puzzling phenomenon. Cattell was interested in how long it took to perceive letters, words, colors, and pictures of objects. In one study, he pasted letters on a revolving drum (see Figure 13.13) and determined the rate at which the letters could be read aloud as they passed by a slit in a screen. Cattell found that it took about twice as long to read unrelated words as it did to read words that formed a sentence. He also found a similar disadvantage for reading unrelated letters compared with letters that formed a word (Cattell, 1886, p. 64). The relative ease with which letters can be read if they are embedded in a word rather than presented with unrelated letters is known as the **word superiority effect.**

Since Cattell's original report, dozens of follow-ups have confirmed the original finding. But what causes word superiority? One possibility is that the surrounding letters of a word make it easier to derive the remaining letters. For example, once you've seen the letters "LABE," the chances are good that the next letter will be "L."

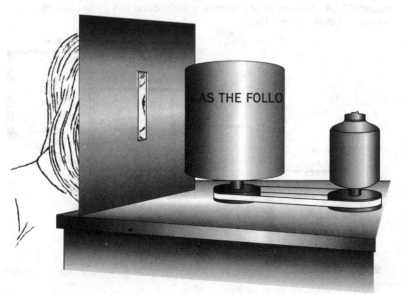

FIGURE 13.13 Cattell's apparatus for testing the word superiority effect.

In this case, the letter recognition might be expedited because the prior letters reduced the need to spend much time on the last letter.

Various studies have used methods more sophisticated than Cattell's to demonstrate that the word superiority effect cannot be chalked up entirely to deduction (Reicher, 1969; Wheeler, 1970). These studies instead suggest that familiarity directly affects the process of extracting visual information. In one study (Johnston and McClelland, 1973), observers were given a brief presentation of either a word or a single letter. In either case, this test stimulus was followed by a patterned masker that obliterated any afterimage (see Figure 13.14). After this sequence of events, the observer was given two alternatives and had to pick the one that corresponded to the test stimulus. For example, if the word "COIN" had been the test stimulus, the observer might have to choose between the alternatives "COIN" and "JOIN." Since either "C" or "J" could form a word with the remaining three letters ("OIN"), the observer could not use the other letters to deduce the correct answer. Instead, a correct answer required actually being able to see the first letter clearly enough to decipher whether it was

a "C" or a "J." The letter that distinguished the two alternatives could occupy any position in those words (for example, "BENT" or "BUNT"). Thus the observer could not just attend to one particular position in a test word. When the test stimulus consisted of a single letter, such as "J," the observer again had to choose from two alternatives, such as "C" and "J." Again, the observer could not do better than chance unless he or she had seen the letter.

The results were typical of many word superiority studies. Observers were more accurate in choosing between "COIN" and "JOIN" than they were in choosing between "C" and "J." Although trials with single letters presumably required less processing, observers were nonetheless more accurate on trials on which they had to process all four letters (Johnston and McClelland, 1973). This finding demonstrates that when you see a word, you do not process each letter separately and in isolation from the rest. In fact, observers who try to restrict their attention to just one letter of a word are less accurate in perceiving that letter than when they do attend to the word within which the letter was embedded (Johnston and McClelland, 1974). A large unit (such as a

FIGURE 13.14 The sequence of events seen by observers in the study by Johnston and McClelland (1973).

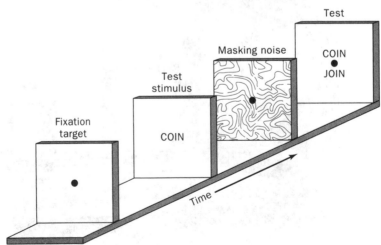

word) may be perceived more accurately than any of its isolated component parts (such as a letter).*

What, though, is the origin of this effect? Though many experiments have attempted to answer this question, the matter is still unclear. From his own experiments and those of others, William Prinzmetal (1992) argues that several different fac-

tors may actually be at work. Prinzmetal, incidentally, showed that the word superiority effect can be produced without resort to brief presentations. Figure 13.15, which shows a stimulus adapted from one used in his studies, allows you to experience the word superiority effect for yourself.

Object Superiority. The perceptual advantage that larger, meaningful stimuli enjoy over their smaller, constituent elements is not restricted to words. In fact, James Pomerantz reviewed many analogous studies using figural units and groupings rather than words. Here's one example from

---

* McClelland and Rumelhart (1981) presented an explicit model of processes that could produce a word superiority effect. Their model took the form of a network of interacting elements arranged in layers. The elements represent the features of various letters, the letters themselves, and four-letter words.

FIGURE 13.15 Demonstration of word superiority effect. Alongside each panel are two potential targets; only one is actually present, near the center of the panel, though somewhat obscured by the panel's squiggles. Compare the relative ease of deciding for the first and third panels whether the target is "WIND" or "WILD"; for the second panel, whether the target is "N" or "L"; and for the fourth panel, whether the target is ##N# or ##L#. (After Prinzmetal, 1992.)

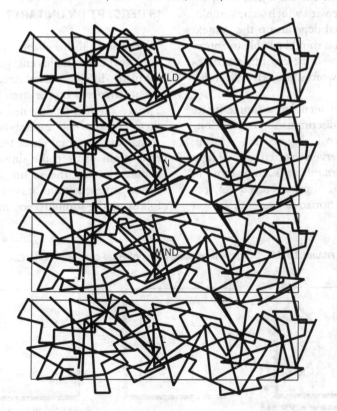

Pomerantz's (1981) research. Observers were shown a set of slanted lines such as those in panel A of Figure 13.16. The observers had to identify the single item that was perceptually distinct from the other three. For each presentation, Pomerantz measured how long it took to make this judgment. On average, observers took 1.9 seconds to spot the odd element in stimuli such as those shown in panel A (here, the negative diagonal at the lower right). Next, Pomerantz created a more complicated stimulus by adding to each diagonal an L-shaped figure (see panel B). This addition produced the stimuli shown in panel C. When observers had to spot the odd item in this new set, they took only 0.75 second—65 percent faster than with the "simpler" stimuli. Pomerantz called this improvement in performance a **configural superiority effect.** A related study (Weisstein and Harris, 1974) found that it is easier to identify a briefly flashed line when that line is part of a drawing of a three-dimensional object. Both results imply that the ease with which some stimulus component is processed depends on the context of that component. You should be able to appreciate the analogy between these configural superiority effects and the word superiority effect discussed earlier.

However, adding elements to a simple figure does not always make discrimination easier. Consider the stimuli shown in Figure 13.17. Again, when Pomerantz's observers selected the odd item from a set of single parentheses such as those in the left panel, response times averaged 2.4 seconds. When a single, horizontal parenthesis was added to each vertical one, the stimulus in the right panel was created. When observers had to select the odd item in this new set, they took 23 percent longer. These conditions, rather than producing a configural superiority effect, produce the opposite. Pomerantz suggests that because the added horizontal elements did not form perceptual groups with the vertical ones, no new features emerged to aid perception.

* * *

This completes our survey of findings on knowledge's effects on perception, organized around four complementary modes of influence. In these final, closing sections, we consider several general issues that have been threaded throughout the earlier chapters. These issues concern the nature of perception and its relation to other cognitive activities, including memory and imagination.

IS PERCEPTION UNITARY?

You've seen in this chapter and elsewhere in the book that any stimulus engages (produces activity in) many different neural structures. The array of events triggered by the stimulus courses through a maze of interlocking neural circuits. Because these neural events are elaborated over time, the spatial and temporal character of the neural representation of even the simplest stimulus is dynamic. Because the nature and distribution of neural representations fluctuate in the short time following the stimulus, you might expect the re-

FIGURE 13.16 Displays producing the configural superiority effect.

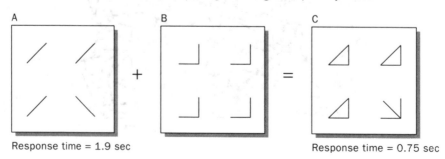

Response time = 1.9 sec   Response time = 0.75 sec

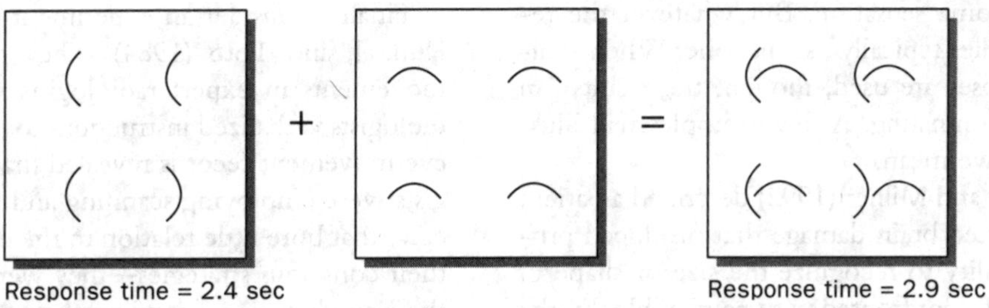

Response time = 2.4 sec   Response time = 2.9 sec

FIGURE 13.17 Displays producing a configural inferiority effect.

sulting percepts to vary correspondingly. In the extreme, these many changing representations might provide conflicting accounts of the stimulus, perhaps even provoking multiple incompatible percepts. This possibility is certainly supported by the demonstration just cited of prosopagnosics' unconscious recognition of otherwise "unrecognizable" faces. What are the implications of this possibility for studying perception?

Behavioral studies of perception must use some response as an index of the internal state called perception. This requirement could encourage an investigator to assume that at any one moment there is just one perceptual state to be studied. But this assumption would often be wrong. The portrayal of the sensory world found in conscious perception is not the only portrayal being produced within the nervous system. Much information processing subserves aspects of perception that fail to achieve conscious experience (see Loftus and Kliner, 1992). For example, a grating stimulus rendered invisible by binocular rivalry can still alter the appearance of subsequently viewed patterns (Blake, Westendorf, and Overton, 1980). In other words, observers need not consciously experience the presence of the grating for it to generate visual aftereffects. This occurs because the neural representation of that grating occurs at a level of processing that we may characterize as "preconscious."

This idea that stimuli have multiple effects was put forcefully by Anthony Marcel about a decade ago (Marcel, 1983). Daniel Dennett (1991) bound Marcel's notion and other related ideas into an intriguing theory of mental processes. Dennett argues that mental activity, including perception, is accomplished by elaboration and interpretation that proceeds on various parallel tracks. (This idea of parallel processing in perception should be familiar from previous chapters of this book.)

In this view it is wrong to think that a stimulus has just a single effect or even a single straight-line series of effects. It is also erroneous to imagine there is one place in the brain or one moment in time at which the information conveyed by a stimulus blossoms, Cinderella-like, from nonperception into perception. Instead, the battery of signals initiated by that stimulus are elaborated simultaneously along many different pathways of the brain, each with its own characteristics and connections. The elaboration takes time (on the order of hundreds of milliseconds), and the nature of the representations can change significantly during that elaboration (A. Sekuler and Palmer, 1992).

If we had a way to probe the diverse pathways, or the means to tap the elaboration at various points in its development, we might uncover a whole range of idiosyncratic accounts of the initiating stimulus. The theories of Marcel (1983) and Dennett (1991) tell us to expect precisely such idiosyncratic and, perhaps, conflicting accounts. The existence of these predicted effects goes unnoticed because we usually have no way to capture more than one perception at a time. Behavioral studies can potentially use many different kinds of responses, anything from a verbal judgment of "Yes, I see it" or "No, I don't see it," a button press to signal that a tone has become audible, to a numerical value that reflects the magnitude of some sensation. But whatever the response, studies typically use just one. When multiple responses are used, though, the results can be truly illuminating. A few examples will illustrate what we mean.

Goodale and Milner (1992) described a patient with restricted brain damage that produced profound inability to recognize the size or shape of seen objects. Confronted with pairs of blocks, the patient could not tell one from the other. She also could not comply with instructions to adjust the gap between thumb and index finger to match the size of a block. However, when she casually reached out in order to grasp an object, she showed perfectly normal preshaping of the grasping hand. In other words, like the hand of a normal subject, before it touched the object, her hand had assumed just the right shape to accommodate the object. Clearly, the size and shape of seen objects were being registered.

In another demonstration of dissociation between indicator responses, Kunst-Wilson and Zajonc (1980) used normal observers and pitted a measure of stimulus detectability against a measure of stimulus preference. In their study, ten irregular octagons were presented several times each for such short times, and at such low light levels, that they were not visible. These ten octagons had been selected randomly from a larger set of twenty octagons. Later, individuals were shown all twenty octagons, two at a time, at sufficiently long durations that the octagons could be seen quite clearly. An observer was given two different tasks. First, for each pair of octagons, the person tried to recognize which one had been presented earlier in the experiment. Additionally, the person stated which of the two shapes he liked better. Recognition judgments were at chance (47 percent), but the other, preference judgments showed a significant preference for the octagons that had been presented earlier (60 percent). This result has been confirmed and extended several times since (Bonnano and Stilling, 1986; Mandler, Nakamura, and Shebo van Zandt, 1987). A similar dissociation between recognition and expressed preference was demonstrated with prosopagnosic patients (Greve and Bauer, 1990).

Finally, consider an experiment by Carmody, Kundel, and Toto (1984). They measured eye movements in expert radiologists while the radiologists verbalized instructions to residents. The eye movement records revealed that the radiologists were employing scanning and fixation strategies that bore little relation to the descriptions of their conscious strategies—they were unaware of the knowledge base guiding their perceptual decisions (see Reber, 1992, for further discussion of unconsciously registered information).

These and similar findings force us to rethink what we mean by "see" or "recognize." If one asks, did the observers see the stimulus, the answer necessarily varies with the indicator response. Presumably, each indicator response probes a different aspect of perception's rich and complex streams.

TIME, PERCEPTION, AND MEMORY

Throughout the chapter, we've talked about knowledge's impact on perception. Knowledge is clearly related to memory; without the capacity to store and retrieve information, knowledge is impossible. This relationship raises an important theoretical issue: When does perception end and memory begin? Looking about your surroundings you see the relative locations of objects (that is, their spatial layout) as well as the shapes and colors of those objects. Everyone agrees that this experience, grounded in the present, constitutes perception. Now, suppose we ask you to envision your bedroom where you lived when you were 12 years old. If you're like most people, you're able to visualize the room's key features with some degree of success. Are you perceiving your bedroom or remembering it? Everyone would agree that this experience, drawn from the past, is an instance of memory.

Time, then, seems to be a factor that distinguishes perception from memory. Yet how far back in time do we go before perception dissolves into memory? As Gibson (1966) argued, this question may be meaningless, just as may be the distinction between perception and memory. Perception of events necessarily involves transformation of objects over time. Consider, for instance, a rapidly approaching train that you're watching while standing on the railroad tracks. (Do not attempt to carry out this hypothetical experiment.) At any given moment, the size of the image of the train on your retina is some particular value (dependent on the size of the train and its current distance from you). But as you stare at the oncoming train, its image size changes continuously (expanding, in this case). You know from Chapter 8 that this change in image size specifies the train's approach and its time to collision with you. How do you arrive at this impression of the train's looming approach? Do you integrate the present image size with remembered sizes from the past? In a sense, the brain must be performing some type of integration, but do we gain anything by saying that the brain integrates past representations of the train's size (memories) with the present? Gibson argues no. Just as the visual system integrates information over space, allowing us to perceive the spatial relations of objects in our environment, it also integrates information over time, allowing us to perceive events as they unfold temporally. And this integration does not entail simply adding together discrete samples collected over time. Rather, the perception of temporal order (succession) is like the perception of spatial order (adjacency)—both involve the registration of relational information.

As stressed throughout the book, perception is often keenest when things do change over time. We inspect an object visually by moving our eyes over the object's surface to pick up details about its shape and texture; we rub our fingers over the surface of an object to glean information about its size and consistency; we turn our heads in various directions when sniffing the air to identify the location of an odor. All these are examples of the active nature of perception. We purposefully create transformations of the stimulus, to potentiate perception. Hearing, of course, is temporal by its very nature—only by integrating sounds over time can we appreciate the nature and the source of a sound, such as a friend's voice.

Note, too, that this characterization of temporal order as a primary stimulus to perception obviates the need to invoke special processes to explain object constancy. Imagine a ball rolling across the floor and passing temporarily behind a piece of furniture, only to reemerge once again. We continue to perceive the ball and its trajectory even when it is temporarily out of view, or occluded; this is what is meant by the term **object constancy.** Rather than claiming that we "remember" the ball while it is out of the field of view, Gibson would argue that we literally "see" the ball because the stimulus information for this event unfolds continuously over time. Successive images aren't collected in memory over time; a single "image" is created over space and time. Gibson's solution to the perception/memory question is appealing in its simplicity, but can it explain how you're able to visualize the layout of your bedroom at home? No one, including Gibson, believes that the continuity of perception stretches back in time over years. Instead, the gap is bridged by mental images, experiences created entirely within our heads. We shall close this chapter with some discussion of this fascinating topic, imagery.

IMAGERY: PERCEPTION IN REVERSE?

Think back to the question about the bedroom you occupied when you were 12 years old. With coaxing, most people can give at least a rough answer to these kinds of questions, and those answers usually bear some relation to reality (Chambers and Reisberg, 1992). In this closing section, we're concerned less with the accuracy of images than with the process that creates them: How does one generate an answer to questions like the one about the bedroom? Typically, one first constructs a mental image of the room and then, with that image firmly in place, surveys its contents. Mental images have fascinated and mystified people through the ages and for years have eluded efforts to understand what they were. Recently, though, researchers have devised ways to study mental images by means of rigorous experimental methods (for example, Shepard and Cooper, 1982; Kosslyn, 1980). These efforts have yielded a start toward understanding images' properties, limitations, neural bases, and relation to perception.

From one perspective, imagery and perception can be seen as two sides of a single coin. Some investigators treat imagery as perception that happens to be running in reverse. This approach comes from the fact that perception begins with an object and can lead to the production of that object's name, while imagery starts with the object's name and produces a visual surrogate for the object (Kosslyn and Koenig, 1992). Sometimes, the resultant surrogate resembles its object so strongly that the two are mistaken for one another.

One of the most original demonstrations of confusion between imagery and perception is found in work by the pioneer female experimental psychologist, Cheves Perky (1910). While seated in a completely dark room, Perky's observers stared steadily at a screen some distance away. On a signal from Perky, an observer conjured up a mental image of some particular object, such as a banana. While the observer generated the requested image, Perky surreptitiously cast on the screen a dim image matching the object that the observer was trying to imagine. For instance, when an observer was told to imagine a banana, a banana-shaped, yellow image was cast on the screen. Prior testing by Perky had indicated that this image would be just barely visible. To further mimic a mental image, the real image on the screen was jiggled slightly, producing a shimmering quality. (If all this sounds complicated, it's because it was; three people were required to run Perky's apparatus.)

Twenty-seven observers were asked to describe various "imagined" shapes. Twenty-four of the twenty-seven never realized that they were seeing things, not just imagining them. (An experimenter's error allowed the other three observers to catch on to Perky's deception.) When the experiment was finished, "the observer was asked if he was 'quite sure that he had imagined all these things.' The question almost always aroused surprise, and other times indignation"

(Perky, 1910, p. 431). The observers' descriptions of their "imaginings" are remarkable. One person volunteered, "I can get it [the image] steadily so long as I keep my mind absolutely on it" (p. 432). Another commented, "The banana is up on end; I must have been thinking of it growing" (p. 432). Many observers unwittingly combined what they saw with what they imagined: one reported seeing a lemon (the real image) lying on a table (a mental image); another reported seeing a leaf (a real image) covered with red veins (a mental image). Even after they were shown the entire setup and told about having been fooled, many observers still refused to believe that they had actually seen something real and argued steadfastly that they had imagined it all. More recently, some of Perky's findings have been followed up (see Segal and Fusella, 1970; Reeves, 1981).

WHAT DOES VISUAL IMAGERY LOOK LIKE?

Perky's study suggests an intriguing equivalence between vision and imagery. Clearly, imagery does look something like the thing being imaged, but how close is their resemblance? This is a question that people have been trying to answer ever since Perky's own experiments. For example, one of Perky's contemporaries, Lillien J. Martin, studied imagery by asking people to form a mental image of a real object, project the image alongside the real object, and then describe the differences between image and object (cited in Harvey, 1986). One impediment to this direct approach is the difficulty of finding descriptor words perfectly suited to the unusual task.

In a modern study of imagery, Lewis Harvey (1986) extended Martin's basic procedure, but avoided the problem of reliance on observers' word pictures. Harvey investigated observers' mental images of a face, using two techniques mentioned earlier, multidimensional scaling (mentioned in Chapter 12 and detailed in the Appendix) and spatial frequency analysis (see Chapter 5). Observers used a standard rating scale of 1 through 7 to express perceived similarity. From his own previous research, as well as that of

Martin, Harvey believed that a mental image of a face would have reduced detail (that is, less high spatial frequency content) compared with the original. To test this idea and to quantify the image's appearance, Harvey created a set of photographs. Each showed the face with a different set of spatial frequencies removed.

Observers studied the original, unfiltered photograph of the face in order to form a clear visual image. They then made two kinds of similarity judgments. In one, they saw pairs of filtered photographs and rated how similar one was to the other. For the second kind of judgment, just one filtered photograph was shown at a time and the observer rated how similar it was to the mental

image of the original. The similarity judgments, analyzed by multidimensional scaling, confirmed that the visual image most closely resembled a face from which a certain set of high spatial frequencies had been removed, reducing the sharpness of edges and borders. The top panels of Figure 13.18 show photographs of two faces; the bottom panels show the photographs after they've been transformed to match the mental images that a person might have of the originals.

Incidentally, Harvey offers intriguing speculation about the apparent character of mental images. Basically, he suggests that we don't need to store much detail in the image because detail can be encoded by means of words. According to

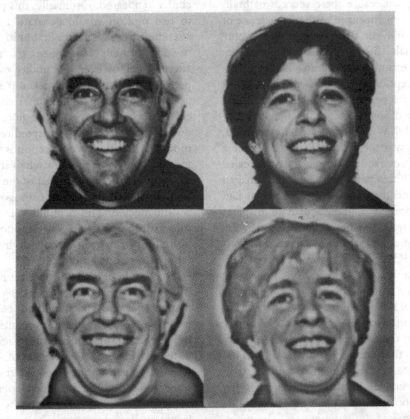

FIGURE 13.18 Upper panels: Photos of a male and female. Lower panels: The photos transformed so that they would match a subject's mental image of the originals. (Photographs and computer image processing courtesy of Lewis Harvey.)

Harvey, reliance on words as a medium for storing visual detail may also reflect a developmental co-incidence: human infants develop full capacity to see visual detail just about the same time that they learn to speak.

WHERE DOES VISUAL IMAGERY COME FROM?

These and other findings show strong parallels between the phenomenology of imagery and the phenomenology of vision (Finke, 1985). But these parallels do not prove that imagery and vision actually share a common neural basis (for example, Pylyshyn, 1981; Morgan, 1983). Martha Farah and her colleagues have pursued this issue vigorously and with interesting results (Farah, Peronnet, Gonon, and Giard, 1988). In one general approach, Farah and her group recorded from the scalp electrical brain activity while a person performed various tasks, including the generation of visual images. Because these records of brain activity can be synchronized to the occurrence of some stimulus or event, these are known as event-related potentials (ERPs). Farah and colleagues used ERPs to examine interactions between imagery and perception.

In one study, a person began a trial by forming a mental image of some letter of the alphabet, say, an "H" or a "T." With the imaged letter in mind, the individual was then shown a real "H" or a real "T." ERPs evoked by the real letters revealed form-specific interactions between the imaged letter's form and the form of the letter that had actually been presented. In particular, an image of one letter greatly altered the ERP provoked by the actual presentation of that same letter, but had less effect on the ERP provoked by other letters. This form-specific interaction led Farah and colleagues to conclude that real and imaged letters engage at least one neural site in common and that within this site, form information is preserved. Subsidiary evidence, from the time course of these interactions, points to the extrastriate visual cortex as the site of the interaction. Together with Farah's other studies using ERPs, this result suggests that visual perception and the generation of visual imagery share some of the same areas of the brain.

Presumably, this sharing facilitates strong interactions between perception and imagery.

Gilden, Blake, and Hurst (1992) employed a somewhat more indirect technique to get at the same question as Farah, namely the neural basis of imagination. In their study, observers saw a spot of light move across a video monitor at a fixed speed. Toward the middle of its travel, the spot disappeared for a short time and then reappeared at the location where it would have been had it remained visible throughout; perceptually, the dot seemed to move behind an opaque occluder. On some trials the spot didn't reappear, but the observer's task was to indicate by tapping a key when the spot would have reemerged from behind the occluder—this task, then, required the observer to imagine the continued motion of the invisible spot. Observers performed this task after being exposed for some time to real motion within the region of the display where the "occluder" appeared. Ordinarily, this prior exposure to real motion would generate a vivid motion aftereffect (recall Chapter 8), but in Gilden's study no real stimulus was present to create such an aftereffect. However, the ability of observers to perform the imagination task *was* influenced by prior motion adaptation, as inferred from observers' time judgments: the imagined spot slowed down as it "crossed" the adapted region when its motion was in the same direction as the adaptation motion, but it speeded up when its motion was in the direction opposite that of the adapting motion. Imagined motion in orthogonal directions was unaffected. This is exactly the pattern of results expected if the imagined motion entailed the utilization of neurons ordinarily involved in the registration of real motion.

So we close with the interesting speculation that imagery and perception engage common neural processes. This would not be so surprising, for imagery—like perception—can serve to guide our actions within the world. Imagination allows us to envision the consequences of some behavior without actually going through the motions. In some instances, the imagined consequence encourages us to act; other times, we're better off leaving it to imagination.

SUMMARY

This chapter has emphasized the important role that knowledge plays in shaping perceptual experience. William James made this point well when he wrote, "Whilst part of what we perceive comes through our senses from the object before us, another part (and it may be the larger part) always comes . . . out of our own head" (1890, vol. 2, p. 103). The knowledge that influences perception takes many forms that, together, maximize the effectiveness of actions that perception dictates. As stated in the first chapter of this book, perception's chief role is to guide one's actions within the world. In this chapter, we've seen that knowledge of the world not only shapes perception but also imbues perception with value and utility.

KEY TERMS

agnosias
attention
autokinetic effect
bottom-up
configural superiority effect

geons
object constancy
perceptual differentiation
phonemic restoration effect
prosopagnosia

pulvinar
Rorschach test
top-down
word superiority effect

Behavioral Methods for Studying Perception

Members of our species have long been curious about perception. Our ancestors probably asked, "Why do colors disappear at night?" or "Why has it become increasingly difficult for me to hear the sweet sound of birds at dawn?" To derive answers to these and similar questions, they relied on their introspective reflections—analysis of the content of their own perceptual experiences. Today, too, introspection guides our intuitions about perception, but the field of perception would not have advanced to its current level of sophistication if introspection were the only available tool for investigation. This Appendix outlines some of the other, more sophisticated techniques that have evolved for quantifying sensory judgments. Keep in mind, though, that the results from these newer techniques must ultimately be consonant with our introspective experiences.

THE BIRTH OF PSYCHOPHYSICS

As science and commerce flourished, a need arose for greater reliability and accuracy in sensory judgments. This need, in turn, fostered the development of more formal methods. In 1860, Gustav Theodor Fechner, a German physicist and philosopher, published a book in which he formalized behavioral methods that others had developed to study perception (Fechner, 1860/1966). Formalizing the "rules" of a method allowed people to compare different sets of observations.

Fechner's methods continue to be important today, and many of the results described in our book came from application of those methods. We will go over those methods and some of their modern variants. Though Fechner proved to be very farsighted, he could not anticipate all the many methods that are currently used. Some of these newer methods are described at various places in the text itself. These include preferential looking (Chapters 5, 6, and 7), multidimensional scaling (Chapters 12 and 13), magnitude estimation (Chapters 10 and 12), reaction time (Chapters 5 and 13), and the various methods used to study animal perception (Chapters 4, 5, 8, 11, 12, and 13). In addition, we examine research that exploits concurrent behavioral and physiological measurements, a very new but promising method (Chapters 1, 4, 8, 11, and 13).

Note that we do not present any method in elaborate detail; instead, we summarize key features. To develop such detail would require a volume of its own. Incidentally, we have an unimpeachable precedent for keeping details to a minimum while emphasizing the major concepts. Fechner himself wrote:

Had I wished . . . to set forth here all the special methods of experimentation and calculation that have to be taken into account in more detailed investigations, or had I wanted to provide a theoretical basis and experimental proof for all the rules that are applicable, I would have disturbed the flow of the argument, interfering with the interests of those who are more concerned with the general understanding of the methods than with their use by themselves. (1860/1966, p. 60)

Where should we start? When archaeologists unearth an ancient tool, they first seek to understand what the tool was used for. Similarly, to understand the methods Fechner presented in his book, one must inquire first about the purposes Fechner had in mind for those methods. In other words, why did he want to measure perception?

An amateur philosopher with considerable training in physics, Fechner was interested in establishing a new science, which he termed **psychophysics.** Psychophysics, as envisioned by Fechner (1860/1966), was to be "an exact theory of the . . . relations of body and soul or, more generally, of the material and the mental, of the physical and psychological worlds" (p. 7). Appropriately enough, Fechner called his book *Elements of Psychophysics*. Part of Fechner's program depended on an ability to measure the sensations that physical stimuli evoke in human observers. Since these sensations arise from an interaction between the physical and psychological worlds, Fechner believed that if he could quantify the sensations evoked by various stimuli, he would be able to develop equations that would tie the two worlds together.

Suppose that you, like Fechner, wished to write a simple psychophysical equation that would relate the quantity of sensation to the intensity of some stimulus. To portray such an equation, you might produce a graph relating sensation and intensity, with stimulus intensity on the horizontal axis and sensation magnitude on the vertical. For a psychophysical equation that is described by a straight line, you'd need to find out only two things before you could draw such a graph. First, you'd need to determine the minimum stimulus value that evoked any sensation whatever. This value would define the point at which the straight line intersected the horizontal axis. Second, you'd need to determine the rate at which the sensation grew as you increased stimulus intensity. Graphically, this rate of growth would correspond to the slope of the psycho-

physical equation. The first of these values (the intercept) is known as the **absolute threshold**—the stimulus intensity defining the transition between undetectable and detectable; the absolute threshold, in other words, is the intensity that an observer can just barely detect. The second of these values is known as the **difference threshold**—the minimum amount by which stimulus intensity must be changed in order to produce a noticeable change in the sensation. With certain assumptions (described below), knowledge of these two values—the absolute threshold and the difference threshold—would enable you to write the desired psychophysical equation. And this is what Fechner tried to do.

One assumption crucial to Fechner's enterprise was that the difference threshold would be constant. If the difference threshold changed in value—say, from when you were working with weak stimuli to when you were working with strong stimuli—there would be no single value that could be used to estimate the slope of the psychophysical equation; instead, the slope itself would change from one part of the line to another, implying that the corresponding equation is more complex than that for a straight line. And, in fact, the difference threshold is most certainly *not* constant. Suppose, for example, you initially present to an observer a spot of light whose intensity is 100 units, a value that is easily visible. Now suppose you increase the light's intensity until the observer first notices a change from the initial level. Imagine that this new level had to be 110 units. The difference threshold here would be 110 − 100, or 10 units. If you repeated the process, beginning now with a light of 1,000 units, you would find that the observer did not notice a change of just 10 units, as before. Instead, a much larger change would be required to produce a just noticeable change—say, a change from 1,000 to 1,100 units. So in this second case, the difference threshold would be 1,100 − 1,000, or 100 units.

From the work of his contemporary Ernst Weber, Fechner knew that although the difference threshold itself was not constant, it tended to be a constant *proportion* of the initial stimulus value. In the hypothetical examples just described, both difference thresholds were 10 percent of the initial stimulus. Using various stimuli, Weber had shown that a fixed-proportion increase in stimulus intensity was sufficient to produce a just noticeable change in sensation. To honor him, Fechner called this constancy **Weber's Law.** As we've just seen, Weber's Law states that

$$\Delta I / I = k$$

where ΔI ("delta I") signifies the difference threshold (the amount by which stimulus intensity must be changed in order to produce a just noticeable change), I signifies the initial stimulus intensity, and k signifies that the proportion on the left side of the equation is a constant despite changes in I.

Some of the methods developed by Fechner, which are the focus of this Appendix, were designed to measure just noticeable differences. Using these methods, others have ascertained that Weber's Law holds only approximately, thereby undermining Fechner's aim. However, the methods Fechner systematized continue in use today. Since they play such a key role in the study of perception, it's worth spending some time summarizing them here. But Fechner's methods aren't the only important behavioral methods in use today. So after we've summarized Fechner's major methods, we'll turn to some modern variants of those methods. Finally, we'll consider some methods that represent important new departures in the behavioral methods used to study perception.

In most of the examples given below, we'll assume that the thresholds of interest are visual thresholds; however, any of these methods could be adapted for studying hearing, smell, or taste as well. Within our visual framework, the absolute threshold is the minimum intensity of a flash of light that an observer can see; lesser intensities produce no sensation. The difference threshold is the smallest perceivable difference in intensity between two flashes of light; smaller differences cannot be discerned.

Before we turn to the various ways for measuring absolute and difference thresholds, you should know that Fechner himself doubted how well one could measure a threshold that truly merited the description "absolute." He observed (1860/1966) that even when no light whatever was present, observers in complete darkness tended to experience a dim, vague light that arose from what he termed an "inner source of light sensation" (p. 108). Today, we call this source of light **intrinsic light** or, more poetically, **dark light.** Fechner realized that intrinsic light would cause problems for an observer who tried to determine whether a stimulus did produce *some* sensation or whether the stimulus produced *no* sensation whatever. The problem, he realized, is that observers are liable to confuse this inner source of light with the real thing. This confusion would prevent the observer from making absolute judgments about the dim light alone; instead, the observer would have to discriminate the effects of a real, dim light from the effects of intrinsic light. In this sense, even the absolute threshold involves judging differences: the effect of real light adds to the effect associated with dark light. And if the effect of dark light varies from moment to moment (which it probably does), the judgment becomes even more complicated. Various studies have borne out Fechner's concern about intrinsic light, showing that this intrinsic light affects vision and psychophysical judgments in important ways (Barlow and Sparrock, 1964; Rushton, 1965).

FECHNER'S THREE METHODS

To measure thresholds, Fechner proposed three different behavioral methods, known today as the **method of limits,** the **method of constant stimuli,** and the **method of adjustment** (over the years, they have been known by a variety of names). Since Fechner wanted to measure both absolute thresholds and difference thresholds, he had to formulate two slightly different versions of each method—one version for each type of threshold that he needed to measure. Here, we'll present both versions for the method of limits and for the method of constant stimuli. Since the method of adjustment is used primarily to measure absolute thresholds, we'll describe only that version of the method.

Although the three methods differ in their details, they share some things in common. For example, all the methods restrict observers to one of two responses on each trial ("yes" versus "no" for absolute thresholds; "stronger" versus "weaker" for difference thresholds). Also, to measure an absolute threshold, all the methods specify presenting just one stimulus at a time; the observer's task is to report whether that stimulus elicited any sensation at all. To measure a difference threshold, all the methods specify presenting two stimuli at a time; here, the observer's task is to compare the sensations elicited by the two and report which is greater. So, to measure the absolute threshold, stimuli are weak, and the responses are either "Yes, I see it" or "No, I don't see it." To measure difference thresholds, the intensity of one stimulus, the *standard stimulus,* is greater than zero, and the intensity of the other stimulus, the *comparison stimulus,* may be either more intense or less intense than the standard; the response categories are "brighter" and "dimmer." There are many variations on these methods, but these three basic formats are recognizable in a great many studies (Woodworth and Schlosberg, 1954, p. 195).

THE METHOD OF CONSTANT STIMULI

With this method, each of a fixed set of stimuli is presented multiple times in a quasi-random order. The frequency with which each stimulus elicits each of the two responses is tallied and used to plot what is known as a **psychometric function.** The threshold is the stimulus intensity that evokes a particular proportion of the two responses.

Absolute Threshold. The experimenter begins by selecting a set of light intensities varying from very weak (or zero intensity) to reliably visible (typically, somewhere between four and seven intensities are tested). Stimuli are presented one at a time in a quasi-random order that ensures each

will occur equally often. After every presentation, the observer reports whether or not the light was seen. Once each light intensity has been presented many times (at least 20 to 25 times), the proportion of "yes, seen" and "no, not seen" responses is calculated for each light level and plotted in a graphic format with "intensity" along the abscissa and "percentage seen" along the ordinate; this format constitutes a psychometric function. Now, if there were a fixed absolute threshold for detection, the psychometric function should look like the solid line in the left-hand graph in Appendix Figure 1—the abrupt transition from "not seen" to "seen" would occur at this threshold intensity. In fact, however, psychometric functions never conform to this idealized representation. Instead, the curve increases gradually in a manner depicted by the curved line in the right-hand graph in Appendix Figure 1. More intense lights evoke greater proportions of "seen" responses. This pattern of results means, therefore, that light intensities in the intermediate region (between "never seen" and "always seen") are visible on some trials but not on others. The threshold, in other words, seems to vary within limits. Consequently, the definition of "threshold intensity" must be a statistical one. By convention, the absolute threshold measured with the method of constant stimuli is defined as the intensity value eliciting "seen" responses on 50 percent of the trials. This 50 percent value can be estimated graphically, as shown in Appendix Figure 1. There are various reasons why the psychometric function has this characteristic "S" shape and not an idealized step function. Among those are the constant fluctuations in sensitivity of any biological sensory system (including the dark light mentioned earlier). Those inherent fluctuations mean that the background level of activity within the system is changing, and it is against that background that an observer must detect activity associated with actual stimulation. Other contributing factors will be discussed later in this Appendix.

Difference Threshold. Two stimuli are presented on each trial. One of these, the standard stimulus, has a fixed intensity; the other, the com-

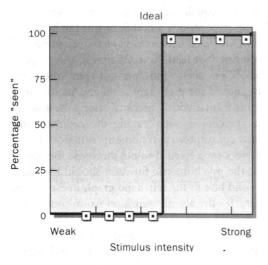 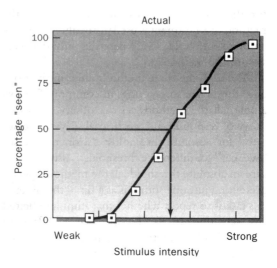

APPENDIX FIGURE 1   Ideal (left) and actual (right) results of an absolute threshold experiment using the method of constant stimuli.

parison stimulus, is selected randomly from a set of stimuli whose different intensities bracket the standard. On each trial the observer judges whether the intensity of the comparison stimulus was stronger or weaker than that of the standard. Many such judgments are obtained for all pairs of comparison and standard stimuli.

Results are summarized by plotting the proportion of trials on which each comparison stimulus is judged to be stronger than the standard, yielding another type of psychometric function. These proportions are then used to identify comparison stimulus intensities that are just noticeably different from the standard. Two just noticeably different comparison stimuli are identified: one of these is the comparison stimulus that is just noticeably *weaker* than the standard; the other is the comparison stimulus that is just noticeably *stronger* than the standard. Here, too, we find that performance is more variable than the ideal: a given stimulus difference may be discriminable on one trial but not on the next. So, again, we must define the difference threshold statistically. By convention, a comparison stimulus that 75 percent of the time is judged weaker than the standard is considered to be just noticeably *weaker* than

that standard; also, a comparison stimulus that 75 percent of the time is judged stronger than the standard is considered to be just noticeably *stronger* than that standard. Once these two just noticeably different stimuli are identified, the threshold is calculated by averaging the absolute difference in intensity between the standard and each of the stimuli that are just noticeably different from the standard.

THE METHOD OF LIMITS

One drawback to the method of constant stimuli is the need to collect lots of observations for each stimulus (absolute threshold) or for each set of stimulus pairings (difference threshold). The method of limits offers a shortcut, where on each trial the stimulus is changed gradually until the observer's response changes. The threshold is defined as that intensity of light at which the response changes.

Absolute Threshold. A single flash of light is changed in successive, discrete steps, and the observer's response to each is recorded. Suppose the light is initially so weak (or altogether absent) that the observer responds, "No, I don't see it." In this case, the light is increased in steps until the observer *can* see it. The light intensity at which the observer's response changes is taken as an estimate of the threshold. Or the light may initially be intense enough that the observer responds, "Yes, I see it." In this case, the light is decreased in steps until the observer can*not* see it. Again, the intensity of light at which the response changes provides an estimate of the threshold. A series of light flashes that approaches the threshold from below (starting with very weak stimuli) is called an *ascending series;* a series that approaches the threshold from above is called a *descending series.* Often, ascending and descending series yield systematically different estimates of the threshold, so most experimenters use both types of series in alternation and then average the results. Moreover, the threshold estimates from a series of, say, ascending trials may differ. This variability stems from the same sources that produce the variability in the method of constant stimuli discussed above. In principle, the stimulus threshold estimated with the method of limits should correspond to the intensity value associated with the 50 percent point on a psychometric function obtained with the method of constant stimuli. In practice, this may or may not be true.

Difference Threshold. On each trial, two flashes of light are presented—one called the "standard," the other called the "comparison"; the pair may be presented either simultaneously, one next to the other, or successively, one after the other. The intensity of the standard light remains constant, and the intensity of the comparison light is changed in a series of steps. After each change, the observer judges the comparison stimulus as "brighter" or "dimmer" than the standard. In an ascending series, the comparison stimulus is initially weaker than the standard and it increases from trial to trial; in a descending series, the comparison stimulus is initially stronger than the standard and it decreases. A series terminates when the observer's response changes from "dimmer"

to "brighter" (in an ascending series), or from "brighter" to "dimmer" (in a descending series). The threshold, then, is the absolute value of the difference between the lights at the time the response changed. As before, ascending and descending series may be alternated and the threshold estimates averaged.

THE METHOD OF ADJUSTMENT

In an even more efficient variant of the method of limits, the observer is given control over the intensity of the stimulus and instructed to adjust it so that it is just visible (absolute threshold) or appears to match some other, standard light (difference threshold).

Absolute Threshold. The experimenter provides the observer with the means to vary the intensity of a light. The observer now adjusts the intensity so that the light changes from invisible to just barely visible, providing one estimate of the absolute threshold. The observer also adjusts the light from visible to just barely invisible, providing another estimate of threshold. Typically, the two kinds of estimates are repeated several times and the results averaged. Observers report that they find this method easier to use than the method of limits, even though the two clearly resemble each other. Probably observers find it easier to judge the stimulus on the basis of continuous trial and error (method of adjustment) than when they see just one stimulus at a fixed value (method of limits).

MODIFICATIONS OF FECHNER'S METHODS

Over the years, researchers have introduced various modifications to each of Fechner's methods as the need arose. Sometimes these modifications were shaped by the apparatus and stimuli that were available to a particular researcher. Other times, the modifications were designed to minimize some deficiency of the method or to promote efficiency. We'll consider two modifications that are particularly important.

THE STAIRCASE METHOD: A MODIFICATION OF THE METHOD OF LIMITS

The method of limits has several limitations that were apparent almost from its inception. As you'll recall, this method requires that a series of stimuli be presented, all of which elicit the same response—such as, "Yes, I see it." Moreover, the method often involves presenting many stimuli that are far from the observer's actual threshold. The inclusion of these stimuli reduces the efficiency of the basic method of limits, since such stimuli contribute little to the estimate of threshold. A variant of the method of limits, the so-called **staircase method,** offers enhanced efficiency (Cornsweet, 1962). In a typical staircase, the experimenter begins with an intensity well above the threshold and decreases it until the observer declares it invisible. As soon as the response changes, the direction of stimulus change is reversed. Now intensity increases until the response changes again, following which the intensity decreases once more. In a typical staircase, these alternations in the direction of stimulus change continue until six or seven "reversals" have occurred (see Appendix Figure 2). The threshold is then estimated by finding the average of all the

stimulus intensities at which the observer's responses changed. With this staircase procedure, most of the stimulus values are concentrated in the threshold region, making it a more efficient procedure.

There's a problem, though, with this simple staircase procedure. Like the basic method of limits, a simple staircase allows the observer to become aware of the scheme that governs stimulus presentation. The observer's responses are then liable to be influenced by that knowledge. For example, an observer may anticipate that the threshold is being approached and change the response prematurely. To overcome this problem, Cornsweet (1962) introduced a procedure that retains the efficiency of a staircase but minimizes the observer's knowledge of the direction from which the threshold is being approached. Cornsweet's idea was to interleave two or more concurrent staircases.

Appendix Figure 3 illustrates a simple case of two interleaved staircases and *strict alternation* between them. On trial 1, staircase A begins with a stimulus that is expected to be above threshold, and the observer reports seeing it. On trial 2, staircase B starts with a stimulus that is expected to be below threshold, and the observer reports not seeing it. On trial 3, the next stimulus from staircase A is presented—at a lower intensity than before, since the observer saw it the first time. On

APPENDIX FIGURE 2 The results of a staircase experiment.

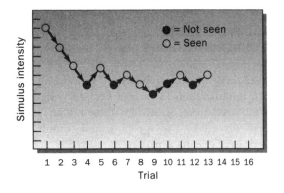

APPENDIX FIGURE 3 The results of an experiment using two interleaved staircases.

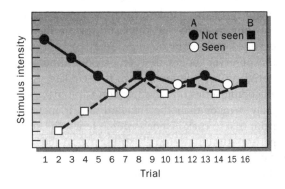

trial 4, the next stimulus from staircase B is presented, and so on. As Appendix Figure 3 shows, over the course of trials both staircases converge and the stimulus intensities tend to be concentrated about a single value, the threshold. A further improvement developed by Cornsweet involves *randomly* interleaving the two staircases so that the observer can never figure out which staircase to expect from trial to trial.

MODIFICATIONS OF THE METHOD OF CONSTANT STIMULI

Although constant stimuli's random presentation of stimuli precludes the problems associated with limits' serial ordering of stimuli, constant stimuli, like limits, is inefficient. In particular, many of the stimuli presented are far enough away from the threshold to be of relatively little use. For instance, little information is gained from presenting light intensities that are always detectable or light intensities that can never be detected. This inefficiency can be avoided by pretesting, which allows the stimuli to be carefully tailored to the capacities of the observer. Alternatively, various methods have been developed to adapt or modify the stimulus set while the experiment itself is in progress (Andrews and Miller, 1978; Watt and Andrews, 1981; Watson and Pelli, 1983). This latter approach is preferable over pretesting because, as we've pointed out, the observer's sensitivity fluctuates somewhat during an experiment. As a result, a stimulus set optimized during pretesting might not be optimal for the entire experiment. The most sophisticated and efficient versions of these adaptive strategies require the use of a computer, but the gain—in efficiency and accuracy— seems well worth the effort.

There is another reason that many researchers consider the method of constant stimuli to be inefficient, at least for measuring difference thresholds: the method requires two stimuli per trial—a standard and a comparison—rather than just one. And, naturally, it takes longer to present two stimuli than it does to present just one. Fortunately, the standard is probably superfluous in many circumstances. Usually, an observer's judgments are just as precise in the absence of a standard as they are in the presence of one (Woodworth and Schlosberg, 1954, pp. 217–218).

To appreciate what omitting the standard entails, consider an experiment by Suzanne McKee (1981). To measure the difference threshold for visual velocity—the smallest difference in speed that an observer can discriminate—McKee used the method of constant stimuli but with the standard omitted. On each trial, a computer caused a single vertical line to move across a television display; only one line was presented per trial. The line's velocity on each trial was chosen randomly from a set of seven highly similar velocities. The observer watched a line pass by and judged whether its velocity was faster or slower than the mean of all seven velocities.

Note that McKee never actually had to show the observers which velocity was the mean; instead, by watching a few presentations of all the velocities, the observers built up a highly accurate mental representation of the mean velocity. It should not surprise you that observers can make accurate perceptual comparisons even when there is no explicit standard present. After all, the method merely requires an observer to do what he or she does many times every day: combine separate samples of perceptual information into an accurate overall perceptual impression. (For a quantitative treatment of the integration of separate perceptual samples, see Helson, 1964.)

FORCED-CHOICE, OBJECTIVE METHODS

The methods discussed so far rely on the observer's own, subjective report of what is or is not seen. These reports are termed "subjective" because an experimenter cannot judge whether the observer was correct or incorrect. For instance, when an observer reports, "I see it," we must take that report at face value; it cannot be disputed or verified. In a moment we'll mention why this may be a problem. But first let's consider an effective solution.

In recent years, an alternative, objective approach—the **forced-choice method**—has gained considerable popularity. In an experiment using a forced-choice method, the observer must *prove* that he or she can detect the stimulus, and the observer's claims can be checked.* The observer gives proof by identifying some characteristic of the light other than its intensity. For example, the experimenter might arrange to present a dim light either to the right or to the left of a fixation point. The observer does not have to say whether the light was visible but instead merely identifies the light's position—responding either "left" or "right." In modern times, the forced-choice method was introduced by Blackwell (1946). However, the method was probably devised by Bergmann in 1852, nearly 100 years before Blackwell (Fechner, 1860/1966, p. 242). In order to measure visual acuity, Bergmann used a forced-choice method with grating patterns. He devised a way to vary the orientation of a test grating (recall Chapter 5), and instead of asking the observer whether a particular grating was visible, Bergmann forced the observer to identify the grating's orientation. [Incidentally, Bergmann not only devised the forced-choice method, he also discovered that stimulus uncertainty reduces detectability (see Chapter 5) and that some orientations are easier to see than others—the oblique effect (see Chapter 4).]

But what has been learned from the use of forced-choice methods that wasn't known before? For one thing, these methods show that the nervous system registers more sensory information than one is ordinarily aware of. Putting this another way, forced-choice research shows that people can discern lights so dim or sounds so weak that people claim they cannot see or hear them. Here's a typical demonstration of this remarkable fact. Suppose that you begin by using one of Fechner's methods, say, the method of adjustment, to measure an absolute threshold. After running many trials, you determine a light intensity that the observer says is "just barely visible." You then take that same "threshold" light intensity and present it to the same observer in a forced-choice experiment. The dim light is flashed either to the left or to the right of a fixation point while the observer tries to identify its location. Although such comments are not part of the actual data-collection procedure, the observer may frequently volunteer that his responses are mere guesses and that nothing was actually visible. After many trials, you tally up the number of times the observer was correct. Despite the observer's claims, you find that he was correct 100 percent of the time. Next you decrease the light's intensity to a level *below* the threshold value previously determined by the method of adjustment. When you repeat the forced-choice testing with this new, even dimmer light, the observer protests even more strongly, insisting after every trial that he hadn't seen the light and that he was only guessing about its location. Surprisingly, though, the observer continues to do well—perhaps getting 70 to 75 percent of the choices right. Note that this is well above chance level; if the observer were really just guessing, on average only 50 percent of the responses would be correct.

Similar results have been obtained in studies of the other senses. Typically, forced-choice testing confirms that stimuli can be discerned whose intensities are well below the absolute thresholds defined by Fechner's subjective methods. Don't misconstrue the import of this observation—people aren't lying when they make subjective threshold settings; they are relying on information necessary to generate a conscious experience of the stimulus, and the amount of information needed to support that decision appears to be greater than that required for forced-choice performance (where conscious experience is not a necessary component of the judgment).

---

* The term "forced-choice" does not mean simply that the observer is forced to say something besides "I don't know." Rather, this procedure involves structuring stimulus presentations so that accuracy can be objectively verified—if the experimenter can unequivocally provide error feedback, the procedure is properly called "forced-choice." Note, responses based on subjective impression—for instance, "this is louder than that"—even if responses are required after each stimulus presentation, are not genuinely forced-choice. When a listener reports that one tone is louder than another, how can you argue?

Forced-choice testing is also useful for eliminating extraneous (nonsensory) differences among observers. In subjective (nonforced-choice) experiments, results can be strongly influenced by the criterion that the observer uses for saying whether or not a light was visible. The **criterion** is the implicit rule that the observer uses to convert sensory information into overt responses. For example, one observer may have a strict criterion; she will not report "seeing" a stimulus unless the sensory evidence is quite strong. Another observer may have a more lax criterion; she is satisfied with weaker sensory evidence. The first observer's responses might lead you to conclude that the observer's threshold was considerably higher than the second observer's when, in fact, their apparent differences could have been caused by criterion differences alone.

Forced-choice methods, then, should be employed whenever you want to factor out possible criterion differences among observers. The same holds true if you are dealing with groups of observers whose criteria are likely to differ. Since elderly people tend to be more reluctant about saying "Yes, I detect it" (Rees and Botwinick, 1971), forced-choice methods are useful in comparing the sensory capacities of older and younger observers. Let's take another example. Hospitalized schizophrenics may be reluctant to admit that they see anything that they are not absolutely sure about. So forced-choice methods are important in comparing the vision of schizophrenic and normal observers. In these comparisons and others, if *criterion* differences cannot be ruled out, it is impossible to evaluate conclusively possible differences in *sensory* capacities. More commonly, researchers have to worry about the constancy of a single observer's criterion from one test to another. This would be important if one is interested in whether some treatment—such as perceptual training—changes an observer's ability to see, or whether the training had affected only the observer's willingness to *say* she sees something.

Before concluding this outline of forced-choice methods, we should note that some of Fechner's original methods can be converted into forced-choice versions. You can devise a forced-choice method of limits or a forced-choice method of constant stimuli. In fact, forced-choice staircases have become particularly popular, with the correctness or incorrectness of a person's responses determining whether the stimulus is increased or decreased from trial to trial (Heinemann, 1961).

SENSORY DECISION THEORY

There's another important topic that must be included in any survey of psychophysical methods. That topic is **sensory decision theory (SDT),** a term that covers both a set of procedures as well as a sophisticated psychophysical theory (Green and Swets, 1966). SDT, also sometimes called **signal detection theory** in recognition of its origins in electrical engineering, offers psychophysics two distinct but complementary benefits. One benefit comes from SDT's procedures for expressing precisely and quantitatively what information is contained in some stimulus. In a visual stimulus, for example, the information includes the spatial distribution of light from different parts of the stimulus and a description of how that distribution changes with time. Characterizing the stimulus so allows one to determine the efficiency with which a human observer uses the potential information. Defining the potential information in a stimulus specifies an upper theoretical limit to observer performance. Knowing that theoretical limit makes it possible to compare the performance of a human observer against the performance of an ideal or perfect observer, that is, one who uses all the stimulus's information. If, as usually happens, information were lost by the eye or by other parts of the visual system, performance would be less than ideal. Take one example. Some light incident on the eye's cornea is either absorbed or reflected rather than transmitted into the eye itself. This loss of light, which is governed by the cornea's structure, reduces the amount of information potentially available in the stimulus. The eye's detection performance is limited, then, because the visual system never gets access to the information lost to absorption or reflection. With appropriate calculations, one can define precisely how much reduction in performance is mandated by this or any other information loss. Geisler (1989) puts this aspect of SDT to excellent use in a psychophysical analysis of the stages in visual processing.

SDT's other benefit to psychophysics is its explicit recognition that perceptual measurements are influenced by the motivational state as well as the sensory capacities of the observer. As a result, SDT's procedures can distinguish the two influences, providing separate measures of sensory and nonsensory influences (McNicol, 1972; Mac-Millan and Creelman, 1991). At the completion of an SDT experiment, one has two measures of an observer's performance. One measure, d', reflects the observer's sensory capacity; the other measure, β, reflects the observer's criterion for acting on the information provided by the senses.*

As we've said, SDT recognizes that the response "Yes, I see it" depends on two factors—sensory capacity and motivation. To distinguish the two, SDT compares the frequency with which the observer says "yes" when some dim light *has* been presented and the frequency with which the observer says "yes" when *no* light has been presented. Take an example. Suppose some observer says "yes" every single time a very dim light is presented. You might think his eyes are very sensitive. However, you discover that the same observer also says "yes" when no light whatever is presented. Clearly, you should not take every "yes" at face value.

To achieve its goals, SDT must always compare the observer's responses in two different circumstances. When vision is being assessed, SDT determines the observer's responses to a weak light (called "signal") as well as to no light (called "noise"). Typically, these signal and noise trials are randomly intermixed. After each trial, the observer responds "yes" or "no." A "yes" response on a signal (that is, a trial involving presentation of light) is termed a "hit" (because the observer was correct, or made a hit); a "yes" response on a noise trial (that is, one *without* a light) is termed a "false alarm" (because the observer erred, saying he saw something when nothing had been presented). After presenting multiple signal and noise trials, the experimenter tallies the proportion of signal trials on which the observer responded "yes" and the proportion of noise trials on which the observer responded "yes."

The two proportions, the hit rate and false alarm rate, can be plugged into equations to get the sought-after values of d' and β. It's not necessary to work through the details of these calculations here; in fact, researchers generally rely on published tables to convert their hit and false alarm rates into d'.

To make sure that you've got the idea of SDT, consider the outcome of a hypothetical experiment. Suppose that two observers are tested with the same dim light and that both achieve the same hit rate. However, one observer produces a higher false alarm rate than the other. Which observer has the higher sensitivity to the dim light? The answer is, the observer whose false alarm rate is lower—her responses indicate that she was superior in discriminating the presence of light from the absence of light. Sensory decision theory treats all tests of detection as tests of an observer's ability to discriminate the presence of a stimulus from its absence (recall Fechner's "inner source of light sensation"). Good discrimination is shown by the combination of a high hit rate and a low false alarm rate. A large difference between an observer's responses when there is a light and when there isn't a light signifies that she can distinguish between the two. Poor discrimination is evidenced when the hit and false alarm rates are equal or

---

* One sensory area to which SDT has been applied is the question of whether acupuncture truly reduces the sensation of pain or merely makes a patient less willing to report the presence of pain. Experimental results with SDT are mixed: some data suggest a change only in the patient's criterion for reporting pain (Clark and Yang, 1974); other data suggest a genuine sensory change (Chapman, Chen, and Bonica, 1977).

SDT has also been applied to problems in a wide variety of nonsensory areas. These include the study of memory (Banks, 1970; Swets, 1973), anxiety (Grossberg and Grant, 1978), medical diagnosis (Emmerich and Levine, 1970; Swets, 1979), identification in police lineups (Wells, Lindsay, and Ferguson, 1979), perception of hazards in mine shafts (Blignaut, 1979), and other problems as well. In each, SDT has been useful because of its ability to separate informational and motivational influences on judgments.

nearly equal. In the extreme, when the two rates are equal, you know that the observer has completely failed to distinguish between the absence and presence of a light—performance is at chance level, no matter how high the hit rate might be.

Our discussion of the observer's criterion for reporting sensory information has emphasized differences among observers. But you should recognize that any single observer's criterion varies, depending on a number of factors. SDT specifies how an observer's criterion is likely to change along with changes in the relative importance of hits and false alarms. If an observer is in a situation where it is vital to detect *all* the stimuli and the cost of making a few false alarms is trivial, then SDT predicts the observer will adopt a liberal criterion. This is exemplified in the situation of a radar operator who must monitor the radar for any sign of approach by an enemy. The operator must not miss any possible enemy intrusions whatever. However, if false alarms are costly—in monetary terms or in psychological terms—the observer should adopt a stricter criterion. This is exemplified in the situation of a person who on several successive nights has imagined the sound of a burglar and therefore called the police. He must be very cautious about sounding yet another false alarm.

SDT also specifies how the criterion might change along with changes in the probability that a stimulus will occur. If the observer knows ahead of time that a stimulus is very likely to occur, then optimally she should adopt a liberal criterion for reporting the presence of the stimulus. However, if the observer knows that a stimulus is very unlikely, the optimal strategy is to adopt a strict criterion (that is, to require more powerful evidence before reporting that the very unlikely event has actually occurred).

PSYCHOPHYSICAL FUNCTIONS FROM PSYCHOMETRIC DATA

Each technique described in the previous sections produces a measure of the threshold, either an absolute threshold or a difference threshold. Any of these techniques generates data that specify how performance changes with some stimulus variable that is scaled along an intensive dimension. For instance, Appendix Figure 1 plots the percentage of "seen" responses against light intensity. Curves of this form, as mentioned earlier, are called psychometric functions, and from such a curve we may derive a single intensity value as an estimate of the threshold.

In studying perception we often are interested in how the threshold changes with some stimulus variable. This requires that we measure the threshold repeatedly, over a range of values along some stimulus dimension. For instance, the visual threshold for detecting a spot of light varies depending on the wavelength of that light (recall Figure 3.22); the contrast threshold for detecting a grating pattern varies with the spatial frequency of the pattern (recall Figure 5.17). Likewise, in hearing, the threshold intensity for detecting a tone varies with the tone's frequency (recall Figure 10.1). These represent measurements of absolute thresholds as the function of different values along a stimulus dimension of interest (for instance, spatial frequency). These kinds of curves— plots of threshold as the function of some stimulus variable—are called **psychophysical functions.** A psychophysical function represents a family of thresholds, not just a single threshold value. Thus, a psychophysical function more completely summarizes the operation of a sensory system than does a single threshold point from that function.

The examples given above are psychophysical functions for detection thresholds. It is also possible to generate a psychophysical function showing how a difference threshold varies with some stimulus variable. Imagine, for example, measuring the smallest difference in wavelength that can just be discriminated from some standard wavelength value—this would constitute a wavelength discrimination threshold. This procedure could be repeated for a number of different standard wavelengths, thus generating a family of wavelength discrimination thresholds. The individual difference thresholds would then be plotted on a graph showing the magnitude of the difference threshold along the vertical axis and wavelength along the horizontal axis. Such a curve would constitute a psychophysical function.

You can think of a psychophysical function as a curve summarizing the data from a family of psychometric functions. Each data point on the psychophysical function is a threshold derived from a psychometric function. This relation is illustrated in Appendix Figure 4, a schematic audibility function (see Chapter 10) and a sample of the associated psychometric functions. Each data point in the lower part of the figure is an intensity threshold just sufficient to detect a tone of given frequency. Also shown in schematic form are three psychometric functions associated with three of the thresholds; not shown are the psychometric functions for the other threshold values. All the psychometric functions would, incidentally, represent thresholds measured using a method of constant stimuli (recall Appendix Figure 1). One could, of course, measure the family of thresholds using, say, a method of adjustment, in which case there would be no associated psychometric function. Still, the psychophysical function would be that family of thresholds obtained by repeating the method of adjustment for a number of different stimulus values.

MAGNITUDE ESTIMATION AND THE POWER LAW

You've probably seen judges award points to athletes, such as divers or figure skaters, as a rating of their performance. Or maybe you've watched talent shows on television where audience members register their "votes" for contestants on an ap-

APPENDIX FIGURE 4 Construction of a psychophysical function from psychometric functions. Insets show three different psychometric functions that yield data points for the psychophysical function.

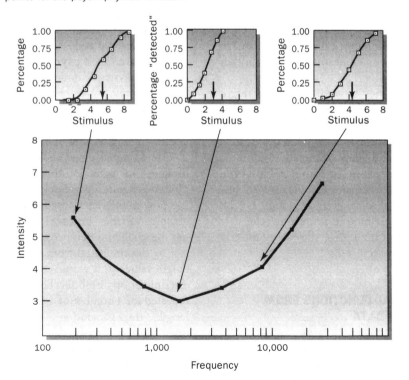

plause meter, the winner being the individual who gets the loudest applause. Perhaps you've been asked to rate how well you like different songs by assigning numbers to them, higher numbers indicating greater liking. In each of these instances, the individual doing the rating behaves like a measuring gauge—that person estimates the magnitude of some quality present in a given object, person, or event, where "quality" refers to some psychological factor, such as gracefulness, appeal, and so forth.

This same strategy can be applied to the measurement of subjective sensory experiences such as the loudness of a sound or the brightness of a light. Used in this manner, such strategies fall under the rubric of **direct scaling techniques.** These techniques are called "direct" because the judgments people make presumably directly reflect the magnitude of some sensation they are experiencing; and those judgments, according to the advocates of direct scaling techniques, are just as valid as the reading of sound levels taken with a meter. In a way, direct scaling is similar to introspection (recall Chapter 1), in that a person's subjective report is supposed to reflect the contents of conscious experiences such as loudness. However, in the case of direct scaling, the person's ratings are constrained in ways that make it possible to quantify the rating, thereby revealing regularities between the judgments of different people.

The person most responsible for the development of direct scaling techniques was S. S. Stevens. The various techniques he devised for studying the intensity of sensations associated with seeing, hearing, taste, smell, and touch are summarized in Stevens (1960). His most popular technique was magnitude estimation, the technique described in Chapters 10 and 12 as it is applied to loudness and to odor intensity. According to Stevens, the idea of assigning numbers to gauge the strength of a sensation came from a friendly challenge:

It all started from a friendly argument with a colleague who said, "You seem to maintain that each loudness
has a number and that if someone sounded a tone I should be able to tell him the number." I replied, "That's an interesting idea. Let's try it." (1956, p. 2)

Stevens responded to this challenge by setting up an experiment and instructing participants as follows:

You will be presented with a series of stimuli in irregular order. Your task is to tell how intense they seem by assigning numbers to them. Call the first stimulus any number that seems appropriate to you. Then assign successive numbers in such a way that they reflect your subjective impression. There is no limit to the range of numbers that you may use. You may use whole numbers, decimals or fractions. Try to make each number match the intensity as you perceive it. (1975, p. 30)

As a rule, the stimuli to be rated are presented several times each, in an irregular order. No training is necessary, so it is possible to test a person in a relatively short time; this is one reason for the method's popularity. Stevens used magnitude estimation to study all the senses. He discovered that for each sense modality, the *perceived* strength of a stimulus increased in proportion to the stimulus's *physical* intensity raised to some power, or exponent. (This is the power law mentioned in Chapter 10.) Each sense modality has its own characteristic power, or exponent, and some of these values are summarized in Appendix Figure 5. Note that the exponent for brightness is 0.3. This rather small value indicates that large increases in light intensity produce relatively small increases in brightness. In contrast, look at the exponent and graph line for electric shock—here's a sensation that grows much faster than the intensity of the stimulus. In the case of electric shock, doubling the intensity causes about a tenfold change in the perceived strength of that shock. Interestingly, perceived length has an exponent of 1.0, indicating that perceived length corresponds almost perfectly with actual length.

Stevens and other proponents of his ideas developed methods besides magnitude estimation to

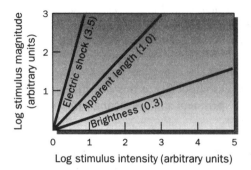

APPENDIX FIGURE 5 Power functions for three different sensory judgments.

measure sensation (see Gescheider, 1976). One of the more clever methods, called **cross-modality matching,** requires a person to equate the strengths of sensations arising from the stimulation of different sense modalities. To illustrate: a person might be asked to adjust the loudness of a sound until its strength matched the brightness of a light. At first glance, this kind of judgment sounds strange, but people actually have no trouble doing it. Probably, cross-modality matching is not so different from deciding how well you enjoyed a performance and clapping by an amount that reflects your enjoyment.

The matches produced across modalities conform to predictions derived from the power law. For example, to match a small increase in the intensity of an electric shock, a person requires a large increase in the intensity of a sound; this merely reflects the fact that perceived shock intensity grows much more rapidly than loudness.

These scaling techniques, particularly magnitude estimation, have recently been applied to psychological attributes other than sensory judgments. The seriousness of various crimes, the beauty of artworks, and the perceived status of various occupations—these are some of the psychological attributes that have been quantified by means of direct scaling. Though it's still in its infancy, this approach holds great promise for helping clarify what is meant by otherwise vague concepts such as "attractiveness" or "competence." In the future, perhaps it might even be possible to dispense with the election of public officials, substituting some scaling process in its stead. In such a scheme, desirable attributes for various offices would first be identified, then different candidates scaled for those attributes.

MULTIDIMENSIONAL SCALING

The procedures described so far have focused on the detection or discrimination of small differences in sensory stimulation or the growth in sensation with intensity. Now we turn to a rather different procedure—**multidimensional scaling (MDS)**—designed to quantify the degree to which arrays of stimuli are comparable along some dimension or set of dimensions. Unlike the methods described above, MDS is typically applied to complex stimuli that are easily discriminable from one another. The goal with MDS is to construct a pictorial representation of the similarities among stimuli (Schiffman, Reynolds, and Young, 1981). Technically speaking, MDS mathematically generates an n-dimensional space, or map, into which all stimuli under study will fit. The number of dimensions required to construct that space provides revealing information about the similarities among the stimuli.

The stimuli in an MDS study can be almost anything—perfumes, cola drinks, beers, taste chemicals, colors, U.S. senators, food flavors, and so on. Regardless of what the stimuli are, though, an MDS study begins by asking people to judge how similar the stimuli are to one another.

Sometimes, a researcher does not know what basis people will use to make their similarity judgments. For example, if they're judging the similarity of a Chevrolet Corvette and a Mazda RX7, they might respond to the fact that both are sports cars (and judge them "similar") or to the fact that they come from different countries (and judge them "dissimilar"). This can be a problem if the researcher wants to avoid biasing people's judgments. With taste and smell, it's very hard to know the basis for perceptions of similarity and dissimilarity. Here MDS comes in extra handy, helping define the perceptual basis for the judgments (even though the researcher doesn't know that basis ahead of time).

Let's start with a simple experiment. Suppose we concoct four different concentrations of sodium chloride (salt) in water. We give them two at a time to people who sip them and then make a numerical judgment of how similar the two are. Suppose they rate similarity on a scale from 100 meaning "perfect identity between the two," all the way to 0 for "absolutely no similarity whatever" (other judgment schemes can also be used; see Schiffman, Reynolds, and Young, 1981).

In our hypothetical study, salt solutions A and C are judged most similar; solutions A and B least similar; and the other pairs, as somewhere in between. How does one make a spatial map that corresponds to these judgments? The goal is to make a map with four points, A, B, C, and D; the distances between the points should correspond to the judgments of similarity—similar salt solutions should be close together and dissimilar ones far apart. For convenience, we start with the pair A and B. Since these two solutions are judged least alike, their corresponding spots on the map should be far apart. Arbitrarily, we can position A at the left and B way to the right. Since D is judged equally similar to A and B, D should go about halfway between A and B. Finally, because A and C are judged quite similar, we know that C goes somewhere close to A; but we don't know whether to left or right. We get the answer by comparing judgments of A and B, on the one hand, with judgments of B and C, on the other. Since C and B are judged more similar than A and B, we know that C must lie somewhere between A and B. The complete arrangement is shown in panel A of the diagram in Appendix Figure 6. To validate our map, we can look at similarity judgments and corresponding points that we haven't used thus far. On the map, C is closer to A than to D; this is consistent with the fact that C is judged more similar to A than it is to D.

When the stimuli can be represented along a single straight line, it indicates judgments were

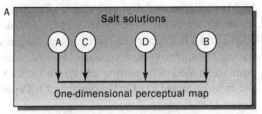

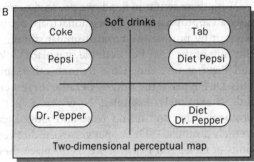

APPENDIX FIGURE 6 Maps depicting dimensions derived from multidimensional scaling.

made on the basis of a single aspect, or "dimension," of the stimuli—in this case, probably the intensity of the salt taste. Thus the study with salt solutions led to a map that was a one-dimensional representation. In this hypothetical example involving salt solutions, a one-dimensional map makes sense because the solutions differed in only one way. With more complex stimuli, however, a one-dimensional map may be inadequate because people rely on more than one dimension to derive their similarity judgments. In such cases, a map of two or three dimensions might be needed. Let's take a simple example, based on an actual experiment (Schiffman, Reynolds, and Young, 1981).

Suppose we take six brands of carbonated soft drinks (with brand identifications hidden): Coca-Cola, Pepsi-Cola, Dr Pepper, Tab (a diet cola similar to Coca-Cola), Diet Pepsi-Cola, and Diet Dr Pepper. As before, we allow people to sip pairs of the drinks and then ask for numerical judgments of how similar the two are. These similarity judgments are the data from which we will try to produce our perceptual map. Here are the hypothetical results. Coke and Pepsi are judged highly similar in taste, but each one is judged quite dissimilar from Dr Pepper. In addition, Coke, Pepsi, and Dr Pepper are each judged dissimilar to their respective diet versions. Finally, some pairs are judged to be particularly *dis*similar: Coke (or Pepsi) versus Diet Dr Pepper, and Dr Pepper versus Diet Pepsi or Tab.

With these results in hand, we proceed to produce an appropriate one-dimensional map. Again, we start by putting the most dissimilar stimuli at the ends of the line. For example, we place Coke and Pepsi at one end (close to each other) and Diet Dr Pepper at the other—because these were judged extremely dissimilar. Now we've got a problem; other soft drinks were also judged extremely dissimilar—Dr Pepper versus the diet versions of Coke and Pepsi. If we try to place these on the same line we used for Diet Dr Pepper, Coke, and Pepsi, the map will necessarily contradict some of the similarity judgment data we collected. Try it for yourself. The solution is to make a two-dimensional map such as the one shown in panel B of the diagram in Appendix Figure 6. The arrangement of the stimuli on this map is consistent with the idea that people were judging sodas on the basis of two criteria—whether they had a *cherry* taste (like Dr Pepper) and whether they had

a *diet* taste. Note that the data themselves forced us to describe the perceptions in two dimensions.

Incidentally, it was fairly easy to create the maps in our two examples because both examples involved a small number of stimuli. Most real MDS experiments, though, use a dozen or more stimuli, making it quite difficult to produce the right map "by hand." In those cases, the researcher could use a computer program containing sophisticated trial-and-error schemes for making the map. Programs available for this task are described in the excellent introduction to MDS by Schiffman and her colleagues (Schiffman, Reynolds, and Young, 1981). These researchers also describe a whole series of uses of MDS, including the development of new consumer products.

* * *

This concludes our discussion of psychophysical methods used in perception research. Though Fechner's goals for psychophysics—an exact science of the relation between mind and body—have not been completely realized, there can be little doubt about the value of his contributions. As a result, today many people all over the world celebrate October 22, called by some "Fechner Day" (Boring, 1961). For on that date in 1850, Fechner first got the idea for his psychophysics.

K E Y   T E R M S

absolute threshold	forced-choice method	psychometric function
β	intrinsic light	psychophysical functions
criterion	method of adjustment	psychophysics
cross-modality matching	method of constant	sensory decision theory
d'	stimuli	(SDT)
dark light	method of limits	signal detection theory
difference threshold	multidimensional scaling	staircase method
direct scaling techniques	(MDS)	Weber's Law

Glossary

The number in parentheses following each term refers to the page number on which that term is introduced.

Abney's Law (96)   The principle that the visual effectiveness of a light composed of different wavelengths can be predicted from the sum of the responses to the wavelengths considered separately.

absolute distance (216)   The distance from an observer to an object. See *relative distance*.

absolute threshold (489)   The minimum stimulus intensity that a person can detect. See *difference threshold*.

accommodation (38, 217)   The variation in the eye's optical power brought about by temporary changes in the shape of the lens.

achromatic system (203)   In the opponent-process view of color vision, the pathway that generates and transmits information about an object's lightness. See *chromatic system*.

acoustic energy (293)   The variations in air pressure produced by the vibration of an object.

acoustic reflex (304)   Muscular contractions within the middle ear that damp sound vibrations by stiffening the eardrum and restricting the movements of the ossicles.

acoustics (294)   The branch of physics concerned with sound.

action potentials (66)   Brief electrical discharges that are generated by a neuron and that represent the "vocabulary" of communication within the nervous system. See *axon*.

adaptation (134, 323, 446)   A reduction in the responsiveness of neurons, produced by prolonged stimulation.

additive color mixture (190)   A color that results when several component colors are combined in such a way that each component contributes a portion to the spectral composition of the combination. See *subtractive color mixture*.

aerial perspective (240)   The tendency for objects at a distance to appear less distinct, since light reflected from those objects must travel through atmosphere containing particles of dirt and water.

afterimage (30, 202)   A visual sensation that persists after exposure to some intense stimulus; also, an illusory color produced by exposure to an intense stimulus.

agnosias (457)   Neurological conditions in which people cannot recognize objects; depending on the sense involved, an agnosia is said to be visual, auditory, or tactile. See *prosopagnosia*.

aliasing (60)   Creation of spurious low-frequency information when high-frequency information is undersampled, as by photoreceptor mosaic.

ambient system (273)   The aspect of vision responsible for spatial orientation; uses information from peripheral as well as central vision. See *focal system*.

ambiguity problem (133)   Because several stimulus variables jointly determine the response of any sensory neuron, a single neuron's response is ambiguous with respect to stimulus conditions.

Ames room (235) A specially constructed room in which the floor-to-ceiling heights as well as the sizes and shapes of the doors and windows have been distorted to make the room appear rectangular when viewed from one specific vantage point. To an observer looking into the room through a peephole, people of identical heights standing in different parts of the room look dramatically different in height. The Ames room illustrates how perceived distance influences perceived size.

amodal completion (233) Perception of an object's occluded region(s).

amplitude (296) The property of sound waves that is related to the magnitude of the change in air pressure produced by a sound source. This property, sometimes referred to as *intensity,* is related to loudness. See *intensity.*

analytic introspection (143) A method for studying perception in which trained people attend to and describe the experiences evoked by some stimulus.

anomalous myopia (50) A temporary myopia induced by lack of adequate stimuli for accommodation.

anosmia (417) An inability to smell odors. See specific anosmias.

Anton's syndrome (15) A neurological condition in which a cortically blind person denies his or her blindness.

anvil (incus) (301) The middle member of the three ossicles within the middle ear; it relays sound vibrations from the hammer to the stirrup.

apparent motion (284) The illusory impression, created by the rapid alternation of objects presented at different spatial locations, that the objects have moved smoothly from one location to the other. See *element movement, group movement.*

aqueous humor (36) A watery fluid, produced by the ciliary body, that nourishes structures within the eye's anterior chamber and helps maintain the eye's shape.

astigmatism (52) An error in refraction caused by variation in optical power along various meridians of the cornea.

attention (459) A selective process that amplifies the effectiveness of some stimuli and diminishes the effectiveness of others.

audibility function (AF) (329) In hearing, a graph portraying threshold intensity as a function of the frequency of the test tone.

auditory canal (300) The hollow cavity leading from the pinna to the eardrum, which in humans is about 2.5 cm long and 7 mm in diameter.

auditory cortex (326) A region of the cortex devoted to analysis of complex sound information, including biologically relevant sounds involved in communication.

auditory image (355) With a complex sound field arising from several different auditory events, the information associated with just one of those events.

auditory nerve (318) The bundle of nerve fibers innervating the cochlea and carrying information from the ear to higher stages of the auditory system. Also known as the *eighth cranial nerve.*

autokinetic effect (466) The illusory impression of motion created when a small stationary target is seen in a homogeneous dim field.

axon (72) The portion of a neuron over which action potentials are conducted. A group of axons constitute a *nerve* or a *tract.* See *action potential.*

bandpass noise (343) Noise containing a restricted, contiguous band of frequencies.

basilar membrane (305) The thin sheet of tissue separating the tympanic canal and the cochlear duct.

beta (β) (498) In sensory decision theory, a measure of the observer's bias.

binaural (323) Listening with two ears. See *monaural.*

binaural cues (323) Sources of sound information for localizing a sound source by comparing the sounds received by the two ears.

binaural unmasking (368) A reduction in the

ability of masking noise heard with both ears to mask another sound heard by one ear only. See *masking*.

binocular (123) Seeing with two eyes. See *monocular*.

binocular cell (123) A visual cortical cell receiving excitatory input from both eyes.

binocular rivalry (225) The alternation of a percept over time between one eye's view and the other eye's view when the two eyes view very different stimuli.

blindsight (117) The ability of some cortically blind people to point to the location of a light that they cannot see.

blobs (125) Clusters of color-opponent cells in the upper layers of the visual cortex. Cells within these clusters, often referred to as blob cells, receive input from color-selective cells of the parvocellular pathway.

Bloch's Law (88) The principle that all stimuli in which the product of time and intensity is constant will be equally detectable.

blue-yellow cells (206) Neurons showing a polarized response to spectral lights, which increases over one portion of the spectrum and decreases over another portion; the transition between the two types of responses occurs between the regions of the spectrum called blue and yellow. See *red-green cells*.

bone conduction (331) The transmission of sound wave vibrations through the bones of the skull to the cochlea. A procedure for testing the integrity of the cochlea in the presence of middle-ear damage.

bottom-up (453) A tendency for perception to be shaped by the flow of information from the receptors to higher nervous centers. See *top-down*.

Braille (385) System of writing in which letters or characters are represented by patterns of tangible dots.

brightness (182) The dimension of color experience related to the amount of light emitted by an object. See *hue, saturation*.

broadband noise (343) Noise whose energy covers a wide range of frequencies.

CAT scan (20) An image of the brain, or other structure, that is created by means of computer-assisted tomography.

cataract (39) Clouding that reduces the lens's transparency and, hence, degrades the quality of the retinal image.

center frequency (343) The frequency lying at the center of the range of frequencies contained in bandpass noise.

choroid (36) A dark, spongy structure containing blood vessels that supply nourishment to the retina; because of its heavy pigmentation, the choroid absorbs scattered light.

chromatic system (203) In the opponent-process view of color vision, the pathway that generates and transmits information about an object's color. See *achromatic system*.

cilia (308, 421) A tiny tuft of thin hairs projecting out of each olfactory receptor cell and extending through the mucous layer into the nasal cavity; thought to be the site where odorous molecules trigger electrical changes in the olfactory receptor cell.

ciliary body (36) Located in the eye, a spongy network of tissue that manufactures aqueous humor.

closure (145) The Gestalt principle of organization referring to the tendency of the visual system to obscure small breaks or gaps in objects. See *proximity, similarity*.

cochlea (305) A coiled, fluid-filled chamber in the inner ear containing the specialized organ for hearing, the basilar membrane.

cochlear emissions (315) Sounds that are generated entirely from within the cochlea.

cochlear nucleus (323) A structure receiving input from the auditory nerve; its cells exhibit a high degree of frequency tuning.

cocktail party effect (368) The ability to attend selectively to the speech of one person in the midst of many other speakers.

collector cells (40) Specialized neurons within the eye that receive and process information from the photoreceptors.

color constancy (189) The tendency of an object's color to remain unchanged despite changes in the spectrum of light falling on— and reflected by—that object.

color contrast (201)   A change in color appearance brought about by juxtaposing particular color pairs.

color deficiency (209)   In humans, a departure from normal trichromatic color vision; takes various forms, including anomalous trichromacy, dichromacy, and monochromacy.

common chemical sense (432)   An aspect of olfaction responsible for the detection of strong concentrations of potentially dangerous substances; responsible for the "feeling" in the nose produced by certain substances.

complementary (185)   Describing two colors that can be mixed to form white.

complex cells (119)   Visual cortical cells that do not exhibit clearly defined ON and OFF regions within their receptive fields, making it difficult to predict what stimulus will produce the largest response. See *simple cells*.

composite light (183)   According to Newton, any light that is made up of several different color components. See *pure light*.

computer vision (178)   The ability of machines, notably computers, to perceive and interpret a visual scene.

conditioned taste aversion (449)   Learned avoidance of certain taste substances, usually following nausea from ingesting the substance.

conduction loss (331)   A form of hearing loss attributable to a disorder in the outer or middle ear; it typically involves an overall loss in sensitivity at all sound frequencies. See *sensory/ neural loss*.

cone of confusion (362)   The set of points in space that potentially could have given rise to any one interaural time difference or interaural intensity difference.

cones (55)   Photoreceptors that are specialized for daylight and color vision. See *rods*.

configural superiority effect (480)   The finding that, under some circumstances, a complex figure, or part of a complex figure, may be seen more readily than one of its parts presented in isolation.

conjunctive (33)   Referring to those move-

ments of the eye in which both eyes move in the same direction. See *vergence*.

contralateral fibers (103)   In the case of vision, those optic nerve fibers that project from one eye to the opposite side of the brain. See *ipsilateral fibers*.

contrast (153)   The difference in light intensity between an object and its immediate surroundings; also, the intensity difference between adjacent bars in a grating.

contrast sensitivity function (CSF) (159)   A graph depicting a person's ability to see targets of various spatial frequency; on the x-axis is the spatial frequency of the test target; on the y-axis is sensitivity, the reciprocal of the minimum contrast needed to see the test target.

contrast threshold (151)   The minimum contrast needed to see some target.

convergence (217)   The ability of the eyes to turn inward, toward each other, in order to fixate a nearby object.

convergence insufficiency (231)   Difficulty with turning the eyes inward to fixate a nearby object.

cornea (36)   The transparent portion of the eye's front surface, which refracts light and allows it to pass into the eyeball.

cortical deafness (328)   Impaired hearing that results from damage to the auditory cortex.

cortical magnification (111)   The mapping of the retina onto the visual cortex so that the representation of the fovea is exaggerated or magnified.

criterion (497)   The implicit rule used by an observer in order to convert sensory information into overt responses.

critical band (344)   The restricted range of frequencies that mask a given test frequency. The critical band reflects the frequency tuning of the neurons that detect the test frequency.

critical flicker frequency (CFF) (252)   The highest perceptible rate of temporal variation in light intensity.

cross-adaptation (435)   A temporary loss in sensitivity to one odor following exposure to a different odor.

cross-fiber theory (443)   The idea that taste

qualities are represented by the pattern of neural activity among an ensemble of neurons; also has application in vision, hearing, and smell.

cross-modality matching (502) A psychophysical procedure in which one sort of stimulus (for instance, a light) is adjusted so that the sensation the stimulus produces matches the sensation produced by a different sort of stimulus (for instance, a sound).

crowding effect (93) The tendency for small letters to be difficult to read when they are in close proximity to one another.

crystalline lens (38) The elliptical optical element located immediately behind the iris of the eye. Temporary variations in thickness alter the eye's accommodation, or optical power.

cutoff frequency (157) The spatial frequency at which a lens's transfer function falls to zero; the highest frequency that a lens can image; the highest frequency to which a visual system can respond.

d' (498) In sensory decision theory, a measure of sensitivity.

dark adaptation (95) The increase in visual sensitivity that accompanies time in darkness following exposure to light.

dark light See *intrinsic light*.

decibel (dB) (296) A unit for expressing sound amplitude.

delay line (325) Key element in a theory designed to explain binaural cells' sensitivity to interaural time differences. The delay line retards the arrival of signals from one ear relative to those from the other ear.

depth of field (38) The range of distances over which the image of a scene remains sharply focused; varies with pupil size.

depth perception (215) The ability to perceive the three-dimensional locations of objects in relation to the perceiver's position in space. Besides specifying distance, depth perception allows a perceiver to segregate objects from their backgrounds and to discern the three-dimensional shapes of objects.

detection (141, 181) The process by which an object is picked out from its surroundings; also, the process by which the presence of some object is perceived.

dichromatic (195) Referring to a person whose eye contains two types of cone photopigments.

difference threshold (489) The minimum amount by which stimulus intensity must be changed in order to produce a just noticeable change in sensation. See *absolute threshold*.

diffuse fibers (392) In touch system, first-order afferent neurons having large receptive fields with poorly defined borders.

diplesthesia (406) In touch, the illusory experience of two objects when only one is actually present.

diplopia (230) Double vision, a condition that results when images from the two eyes are seen separately and simultaneously.

direct scaling techniques (501) A set of psychophysical procedures for measuring subjective sensory experiences such as loudness or brightness; these procedures are based on the assumption that people can rate sensory magnitude.

direction-selective cell (276) A neuron in the visual cortex that responds most vigorously to a particular direction of target movement.

direction selectivity (122) A tendency of some neurons in the visual system to respond most strongly to objects that move in a particular direction.

discrimination (141, 181) The process by which one object is distinguished from another.

discrimination threshold (347) The minimum physical difference, usually an intensity difference, that allows two objects to be distinguished from each other.

disparity-selective cells (227) Cells in the visual cortex that receive input from both eyes and that respond only when an object is situated at a particular distance from the two eyes. See *stereoblindness*.

distance senses See *far senses*.

divergent (45) Referring to light whose wavefronts spread outward, usually as the light proceeds away from its source.

dualism (5)   The philosophical view that mental events need not be associated with neural events. See *materialism*.

duplex (861)   Referring to the co-existence within the eye of two different systems, scotopic and photopic. The scotopic system provides high sensitivity in dim light; the photopic system provides high resolution under daylight conditions.

duplex theory (363)   In hearing, the idea that the interaural time difference (ITD) is used to localize low-frequency sounds and the interaural intensity difference (IID) is used to localize high-frequency sounds.

dynamic visual acuity (269)   The finest spatial detail that can be resolved; measured while a target is moving.

eardrum (tympanic membrane) (300)   The thin, oval membrane that covers the end of the auditory canal and separates the outer ear and the middle ear; it vibrates when sound waves strike it.

eccentricity (71)   The distance between the center of the retina and the location of the retinal image cast by an object.

echoes (294)   Reflected sound waves.

efferent fibers (318)   In the auditory system, neural projections from the brain back to the cochlea.

egocentric direction (215)   The direction in which an object is located relative to an observer.

electromagnetic radiation (27)   Energy that is produced by oscillation of electrically charged material; light encompasses a small portion of the electromagnetic spectrum.

element movement (286)   In an ambiguous type of apparent movement, the percept that some of the stimulus's components are stationary while one component moves back and forth. See *apparent motion, group movement*.

emmetropic (46)   Referring to an eye whose focal point, in the absence of accommodation, coincides exactly with the retina.

equal loudness contours (339)   A set of curves describing the sound intensities at which different frequencies all sound equal in loudness. See *loudness matching*.

Eustachian tube (304)   The opening connecting the middle ear and the throat, which maintains air pressure within the middle ear at nearly the same value as the air pressure in the outside environment.

evoked potential (EP) (18)   The electrical response in a collection of neurons that is provoked by a stimulus.

extraocular muscles (32)   In humans, six large muscles attached to the globe of the eye; by rotating the eyeball within the orbit, the coordinated contractions of these muscles control the direction of gaze. See *rectus muscles*.

far senses (distance senses) (6)   Senses, such as vision, that enable an organism to perceive objects or events some distance away. See *near senses*.

fibrous tunic (35)   The strong, leathery outermost layer of the eyeball.

figure/ground organization (146)   The tendency to see part of a scene (the figure) as a solid, well-defined object standing out against a less distinct background (the ground).

flavor (436)   A complex sensation associated with food, based on the food's taste, temperature, texture, and smell.

flicker (252)   Temporal variation in light intensity; also, the percept of such temporal variation.

floaters (40)   Debris that drifts about within the eye's vitreous casting shadows on the retina and producing dark spots that appear to move along with the eye.

focal system (273)   The aspect of vision that is responsible for object identification and discrimination; predominantly uses central, rather than peripheral, vision. See *ambient system*.

forced-choice (117)   Said of a response used in the forced-choice method. See *forced-choice method*.

forced-choice method (496)   A psychophysical procedure in which a person must identify the interval during which a stimulus occurred; in an alternative version, the person must identify the spatial location at which a stimulus was presented.

Fourier analysis (158)   A method for calculating the frequency content of any temporal or spatial signal; can be used to determine the spatial frequency content of a visual scene or other target.

fovea (54)   Pit or depression in the retina; the region of sharpest vision.

free nerve endings (396, 421)   Nerve cells in the olfactory epithelium that mediate the common chemical sense.

frequency theory (310)   The idea that the basilar membrane vibrates as a unit in response to sound, in synchrony with sound pressure changes. See *place theory*.

frequency tuning curve (320)   A graph describing the sensitivity of an auditory neuron to tones of various frequencies.

fundamental frequency (349)   The lowest frequency among the set of frequencies associated with a complex sound.

geons (472)   In one theory of visual recognition, the geometric elements into which seen objects are decomposed. The term is short for *geo*metrical ic*ons*.

Gestalt principles of organization (145)   Certain stimulus properties that control the perceptual grouping of objects. See *closure, good continuation, proximity, similarity*.

glaucoma (37)   A relatively common ocular disorder in which fluid pressure builds up within the eyeball, eventually causing blindness if not corrected.

global motion (283)   The experience of motion in a single direction that arises from a stimulus whose elements move in a variety of different directions.

good continuation (146)   The tendency to see neighboring elements as grouped together when they are potentially connected by straight or smoothly curving lines.

grating (151)   A target consisting of alternating darker and lighter bars, used to study spatial vision. See *sinusoidal grating*.

group movement (286)   In an ambiguous type of apparent movement, the percept that all stimulus components move back and forth *en masse* (as a group). See *apparent motion, element movement*.

grouping (24)   The aggregation of several related elements into a larger coherent unit. A key part of the recognition process.

habituation (208)   The process by which an organism ceases to respond to some stimulus.

hair cells (307)   The ears' receptors. See *inner hair cells, outer hair cells*.

hammer (malleus) (301)   The outermost of the three ossicles within the middle ear; one end of the hammer is attached to the eardrum, and the other end relays sound vibrations to the anvil.

haptics (401)   Sensory information that depends upon both touch and kinesthesis.

harmonics (351)   Acoustic frequencies that are multiples of one another, often occurring in speech and music. Harmonic tones tend to be perceptually grouped in hearing.

Hermann grid (76)   A regular, geometric pattern within which illusory spots are seen; the presence and strength of the illusory spots depend on the spacing of the grid's elements.

hertz (Hz) (298)   A unit for expressing the frequency with which the intensity of a sound or a light varies over time.

horopter (223)   An imaginary plane in visual space that contains objects whose images fall on corresponding points of the retina of the left and right eyes; any object situated on the horopter will be seen as single.

hue (182)   The dimension of color experience that distinguishes among red, orange, yellow, green, blue, and so on; the dimension of color most strongly determined by light's wavelength; commonly used as synonym for *color*. See *brightness, saturation*.

hypercolumn (126)   An aggregation of columns of cortical cells whose receptive fields overlap on the same restricted region of the retina.

hyperopic (46)   Referring to an abnormally short eyeball, in which the image is blurred because the eye's focal point lies behind the retina.

identification (141)   The process of distinguishing a particular object.

illusions (24)   Perceptual errors.

illusory conjunction (132)   Condition in which features that actually belong to separate objects appear to be combined.

image (44)   The spatial distribution of light energy produced by the action of some optical system.

incus   See *anvil*.

induced motion (278)   The illusory impression, created when moving contours are nearby a stationary object, that the stationary object is moving.

inner hair cells (IHCs) (307)   The approximately 3,5 flask-shaped structures situated along the length of the basilar membrane of the human ear. See *outer hair cells*.

intensity (76)   The physical variable expressing the strength or amplitude of a stimulus, such as light or sound. Intensity can be measured by physical devices such as photometers and sound-level meters. See *amplitude*.

interaural intensity difference (IID) (325, 360)   The difference in the intensity of sound arriving at the two ears; one of the sources of information for sound localization. See *interaural time difference*.

interaural time difference (ITD) (324, 361)   The difference in the time of arrival of a sound wave at the two ears; one of the sources of information for sound localization. See *interaural intensity difference*.

interposition (231)   A monocular depth cue based on occlusion of a distant object by a closer one.

intrinsic light (dark light) (490)   The impression, in complete darkness, of a dim cloud of light.

ipsilateral fibers (102)   In the case of vision, those optic nerve fibers that project from one eye to the same side of the brain. See *contralateral fibers*.

iris (37)   The two-layered ring of tissue that gives the eye its characteristic color.

isomorphism (147)   The Gestalt hypothesis that spatial distribution of brain activity evoked by some object bears a topological resemblance to that object.

kinesthesis (401)   Information about the movement and position of a limb that derives from receptors that are in the muscles, tendons, and joints of that limb.

lateral geniculate nucleus (LGN) (105)   A group of nerve cell bodies arranged in layers in the thalamus, each layer receiving input from either the left eye or the right eye; the major relay station between the eye and the visual cortex.

lateral inhibition (69)   Antagonistic neural interaction between adjacent regions of a sensory surface, such as the retina.

lesion (17)   Damage to a restricted region of the body, particularly some portion of the nervous system.

lightness (76)   A perceptual variable that is correlated with light intensity.

lightness constancy (81)   The tendency for the perceived lightness of an object to remain constant despite variation in the level of its illumination.

lightness contrast (80)   An effect in which a fixed physical intensity of light produces different perceived lightnesses depending upon the intensity of the light's background.

linear perspective (237)   The convergence of lines that makes a two-dimensional representation of a scene appear to be three-dimensional.

localization ability (383)   An observer's capacity to identify the position of some stimulus.

loudness (337)   The subjective experience associated with sound intensity.

loudness matching (337)   A psychophysical procedure in which a listener adjusts the intensity of one tone until it sounds as loud as another tone. See *equal loudness contours*.

M cells (72) Retinal ganglion cells characterized by relatively large cell bodies and axons, large receptive fields, strong response to small differences in light levels in receptive field center and surround, and lack of sensitivity to stimulus wavelength. See *P cells*.

Mach bands (75) Illusory spatial gradations in perceived lightness that occur in the absence of corresponding gradations in the actual spatial distribution of light.

macula (42) The small, circular central region of the retina where vision is most acute.

magnitude estimation (337) A psychophysical procedure in which people assign numbers to stimuli in proportion to the perceived intensity of those stimuli.

magnocellular layers (106) In the lateral geniculate nucleus, layers containing large cells; layers 1 and 2.

malleus See *hammer*.

masking (343) A reduction in one stimulus's visibility or loudness as a result of the juxtaposition of another, stronger stimulus. See *binaural unmasking*.

materialism (5) The philosophical view that ascribes all mental experiences to neural events. See *dualism*.

mechanoreceptors (380) Receptors that respond to deformation of the skin.

medial geniculate nucleus (326) A structure in the thalamus that is part of the auditory system.

Meissner corpuscles (394) An encapsulated touch receptor located in the skin's upper layer.

melody contour (356) The rise and fall of successive notes in a musical passage.

meridional amblyopia (120) A loss in visual acuity for lines of a particular orientation.

Merkel disk (394) An unencapsulated touch receptor located at an intermediate depth within the skin.

metamers (171, 193) Two or more objects that appear identical despite acute physical differences.

method of adjustment (490) A psychophysical procedure in which a person adjusts a stimulus so that it is just detectable (absolute threshold) or until a just noticeable change is produced (difference threshold).

method of constant stimuli (490) A psychophysical procedure in which each of a fixed set of stimuli is presented in random order.

method of limits (490) A psychophysical procedure in which the stimulus intensity changes progressively in small steps until the person's response changes, for example, from "No, I don't see it" to "Yes, I do see it."

microelectrode (66) A thin wire that can be inserted into brain tissue in order to record action potentials.

microspectrophotometry (197) A technique for measuring, at various wavelengths, the quantity of light reflected or absorbed by a small object; used to measure cone photopigments.

missing fundamental (351) With a complex series of harmonic tones, the fundamental tone of the series may continue to be heard despite the fact that it has been physically removed.

mixture suppression (436) The strength of odor produced by some substance presented alone may be reduced when that same substance is presented in combination with another.

monaural (323) Listening with one ear. See *binaural*.

monochromat (194) A person whose eye contains just one type of cone photopigment.

monocular (123) Seeing with one eye. See *binocular*.

motion aftereffect (waterfall illusion) (278) The illusory impression, after prolonged viewing of movement in one direction, that a stationary object is moving in the opposite direction.

motion capture (283) An object that moves in one direction over a field of randomly moving elements causes those elements to appear to move in the same direction as the object itself.

motion parallax (241) A source of potent monocular depth information based on differences in relative motion between images of objects located at different distances from an observer.

multichannel model (153) The hypothesis that spatial vision is the product, in part, of sets of neurons responsive to different spatial frequencies.

multidimensional scaling (MDS) (416) A quantitative technique for geometrically representing similarity among stimuli.

myelin (102) A membrane that insulates a neuron's axon and speeds conduction of nerve impulses along that axon.

myopic (46) Referring to an abnormally long eye, in which the retinal image is blurred because the eye's focal point lies in front of the retina.

naive realism (10) The philosophical view that perception accurately portrays all objects and events in the world.

nanometer (62) A unit of length in the metric system corresponding to one-billionth of a meter, used for specifying wavelength of light.

nasal cycle (419) Periodic alternation in which first one then the other nostril is obstructed.

near senses (6) Senses, such as touch, that require close proximity between the perceiver and the object or event to be perceived. See *far senses*.

neon spreading (233) The illusory migration of color from one region into neighboring regions.

neurogram (372) A graph depicting variations over time in the neural activity within a large number of frequency-selective neurons in response to a complex sound.

neutral point (195) In a dichromatic eye, the wavelength of light that appears white (neutral in color).

Newton's color circle (185) A geometric arrangement of colors summarizing the results of mixing varying amounts of different colors.

noise (298) A complex sound whose many constituent frequencies combine to produce a random waveform.

nonspectral colors (187) Colors, such as purple, that are not found in the spectrum.

object constancy (483) An object may continue to be perceived despite its being occluded briefly.

oblique effect (120) The tendency for lines oriented vertically or horizontally to be more visible than lines oriented along a diagonal.

occipital lobe (110) A region of the brain involved in vision; located at the brain's posterior.

ocular dominance (123) The variation in strength of excitatory input from the two eyes to a binocular cell of the visual cortex.

oculomotor cues (217) Kinesthetic cues to depth derived from muscular contractions of the extraocular muscles.

odor adaptation (434) A reduction in odor sensitivity following prolonged exposure to an odorous substance.

odor constancy (431) The tendency of an odor's perceived intensity to remain constant despite variations in the flow rate of air drawn into the nose.

odor hallucinations (433) Odors experienced without any physical stimulus; a phenomenon sometimes associated with brain damage.

olfactory brain (423) A cluster of neural structures that receives projections from the olfactory bulb via the olfactory tract.

olfactory bulb (423) The brain structure that receives input from the olfactory nerve.

olfactory epithelium (419) A patch of tissue situated near the top of the nasal cavity and containing the olfactory receptor cells.

olfactory nerve (421) The bundle of axons from olfactory receptor cells that project to the olfactory bulb, carrying information about odorous substances from the nose to the brain. Also called the *first cranial nerve*.

olfactory receptor cell (419) One of the specialized structures within the olfactory epithelium that registers the presence of odorous substances.

ophthalmoscope (40) An optical device used to visualize the inside of the eye.

optic ataxia (263) A neurological disorder characterized by difficulties in the visual guidance of limb movement.

optic chiasm (102) The point at which nerve

fibers from the two eyes are rerouted to higher visual centers, with some fibers from each eye projecting to the same side of the brain (ipsilateral fibers) and the remainder projecting to the opposite side of the brain (contralateral fibers).

optic disk (42)   The region of the eye where the optic nerve penetrates the retina; also, the region where major blood vessels enter and exit the eye's interior.

optic nerve (102)   The bundle of axons of retinal ganglion cells that carries visual information from the eye to the brain. Also known as the *second cranial nerve*.

optic tracts (103)   The two bundles of axons of retinal ganglion cells formed after the nerve fibers exit the optic chiasm.

orbit (33)   Cavity in the skull that houses the eyeball and its supporting structures.

organ of Corti (306)   The receptor organ for hearing, situated within the cochlear duct.

orientation (153)   The degree of inclination of a contour within a two-dimensional plane.

orientation selectivity (118)   A unique property of visual cortical cells, whereby they respond best to contours of a particular orientation, with the response decreasing as the orientation deviates increasingly from the preferred value.

ossicles (301)   A series of three tiny bones that transmit sound vibrations from the eardrum to the oval window. See *anvil, hammer, stirrup*.

otosclerosis (331)   A disorder of the middle ear involving immobilization of the stirrup.

outer hair cells (OHCs) (308)   The approximately 12,000 cylindrical structures situated along the length of the basilar membrane of the human ear. See *inner hair cells*.

oval window (301)   The small opening into the inner ear, which is covered by a thin membrane and which receives vibrations from the eardrum via the ossicles.

P cells (72)   Retinal ganglion cells characterized by relatively small cell bodies and axons, small receptive fields, weak response to small differences in light levels in receptive field center

and surround, and good sensitivity to stimulus wavelength. See *M cells*.

Pacinian corpuscle (394)   An encapsulated touch receptor located in the skin's lower layer.

papillae (440)   Protuberances distributed over the tongue's surface, the walls of which are lined with taste buds.

parietal cortex (404)   A major division of the cerebral cortex; the parietal cortex covers the upper, rear portion of the side of the brain; receives information from touch system.

parvocellular layers (106)   In the lateral geniculate nucleus, layers containing small cells; layers 3 through 6.

perceived distance (236)   The apparent visual separation between two objects or between an object and the viewer.

perception (1)   The acquisition and processing of sensory information in order to see, hear, taste, smell, or feel objects in the world; also guides an organism's actions with respect to those objects. Perception may involve conscious awareness of objects and events; this awareness is termed a *percept*.

perceptual differentiation (468)   The tendency of exposure to particular stimuli to sharpen one's ability to distinguish among them.

perfect pitch (354)   The comparatively rare ability to identify any musical note played or to reproduce vocally any named note. See *relative pitch*.

perimetry (112)   A procedure for measuring a visual field, which involves determining the positions in visual space where a person can and cannot see a small spot of light.

PET scan (20)   An image of the brain, or other structure, that is created by means of positron emission tomography.

phantom limb (405)   The illusory experience, often painful, that an amputated limb is still attached to the body.

pheromones (412)   Odors that serve as sexual signals.

phonagnosia (377)   Inability to identify speakers by means of their voices.

phoneme (370)   A sound difference that affects

the meaning of an utterance; widely regarded as the fundamental unit of speech.

phonemic restoration effect (465)   The tendency to hear a sound that has actually been deleted from an utterance.

phosphenes (132)   Visual sensations arising entirely from neural events within the visual pathways, in the absence of light stimulation.

photon (88)   The smallest unit of light energy.

photopic (86)   Referring to vision under daylight levels of illumination. See *scotopic*.

photopigment (61)   Light-sensitive molecules within a photoreceptor; light causes the photopigment to isomerize, releasing energy that alters the photoreceptor's electrical potential.

photoreceptors (40)   Specialized nerve cells (rods and cones) in the eye that contain photopigment; absorption of light by these cells triggers changes in the cells' electrical potential.

pigment epithelium (42)   A layer of the retina that helps to dispose of cellular debris.

pinna (300)   The part of the ear projecting from the side of the head; by influencing the frequency composition of sound waves entering the ear, this prominent structure plays a role in sound localization.

pitch (348)   The subjective counterpart to sound frequency.

place theory (311)   The idea that different portions of the basilar membrane vibrate in response to different sound frequencies. See *frequency theory*.

power law (340)   The psychophysical principle that sensation magnitude tends to grow as a power function of stimulus intensity.

presbycusis (322)   In hearing, an age-related gradual loss of sensitivity to high-frequency tones.

presbyopia (51)   A significant decline in accommodative ability beginning in middle age.

primitives (147)   In theories of vision, simple elements that are thought to be building blocks for perception.

profile analysis (348)   The process by which the relative activity of various neurons registers some property of a stimulus.

proprioception (263, 401)   The sense that enables one to feel where one's limbs are.

prosopagnosia (131, 457)   An inability to recognize faces. See *agnosias*.

proximity (145)   The Gestalt principle of organization referring to the perceptual tendency to group together objects that are near one another. See *closure, similarity*.

psychometric function (491)   A graph showing the frequency with which each stimulus elicits each of two possible responses.

psychophysical function (499)   A graph showing the threshold as a function of some stimulus variable.

psychophysics (1, 489)   The branch of perception that is concerned with establishing quantitative relations between physical stimulation and perceptual events.

pulvinar (462)   A structure within the thalamus of the brain; thought to play a key role in attention.

punctate fibers (392)   In touch system, first-order afferent neurons have small receptive fields with sharply defined borders.

pupil (38)   The aperture in the eye formed by two sets of concentric bands of muscle; the constriction and dilation of these muscles vary the diameter of the pupil.

pure light (183)   According to Newton, any light that cannot be broken down into constituent colors. See *composite light*.

pure tones (298)   Sinusoidal variations in sound pressure, such as those produced by striking a tuning fork.

Purkinje shift (94)   Perceptual variation in the relative lightness of different colors as illumination changes from daylight to twilight.

pursuit eye movements (268)   Smooth movements of the eyes that allow them to follow a moving target.

random–dot stereogram (225)   A pair of pictures composed of black and white dots randomly positioned within the pictures; when such pictures are viewed stereoscopically (one picture seen by each eye), a vivid sensation of depth results, making an object appear to stand out from its surroundings.

rapidly adapting (RA) fibers (392)   First-order afferent neurons that respond in a relatively transient manner to sustained deformation of the skin.

receptive field (69)   The area of the retina within which the activity of a neuron can be influenced; sometimes defined in terms of the region of visual space from which a neuron can be influenced.

recognition (24)   The appreciation that some object or event has been encountered previously.

rectus muscles (32)   Four of the extraocular muscles; largely responsible for moving the eyeball back and forth horizontally (medial rectus and lateral rectus) and up and down vertically (superior rectus and inferior rectus). See *extraocular muscles*.

red-green cells (206)   Neurons showing a polarized response to spectral lights, which increases over one portion of the spectrum and decreases over another portion; the transition between the two types of responses occurs between the regions of the spectrum called green and red. See *blue-yellow cells*.

refraction (54)   The bending of light by an optical element such as a lens.

relative distance (216)   The distance between two objects. See *absolute distance*.

relative pitch (354)   The comparatively common ability to identify a tonal interval without necessarily knowing the particular tones that make up that interval. See *perfect pitch*.

resolution (85)   The ability to distinguish spatial details of an object.

resonant frequency (302)   The frequency at which a given object vibrates when set into motion.

reticular activating system (109)   A brain stem structure that governs an organism's general level of arousal.

retina (35)   The innermost layer of the eyeball, where light is detected by photoreceptors and transduced into neural signals that are processed by collector cells.

retinal disparity (220)   A slight difference in lateral separation between objects seen by the left eye and by the right eye; makes stereopsis possible. See *stereopsis*.

retinal ganglion cells (66)   The collector cells that are responsible for the last stage of visual processing within the retina; axons of the retinal ganglion cells constitute the optic nerve.

retinal image (43)   The distribution of light falling on the retina; the quality and overall intensity of this image influence visual perception.

retinotopic map (107)   A neural representation within the visual system that preserves the spatial layout of the retina.

Ricco's Law (89)   The principle that stimuli will be equally detectable if the product of their intensity and area is constant.

rods (55)   Photoreceptors that are specialized for vision under dim light. See *cones*.

Rorschach test (466)   A projective psychological test in which people are shown inkblots and asked to describe what they see.

round window (305)   The thin membrane that covers a small opening into the middle ear; displacement of this membrane compensates for pressure variations within the cochlea.

Ruffini endings (394)   An unencapsulated touch receptor located at an intermediate depth within the skin.

saccades (264)   Rapid, jerky movements of the eyes, which function to change fixation from one location to another.

saturation (182)   The dimension of color experience that distinguishes pale or washed-out colors from vivid colors. See *brightness, hue*.

scale (149)   Relative size or extent.

sclera (36)   The tough, dense material that forms the eye's outermost coat; seen from the front, the sclera is the white of the eye.

sclerosis (39)   The hardening of any living tissue; hardening of the eye's crystalline lens may play a role in presbyopia. See *presbyopia*.

scotoma (111)   A region of blindness within the visual field.

scotopic (86)   Referring to vision under dim levels of illumination. See *photopic*.

segregation (24)   The differentiation of some object from its background or from neighboring elements. A key part of the recognition process.

selective adaptation (167, 277)   A method of studying mechanisms of perception, in which a person's sensitivity to particular targets is depressed by prolonged exposure to one particular target.

sensory decision theory (SDT) (497)   A quantitative treatment of detection and discrimination performance, in which the observer is characterized as a maker of statistical decisions; the system also prescribes techniques that allow the observer's sensitivity to the stimulus to be estimated independently of the observer's criterion, or preference for particular responses. Also called *signal detection theory*.

sensory/neural loss (331)   A form of hearing loss originating within the inner ear or the auditory pathways; may involve selective loss of sensitivity to a limited range of frequencies. See *conduction loss*.

sensory-specific satiety (450)   Eating one particular food may diminish hunger for that food without affecting hunger for other foods.

sensory transduction (1)   The process occurring within sensory receptors by which physical energy (stimulus) is converted into neural signals.

shading (240)   A gradient in the level of reflected light across the surface of a three-dimensional object. This gradient provides a cue to depth, since flat, two-dimensional surfaces don't cast shadows.

shape constancy (177)   The tendency for an object's perceived shape to remain constant despite changes in the shape of the retinal image of that object.

signal detection theory   See *sensory decision theory*.

similarity (145)   The Gestalt principle of organization referring to the perceptual tendency to group together objects that are similar to one another in texture, shape, and so on. See *closure, proximity*.

simple cells (119)   Visual cortical cells that exhibit clearly defined ON and OFF regions within their receptive fields. See *complex cells*.

single cell recording (66)   The use of a microelectrode to record the neural activity of individual nerve cells as they respond to stimulation.

sinusoidal grating (151)   A target in which the intensity of darker and lighter bars varies sinusoidally over space. See *grating*.

size aftereffect (175)   A change in the apparent size of an object following inspection of an object of a different size.

size constancy (248)   The tendency for an object's perceived size to remain constant despite changes in the size of the retinal image of that object as viewing distance varies.

slowly adapting (SA) fibers (392)   First-order afferent neurons that respond in a relatively sustained manner to sustained deformation of the skin.

smooth eye movements (268)   Smooth movements of the eyes, which can function in the pursuit of a moving target.

solipsism (10)   The belief that no one exists other than oneself.

sound localization (359)   Ability to identify the position of some sound stimulus.

sound pressure level (SPL) (297)   A reference level for sound intensity.

spatial frequency (153)   For a grating target, the number of pairs of bars imaged within a given distance on the retina; units of spatial frequency are cycles/mm or, equivalently, cycles/degree of visual angle.

spatial phase (153)   The position of a grating relative to some visual landmark.

spatial summation (86)   The process by which neural signals from neighboring retinal areas are combined, thereby increasing sensitivity. See *temporal summation*.

specific anosmias (417)   Conditions in which

people have normal odor sensitivity for some substances but reduced sensitivity for other substances. See *anosmia*.

specific nerve energies (13)   The doctrine that the qualitative nature of a sensation depends on which particular nerve fibers are stimulated.

spectral colors (183)   Hues that are present in a spectrum created by diffracting white light as, for example, in a rainbow.

spectrogram (370)   A graph depicting the frequency composition of a sound as a function of time.

squint   See *strabismus*.

stabilized retinal images (268)   Images whose location on the retina remains fixed despite movements of the eye.

staircase method (494)   A psychophysical procedure in which the stimulus presentations, governed by a person's responses, are made to bracket the threshold; an interactive variant of the method of limits.

stapes   See *stirrup*.

stereoblindness (228)   The inability to see depth using retinal disparity information, a condition thought to result from a reduction in the number of binocular visual cells in the visual cortex. See *disparity-selective cells*.

stereopsis (219)   Binocular depth perception based on retinal disparity. See *retinal disparity*.

stereoscope (223)   An optical device for presenting pictures separately to the two eyes.

stimulus (1)   The pattern of physical energy set up by an object or event in the environment.

stimulus uncertainty (266)   Lack of knowledge about some property or properties of a stimulus; such uncertainty reduces the stimulus's detectability.

stirrup (stapes) (301)   The innermost of the ossicles within the middle ear; attached to the oval window, it receives sound vibrations from the anvil and sets the oval window into vibration.

strabismus (228)   Squint; a condition in which the two eyes are misaligned, making normal binocular fixation impossible.

structure from motion (SFM) (257)   The impression of an object's shape that derives from the object's motion.

subjective contours (22)   Illusory contours or surfaces, especially like those devised by Kanizsa.

subjective idealism (10)   The view that the physical world is entirely the product of the mind.

subtractive color mixture (190)   A color produced when each of a number of components absorbs a portion of the light's spectrum, thereby subtracting that portion from the reflected spectrum. See *additive color mixture*.

superior colliculus (105)   A subcortical brain structure located in the midbrain; this structure plays a role in the initiation and guidance of eye movements.

synapse (63)   A tiny gap between adjacent nerve cells. See *transmitter substance*.

taste buds (440)   Garlic-shaped structures lining the walls of the papillae on the tongue and containing chemical-sensitive cells that register the presence of taste solutions.

taste hedonics (449)   Judgments of the pleasantness of taste substances.

taste modification (446)   Alteration in the taste of one substance when it is sampled together with another substance.

taste suppression (447)   The reduction in the strength of one taste sensation by another; for example, sugar suppresses the bitter taste of coffee.

tectorial membrane (306)   An awninglike layer of tissue arching over the hair cells within the inner ear.

temporal summation (88)   The process by which signals from a neuron or neurons are cumulated over time, thereby increasing sensitivity. See *spatial summation*.

temporary threshold shift (334)   A short-lived decrease in hearing sensitivity caused by exposure to noise.

texture gradient (239)   A form of perspective in which the density of a surface's texture increases with distance, providing information about the slant of the surface.

threshold intensity (320, 329)   The minimum sound intensity necessary to elicit a neural response from an auditory neuron.

tilt aftereffect (134)   A temporary change in the perceived orientation of lines following adaptation to lines of a similar, but not identical, orientation.

timbre (352)   The quality of sound that distinguishes different musical instruments. See *harmonics*.

tinnitus (317)   An annoying, persistent ringing in the ears.

tip of the nose effect (430)   The phenomenon in which an odor seems familiar though one cannot name it.

tonotopic organization (314)   The orderly layout of preferred frequencies over the length of the basilar membrane.

top-down (453)   A tendency for perception to be shaped by a flow of information from higher nervous centers toward lower ones. See *bottom-up*.

touch acuity (382)   Ability to distinguish a small separation between two closely adjacent stimuli applied to the skin.

transfer function (157)   A graph showing, for various target spatial frequencies, the contrast contained in an image.

transmitter substance (63)   One of several different neurochemicals that diffuse across synaptic gaps between adjacent nerve cells, allowing cells to communicate with one another. See *synapse*.

transparency (233)   The property of a nonopaque object that makes it possible to see other objects located behind the nonopaque one. Transparency implies depth without occlusion.

traveling wave (313)   The movement of the basilar membrane in response to fluctuations in fluid pressure with the cochlea.

trichromatic (195)   Referring to a person whose eye contains three types of cone photopigments.

unilateral neglect (405)   Neurological disorder in which a patient ignores events on one side of the body.

univariance principle (193)   The hypothesis that any photoreceptor's response corresponds to just a single variable, the amount of light absorbed; because photoreceptors obey the univariance principle, the wavelength characteristics of light that stimulate a photoreceptor are not directly represented in the receptor's response.

vascular tunic (35)   The middle layer of the eyeball; responsible for much of the eye's nourishment.

vergence (33)   Referring to eye movements in which the two eyes move in opposite directions. See *conjunctive*.

vestibular (273)   The system responsible for the body's sense of balance.

vestibular eye movements (271)   Eye movements that promote the steadiness of gaze by compensating for movements of the head and body.

vestibule (271)   A chamber in the inner ear involved in vestibular eye movements.

visual acuity (85)   A measure of the smallest detail that a person can resolve.

visual cues (217)   Sources of depth information based on monocular and binocular image properties.

visual field (112)   The extent of visual space over which vision is possible with the eyes held in a fixed position.

visual masking (253)   The reduction of one target's visibility by the presentation of another target nearby in time and space.

vitreous (40)   The thick transparent fluid that fills the eye's largest chamber.

waterfall illusion   See *motion aftereffect*.

wavelength (27)   The distance from the peak of one wave to the peak of the next. For electromagnetic radiation, such as light, wavelength is determined by the rate at which the emitting substance oscillates. This physical property of light, specified in nanometers, is related to the perceptual experience of hue.

Weber's Law (490)   The principle that for various stimulus intensities the difference threshold tends to be a constant fraction of the stimulus.

window of visibility (159)   The range of spatial frequencies that, with sufficient contrast, an observer can see.

word superiority effect (477)   The finding that, under some conditions, an entire word may be read more rapidly (or be seen more easily) than just one of the word's letters.

Young–Helmholtz theory (196)   The theory that human color vision is trichromatic—that is, it depends on the responses of three types of cones.

References

Abadi, R., and **Pascal, E.** (1989) The recognition and management of albinism. Ophthalmic and Physiological Optics, 9, 3–15.

Ackerman, D. (1990) A natural history of the senses. New York: Random House.

Adams, A. J., Wang, L. S., Wong, L., and **Gould, B.** (1988) Visual acuity changes with age: Some new perspectives. American Journal of Optometry and Physiological Optics, 65, 403–406.

Adams, A. J., Zisman, F., Rodic, R., and **Cavender, J.** (1982) Chromaticity and luminosity changes in glaucoma and diabetes. In G. Verriest (ed.), Colour vision deficiencies, VI. Proceedings of the Sixth Symposium of the International Research Group on Colour Vision Deficiencies. The Hague: W. Junk. Pp. 413–416.

Addams, R. (1834/1964) An account of a peculiar optical phaenomenon. In W. Dember (ed.), Visual perception: The nineteenth century. New York: John Wiley & Sons. Pp. 81–83.

Adelson, E. H., and **Movshon, A. J.** (1982) Phenomenal coherence of moving visual patterns. Nature, 300, 523–525.

Adrian, E. D., and **Zotterman, Y.** (1926) The impulses produced by sensory nerve endings: III. Impulses set up by touch and pressure. Journal of Physiology, 61, 465–483.

Ahissar, E., Bergman, H., and **Vaadia, E.** (1992) Encoding of sound-source location and movement: Activity of single neurons and interactions between adjacent neurons in the monkey auditory cortex. Journal of Neurophysiology, 67, 203–215.

Ahlstrom, R., Berglund, R., Berglund, U., Engen, T., and **Lindvall, T.** (1987) A comparison of odor perception in smokers, nonsmokers, and passive smokers. American Journal of Otolaryngology, 8, 1–6.

Ahlstrom, R., Berglund, R., Berglund, U., Lindvall, T., and **Wennberg, A.** (1986) Impaired odor perception in tank cleaners. Scandinavian Journal of Work and Environmental Health, 12, 574–581.

Albano, J. E., Mishkin, M., Westbrook, L. E., and **Wurtz, R. H.** (1982) Visuomotor deficits following ablation of monkey colliclus. Journal of Neurophysiology, 48, 338–351.

Albrecht, D. G., Farrar, S. B., and **Hamilton, D. B.** (1984) Spatial contrast adaptation characteristics of neurones recorded in the cat's visual cortex. Journal of Physiology, 347, 713–739.

Allen, J. B., and **Neely, S. T.** (1992) Micromechanical models of the cochlea. Physics Today, 45, 40–47.

Alpern M. (1981) Color blind color vision. Trends in Neurosciences, 4, 131–135.

Amoore, J. E. (1970) Molecular basis of odor. Springfield, Ill.: Thomas.

Amoore, J. E. (1991) Specific anosmias. In T. V. Getchell, R. L. Doty, L. M. Bartoshuk, and J. B. Snow (eds.), Smell and taste in health and disease. New York: Raven Press. Pp. 655–664.

Andrews, D. P., and **Miller, D. T.** (1978) Acuity for spatial separation as a function of stimulus size. Vision Research, 18, 615–620.

Anholt, R. R. H. (1991) Odor recognition and olfactory transduction: The new frontier. Chemical Senses, 16, 421–427.

Anliker, J. A., Bartoshuk, L., Ferris, A. N., and **Hooks, L. D.** (1991) Children's food preferences and genetic sensitivity to the bitter taste of 6-n-propythiouracil (PROP). American Journal of Clinical Nutrition, 54, 316–320.

Annis, R. C., and **Frost, B.** (1973) Human visual ecology and orientation anisotropies in acuity. Science, 182, 729–731.

Anstis, S. M. (1974) A chart demonstrating variations in acuity with retinal position. Vision Research, 14, 589–592.

Anstis, S. M. (1978) Apparent movement. In R. Held, H. W. Leibowitz, and H.-L. Teuber (eds.), Handbook of sensory physiology, vol. 8. Berlin: Springer-Verlag. Pp. 655–673.

Appelle, S. (1972) Perception and discrimination as a function of stimulus orientation: The oblique effect in man and animals. Psychological Bulletin, 78, 266–278.

Applegate, W. B., Miller, S. T., Elam, J. T., Freeman, J. M., Wood, T. O., and **Gettlefinger, T. C.** (1987) Impact of cataract surgery with lens implantation on vision and physical function in elderly patients. Journal of the American Medical Association, 257, 1064–1066.

Arezzo, J. C., Schaumburg, H. H., and **Petersen, C. A.** (1983) Rapid screening for peripheral neuropathy: A field study with the Optacon. Neurology, 33, 626–629.

Ashmead, D. H., LeRoy, D., and **Odom, R.** (1990) Perception of the relative distances of nearby sound sources. Perception & Psychophysics, 47, 326–331.

Aslin, R. N. (1981) Development of smooth pursuit in human infants. In D. F. Fisher, R. A. Monty, and J. W. Senders (eds.), Eye movements: Cognition and visual perception. Hillsdale, N.J.: Erlbaum. Pp. 31–51.

Atkinson, J., Braddick, O. J., and **Moar, K.** (1977) Contrast sensitivity of the human infant for moving and stationary patterns. Vision Research, 17, 1045–1047.

Axelsson, A., and **Lindgren, F.** (1978) Hearing in pop musicians. Acta Otolaryngology, 85, 225–231.

Bahill, A. T., and **LaRitz, T.** (1984) Why can't batters keep their eyes on the ball? American Scientist, 72, 249–253.

Baird, J. C. (1982) The moon illusion: II. A reference theory. Journal of Experimental Psychology: General, 111, 304–315.

Baird, J. C., and **Wagner, M.** (1982) The moon illusion: I. How high is the sky? Journal of Experimental Psychology: General, 111, 296–303.

Baker, C. L., and **Braddick, O. J.** (1982) Does segregation of differently moving areas depend on relative or absolute displacement? Vision Research, 22, 851–856.

Baldwin, W. R. (1981) A review of statistical studies of relations between myopia and ethnic, behavioral, and physiological characteristics. American Journal of Optometry and Physiological Optics, 58, 516–527.

Ball, K., and **Sekuler, R.** (1981) Cues reduce direction uncertainty and enhance motion detection. Perception & Psychophysics, 30, 119–128.

Ballantyne, J. C. (1977) Deafness (3rd ed.). Edinburgh: Churchill Livingstone.

Banks, M. S. (1982) The development of spatial and temporal contrast sensitivity. Current Eye Research, 2, 191–198.

Banks, M. S., Aslin, R. N., and **Letson, R. D.** (1975) Sensitive period for the development of human binocular vision. Science, 190, 675–677.

Banks, M. S., and **Bennett, P. J.** (1988) Optical and photoreceptor immaturities limit the spatial and chromatic vision of human neonates. Journal of Optical Society of America A, 5, 2059–2079.

Banks, M. S., and **Salapateck, P.** (1978) Acuity and contrast sensitivity in 1-, 2-, and 3-month-old human infants. Investigative Ophthalmology & Visual Science, 17, 361–365.

Banks, W. P. (1970) Signal detection theory and human memory. Psychological Bulletin, 74, 81–99.

Barac-Cikoja, D., and **Turvey, M. T.** (1991) Perceiving aperture size by striking. Journal of Experimental Psychology: Human Perception and Performance, 17, 330–346.

Barlow, H. B. (1972) Single units and sensation: A neuron doctrine for perceptual psychology? Perception, 1, 371–395.

Barlow, H. B. (1982) What causes trichromacy? A theoretical analysis using comb-filtered spectra. Vision Research, 22, 635–644.

Barlow, H. B., Blakemore, C., and **Pettigrew, J. D.** (1967) The neural mechanism of binocular depth discrimination. Journal of Physiology, 193, 327–342.

Barlow, H. B., Fitzhugh, R., and **Kuffler, S. W.** (1957) Change of organization in the receptive fields of the cat's retina during dark adaptation. Journal of Physiology, 137, 327–337.

Barlow, H. B., and **Hill, R. M.** (1963) Evidence for a physiological explanation of the waterfall illusion. Nature, 200, 1345–1347.

Barlow, H. B., and **Sparrock, J. M. B.** (1964) The role of afterimages in dark adaptation. Science, 144, 1309–1314.

Barsky, A. J., Goodson, J. D., Lane, R. S., and **Cleary, P. D.** (1988) The amplification of somatic symptoms. Psychosomatic Medicine, 50, 510–519.

Bartoshuk, L. M. (1974) Taste illusions: Some demonstrations. Annals of the New York Academy of Sciences, 237, 279–285.

Bartoshuk, L. M. (1975) Taste mixtures: Is mixture suppression related to compression? Physiology & Behavior, 14, 643–649.

Bartoshuk, L. M. (1978) History of taste research. In E. C. Carterette and M. P. Friedman (eds.), Handbook of perception, vol. 6A. New York: Academic Press. Pp. 3–18.

Bartoshuk, L. M. (1980) Separate worlds of taste. Psychology Today, 14, 48–63.

Bartoshuk, L. M., Dateo, G. P., Vandenbelt, D. J., Buttrick, R. L., and **Long, L.** (1969) Effects of Gymnema sylvestra and Synsepalum dulcificum on taste in man. In C. Pfaffmann (ed.), Olfaction and taste, vol. 3. New York: Rockefeller University Press. Pp. 436–444.

Batteau, D. W. (1967) The role of the pinna in human localization. Proceedings of the Royal Society of London, Series B, 168, 158–180.

Bauer, R. M. (1984) Autonomic recognition of names

and faces in prosopagnosia: A neuropsychological application of the Guilty Knowledge Test. Neuropsychologia, 22, 457–469.

Beattie, G. W., Cutler, A., and **Pearson, M.** (1982) Why is Mrs. Thatcher interrupted so often? Nature, 300, 744–747.

Bechtel, W., and **Abrahamsen, A.** (1991) Connectionism and the mind, an introduction to parallel processing in networks. Cambridge: Basil Blackwell.

Beck, J., Prazdny, K., and **Rosenfeld, A.** (1983) A theory of textural segmentation. In J. Beck, B. Hope, and A. Rosenfeld (eds.), Human and machine vision. New York: Academic Press. Pp. 1–38.

Bedichek, R. (1960) The sense of smell. Garden City, N.Y.: Doubleday.

Beidler, L. M. (1978) Biophysics and chemistry of taste. In E. C. Carterette and M. P. Friedman (eds.), Handbook of perception, vol. 6A. New York: Academic Press. Pp. 21–49.

Beidler, L. M., and **Smallman, R. L.** (1965) Renewal of cells within taste buds. Journal of Cell Biology, 27, 263–272.

Bekesy, G. von (1960) Experiments in hearing. New York: McGraw-Hill.

Bekesy, G. von, and **Rosenblith, W. A.** (1951) The mechanical properties of the ear. In S. S. Stevens (ed.), Handbook of experimental psychology. New York: John Wiley & Sons. Pp. 1075–1115.

Belendiuk, K., and **Butler, R. A.** (1978) Directional hearing under progressive impoverishment of binaural cues. Sensory Processes, 2, 58–70.

Benedetti, F. (1985) Processing of tactile spatial information with crossed fingers. Journal of Experimental Psychology: Human Perception and Performance, 11, 517–525.

Benedetti, F. (1986) Tactile diplopia (diplesthesia) on the human fingers. Perception, 15, 83–91.

Benedetti, F. (1991) Reorganization of tactile perception following the simulated amputation of one finger. Perception, 20, 687–692.

Benton, A. L. (1980) The neuropsychology of facial recognition. American Psychologist, 35, 176–186.

Berglund, B., Berglund, U., Engen, T., and **Lindvall, T.** (1971) The effect of adaptation on odor detection. Perception & Psychophysics, 9, 435–438.

Bergman, M. (1966) Hearing in the Mabaans. Archives of Otolaryngology, 81, 75–79.

Berkeley, G. (1709/1950) A new theory of vision. London: Dent.

Berkley, M. A., and **Watkins, D. W.** (1971) Visual acuity of the cat estimated from evoked cerebral potentials. Nature, 234, 91–92.

Berlin, B., and **Kay, P.** (1969) Basic color terms: Their universality and evolution. Berkeley: University of California Press.

Bertenthal, B. I. (1992) Infants' perception of biome-chanical motions: Intrinsic image and knowledge-based constraints. In C. Granrud (ed.), Visual perception and cognition in infancy. Hillsdale, N.J.: Erlbaum. Pp. 175–214.

Bertino, M., and **Chan, M. M.** (1986) Taste perception and diet in individuals with Chinese and European ethnic backgrounds. Chemical Senses, 11, 229–241.

Bexton, W. H., Heron, W., and **Scott, T. H.** (1954) Effects of decreased variation in the sensory environment. Canadian Journal of Psychology, 8, 70–76.

Biederman, I. (1987) Recognition-by-components: A theory of human image understanding. Psychological Review, 94, 115–147.

Biederman, I. (1990) Higher-level vision. In D. N. Osherson, S. Kosslyn, and J. Hollerbach (eds.), An invitation to cognitive science: Visual cognition and action. Cambridge: M.I.T. Press. Pp. 41–72.

Biederman, I., Glass, A. L., and **Stacey, E. W., Jr.** (1973) Searching for objects in real-world scenes. Journal of Experimental Psychology, 97, 22–27.

Biederman, I., Mezzanotte, R. J., Rabinowitz, J. C., Francolini, C. M., and **Plude, D.** (1981) Detecting the unexpected in photointerpretation. Human Factors, 23, 153–164.

Biederman, I., Rabinowitz, J. C., Glass, A. L., and **Stacey, E. W., Jr.** (1974) On the information extracted from a glance at a scene. Journal of Experimental Psychology, 103, 597–600.

Birch, J., Chisholm, I. A., Kinnear, P., Marre, M., Pinckers, A. J. L. G., Pokorny, J., Smith, V., and **Verriest, G.** (1979) Acquired color vision defects. In J. Pokorny, V. Smith, G. Verriest, and A. J. L. G. Pinckers (eds.), Congenital and acquired color vision defects. New York: Grune and Stratton. Pp. 243–348.

Birren, F. (1941) The story of color: From ancient mysticism to modern science. Westport, Conn.: Crimson Press.

Birren, F. (1978) Color and human response. New York: Van Nostrand Reinhold.

Blackwell, H. R. (1946) Contrast thresholds of the human eye. Journal of the Optical Society of America, 36, 624–643.

Blake, R. (1978) Strategies for assessing visual deficits in animals with selective neural deficits. In R. B. Aslin, J. R. Alberts, and M. R. Petersen (eds.), Development and perception. New York: Academic Press. Pp. 95–112.

Blake, R. (1988a) Cat spatial vision. Trends in Neurosciences, 11, 78–83.

Blake, R. (1988b) Dichoptic reading: The role of meaning in binocular rivalry. Perception & Psychophysics, 44, 133–141.

Blake, R. (1993) Cats perceive biological motion. Psychological Science, 4, 54–57.

Blake, R., and **Fox, R.** (1972) Interocular transfer of adaptation to spatial frequency during retinal ischaemia. Nature, 240, 76–77.

Blake, R., and **Hirsch, H. V. B.** (1975) Deficits in binocular depth perception in cats after alternating monocular deprivation. Science, 190, 1114–1116.

Blake, R., Westendorf, D. H., and **Overton, R.** (1980) What is suppressed during binocular rivalry? Perception, 9, 223–232.

Blake, R., and **Wilson, H. R.** (1991) Neural models of stereoscopic vision. Trends in Neurosciences, 14, 445–452.

Blakemore, C. (1976) The conditions required for the maintenance of binocularity in the kitten's visual cortex. Journal of Physiology, 261, 423–444.

Blakemore, C., and **Campbell, F. W.** (1969) On the existence of neurones in the human visual system selectively sensitive to the orientation and size of retinal images. Journal of Physiology, 203, 237–260.

Blakemore, C., Muncey, J. P. J., and **Ridley, R. M.** (1973) Stimulus specificity in the human visual system. Vision Research, 13, 1915–1931.

Blakemore, C., Nachmias, J., and **Sutton, P.** (1970) The perceived spatial frequency shift: Evidence for frequency selective neurones in the human brain. Journal of Physiology, 210, 727–750.

Blignaut, C. J. H. (1979) The perception of hazard: II. The contribution of signal detection to hazard perception. Ergonomics, 22, 1177–1183.

Bliven, B., Jr. (1976) Annals of architecture: A better sound. New Yorker, 52, 51–135.

Bloom, H. S., Criswell, E. L., Pennypacker, H. S., Catania, A. C., and **Adams, C. K.** (1982) Major stimulus dimensions determining detection of simulated breast lesions. Perception & Psychophysics, 32, 251–260.

Bobrow, N. A., Money, J., and **Lewis, V. G.** (1971) Delayed puberty, eroticism, and sense of smell: A psychological study of hypogonadotropism, osmatic and anosmatic (Kallmann's syndrome). Archives of Sexual Behavior, 1, 329–344.

Bodis-Wollner, I. (1972) Visual acuity and contrast sensitivity in patients with cerebral lesions. Science, 178, 769–771.

Boll, F. (1877/1977) On the anatomy and physiology of the retina. Vision Research, 17, 1253–1267.

Bonnano, G. A., and **Stilling, N. A.** (1986) Preference, familiarity, and recognition after repeated brief exposures to random geometric shapes. American Journal of Psychology, 99, 403–415.

Bonnet, C. (1982) Thresholds of motion perception. In A. Wertheim, W. Wagenaar, and H. W. Leibowitz (eds.), Tutorials in motion perception. New York: Plenum Press. Pp. 41–79.

Boorstin, D. J. (1985) The discoverers. New York: Vintage Books.

Borg, E., and **Counter, S. A.** (1989) The middle-ear muscles. Scientific American, 261, 74–80.

Boring, E. G. (1930) A new ambiguous figure. American Journal of Psychology, 42, 444.

Boring, E. G. (1942) Sensation and perception in the history of experimental psychology. New York: Appleton-Century-Crofts.

Boring, E. G. (1961) Fechner: Inadvertent founder of psychophysics. Psychometrika, 26, 3–8.

Bornstein, M. H., Kessen, W., and **Weiskopf, S.** (1976) The categories of hue in infancy. Science, 191, 201–202.

Bough, E. W. (1970) Stereoscopic vision in macaque monkey: A behavioural demonstration. Nature, 225, 42–44.

Bowmaker, J. K. (1983) Trichromatic colour vision: Why only three receptor channels? Trends in Neurosciences, 6, 41–43.

Boyce, P. R. (1981) Human factors and lighting. New York: Macmillan.

Boynton, R. M. (1979) Human color vision. New York: Holt, Rinehart & Winston.

Boynton, R. M. (1982) Spatial and temporal approaches for studying color vision: A review. In G. Verriest (ed.), Colour vision deficiences, VI. Proceedings of the Sixth Symposium of the International Research Group on Colour Vision Deficiences. The Hague: W. Junk. Pp. 1–14.

Boynton, R. M., and **Gordon, J.** (1965) Bezold-Brücke hue shift measured by color naming technique. Journal of the Optical Society of America, 55, 78–86.

Boynton, R. M., and **Olson, C. X.** (1987) Locating basic colors in the OSA space. Color Research and Applications, 12, 94–105.

Bracewell, R. N. (1989) The Fourier transform. Scientific American, 260, 86–95.

Bradley, R. M. (1979) Effects of aging on the sense of taste: Anatomical considerations. In S. S. Han and D. H. Coons (eds.), Special senses in aging: A current biological assessment. Ann Arbor, Mich.: Institute of Gerontology, University of Michigan. Pp. 3–8.

Bradley, R. M. (1991) Salivary secretion. In T. V. Getchell, R. L. Doty, L. M. Bartoshuk, and J. B. Snow (eds.), Smell and taste in health and disease. New York: Raven Press. Pp. 127–144.

Brammer, A. J., and **Verrillo, R. T.** (1988) Tactile changes in hands occupationally exposed to vibration. Journal of the Acoustical Society of America, 84, 1940–1941.

Braunstein, M. L. (1976) Depth perception through motion. New York: Academic Press.

Braunstein, M. L., and **Payne, J. W.** (1969) Perspective and form ratio as determinants of relative slant judgments. Journal of Experimental Psychology, 81, 584–590.

Braunstein, M. L., and **Stern, K. R.** (1980) Static and dynamic factors in the perception of rotary motion. Perception & Psychophysics, 27, 313–320.

Bravo, M., Blake, R., and **Morrison, S.** (1988) Cats see subjective contours. Vision Research, 28, 861–865.

Bregman, A. S. (1990) Auditory scene analysis. Cambridge: M.I.T. Press.

Bregman, A. S., and **Mills, M. I.** (1982) Perceived movement: The Flintstone constraint. Perception, 11, 201–206.

Bregman, A. S., and **Pinker, S.** (1978) Auditory streaming and the building of timbre. Canadian Journal of Psychology, 31, 151–159.

Breitmeyer, B. G. (1975) Simple reaction time as a measure of the temporal response properties of transient and sustained channels. Vision Research, 15, 1411–1412.

Breitmeyer, B. G. (1984) Visual Masking. Oxford, England: Oxford University Press.

Brindley, G. S. (1970) Physiology of the retina and visual pathway. Baltimore: Williams & Wilkins.

Brindley, G. S., and **Lewin, W. S.** (1968) The sensations produced by electrical stimulation of the visual cortex. Journal of Physiology, 196, 479–493.

Broadbent, D. E. (1977) The hidden preattentive process. American Psychologist, 32, 109–118.

Brouwer, J. N., Glaser, D., Segerstad, C. H. A., Hellekant, G., Ninomiya, Y., and **van der Wel, H.** (1983) The sweetness-inducing effect of miraculin: Behavioral and neurophysiological experiments in the rhesus monkey, Macaca mulatta. Journal of Physiology, 337, 221–240.

Brown, J. F. (1931) The visual perception of velocity. Psychologische Forschung, 14, 199–232.

Brown, J. L, and **Mueller, C. G.** (1965) Brightness discrimination and brightness contrast. In C. H. Graham (ed.), Vision and visual perception. New York: John Wiley & Sons. Pp. 208–250.

Brown, J. M., and **Weisstein, N.** (1988) A spatial frequency effect on perceived depth. Perception & Psychophysics, 44, 157–166.

Bruner, J. S., and **Potter, M. C.** (1964) Interference in visual recognition. Science, 144, 424–425.

Bruno, N., and **Cutting, J. E.** (1988) Minimodularity and the perception of layout. Journal of Experimental Psychology: General, 117, 161–170.

Buchsbaum, G., and **Gottschalk, A.** (1983) Trichromacy, opponent colours coding, and the optimum colour information in the retina. Proceedings of the Royal Society of London, Series B, 220, 89–113.

Buck, L. B. (1992) The olfactory multigene family. Current Opinion in Neurobiology, 2, 282–288.

Burger, J. F. (1958) Front-back discrimination of the hearing system. Acustica, 8, 302–310.

Burke, W., and **Cole, A. M.** (1978) Extra-retinal influences on the lateral geniculate nucleus. Review of

Physiology, Biochemistry, and Pharmacology, 80, 105–166.

Burr, D. C., and **Ross, J.** (1982) Contrast sensitivity at high velocities. Vision Research, 22, 479–484.

Butler, R. A. (1986) The bandwidth effect on monaural and binaural localization. Hearing Research, 21, 67–73.

Butler, R. A., Humanski, R. A., and **Musicant, A. D.** (1990) Binaural and monaural localization of sound in two-dimensional space. Perception, 19, 241–256.

Butterworth, G., and **Castillo, M.** (1976) Coordination of auditory and visual space in newborn infants. Perception, 5, 155–160.

Cain, W. S. (1977) Differential sensitivity for smell: Noise at the nose. Science, 195, 796–798.

Cain, W. S. (1978) The odoriferous environment and the application of olfactory research. In E. C. Carterette and M. P. Friedman (eds.), Handbook of perception, vol. 7. New York: Academic Press. Pp. 277–304.

Cain, W. S. (1982) Odor identification by males and females: Predictions versus performance. Chemical Senses, 7, 129–142.

Cain, W. S., and **Engen, T.** (1969) Olfactory adaptation and the scaling of odor intensity. In C. Pfaffmann (ed.), Olfaction and taste, vol. 3. New York: Rockefeller University Press. Pp. 127–157.

Cain, W. S., and **Gent, J. F.** (1991) Olfactory sensitivity: Reliability, generality, and association with aging. Journal of Experimental Psychology: Human Perception and Performance, 17, 382–391.

Cain, W. S., and **Murphy, C. L.** (1980) Interaction between chemoreceptive modalities of odour irritation. Nature, 284, 255–257.

Cain, W. S., and **Turk, A.** (1985) Smell of danger: An analysis of LP-gas odorization. American Industrial Hygiene Association Journal, 46, 115–126.

Calis, G., and **Leeuwenberg, E.** (1981) Grounding the figure. Journal of Experimental Psychology: Human Perception and Performance, 7, 1386–1397.

Campbell, D. T. (1974) Evolutionary epistemology. In P. A. Schlipp (ed.), The philosophy of Karl Popper. LaSalle, Ill.: Open Court. Pp. 413–463.

Campbell, F. W., and **Kulikowski, J. J.** (1972) The visual evoked potential as a function of contrast of a grating pattern. Journal of Physiology, 222, 345–356.

Campbell, F. W., and **Maffei, L.** (1981) The influence of spatial frequency and contrast on the perception of moving patterns. Vision Research, 21, 713–721.

Campbell, F. W., and **Robson, J. G.** (1968) Application of Fourier analysis to the visibility of gratings. Journal of Physiology, 197, 551–566.

Campion, J., Latto, R., and **Smith, Y. M.** (1983) Is blindsight an effect of scattered light, spared cortex, and near-threshold vision? Behavioral and Brain Sciences, 6, 423–486.

Carey, S., and **Diamond, R.** (1977) From piecemeal to configurational representation of faces. Science, 195, 312–314.

Carlson, M., and **Burton, H.** (1988) Recovery of tactile function after damage to primary or secondary somatic sensory cortex in infant Macaca mulatta. Journal of Neuroscience, 8, 833–859.

Carlsson, L., Knave, B., Lennerstrand, G., and **Wibom, R.** (1984) Glare from outdoor high mast lighting: Effects on visual acuity and contrast sensitivity in comparative studies of different floodlighting systems. Acta Ophthalmologica, 62, 84–93.

Carmody, D. P., Kundel, H. L., and **Toto, L. C.** (1984) Comparison scans while reading chest images: Taught, but not practiced. Investigative Radiology, 19, 462–466.

Carmody, D. P., Nodine, C. F., and **Kundel, H. L.** (1980) An analysis of perceptual and cognitive factors in radiographic interpretation. Perception, 9, 339–344.

Carpenter, P. A., and **Daneman, M.** (1981) Lexical access and error recovery in reading: A model based on eye fixations. Journal of Verbal Learning and Verbal Behavior, 20, 137–160.

Carpenter, R. H. S. (1992) Turning vision into action. Current Biology, 2, 288–290.

Carr, C. E., and **Konishi, M.** (1988) Axonal delay lines for time measurement in the owl's brainstem. Proceedings of the National Academy of Science, 85, 8311–8315.

Carter, J. H. (1982) The effects of aging upon selected visual functions: Color vision, field of vision, and accommodation. In R. Sekuler, D. Kline, and K. Dismukes (eds.), Aging and human visual function. New York: Liss. Pp. 120–130.

Cattell, J. M. (1886) The inertia of the eye and brain. Brain, 8, 295–312.

Chambers, D., and **Reisberg, D.** (1992) What an image depicts depends on what an image means. Cognitive Psychology, 24, 145–174.

Chapman, C. R., Chen, A. C., and **Bonica, J. J.** (1977) Effects of intrasegmental electrical acupuncture on dental pain: Evaluation by threshold estimation and sensory decision theory. Pain, 3, 213–227.

Chapman, S. (1968) Catching a baseball. American Journal of Physics, 36, 868–870.

Chevreul, M. (1839/1967) The principles of harmony and contrast of colors. F. Birren (ed.). New York: Reinhold.

Churchland, P. M. (1986) Matter and consciousness: A contemporary introduction to the philosophy of mind (revised edition). Cambridge: M.I.T. Press.

Cicerone, C. M., and **Nerger, J. L.** (1989) The relative number of long-wavelength-sensitive to middle-wavelength-sensitive cones in the human fovea centralis. Vision Research, 29, 115–128.

Clark, W. C., and **Yang, J. C.** (1974) Acupunctural analgesia? Evaluation by signal detection theory. Science, 184, 1096–1098.

Claus, R., Hoppen, H. O., and **Karg, H.** (1981) The secret of truffles: A steroidal pheromone? Experientia, 37, 1178–1179.

Cohen, J. (1969) Sensation and perception: II. Audition and the minor senses. Chicago: Rand McNally.

Cohn, T. E., and **Lasley, D. L.** (1974) Detectability of a luminance increment: Effect of spatial uncertainty. Journal of the Optical Society of America, 64, 1715–1719.

Coles, R. R. A., and **Hallam, R. S.** (1987) Tinnitus and its management. British Medical Bulletin, 43, 983–998.

Collewijn, H., Martins, A. J., and **Steinman, R. M.** (1983) Compensatory eye movements during active and passive head movements: Fast adaptation to changes in visual magnification. Journal of Physiology, 340, 259–286.

Collings, V. B. (1974) Human taste response as a function of locus on the tongue and soft palate. Perception & Psychophysics, 16, 169–174.

Collins, B. L., and **Worthey, J. A.** (1984) The role of color in lighting for meat and poultry inspection. U.S. Department of Commerce, National Bureau of Standards Report No. 84-2829. Washington, D.C.

Cometto-Muniz, J. E., and **Cain, W. S.** (1982) Perception of nasal pungency in smokers and nonsmokers. Physiology & Behavior, 29, 727–731.

Cometto-Muniz, J. E., and **Cain, W. S.** (1984) Temporal integration of pungency. Chemical Senses, 8, 315–327.

Corbetta, M., Miezin, R. M., Dobmeyer, S., Shulman, G. L., and **Petersen, S. E.** (1991) Selective and divided attention during visual discriminations of shape, color, and speed: Functional anatomy by positron emission tomography. Journal of Neuroscience, 11, 2382–2402.

Corbin, A. (1986) The foul and the fragrant: Odor and the French social imagination. Cambridge: Harvard University Press.

Corcoran, D. W. J., and **Rouse, R. O.** (1970) An aspect of perceptual organization involved in reading typed and handwritten words. Quarterly Journal of Experimental Psychology, 22, 526–530.

Coren, S., and **Girgus, J. S.** (1978) Visual illusions. In R. Held, H. W. Leibowitz, and H.-L. Teuber (eds.), Handbook of sensory physiology, vol. 8. Berlin: Springer-Verlag. Pp. 551–568.

Corina, D. P., Vaid, J., and **Bellugi, U.** (1992) The linguistic basis of left hemisphere specialization. Science, 255, 1258–1260.

Cornsweet, T. N. (1962) The staircase-method in psychophysics. American Journal of Psychology, 75, 485–491.

Cornsweet, T. N. (1970) Visual perception. New York: Academic Press.

Corso, J. F. (1981) Aging sensory systems and perception. New York: Praeger.

Cowart, B. J. (1981) Development of taste perception in humans: Sensitivity and preference throughout the life span. Psychological Bulletin, 90, 43–73.

Cowey, A., and **Stoerig, P.** (1991) The neurobiology of blindsight. Trends in Neurosciences, 14, 140–145.

Craig, J. C. (1985) Attending to two fingers: Two hands are better than one. Perception & Psychophysics, 38, 496–511.

Craver-Lemley, C., and **Reeves, A.** (1992) How visual imagery interferes with vision. Psychological Review, 99, 633–649.

Critchley, M. (1979) The divine banquet of the brain and other essays. New York: Raven Press.

Crocker, E. C., and **Henderson, L. F.** (1927) Analysis and classification of odors. American Perfumer and Essential Oil Review, 22, 325–327.

Crowe, S. J., Guild, S. R., and **Polvost, L. M.** (1934) Observations on the pathology of high-tone deafness. Bulletin of the Johns Hopkins Hospital, 54, 315–379.

Cutting, J. E. (1978) Generation of synthetic male and female walkers through manipulation of a biomechanical invariant. Perception, 7, 393–405.

Cutting, J. E. (1986) Perception with an eye to motion. Cambridge: M.I.T. Press.

Cutting, J. E., and **Proffitt, D. R.** (1981) Gait perception as an example of how we may perceive events. In R. Walk and H. L. Pick (eds.), Intersensory perception and sensory integration. New York: Plenum Press. Pp. 249–273.

Dabak, A. G., and **Johnson, D. H.** (1992) Function-based modeling of binaural processing: Interaural phase. Hearing Research, 58, 200–212.

Dallos, P. (1981) Cochlear physiology. Annual Review of Psychology, 32, 153–190.

Dallos, P. (1984) Peripheral mechanisms of hearing. In I. Darian-Smith (ed.), Handbook of physiology, vol. 3, part 2. Bethesda, Md.: American Physiological Society. Pp. 595–637.

Dallos, P. (1985) The role of outer hair cells in cochlear function. In M. J. Correia and A. A. Perachi (eds.), Contemporary sensory neurobiology. New York: Liss. Pp. 207–230.

Dallos, P. (1988) Cochlear neurobiology: Revolutionary developments. ASHA, 30, 50–56.

Dallos, P. (1992) The active cochlea. Journal of Neuroscience, 12, 4575–4585.

Dallos, P., and **Cheatham, M. A.** (1976) Production of cochlear potentials by inner and outer hair cells. Journal of the Acoustical Society of America, 60, 510–512.

Dalton, J. (1798/1948) Extraordinary facts relating to the vision of colour: With observations. In W. Dennis (ed.), Readings in the history of psychology. New York: Appleton-Century-Crofts. Pp. 102–111.

Damasio, A. R. (1985) Prosopagnosia. Trends in Neurosciences, 8, 132–135.

Damasio, A. R. (1989) Time-locked multiregional retroactivation: A systems-level proposal for the neural substrates of recall and recognition. Cognition, 33, 25–62.

Damasio, A. R., and **Benton, A. L.** (1979) Impairment of hand movements under visual guidance. Neurology, 29, 170–178.

Damasio, A. R., Damasio, H., and **van Hoesen, G. W.** (1982) Prosopagnosia: Anatomic basis and behavioral mechanisms. Neurology, 32, 331–341.

Damasio, A. R., Tranel, D., and **Damasio, H.** (1990) Face agnosia and the neural substrates of memory. Annual Review of Neuroscience, 13, 89–109.

Daniel, P. M., and **Whitteridge, D.** (1961) The representation of the visual field on the cerebral cortex in monkeys. Journal of Physiology, 159, 203–221.

Dannemiller, J. L. (1989) Computational approaches to color constancy: Adaptive and ontogenetic considerations. Psychological Review, 96, 255–266.

Dannenbaum, R. M., and **Dykes, R. W.** (1988) Sensory loss in the hand after sensory stroke: Therapeutic rationale. Archives of Physical Medicine and Rehabilitation, 69, 833–839.

Dannenbring, G. L. (1976) Perceived auditory continuity with alternately rising and falling frequency transitions. Canadian Journal of Psychology, 30, 99–114.

Darian-Smith, I. (1984) The sense of touch: Performance and peripheral neural processes. In I. Darian-Smith (ed.), Handbook of physiology, vol. 3, part 2. Bethesda, Md.: American Physiological Society. Pp. 739–788.

Darian-Smith, I., Goodwin, A., Sugitani, M., and **Heywood, J.** (1984) The tangible features of textured surfaces: Their representation in the monkey's somatosensory cortex. In G. Edelman, W. E. Gall, and M. W. Cowan (eds.), Dynamic aspects of neocortical function. New York: John Wiley & Sons. Pp. 475–500.

Dartnall, H. J. A., Bowmaker, J. K., and **Mollon, J. D.** (1983) Human visual pigments: Microspectrophotometric results from the eyes of seven persons. Proceedings of the Royal Society of London, Series B, 220, 115–130.

Daum, K. M. (1983) Accommodative dysfunction. Documenta Ophthalmologica, 55, 177–198.

Davidoff, J. B. (1975) Differences in visual perception: The individual eye. New York: Academic Press.

Davis, H., Deatherage, B. H., Rosenblut, B., Fernandez, C., Kimura, R., and **Smith, C. A.** (1958)

Modification of cochlear potentials produced by streptomycin poisoning and by extensive venous obstructions. Laryngoscope, 68, 596–627.

Davis, H., and **Silverman, S. R.** (1960) Hearing and deafness. New York: Holt, Rinehart & Winston.

Davis, L. B., and **Porter, R. H.** (1991) Persistent effects of early odor exposure on human neonates. Chemical Senses, 16, 169–174.

Davis, R. G. (1977) Acquisition of verbal associations to olfactory and abstract visual stimuli of varying similarity. Journal of Experimental Psychology: Human Learning and Memory, 3, 37–51.

Davis, R. G. (1981) The role of nonolfactory context cues in odor identification. Perception & Psychophysics, 30, 83–89.

de Boer, I. (1956) Pitch of inharmonic signals. Nature, 178, 535–536.

de Monasterio, F. M., and **Gouras, P.** (1975) Functional properties of ganglion cells of the rhesus monkey retina. Journal of Physiology, 251, 167–195.

DeCasper, A. J., and **Fifer, W. P.** (1980) Of human bonding: Newborns prefer their mothers' voices. Science, 208, 174–176.

Dennett, D. C. (1991) Consciousness explained. Boston: Little, Brown.

Denton, G. G. (1980) The influence of visual pattern on perceived speed. Perception, 9, 393–402.

Derby, C. D., Ache, B. W., and **Kennel, E. W.** (1985) Mixture suppression: Electrophysiological evaluation of the contribution of peripheral and central neural components. Chemical Senses, 10, 301–316.

Desimone, R. (1991) Face-selective cells in the temporal cortex of monkeys. Journal of Cognitive Neuroscience, 3, 1–8.

Desor, J. A., and **Beauchamp, G. K.** (1974) The human capacity to transmit olfactory information. Perception & Psychophysics, 16, 551–556.

Detwiler, P. B., Hodgkin, A. L., and **McNaughton, P. A.** (1980) Temporal and spatial characteristics of the voltage response of rods in the retina of the turtle. Journal of Physiology, 300, 213–250.

DeValois, R. L., and **DeValois, K. K.** (1975) Neural coding of color. In E. C. Carterette and M. P. Friedman (eds.), Handbook of perception, vol. 5. New York: Academic Press. Pp. 117–166.

DeValois, R. L., and **DeValois, K. K.** (1988) Spatial vision. New York: Oxford University Press.

DeValois, R. L., Smith, C. J., Kitai, S. T., and **Karoly, A. J.** (1958) Responses of single cells in different layers of the primate lateral geniculate nucleus to monochromatic light. Science, 127, 238–239.

DeYoe, E. A., and **van Essen, D. C.** (1988) Concurrent processing streams in monkey visual cortex. Trends in Neurosciences, 11, 219–226.

Dewson, J., Pribram, K., and **Lynch, J.** (1969) Effects of ablations of temporal cortex upon speech sound discrimination in the monkey. Experimental Neurology, 24, 579–591.

Di Lorenzo, P. M. (1989) Across unit patterns in the neural response to taste: Vector space analysis. Journal of Neurophysiology, 62, 823–833.

Dichgans, J., and **Brandt, T.** (1978) Visual-vestibular interaction: Effects on self-motion perception and postural control. In R. M. Held, H. W. Leibowitz, and H.-L. Teuber (eds.), Handbook of sensory physiology, vol. 8. Berlin: Springer-Verlag. Pp. 756–804.

Doane, M. G. (1980) Interaction of eyelids and tears in corneal wetting and the dynamics of the normal human eyeblink. American Journal of Ophthalmology, 89, 507–516.

Dobelle, W. H., and **Mladejovsky, M. G.** (1974) Phosphenes produced by electrical stimulation of human occipital cortex, and their application to the development of a prosthesis for the blind. Journal of Physiology, 243, 553–576.

Dobelle, W. H., Mladejovsky, M. G., Evans, J. R., Roberts, T. S., and **Girvin, J. P.** (1976) "Braille" reading by a blind volunteer by visual cortex stimulation. Nature, 259, 111–112.

Dodd, B. (1977) The role of vision in the perception of speech. Perception, 6, 31–40.

Dodge, R. (1900) The illusion of clear vision during eye movement. Psychological Bulletin, 2, 193–199.

Dosher, B. A., Sperling, G., and **Wurst, S. A.** (1986) Tradeoffs between stereopsis and proximity luminance covariance. Vision Research, 26, 973–990.

Doty, R. L. (1986) Odor-guided behavior in mammals. Experientia, 42, 257–271.

Doty, R. L., Green, P. A., Ram, C., and **Yankell, S. L.** (1982) Communication of gender from human breath odors: Relationship to perceived intensity and pleasantness. Hormones and Behavior, 16, 13–22.

Doty, R. L., Shaman, P., Applebaum, S. L., Giberson, R., Siksorski, L., and **Rosenberg, L.** (1984) Smell identification ability: Changes with age. Science, 226, 1441–1443.

Douek, E. (1974) The sense of smell and its abnormalities. Edinburgh: Churchill Livingstone.

Dowling, J. E. (1966) Night blindness. Scientific American, 215, 78–84.

Dowling, J. E. (1987) The retina: An approachable part of the brain. Cambridge: Harvard University Press.

Dowling, W. J. (1978) Scale and contour: Two components of a theory of memory for melodies. Psychological Review, 85, 341–354.

Dowling, W. J., and **Fujitani, D. S.** (1971) Contour, interval, and pitch recognition in memory for melodies. Journal of the Acoustical Society of America, 49, 524–531.

Drasdo, N. (1977) The neural representation of visual space. Nature, 266, 554–556.

Dreher, B., Fukada, Y., and **Rodieck, R. W.** (1976)

Identification, classification, and anatomical segregation of cells with X-like and Y-like properties in the lateral geniculate nucleus of old-world primates. Journal of Physiology, 29, 433–452.

Drewnowski, A., Bellisle, F., Aimez, P., and **Remy, B.** (1987) Taste and bulimia. Physiology & Behavior, 41, 621–626.

Drewnowski, A., Grinker, J. A., and **Hirsch, J.** (1982) Obesity and flavor perception: Multidimensional scaling of soft drinks. Appetite: Journal of Intake Research, 3, 361–368.

DuBose, C. N., Cardello, A., and **Maller, O.** (1980) Effects of colorants and flavorants on identification, perceived flavor intensity, and hedonic quality of fruit-flavored beverages and cake. Journal of Food Science, 45, 1393–1399, 1415.

Duchamp-Viret, P., Duchamp, A., and **Vigouroux, M.** (1989) Amplifying role of convergence in olfactory system. A comparative study of receptor cell and second-order neuron sensitivities. Journal of Neurophysiology, 61, 1085–1094.

Duhamel, J.-R., Colby, C. L., and **Goldberg, M. E.** (1992) The updating of the representation of visual space in parietal cortex by intended eye movements. Science, 255, 90–92.

Duncker, K. (1929/1938) Induced motion. In W. D. Ellis (ed.), A source book of Gestalt psychology. New York: Humanities Press. Pp. 161–172.

Duncker, K. (1939) The influence of past experience upon perceptual properties. American Journal of Psychology, 52, 255–267.

Durlach, I., and **Colburn, H. S.** (1978) Binaural phenomena. In E. C. Carterette and M. P. Friedman (eds.), Handbook of perception, vol. 4. New York: Academic Press. Pp. 365–466.

Eccles, J. (1979) The human mystery. Berlin: Springer-Verlag.

Edwards, P. A., and **Jurs, P. C.** (1989) Correlation of odor intensities with structural properties of odorants. Chemical Senses, 14, 281–291.

Eimas, P. D., and **Corbit, J. D.** (1973) Selective adaptation of linguistic feature detectors. Cognitive Psychology, 4, 99–109.

Emmerich, D. S., and **Levine, F. M.** (1970) Differences in auditory sensitivity of chronic schizophrenic patients and normal controls determined by use of a forced-choice procedure. Diseases of the Nervous System, 31, 552–557.

Engen, T. (1960) Effects of practice and instruction on olfactory thresholds. Perceptual and Motor Skills, 10, 195–198.

Engen, T. (1982) The perception of odors. New York: Academic Press.

Engen, T. (1987) Remembering odors and their names. American Scientist, 75, 497–503.

Enright, J. T. (1989) Manipulating stereopsis and vergence in an outdoor setting: Moon, sky and horizon. Vision Research, 29, 1815–1824.

Enroth-Cugell, C., Hertz, B. G., and **Lennie, P.** (1977) Convergence of rod and cone signals in the cat's retina. Journal of Physiology, 269, 297–318.

Epstein, W. (1963) The influences of assumed size on apparent distance. American Journal of Physiology, 76, 257–265.

Erickson, R. P. (1963) Sensory neural patterns and gustation. In Y. Zotterman (ed.), Olfaction and taste. Oxford, England: Pergamon Press. Pp. 205–214.

Erickson, R. P. (1968) Stimulus coding in topographic and nontopographic afferent modalities: On the significance of the activity of individual sensory neurons. Psychological Review, 75, 447–465.

Erickson, R. P. (1982) Studies on the perception of taste: Do primaries exist? Physiology & Behavior, 28, 57–62.

Erickson, R. P. (1984) On the neural bases of behavior. American Scientist, 72, 233–241.

Eriksson-Mangold, M. M., and **Erlandsson, S. I.** (1984) The psychological importance of nonverbal sounds. Scandinavian Audiology, 13, 243–249.

Evans, E. F. (1974) Neural processes for the detection of acoustic patterns and for sound localization. In F. C. Schmitt and F. G. Worden (eds.), The neurosciences: Third study program. Cambridge: M.I.T. Press. Pp. 131–145.

Evans, E. F. (1982a) Functional anatomy of the auditory system. In H. B. Barlow and J. D. Mollon (eds.), The senses. Cambridge, England: Cambridge University Press. Pp. 251–306.

Evans, E. F. (1982b) Functions of the auditory system. In H. B. Barlow and J. D. Mollon (eds.), The senses. Cambridge, England: Cambridge University Press. Pp. 307–331.

Exner, S. (1888) Über optische Bewegungsempfindungen. Biologisches Centralblatt, 8, 437–448.

Fantz, R. L. (1961) The origin of form perception. Scientific American, 204, 66–72.

Farah, M. J. (1992) Agnosia. Current Opinion in Neurobiology, 2, 162–164.

Farah, M. J., Peronnet, R., Gonon, M. A., and **Giard, M. H.** (1988) Electrophysiological evidence for a shared representational medium for visual images and visual percepts. Journal of Experimental Psychology: General, 117, 248–257.

Fay, R. R. (1988) Comparative psychoacoustics. Hearing Research, 34, 295–306.

Fechner, G. T. (1860/1966) Elements of psychophysics. D. H. Howes and E. G. Boring (eds.), H. E. Adler (trans.). New York: Holt, Rinehart & Winston.

Federal Railroad Administration. (1992) Rail-highway crossing accident/incident inventory bulletin, calendar year 1991. Washington, D.C.: U.S. Department of Transportation.

Felleman, D. J., and **Van Essen, D. C.** (1991) Distributed hierarchical processing in the primate cerebral cortex. Cerebral Cortex, 1, 1–47.

Ferster, D. (1981) A comparison of binocular depth mechanisms in areas 17 and 18 of the cat visual cortex. Journal of Physiology, 311, 623–655.

Field, D. J. (1987) Relations between the statistics of natural images and the response properties of cortical cells. Journal of the Optical Society of America A, 4, 2379–2394.

Finke, R. (1985) Theories relating mental imagery to perception. Psychological Bulletin, 98, 236–259.

Finlay, D. (1982) Motion perception in the peripheral visual field. Perception, 11, 457–462.

Fischer, R., Griffin, F., England, S., and **Carn, S. M.** (1961) Taste thresholds and food dislikes. Nature, 191, 1328.

Fletcher, H. (1940) Auditory patterns. Review of Modern Physics, 12, 47–65.

Fletcher, H. F., and **Munson, W. A.** (1933) Loudness, its definition, measurement, and calculation. Journal of the Acoustical Society of America, 5, 82–108.

Fletcher, S. W., O'Malley, M. S., and **Bunce, L. A.** (1985) Physicians' abilities to detect lumps in silicone breast models. Journal of the American Medical Association, 253, 2224–2228.

Foley, J. M. (1980) Binocular distance perception. Psychological Review, 87, 411–434.

Foster, D. H., Thorson, J., McIlwain, J. T., and **Biederman-Thorson, M.** (1981) The fine-grain movement illusion: A perceptual probe of neuronal connectivity in the human visual system. Vision Research, 21, 1123–1128.

Fox, R. (1978) Visual masking. In R. Held, H. W. Leibowitz, and H.-L. Teuber (eds.), Handbook of sensory physiology, vol. 8. Berlin: Springer-Verlag. Pp. 629–653.

Fox, R., Aslin, R. N., Shea, S. L., and **Dumais, S. T.** (1980) Stereopsis in human infants. Science, 207, 323–324.

Fox, R., and **Check, R.** (1968) Detection of motion during binocular suppression. Journal of Experimental Psychology, 78, 388–395.

Fox, R., Lehmkuhle, S. W., and **Bush, R. C.** (1977) Stereopsis in the falcon. Science, 197, 79–81.

Fox, R., and **McDaniel, C.** (1982) The perception of biological motion by human infants. Science, 218, 486–487.

Frank, M. (1973) An analysis of hamster afferent taste nerve response functions. Journal of General Physiology, 61, 588–618.

Freeman, R. D., and **Pettigrew, J. D.** (1973) Alteration of visual cortex from environmental asymmetries. Nature, 246, 359–360.

Freeman, W. J. (1991) The physiology of perception. Scientific American, 264, 78–85.

Freud, S. (1910/1938) The psychopathology of everyday life. In A. A. Brill (ed. and trans.), The basic writings of Sigmund Freud. New York: Modern Library. Pp. 35–178.

Freud, S. (1930/1961) Civilization and its discontents. New York: W. W. Norton.

Freytag, E., and **Sachs, J. S.** (1968) Abnormalities of the central visual pathways contributing to traffic accidents. Journal of the American Medical Association, 204, 871–873.

Frisby, J. P. (1980) Seeing. Oxford, England: Oxford University Press.

Frisby, J. P., and **Clatworthy, J. L.** (1975) Learning to see complex random-dot stereograms. Perception, 4, 173–178.

Frisby, J. P., and **Mayhew, J. E. W.** (1976) Rivalrous texture stereograms. Nature, 264, 53–56.

Fry, G. A., Bridgman, C. S., and **Ellerbrock, V. J.** (1949) The effect of atmospheric scattering on binocular depth perception. American Journal of Optometry, 26, 9–15.

Frye, R. E., Doty, R. L., and **Schwartz, B.** (1989) Influence of cigarette smoking on olfaction: Evidence for a dose-response relationship. Journal of the American Medical Association, 263, 1233–1236.

Fuchs, A., and **Binder, M. D.** (1983) Fatigue resistance of human extraocular muscles. Journal of Neurophysiology, 49, 28–34.

Fullard, J. H., and **Barclay, R. M. R.** (1980) Audition in spring species of arctiid moths as a possible response to differential levels of insectivorous bat predation. Canadian Journal of Zoology, 58, 1745–1750.

Furchtgott, E., and **Friedman, M. P.** (1960) The effect of hunger and taste on odor RLs. Journal of Comparative and Physiological Psychology, 53, 576–581.

Gamble, E. A. M. C. (1921) Review of Der Geruch by Hans Henning. American Journal of Psychology, 32, 290–295.

Garb, J., and **Stunkard, A. J.** (1974) Taste aversions in man. American Journal of Psychiatry, 131, 1204–1207.

Garcia, J., and **Koelling, R. A.** (1966) Relation of cue to consequences in avoidance learning. Psychonomic Science, 4, 123–124.

Garcia-Medina, M. R., and **Cain, W. S.** (1982) Bilateral integration in the common chemical sense. Physiology & Behavior, 29, 349–353.

Gardner, R. J. M., and **Sutherland, G. R.** (1989) Chromosome abnormalities and genetic counseling. Oxford: Oxford University Press.

Garfield, E. (1983) The tyranny of the horn—Automobile, that is. Current Contents, 26, 5–11.

Garner, W. R. (1962) Uncertainty and structure as psychological concepts. New York: John Wiley & Sons.

Geisler, W. S. (1989) Sequential ideal-observer analysis of visual discriminations. Psychological Review, 96, 267–314.

Gelb, A. (1929) Die Farbenkonstanz der Sehdinge. In A. Bethe et al. (eds.), Handbuch der normalen und pathologischen physiologie, vol. 12. Berlin: Springer-Verlag. Pp. 594–678.

Geldard, F. A. (1972) The human senses. New York: John Wiley & Sons.

Geldard, F. A., and **Sherrick, C. E.** (1986) Space, time and touch. Scientific American, 255, 90–95.

Gescheider, G. A. (1976) Psychophysics: Method and theory. Hillsdale, N.J.: Erlbaum.

Gescheider, G. A., Sklar, B. F., Van Doren, C. L., and **Verrillo, R. T.** (1985) Vibrotactile forward masking: Psychophysical evidence for a triplex theory of cutaneous mechanoreception. Journal of Acoustical Society of America, 78, 534–543.

Gesteland, R. C. (1978) The neural code: Integrative neural mechanisms. In E. C. Carterette and M. P. Friedman (eds.), Handbook of perception, vol. 6A. New York: Academic Press. Pp. 259–276.

Gesteland, R. C. (1986) Speculations on receptor cells as analyzers and filters. Experientia, 42, 287–291.

Getchell, T. V., Doty, R. L., Bartoshuk, L. M., and **Snow, J. B. (eds.).** (1991) Smell and taste in health and disease. New York: Raven Press.

Geyer, L. H., and **DeWald, C. G.** (1973) Feature lists and confusion matrices. Perception & Psychophysics, 14, 471–482.

Gibson, E. J. (1965) Learning to read. Science, 148, 1066–1072.

Gibson, E. J. (1969) Principles of perceptual learning. New York: Appleton-Century-Crofts.

Gibson, J. J. (1947) Motion picture testing and research. AAF Aviation Psychology Report No. 7. Washington, D.C.: U.S. Army Air Force.

Gibson, J. J. (1950) The perception of the visual world. Boston: Houghton-Mifflin.

Gibson, J. J. (1966) The senses considered as perceptual systems. Boston: Houghton-Mifflin.

Gibson, J. J. (1979) The ecological approach to visual perception. Boston: Houghton-Mifflin.

Gilchrist, A. L. (1977) Perceived lightness depends on perceived spatial arrangement. Science, 195, 185–187.

Gilchrist, A. L. (1988) Lightness contrast and failures of constancy: A common explanation. Perception & Psychophysics, 43, 415–424.

Gilden, D. L., Blake, R., and **Hurst, J.** (1992) Imagined motion is influenced by adaptation. Thirty-third annual meeting of the Psychonomic Society, St. Louis.

Gilinsky, A. S. (1955) The effect of attitude upon the perception of size. American Journal of Psychology, 68, 173–192.

Gillan, D. J. (1982) Mixture suppression: The effect of spatial separation between sucrose and NaCl. Perception & Psychophysics, 32, 504–510.

Gillan, D. J. (1984) Evidence for peripheral and central

processes in taste adaptation. Perception & Psychophysics, 35, 1–4.

Ginsberg, M. D., Yoshii, F., Vibulsresth, S., Chang, J. Y., Durara, R., Barker, W. W., and **Boothe, T. E.** (1987) Human task-specific somatosensory activation. Neurology, 37, 1301–1308.

Ginsburg, A. P., Evans, D. W., Sekuler, R., and **Harp, S. A.** (1982) Contrast sensitivity predicts pilots' performance in aircraft simulators. American Journal of Optometry and Physiological Optics, 59, 105–108.

Gittleman, J. L., and **Harvey, P. H.** (1980) Why are distasteful prey not cryptic? Nature, 286, 149–150.

Glanville, E. V., and **Kaplan, A. R.** (1965) Food preference and sensitivity of taste for bitter compounds. Nature, 205, 851–853.

Glickstein, M. (1988) The discovery of the visual cortex. Scientific American, 259, 118–127.

Glista, G. G., Frank, H. G., and **Tracey, F. W.** (1983) Video games and seizures. Archives of Neurology, 40, 588.

Goethe, J. W. von. (1840/1970) Theory of colours. C. L. Eastlake (trans.). Cambridge: M.I.T. Press.

Gogel, W. C., and **Mershon, D. H.** (1969) Depth adjacency in simultaneous contrast. Perception & Psychophysics, 12, 13–17.

Goldberg, M. E., and **Wurtz, R. H.** (1972) Activity of superior colliculus in behaving monkey: I. Visual receptive fields of single neurons. Journal of Neurophysiology, 35, 542–559.

Goldman, A. I. (1976) Discrimination and perceptual knowledge. Journal of Philosophy, 73, 771–791.

Goodale, M. A., and **Milner, A. D.** (1992) Separate visual pathways for perception and action. Trends in Neurosciences, 15, 20–25.

Goodale, M. A., Pelisson, D., and **Prablanc, C.** (1986) Large adjustments in visually guided reaching do not depend on vision of the hand or perception of target displacement. Nature, 320, 748–750.

Gordon, B. (1972) The superior colliculus of the brain. Scientific American, 227, 72–82.

Gouk, P. (1988) The harmonic roots of Newtonian science. In J. Fauvel, R. Flood, M. Shortland, and R. Wilson (eds.), Let Newton be! A new perspective on his life and works. Oxford, England: Oxford University Press. Pp. 100–125.

Gouras, P., and **Zrenner, E.** (1981) Color coding in the primate retina. Vision Research, 21, 1591–1598.

Graham, C. A., and **McGrew, W. C.** (1980) Menstrual synchrony in female undergraduates living on a co-educational campus. Psychoneuroendocrinology, 5, 253–259.

Graham, C. H. (1965) Visual space perception. In C. H. Graham (ed.), Vision and visual perception. New York: John Wiley & Sons. Pp. 504–547.

Grant, V. W. (1942) Accommodation and convergence

in visual space perception. Journal of Experimental Psychology, 31, 89–104.

Graziadei, P. P. C. (1973) Cell dynamics in the olfactory mucosa. Tissue and Cell, 5, 113–131.

Green, D. M. (1982) Profile analysis: A different view of auditory intensity discrimination. American Psychologist, 38, 133–142.

Green, D. M., Kidd, G., Jr., and **Picardi, M. C.** (1983) Successive versus simultaneous comparison in auditory discrimination. Journal of the Acoustical Society of America, 73, 639–643.

Green, D. M., and **Nguyen, Q. T.** (1988) Profile analysis. Detecting dynamic spectral changes. Hearing Research, 32, 147–164.

Green, D. M., and **Swets, J. A.** (1966) Signal detection theory and psychophysics. New York: John Wiley & Sons.

Green, J. A., Jones, L. E., and **Gustafson, E. E.** (1987) Perception of cries by parents and nonparents: Relation to cry acoustics. Developmental Psychology, 23, 370–382.

Green, K. P., Kuhl, P. K., Meltzoff, A. N., and **Stevens, E. B.** (1991) Integrating speech information across talkers, gender, and sensory modality: Female faces and male voices in the McGurk effect. Perception & Psychophysics, 50, 524–536.

Green, M. (1980) Orientation-specific adaptation: Effects of checkerboards on the detectability of gratings. Perception, 9, 369–377.

Greenberg, D. P. (1989) Light reflection models for computer graphics. Science, 244, 166–173.

Greenhouse, D. S., and **Cohn, T. E.** (1991) Saccadic suppression and stimulus uncertainty. Journal of the Optical Society of America A, 8, 587–595.

Greenwald, A. G., Spangenberg, E. R., Pratkanis, A. R., and **Eskenazi, J.** (1991) Double-blind tests of subliminal self-help audiotapes. Psychological Science, 2, 119–122.

Greer, C. A. (1991) Structural organization of the olfactory system. In T. V. Getchell, R. L. Doty, L. M. Bartoshuk, and J. B. Snow (eds.), Smell and taste in health and disease. New York: Raven Press. Pp. 65–81.

Gregory, R. L. (1961) The brain as an engineering problem. In W. H. Thorpe and O. L. Zangwill (eds.), Current problems in animal behaviour. Cambridge, England: Cambridge University Press. Pp. 307–330.

Gregory, R. L. (1970) The intelligent eye. New York: McGraw-Hill.

Gregory, R. L. (1978) Eye and brain: The psychology of seeing (3rd ed.). New York: McGraw-Hill.

Gregory, R. L. (1979) The aesthetics of anaesthetics. Perception, 8, 123–124.

Gregory, R. L. (1992) How can perceptual science help the handicapped? Perception, 21, 1–6.

Gregory, R. L., and **Drysdale, A. E.** (1976) Squeezing speech into the deaf ear. Nature, 264, 748–751.

Greve, K. W., and **Bauer, R. M.** (1990) Implicit learning of new faces in prosopagnosia: An application of the mere-exposure paradigm. Neuropsychologia, 28, 1035–1042.

Griffin, D. (1959) Echoes of bats and men. New York: Doubleday/Anchor.

Grinker, J., and **Hirsch, J.** (1972) Metabolic and behavioral correlates of obesity. In K. Porter and J. Knight (eds.), Physiology, emotion, and psychosomatic illness. Amsterdam: Elsevier. Pp. 349–374.

Grossberg, J. M., and **Grant, B. F.** (1978) Clinical psychophysics: Applications of ratio scaling and signal detection methods to research on pain, fear, drugs, and medical decision making. Psychological Bulletin, 85, 1154–1176.

Gross-Isseroff, R., and **Lancet, D.** (1988) Concentration-dependent changes of perceived odor quality. Chemical Senses, 13, 191–204.

Grosslight, J. H., Fletcher, H. J., Masterton, R. B., and **Hagen, R.** (1978) Monocular vision and landing performance in general aviation pilots: Cyclops revisited. Human Factors, 20, 27–33.

Gruber, H. E., and **Dinnerstein, A. J.** (1965) The role of knowledge in distance perception. American Journal of Psychology, 78, 575–581.

Guski, R. (1990) Auditory localization: Effects of reflecting surfaces. Perception, 19, 819–830.

Guth, S. K. (1981) The science of seeing—A search for criteria. American Journal of Optometry and Physiological Optics, 58, 870–885.

Gwosdow, A. R., Steven, J. C., Berglund, L. G., and **Stolwijk, J. A. J.** (1986) Skin friction and fabric sensations in neutral and warm environments. Textile Research Journal, 56, 574–580.

Hackney, C. M. (1987) Anatomical features of the auditory pathway from cochlea to cortex. British Medical Bulletin, 43, 780–801.

Haenny, P. E., Maunsell, J. H. R., and **Schiller, P. H.** (1988) State dependent activity in monkey visual cortex: II. Retinal and extraretinal factors in V4. Experimental Brain Research, 69, 245–259.

Hall, M. J., Bartoshuk, L. M., Cain, W. S., and **Stevens, J. C.** (1975) PTC taste blindness and taste of caffeine. Nature, 253, 442–443.

Halpern, B. P. (1983) Tasting and smelling as active, exploratory sensory processes. American Journal of Otolaryngology, 4, 246–249.

Halpern, D. L., Blake, R., and **Hillenbrand, J.** (1986) Psychoacoustics of a chilling sound. Perception & Psychophysics, 39, 77–80.

Halsey, R. M., and **Chapanis, A.** (1951) On the number of absolutely identifiable spectral hues. Journal of the Optical Society of America, 41, 1057–1058.

Hammond, P., and **MacKay, D. M.** (1977) Differential responsiveness of simple and complex cells in cat striate cortex to visual texture. Experimental Brain Research, 30, 275–296.

Hammond, P., Movat, G. S. V., and **Smith, A. T.** (1985) Motion after-effects in cat striate cortex elicited by moving gratings. Experimental Brain Research, 60, 411–416.

Handel, S. (1989) Listening: An introduction to the perception of auditory events. Cambridge: M.I.T. Press.

Hanson, D. R., and **Fearn, R. W.** (1975) Hearing acuity in young people exposed to pop music and other noise. Lancet, 2, 203–205.

Hari, R., Hämäläinen, M., Kaukoranta, E., Mäkelä, J., Joutsiniemi, S.-L., and **Tiihonen, J.** (1989) Selective listening modifies activity of the human auditory cortex. Experimental Brain Research, 74, 463–470.

Harlow, H. F., and **Harlow, M. K.** (1966) Learning to love. Scientific American, 54, 244–272.

Harmon, L. D. (1973) The recognition of faces. Scientific American, 229, 70–82.

Hartline, H. K. (1938) The response of single optic nerve fibers of the vertebrate eye to illumination of the retina. American Journal of Physiology, 121, 400–415.

Harvey, L. O., Jr. (1986) Visual memory: What is remembered? In F. Klix and H. Hagendorf (eds.), Human memory and cognitive capabilities. The Hague: Elsevier. Pp. 173–187.

Harvey, L. O., Jr., and **Doan, V. V.** (1990) Visual masking at different polar angles in the two-dimensional Fourier plane. Journal of the Optical Society of America A, 7, 116–127.

Harvey, L. O., Jr., Roberts, J. O., and **Gervais, M. J.** (1983) The spatial frequency basis of internal representations. In H.-G. Geissler, H. F. J. M. Buffart, E. L. J. Leeuwenberg, and V. Sarris (eds.), Modern issues in perception. Rotterdam: North-Holland. Pp. 217–226.

Hatsopoulos, N. G., and **Warren, W. H., Jr.** (1991) Visual navigation with a neural network. Neural Networks, 4, 303–317.

Hawkins, J. E., Jr. (1988) Auditory physiological history: A surface view. In A. F. Jahn and J. Santos-Sacci (eds.), Physiology of the ear. New York: Raven Press. Pp. 1–28.

Haxby, J. V., Grady, C. L., Horowitz, B., Ungerleider, L. G., Mishkin, M., Carson, R. E., Herscovitch, P., Schapiro, M. B., and **Rapoport, S. C.** (1991) Dissociation of object and spatial visual processing pathways in human extrastriate cortex. Proceedings of National Academy of Sciences, 88, 1621–1625.

Hebb, D. O. (1949) The organization of behavior. New York: John Wiley & Sons.

Hecht, S., Shlaer, S., and **Pirenne, M. H.** (1942) Energy, quanta, and vision. Journal of General Physiology, 25, 819–840.

Heffner, R. S., and **Heffner, H. E.** (1985) Hearing in mammals: The least weasel. Journal of Mammalogy, 66, 745–755.

Heffner, R. S., and **Heffner, H. E.** (1992) Visual factors in sound localization in mammals. Journal of Comparative Neurology, 317, 219–232.

Heinemann, E. G. (1961) The relation of apparent brightness to the threshold for differences in luminance. Journal of Experimental Psychology, 61, 389–399.

Heinemann, E. G., Tulving, E., and **Nachmias, J.** (1959) The effect of oculomotor adjustments on apparent size. American Journal of Psychology, 72, 32–45.

Held, R. (1979) Development of visual resolution. Canadian Journal of Psychology, 33, 213–221.

Heller, M. A. (1986) Central and peripheral influences on tactual reading. Perception & Psychophysics, 39, 197–204.

Helmholtz, H. L. F. von (1909/1962) Treatise on physiological optics (3rd ed.). J. P. C. Southall (ed.). New York: Dover.

Helmholtz, H. L. F. von (1877/1954) On the sensation of tone as a psychological basis for the theory of music (2nd ed.). A. J. Ellis (trans. and ed.). New York: Dover.

Helson, H. (1964) Current trends and issues in adaptation level theory. American Psychologist, 19, 26–38.

Henkin, R. I. (1982) Olfaction in human disease. In G. B. English (ed.), Looseleaf series in otolaryngology. New York: Harper & Row. Pp. 1–39.

Henning, H. (1916) Der Geruch. Leipzig: Barth.

Hershenson, M. (1989) The moon illusion. Hillsdale, N.J.: Erlbaum.

Hess, E. F. (1965) Attitude and pupil size. Scientific American, 212, 46–54.

Hess, R., Sharpe, L., and **Nordby, K.** (1990) Night vision: Basic, clinical and applied aspects. Cambridge, England: Cambridge University Press.

Heywood, S., and **Ratcliff, G.** (1975) Long-term oculomotor consequences of unilateral colliculectomy in man. In G. Lennerstrand and P. Bach-y-Rita (eds.), Basic mechanisms of ocular motility and their clinical implications. Elmsford, N.Y.: Pergamon Press. Pp. 561–564.

Hickey, T. (1977) Postnatal development of the human lateral geniculate nucleus: Relationship to a critical period for the visual systems. Science, 198, 836–838.

Hikosaka, O., Tanaka, M., Sakamoto, M., and **Iwamura, Y.** (1985) Deficits in manipulative behaviors induced by local injections of muscimol in the first somatosensory cortex of the conscious monkey. Behavior Research, 325, 375–380.

Hildreth, E. (1986) Edge detection. In Encyclopedia of artificial intelligence, vol. 1. New York: John Wiley & Sons. Pp. 257–267.

Hiris, E., and **Blake, R.** (1992) Another perspective on the visual motion aftereffect. Proceedings of the National Academy of Sciences, 89, 9025–9028.

Hirsch, E. D., Jr. (1988) Cultural literacy. New York: Vintage Books.

Hirsch, J., and **Miller, W. H.** (1987) Does cone positional disorder limit resolution? Journal of the Optical Society of America A, 4, 1481–1492.

Hochberg, J. (1971) Perception: I. Color and shape. In J. W. Kling and L. A. Riggs (eds.), Woodworth and Schlosberg's experimental psychology (3rd ed.). New York: Holt, Rinehart & Winston. Pp. 395–474.

Holley, A. (1991) Neural coding of olfactory information. In T. V. Getchell, R. L. Doty, L. M. Bartoshuk, and J. B. Snow (eds.), Smell and taste in health and disease. New York: Raven Press. Pp. 329–344.

Hollo, A. (1977) Age four. In Sojourner microcosms: New and selected poems. Berkeley, Calif.: Blue Wind Press. P. 30.

Holmes, G. (1918) Disturbances of vision by cerebral lesions. British Journal of Ophthalmology, 2, 353–384.

Holway, A. F., and **Boring, E. G.** (1941) Determinants of apparent visual size with distance variant. American Journal of Psychology, 54, 21–37.

Hood, D. C., and **Finkelstein, M. A.** (1986) Sensitivity to light. In K. Boff, L. Kaufman, and J. Thomas (eds.), Handbook of perception and human performance, vol. 1. New York: Wiley-Interscience. Pp. 5.1–5.66.

Hopfield, J. J. (1991) Olfactory computations and object perception. Proceedings of the National Academy of Science, 88, 6462–6466.

Horner, D. G. (1982) Can vision predict baseball players' hitting ability? American Journal of Optometry and Physiological Optics, 59, 69.

Houston, R. A. (1917) Newton and the colours of the spectrum. Science Progress, 12, 250–264.

Howard, I. P., Bergström, S. S., and **Masao, O.** (1990) Shape from shading in different frames of reference. Perception, 19, 523–530.

Howard, M. (1983) The Warner touch. New Republic. 188, 9–12.

Hubel, D. H., and **Wiesel, T. N.** (1962) Receptive fields, binocular interaction, and functional architecture in the cat's visual cortex. Journal of Physiology, 160, 106–154.

Hubel, D. H., and **Wiesel, T. N.** (1970) Stereoscopic vision in macaque monkey. Nature, 225, 41–42.

Hubel, D. H., and **Wiesel, T. N.** (1974a) Uniformity of monkey striate cortex: A parallel relationship between field size, scatter, and magnification factor. Journal of Comparative Neurology, 158, 295–306.

Hubel, D. H., and **Wiesel, T. N.** (1974b) Sequence regularity and geometry of orientation columns in the monkey striate cortex. Journal of Comparative Neurology, 158, 267–294.

Hubel, D. H., and **Wiesel, T. N.** (1977) Functional architecture of macaque monkey visual cortex. Proceedings of the Royal Society of London, 198, 1–59.

Hubel, D. H., and **Wiesel, T. N.** (1979) Brain mechanisms of vision. Scientific American, 241, 150–163.

Hubel, D. H., Wiesel, T. N., and **LeVay, S.** (1977) Plasticity of ocular dominance columns in monkey striate cortex. Philosophical Transactions of the Royal Society of London, Series B, 278, 377–409.

Hubel, D. H., Wiesel, T. N., and **Stryker, M. P.** (1978) Anatomical demonstration of orientation columns in macaque monkey. Journal of Comparative Neurology, 177, 361–380.

Hughes, A. (1977) The topography of vision in mammals of contrasting life style: Comparative optics and retinal organization. In F. Crescitelli (ed.), Handbook of sensory physiology, vol. VII/5. Berlin: Springer-Verlag. Pp. 613–756.

Hume, D. (1739/1963) A treatise of human nature. In V. C. Chappel (ed.), The philosophy of David Hume. New York: Modern Library. Pp. 11–311.

Humphrey, N. K. (1974) Species and individuals in the perceptual world of monkeys. Perception, 3, 105–114.

Humphreys, G. W., and **Quinlan, P. T.** (1987) Normal and pathological processes in object constancy. In G. W. Humphreys and M. J. Riddoch (eds.), Visual object processing: A cognitive neuropsychological approach. Hove, England: Erlbaum. Pp. 43–106.

Hurd, P. D., and **Blevins, J.** (1984) Aging and the color of pills. New England Journal of Medicine, 310, 202.

Hurvich, L. M. (1969) Hering and the scientific establishment. American Psychologist, 24, 497–514.

Hurvich, L. M. (1981) Color vision. Sunderland, Mass.: Sinauer Associates.

Hurvich, L. M., and **Jameson, D.** (1949) Helmholtz and the three-color theory: An historical note. American Journal of Psychology, 62, 111–114.

Hurvich, L. M., and **Jameson, D.** (1966) The perception of brightness and darkness. Boston: Allyn & Bacon.

Iavecchia, J. H., Iavecchia, H. P., and **Roscoe, S. N.** (1983) The moon illusion revisited. Aviation, Space, and Environmental Medicine, 54, 39–46.

Itoh, K., and **Saito, S.** (1988) Effects of acoustical feature parameters on perceptual speaker identity. Review of the Electrical Communications Laboratories, 36, 135–141.

Ittelson, W. H. (1951) Size as a cue to distance: Static localization. American Journal of Psychology, 64, 54–67.

Ittelson, W. H. (1952/1968) The Ames demonstrations in perception. New York: Hafner.

Jacobsen, A., and **Gilchrist, A.** (1988) The ratio principle holds over a million-to-one range of illumination. Perception & Psychophysics, 43, 1–6.

Jacobsen, S. G., Mohindra, I., and **Held, R.** (1983) Monocular form deprivation in human infants. Documenta Ophthalmologica, 55, 199–211.

James, W. (1890) The principles of psychology. 2 vols. New York: Holt.

James, W. (1892) Psychology: A briefer course. New York: Holt.

Jameson, D., and **Hurvich, L. M.** (1978) Dichromatic color language: "Reds" and "greens" don't look alike but their colors do. Sensory Processes, 2, 146–155.

Jameson, D., and **Hurvich, L. M.** (1989) Essay concerning color constancy. Annual Review of Psychology, 40, 1–22.

Jastreboff, P. J. (1990) Phantom auditory perception (tinnitus): Mechanisms of generation and perception. Neuroscience Research, 8, 221–254.

Jeffress, L. A. (1948) A place theory of sound localization. Journal of Comparative and Physiological Psychology, 41, 35–39.

Jeffress, L. A., and **Taylor, R. W.** (1961) Lateralization vs. localization. Journal of the Acoustical Society of America, 33, 482–483.

Jeghers, H. (1937) The degree and prevalence of vitamin A deficiency in adults. Journal of the American Medical Association, 109, 756–762.

Jessell, T. M., and **Kelly, D.** (1991) Pain and analgesia. In E. R. Kandel, J. H. Schwartz, and T. M. Jessell (eds.), Principles of neural science. New York: Elsevier. Pp. 385–399.

Johansson, G. (1975) Visual motion perception. Scientific American, 232, 76–88.

Johansson, G., von Hofsten, C., and **Jansson, G.** (1980) Event perception. Annual Review of Psychology, 31, 27–64.

Johansson, R. S., and **Vallbo, A. B.** (1979) Tactile sensibility in the human hand: Relative and absolute densities of four types of mechanoreceptive units in the glabrous skin. Journal of Physiology, 286, 283–300.

Johansson, R. S., and **Vallbo, A. B.** (1983) Tactile sensory coding in the glabrous skin of the human hand. Trends in Neurosciences, 6, 27–32.

Johns, T., and **Keen, S. L.** (1985) Determinants of taste perception and classification among the Aymara of Bolivia. Ecology of Food and Nutrition, 16, 253–271.

Johnson, D. M., and **Hafter, E. R.** (1980) Uncertain-frequency detection: Cuing and condition of observation. Perception & Psychophysics, 28, 143–149.

Johnson, K. O., and **Hsiao, S. S.** (1992) Neural mechanisms of tactual form and texture perception. Annual Review of Neuroscience, 15, 227–250.

Johnson, K. O., and **Lamb, G. H.** (1981) Neural mechanisms of spatial tactile discrimination: Neural patterns evoked by Braille-like dot patterns in the monkey. Journal of Physiology, 310, 117–144.

Johnson-Laird, P. N. (1988) The computer and the mind: An introduction to cognitive science. Cambridge: Harvard University Press.

Johnston, J. C., and **McClelland, J. L.** (1973) Visual factors in word perception. Perception & Psychophysics, 14, 365–370.

Johnston, J. C., and **McClelland, J. L.** (1974) Perception of letters in words: Seek not and ye shall find. Science, 184, 1192–1194.

Joyce, J. (1922/1934) Ulysses. New York: Random House.

Joyce, J. (1939/1967) Finnegans wake. New York: Viking Press.

Judd, D. B. (1960) Appraisal of Land's work on two-primary color projections. Journal of the Optical Society of America, 50, 254–268.

Julesz, B. (1971) Foundations of cyclopean perception. Chicago: University of Chicago Press.

Julesz, B. (1984) A brief outline of the texton theory of human vision. Trends in Neurosciences, 7, 41–45.

Julesz, B. (1991) Early vision and focal attention. Reviews of Modern Physics, 63, 735–772.

Julesz, B., and **Miller, J. E.** (1975) Independent spatial frequency-tuned channels in binocular fusion and rivalry. Perception, 4, 125–143.

Just, M. A., and **Carpenter, P. A.** (1980) A theory of reading: From eye fixations to comprehension. Psychological Review, 87, 329–354.

Kaas, J. H. (1987) Somatosensory cortex. In G. Adelman (ed.), Encyclopedia of neuroscience, vol. 2. Boston: Birkhauser. Pp. 1113–1117.

Kaas, J. H. (1991) Plasticity of sensory and motor maps in adult mammals. Annual Review of Neuroscience, 14, 137–167.

Kaas, J. H., and **Pons, T. P.** (1988) The somatosensory system of primates. In H. D. Steklis and J. Erwin (eds.), Comparative primate biology, vol. 4: Neurosciences. New York: Liss. Pp. 421–468.

Kaitz, M., Good, A., Rokem, A. M., and **Eidelman, A.** (1987) Mothers' recognition of their newborns by olfactory cues. Developmental Psychobiology, 20, 587–591.

Kalmus, H. (1955) The discrimination by the nose of the dog of individual human odours and in particular the odour of twins. British Journal of Animal Behaviour, 3, 25–31.

Kanizsa, G. (1976) Subjective contours. Scientific American, 234, 48–52.

Kaplan, E., Shapley, R. M., and **Purpura, K.** (1988) Color and luminance contrast as tools for probing the primate retina. Neuroscience Research Supplement 8, S151–S165.

Katz, D. (1925) Der Aufbau der Tastwelt. Zeitschrift fur Psychologie, 11 [see also L. E. Krueger (1970) David Katz' Der Aufbau der Tastwelt (The world of touch): A synopsis. Perception & Psychophysics, 7, 337–341].

Kauer, J. S. (1991) Contributions of topography and parallel processing to odor coding in the vertebrate olfactory pathway. Trends in Neurosciences, 14, 79–85.

Kaufman, L. (1974) Sight and mind: An introduction to visual perception. New York: Oxford University Press.

Kaufman, L., and **Rock, I.** (1962) The moon illusion. Scientific American, 207, 120–132.

Kaukoranta, E., Hari, R., and **Lounasmaa, O. V.** (1988) Responses of the human auditory cortex to vowel onset after fricative consonants. Experimental Brain Research, 69, 19–23.

Keller, H. (1908) Sense and sensibility. Century Magazine, 75, 566–577, 773–783.

Kelling, S. T., and **Halpern, B. P.** (1987) Taste judgments and gustatory stimulus duration: Simple taste reaction times. Chemical Senses, 12, 543–562.

Kellman, P. J., and **Shipley, T. F.** (1991) A theory of visual interpolation in object perception. Cognitive Psychology, 23, 141–221.

Kelly, D. H. (1976) Pattern detection and the two-dimensional Fourier transform: Flickering checkerboards and chromatic mechanisms. Vision Research, 16, 277–289.

Kemp, D. T. (1979) Evidence of mechanical nonlinearity and frequency-selective wave amplification in the cochlea. Archives of Otorhinolaryngology, 224, 37–45.

Kendrick, K. M., Levy, F., and **Keverne, E. B.** (1992) Changes in the sensory processing of olfactory signals induced by birth in sheep. Science, 256, 833–836.

Kenshalo, D. (1972) The cutaneous senses. In J. W. Kling and L. A. Riggs (eds.), Woodworth and Schlosberg's experimental psychology (3rd ed.), vol. 1. New York: Holt, Rinehart & Winston.

Kersten, D. (1987) Predictability and redundancy of natural images. Journal of the Optical Society of America A, 4, 2395–2401.

Kertsa, L. G. (1962) Voice identifications. Nature, 196, 1253–1257.

Keuning, J. (1968) On the nasal cycle. International Rhinology, 6, 99–136.

Keverne, E. B. (1982) Chemical senses. In H. B. Barlow and J. D. Mollon (eds.), The senses. Cambridge: Cambridge University Press. Pp. 428–447.

Kiang, N. Y. S. (1968) A survey of recent developments in the study of auditory physiology. Annals of Otology, Rhinology, and Laryngology, 77, 656–675.

Kiang, N. Y. S. (1975) Stimulus representation in the discharge patterns of auditory neurons. In E. L. Eagles (ed.), The nervous system, vol. 3. New York: Raven Press. Pp. 81–96.

Kinchla, R. A., and **Wolfe, J. M.** (1979) The order of visual processing: "Top-down," "bottom-up," or "middle-out." Perception & Psychophysics, 25, 225–231.

King, A. J., and **Moore, D. R.** (1991) Plasticity of auditory maps in the brain. Trends in Neurosciences, 14, 31–37.

Kinney, J. A., Luria, S. M., Ryan, A. P., Schlicting, C. L., and **Paulson, H. M.** (1980) The vision of submariners and national guardsmen: A longitudinal study. American Journal of Optometry and Physiological Optics, 57, 469–478.

Kirkpatrick, P. (1963) Batting the ball. American Journal of Physics, 31, 606–613.

Klatzky, R. L., Lederman, S. J., and **Metzger, V.** (1985) Identifying objects by touch: An "expert" system. Perception & Psychophysics, 37, 299–302.

Knierim, J. J., and **van Essen, D. C.** (1992) Visual cortex: Cartography, connectivity and concurrent processing. Current Opinion in Neurobiology, 2, 150–155.

Knudsen, E. I., du Lac, S., and **Esterly, S. D.** (1987) Computational maps in the brain. Annual Review of Neuroscience, 10, 41–65.

Knudsen, E. I., and **Konishi, M.** (1978) A neural map of auditory space in the owl. Science, 200, 795–797.

Knudsen, E. I., and **Konishi, M.** (1980) Monaural occlusion shifts receptive-field locations of auditory midbrain units in the owl. Journal of Neurophysiology, 44, 687–695.

Koelega, H. S., and **Koster, E. P.** (1974) Some experiments on sex differences in odor perception. Annals of the New York Academy of Sciences, 237, 234–246.

Koenderink, J. J. (1986) Optic flow. Vision Research, 26, 161–180.

Koenig, W. (1950) Subjective effects in binaural hearing. Journal of the Acoustical Society of America, 22, 61–62.

Koffka, K. (1935) Principles of gestalt psychology. New York: Harcourt, Brace & World.

Köhler, W. (1920/1938) Physical gestalten. In W. D. Ellis (ed.), A source book of gestalt psychology. New York: Humanities Press. Pp. 17–54.

Köhler, W. (1969) The task of gestalt psychology. Princeton: Princeton University Press.

Koretz, J. F., and **Handelman, G. H.** (1988) How the human eye focuses. Scientific American, 259, 92–99.

Kosslyn, S. M. (1980) Image and mind. Cambridge: Harvard University Press.

Kosslyn, S. M., and **Koenig, O.** (1992) Wet mind, the new cognitive neuroscience. New York: The Free Press.

Kowler, E. (1989) Cognitive expectations, not habits, control anticipatory smooth oculomotor pursuit. Vision Research, 29, 1049–1058.

Kowler, E., and **Martins, A. J.** (1982) Eye movements of preschool children. Science, 215, 997–999.

Kramer, M. (1989) Making sense of wine. New York: W. W. Morrow.

Kristensen, S., and **Gimsing, S.** (1988) Occupational hearing impairment in pig-breeders. Scandinavian Audiology, 17, 191–192.

Krueger, L. E. (1975) Familiarity effects in visual information processing. Psychological Bulletin, 82, 949–974.

Kruk, R., and **Regan, D.** (1983) Visual test results compared with flying performance in telemetry-tracked aircraft. Aviation, Space, and Environmental Medicine, 54, 906–911.

Kruk, R., Regan, D., Beverley, K., and **Longridge, T.** (1981) Correlations between visual test results and flying performance on the Advanced Simulator for Pilot Training (ASPT). Aviation, Space, and Environmental Medicine, 52, 455–460.

Kuhl, P. K., and **Meltzoff, A. N.** (1982) The bimodal perception of speech in infancy. Science, 218, 1138–1141.

Kühne, W. (1879/1977) Chemical processes in the retina. Vision Research, 17, 1273–1316.

Kundel, H. L., and **Nodine, C. F.** (1983) A visual concept shapes image perception. Radiology, 146, 363–368.

Kunishima, M., and **Yanase, T.** (1985) Visual effects of wall colours in living rooms. Ergonomics, 28, 869–882.

Künnapas, T. M. (1968) Distance perception as a function of available visual cues. Journal of Experimental Psychology, 77, 523–529.

Kunst-Wilson, W. R., and **Zajonc, R. B.** (1980) Affective discrimination of stimuli that cannot be recognized. Science, 207, 557–558.

Kurtenbach, W., Sternheim, C. E., and **Spillmann, L.** (1984) Change in hue of spectral colors by dilution with white light (Abney effect). Journal of the Optical Society of America A, 1, 365–372.

Kurtz, D., and **Butter, C. M.** (1980) Impairments in visual discrimination performance and gaze shifts in monkeys with superior colliculus lesions. Brain Research, 196, 109–124.

Kuthan, V. (1987) Some contributions of J. E. Purkyne to the visual physiology. Physiologia Bohemoslovaca, 36, 255–267.

LaBerge, D., and **Buchsbaum, M. S.** (1990) Positron emission tomographic measurements of pulvinar activity during an attention task. Journal of Neuroscience, 10, 613–619.

LaBerge, D., Carter, M., and **Brown, V.** (1992) A network simulation of thalamic circuit operations in selective attention. Neural Computation, 4, 318–331.

Ladefoged, P., and **Broadbent, D. E.** (1957) Information conveyed by vowels. Journal of the Acoustical Society of America, 29, 98–104.

Laing, D. G. (1983) Natural sniffing gives optimum odour perception for humans. Perception, 12, 99–118.

Laing, D. G. (1988) Relationship between the differential adsorption of odorants by the olfactory mucus and their perception in mixtures. Chemical Senses, 13, 463–471.

Lancet, D. (1986) Vertebrate olfactory reception. Annual Review of Neuroscience, 9, 329–355.

Lancker, D. R. V., Kreiman, J., and **Cummings, J.** (1989) Voice perception deficits: Neuroanatomical correlates of phonagnosia. Journal of Clinical and Experimental Neuropsychology, 11, 665–674.

Land, E. H. (1959) Experiments in color vision. Scientific American, 200, 84–94, 96, 99.

Landau, B. (1991) Spatial representation of objects in the young blind child. Cognition, 38, 145–178.

Landis, C. (1954) Determinants of the critical flicker fusion threshold. Physiological Review, 34, 259–286.

Lappin, J. S., Doner, J. F., and **Kottas, B. L.** (1979) Minimal conditions for the visual detection of structure and motion in three dimensions. Science, 209, 717–719.

Lawless, H. T., and **Engen, T.** (1977) Association to odors: Interference, memories, and verbal labeling. Journal of Experimental Psychology, 3, 52–59.

Lawless, H. T., Glatter, S., and **Hohn, C.** (1991) Context-dependent changes in the perception of odor quality. Chemical Senses, 16, 349–360.

Lederman, S. J. (1976) The "callus-thenics" of touching. Canadian Journal of Psychology, 30, 82–89.

Lederman, S. J., and **Klatzky, R. L.** (1987) Hand movements: A window into haptic object recognition. Cognitive Psychology, 19, 342–348.

Lederman, S. J., and **Klatzky, R. L.** (1990) Haptic classification of common objects: Knowledge-driven exploration. Cognitive Psychology, 22, 421–459.

Lederman, S. J., Klatzky, R. L., and **Pawluk, D. T.** (1993) Lessons from the study of biological touch for robot haptic sensing. In H. Nicholls (ed.), Advanced tactile sensing for robotics. In World scientific series in robotics and automated systems, vol. 5. Singapore: World Scientific Publishing. Pp. 193–220.

Lederman, S. J., and **Taylor, M. M.** (1972) Fingertip force, surface geometry, and the perception of roughness by active touch. Perception & Psychophysics, 12, 401–408.

Lee, D. N. (1976) A theory of visual control of braking based on information about time-to-collision. Perception, 5, 437–459.

Lee, D. N. (1980) The optic flow field: The foundation of vision. Philosophical Transactions of the Royal Society of London, Series B, 290, 169–179.

Lee, D. N., and **Reddish, P. E.** (1981) Plummeting gannets: A paradigm of ecological optics. Nature, 293, 293–294.

Leehey, S. C., Moskowitz-Cook, A., Brill, S., and **Held, R.** (1975) Orientational anisotropy in infant vision. Science, 190, 900–902.

Leeper, R. W. (1935) A study of a neglected portion of the field of learning—The development of sensory organization. Journal of Genetic Psychology, 46, 41–75.

LeGrand, Y. (1968) Light, colour, and vision (2nd ed.). R. W. G. Hunt and F. R. W. Hunt (trans.). London: Chapman & Hall.

Lehmkuhle, S. W., and **Fox, R.** (1977) Global stereopsis in the cat. Paper presented at the Association for Research in Vision and Ophthalmology, Sarasota, Fla.

Leibowitz, H. W. (1983) A behavioral and perceptual analysis of grade crossing accidents. Operation Lifesaver National Symposium 1982. Chicago: National Safety Council.

Leibowitz, H. W., and **Moore, D.** (1966) Role of changes in accommodation and convergence in the perception of size. Journal of the Optical Society of America, 56, 1120–1122.

Leibowitz, H. W., and **Owens, D. A.** (1975) Anomalous myopias and the intermediate dark focus of accommodation. Science, 189, 646–648.

Leibowitz, H. W., and **Owens, D. A.** (1976) Night myopia: Cause and a possible basis for amelioration. American Journal of Optometry and Physiological Optics, 53, 709–717.

Leibowitz, H. W., Post, R. B., Brandt, T., and **Dichgans, J.** (1982) Implications of recent developments in dynamic spatial orientation and visual resolution for vehicle guidance. In A. Wertheim, W. Wagenaar, and H. W. Leibowitz (eds.), Tutorials in motion perception. New York: Plenum Press. Pp. 231–260.

Lennie, P. (1984) Recent developments in the physiology of color vision. Trends in Neurosciences, 7, 243–248.

Lennie, P., and **D'Zmura, M.** (1988) Mechanisms of color vision. CRC Critical Reviews in Neurobiology, 3, 333–400.

Lennie, P., Krauskopf, J., and **Sclar, G.** (1990) Chromatic mechanisms in striate cortex of macaque. Journal of Neuroscience, 10, 649–669.

Lerner, M. R., Gyorgyi, T. K., Reagan, J., Roby-Shemkovitz, A., Rybczynski, R., and **Vogt, R.** (1990) Peripheral events in moth olfaction. Chemical Senses, 15, 191–198.

Levinson, E., and **Sekuler, R.** (1976) Adaptation alters perceived direction of motion. Vision Research, 16, 779–781.

Levitan, C., and **Kaczmarek, L. K.** (1991) The neuron. Cell and molecular biology. New York: Oxford University Press.

Lewis, A., and **Del Priore, L. V.** (1988) The biophysics of visual photoreception. Physics Today, 41, 38–46.

Li, X., Logan, R. J., and **Pastore, R. E.** (1991) Perception of acoustic source characteristics: Walking sounds. Journal of the Acoustical Society of America, 90, 3036–3049.

Liberman, M. C. (1982) The cochlear frequency map for the cat: Labelling auditory nerve fibers of known characteristics. Journal of the Acoustical Society of America, 72, 1441–1449.

Linder, M. E., and **Gilman, A. G.** (1992) G proteins. Scientific American, 267, 56–65.

Lindsay, P. H., and **Norman, D. A.** (1977) Human information processing (2nd ed.). New York: Academic Press.

Liss, J. M., Weismer, G., and **Rosenbek, J. C.** (1990) Selected acoustic characteristics of speech production

in very old males. Journal of Gerontology: Psychological Sciences, 45, 35–45.

Livingstone, M. S., and **Hubel, D. H.** (1981) Effects of sleep and arousal on the processing of visual information in the cat. Nature, 291, 554–561.

Livingstone, M. S., and **Hubel, D. H.** (1984) Anatomy and physiology of a color system in primate primary visual cortex. Journal of Neuroscience, 4, 309–356.

Livingstone, M., and **Hubel, D. H.** (1988) Segregation of form, color, movement, and depth: Anatomy, physiology, and perception. Science, 240, 740–749.

Locke, J. (1690/1924) An essay concerning human understanding (abridged and edited by A. S. Pringle-Pattison). Oxford, England: Clarendon Press.

Loftus, E. F., and **Kliner, M. R.** (1992) Is the unconscious smart or dumb? The American Psychologist, 47, 761–765.

Loomis, J. M. (1981) Tactile pattern perception. Perception, 10, 5–27.

Loomis, J. M. (1990) A model of character recognition and legibility. Journal of Experimental Psychology: Human Perception and Performance, 16, 106–120.

Loomis, J. M., Klatzky, R. L., and **Lederman, S. J.** (1991) Similarity of tactual and visual picture recognition with limited field of view. Perception, 20, 167–178.

Lu, S. T., Hämäläinen, M. S., Hari, R., Ilmoniemi, R. J., Lounasmaa, O. V., Sams, M., and **Vilkman, V.** (1991) Seeing faces activates three separate areas outside the occipital visual cortex in man. Neuroscience, 43, 287–290.

Ludel, J. (1978) Introduction to sensory processes. New York: W. H. Freeman.

Ludvigh, E., and **Miller, J. W.** (1958) Study of visual acuity during ocular pursuit of moving test objects: I. Introduction. Journal of the Optical Society of America, 48, 799–802.

Lumsden, C. J., and **Wilson, E. O.** (1983) Promethean fire: Reflections on the origin of mind. Cambridge: Harvard University Press.

Lythgoe, J. N. (1979) The ecology of vision. Oxford, England: Clarendon Press.

Macdonald, D., and **Brown, R.** (1985) The smell of success. New Scientist, 106, 10–14.

MacMillan, N. A., and **Creelman, C.** (1991) Detection theory: A user's guide. Cambridge, England: Cambridge University Press.

MacNichol, E. (1964) Three-pigment color vision. Scientific American, 211, 48–56.

Maffei, L., and **Fiorentini, A.** (1972) Retinogeniculate convergence and analysis of contrast. Journal of Neurophysiology, 35, 65–72.

Maffei, L., and **Fiorentini, A.** (1973) The visual cortex as a spatial frequency analyzer. Vision Research, 13, 1255–1267.

Makous, J. C., and **Middlebrooks, J. C.** (1990) Two-dimensional sound localization by human listeners. Journal of the Acoustical Society of America, 87, 2188–2200.

Malcolm, R. (1984) Pilot disorientation and the use of a peripheral vision display. Aviation, Space, and Environmental Medicine, 55, 231–238.

Malpelli, J. G., and **Baker, F. H.** (1975) The representation of the visual field in the lateral geniculate nucleus of Macaca mulatta. Journal of Comparative Neurology, 161, 569–594.

Mandler, G., Nakamura, Y., and **Shebo van Zandt, B. J.** (1987) Nonspecific effects of exposure on stimuli that cannot be recognized. Journal of Experimental Psychology: Learning, Memory, and Cognition, 13(4), 646–648.

Manley, G. A., Koppl, C., and **Konishi, M.** (1988) A neural map of interaural intensity differences in the brain stem of the barn owl. Journal of Neuroscience, 8, 2665–2676.

Mansfield, R. (1974) Neural basis of orientation perception in primate vision. Science, 186, 1133–1135.

Marc, R. E. (1982) Chromatic organization of the retina. In D. S. McDevitt (ed.), Cell biology of the eye. New York: Academic Press. Pp. 435–471.

Marcel, A. J. (1983) Conscious and unconscious perception: An approach to the relation between phenomenal experience and perceptual processes. Cognitive Psychology, 15, 238–300.

Marin, O. S. M. (1976) Neurobiology of language: An overview. Annals of the New York Academy of Sciences, 280, 900–912.

Mariotte, E. (1668/1948) The discovery of the blindspot. In W. Dennis (ed.), Readings in the history of psychology. New York: Appleton-Century-Crofts. Pp. 42–43.

Mark, L. S., and **Todd, J. T.** (1983) The perception of growth in three dimensions. Perception & Psychophysics, 33, 193–196.

Marr, D. (1976) Early processing of visual information. Philosophical Transactions of the Royal Society, Series B, 275, 483–524.

Marr, D. (1982) Vision. New York: W. H. Freeman.

Marron, J. A., and **Bailey, I. L.** (1982) Visual factors and orientation-mobility performance. American Journal of Optometry and Physiological Optics, 59, 413–426.

Marshall, J. C., and **Halligan, P. W.** (1988) Blindsight and insight in visuo-spatial neglect. Nature, 336, 766–767.

Martin, G. (1987) The world through a starling's eye. New Scientist, 114, 49–51.

Martin, K. A. C. (1988) The lateral geniculate nucleus strikes back. Trends in Neurosciences, 11, 192–194.

Masterton, R. B., and **Imig, T. J.** (1984) Neural mechanisms of sound localization. Annual Review of Physiology, 46, 275–280.

Masterton, R. B., Thompson, G. C., Bechtold, J. K., and **Robards, M. J.** (1975) Neuroanatomical basis of binaural phase-difference analysis for sound localization: A comparative study. Journal of Comparative and Physiological Psychology, 89, 379–386.

Mather, G., and **Moulden, B.** (1980) A simultaneous shift in apparent direction: Further evidence for a "distribution-shift" model of direction coding. Quarterly Journal of Experimental Psychology, 32, 325–333.

Matin, L., and **MacKinnon, G. E.** (1964) Autokinetic movement: Selective manipulation of directional components by image stabilization. Science, 143, 147–148.

Mattingly, I. G., and **Liberman, A. M.** (1988) Specialized perceiving systems for speech and other biologically significant sounds. In G. M. Edelman, W. E. Gall, and W. M. Cowan (eds.), Auditory function: Neurobiological bases of hearing. New York: John Wiley & Sons. Pp. 775–793.

Maunsell, J. H. R., and **Newsome, W. T.** (1987) Visual processing in monkey extrastriate cortex. Annual Review of Neuroscience, 10, 363–401.

McAdams, S. (1984) Spectral fusion, spectral parsing, and the formation of auditory images. Paris: IRCAM.

McBurney, D. H. (1974) Are there primary tastes for man? Chemical Senses and Flavor, 1, 17–28.

McBurney, D. H. (1978) Psychological dimensions and perceptual analyses of taste. In E. C. Carterette and M. P. Friedman (eds.), Handbook of perception, vol. 6A. New York: Academic Press. Pp. 125–155.

McBurney, D. H., and **Gent, J. F.** (1979) On the nature of taste qualities. Psychological Bulletin, 86, 151–167.

McBurney, D. H., and **Moskat, L. J.** (1975) Taste thresholds in college-age smokers and nonsmokers. Perception & Psychophysics, 18, 71–73.

McBurney, D. H., Smith, D. V., and **Shick, T. R.** (1972) Gustatory cross adaptation: Sourness and bitterness. Perception & Psychophysics, 11, 228–232.

McCabe, P. A., and **Dey, F. L.** (1965) The effect of aspirin upon auditory sensitivity. Annals of Otology, Rhinology, and Laryngology, 74, 312–325.

McClelland, J. L., and **Rumelhart, D. E.** (1981) An interactive activation model of context effects in letter perception: Part 1. An account of basic findings. Psychological Review, 88, 375–407.

McConkie, G. W., and **Rayner, K.** (1975) The span of the effective stimulus during a fixation in reading. Perception & Psychophysics, 17, 578–586.

McCutcheon, N. B., and **Saunders, J.** (1972) Human taste papilla stimulation: Stability of quality judgments over time. Science, 175, 214–216.

McFadden, D. (1982) Tinnitus: Facts, theories and treatments. Washington, D.C.: National Academy of Sciences Press.

McFadden, D., and **Plattsmier, H. S.** (1983) Aspirin can potentiate the temporary hearing loss induced by intense sounds. Hearing Research, 9, 295–316.

McFadden, D., Plattsmier, H. S., and Pasanen, E. G. (1984) Aspirin-induced hearing loss as a model of sensorineural hearing loss. Hearing Research, 16, 251–260.

McGurk, H., and MacDonald, J. (1976) Hearing lips and seeing voices. Nature, 264, 746–748.

McKee, S. P. (1981) A local mechanism for differential velocity detection. Vision Research, 21, 491–500.

McNicol, D. (1972) A primer of signal detection theory. London: Allen & Unwin.

Meiselman, H. L., and Dzendolet, E. (1967) Variability in gustatory quality identification. Perception & Psychophysics, 2, 496–498.

Melzack, R. (1992) Phantom limbs. Scientific American, 266, 120–126.

Mendelson, J. R. (1992) Neural selectivity for interaural frequency disparity in cat primary auditory cortex. Hearing Research, 58, 47–56.

Merbs, S. L., and Nathans, J. (1992) Absorption spectra of human cone pigments. Nature, 356, 433–435.

Meredith, M. A., and Stein, B. E. (1983) Interactions among converging sensory inputs in the superior colliculus. Science, 221, 389–391.

Merzenich, M. M. (1987) Dynamic neocortical processes and the origins of higher brain functions. In J. P. Changeux and M. Konishi (eds.), Neural and molecular bases of learning. Chichester, England: John Wiley & Sons. Pp. 337–358.

Merzenich, M. M., Nelson, R. J., Kaas, J. H., Stryker, M. P., Jenkins, W. M., Zook, J. M., Cynader, M. S., and Schoppmann, A. (1987) Variability in hand surface representations in Area-3B and Area-1 in adult owl and squirrel monkeys. Journal of Comparative Neurology, 258, 281–296.

Michaels, C. F., and Carello, C. (1981) Direct perception. Englewood Cliffs, N.J.: Prentice-Hall.

Middlebrooks, J. C., and Green, D. M. (1991) Sound localization by human listeners. Annual Review of Psychology 42, 135–159.

Miller, G. (1962) Decision units in the perception of speech. IRE Transactions on Information Theory, 8, 81–83.

Miller, I. J., Jr., and Bartoshuk, L. M. (1991) Taste perception, taste bud distribution, and spatial relationships. In T. V. Getchell, R. L. Doty, L. M. Bartoshuk, and J. B. Snow, Jr. (eds.), Smell and taste in health and disease. New York: Raven Press. Pp. 175–204.

Miller, I. J., Jr., and Reedy, F. E. (1990) Variations in human taste bud density and taste intensity perception. Physiology and Behavior, 47, 1213–1219.

Miller, J. D. (1978) Effects of noise on people. In E. C. Carterette and M. P. Friedman (eds.), Handbook of perception, vol. 4. New York: Academic Press. Pp. 609–640.

Mills, A. W. (1960) Lateralization of high-frequency tones. Journal of the Acoustical Society of America, 32, 132–134.

Mishkin, M., Ungergleider, L. G., and Macko, K. A. (1983) Object vision and spatial vision: Two cortical pathways. Trends in Neurosciences, 6, 414–417.

Mistlin, A. J., and Perrett, D. I. (1990) Visual and somatosensory processing in the macaque temporal cortex: The role of "expectation." Experimental Brain Research, 82, 437–450.

Mitchell, D. E., Freeman, R. D., Millidot, M., and Haegerstrom, G. (1973) Meridional amblyopia: Evidence for modification of the human visual system by early visual experience. Vision Research, 13, 535–558.

Mitchell, D. E., and Ware, C. (1974) Interocular transfer of a visual aftereffect in normal and stereoblind humans. Journal of Physiology, 236, 707–721.

Møller, A. R. (1974) Responses of units in cochlear nucleus to sinusoidally amplitude-modulated tones. Experimental Neurology, 45, 104–117.

Mollon, J. D. (1982) Color vision. Annual Review of Psychology, 33, 41–85.

Mollon, J. D. (1989) "Tho' she kneel'd in that place where they grew . . ." The uses and origins of primate colour vision. Journal of Experimental Biology, 146, 21–38.

Mollon, J. D. (1990) The tricks of colour. In H. Barlow, C. Blakemore, and M. Weston-Smith (eds.), Images and understanding. Cambridge, England: Cambridge University Press. Pp. 61–78.

Moncrieff, R. W. (1956) Olfactory adaptation and odor likeness. Journal of Physiology, 133, 301–316.

Moore, D. R. (1987) Physiology of higher auditory system. British Medical Bulletin, 43, 856–870.

Moore, M. E., Linker, E., and Purcell, M. (1965) Taste sensitivity after eating: A signal detection approach. American Journal of Psychology, 78, 107–111.

Moran, J., and Desimone, R. (1985) Selective attention gates visual processing in the extrastriate cortex. Science, 229, 782–784.

Moray, N. (1959) Attention in dichotic listening: Affective cues and the influence of instructions. Quarterly Journal of Experimental Psychology, 11, 56–60.

Morel, A., and Bullier, J. (1990) Anatomical segregation of two cortical pathways in the macaque monkey. Visual Neuroscience, 7, 555–578.

Morgan, M. J. (1983) Mental rotation: A computationally plausible account of transformation through intermediate steps. Perception, 12, 203–212.

Moskowitz, H. R. (1978) Taste and food technology: Acceptability, aesthetics, and preference. In E. C. Carterette and M. P. Friedman (eds.), Handbook of perception, vol. 6A. New York: Academic Press. Pp. 157–194.

Moulton, D. G. (1974) Dynamics of cell populations in the olfactory epithelium. Annals of the New York Academy of Sciences, 237, 52–61.

Moulton, D. G. (1976) Minimum odorant concentrations detectable by the dog and their implications for olfactory receptor sensitivity. In D. Muller-Schwarze and M. M. Mozell (eds.), Chemical signals in vertebrates. New York: Plenum Press. Pp. 455–464.

Mountcastle, V. B. (1975) The view from within: Pathways to the study of perception. Johns Hopkins Medical Journal, 136, 109–131.

Mountcastle, V. B. (1984) Central nervous mechanisms in mechanoreceptive sensibility. In I. Darian-Smith (ed.), Handbook of physiology: The nervous system, III. Bethesda, Md.: American Physiological Society. Pp. 789–878.

Mountcastle, V. B., Talbot, W. H., and **Kornhuber, H. H.** (1966) The neural transformation of mechanical stimuli delivered to the monkey's hand. In A. V. S. de Reuck and J. Knight (eds.), Touch, Heat and Pain (A CIBA Foundation Symposium). London: Churchill.

Movshon, J. A. (1975) The velocity tuning of single units in cat striate cortex. Journal of Physiology, 249, 445–468.

Movshon, J. A., and **Lennie, P.** (1979) Pattern-selective adaptation in visual cortical neurones. Nature, 278, 850–852.

Mozel, M. M., Smith, B., Smith, P., Sullivan, R., and **Swender, P.** (1969) Nasal chemoreception in flavor identification. Archives of Otolaryngology, 90, 367–373.

Murphy, B. J. (1978) Pattern thresholds for moving and stationary gratings during smooth eye movement. Vision Research, 18, 521–530.

Murphy, C., and **Cain, W. S.** (1986) Odor identification: The blind are better. Physiology & Behavior, 37, 177–180.

Murphy, C., Cain, W. S., and **Bartoshuk, L. M.** (1977) Mutual action of taste and olfaction. Sensory Processes, 1, 204–211.

NRC (1989) Myopia: Prevalence and progression. Washington, D.C.: National Academy Press.

Nadel, L., Culicover, P., Cooper, L. A., and **Harnish, R. M.** (eds.). (1989) Neural connections, mental computations. Cambridge: M.I.T. Press.

Nagel, T. (1991) What is it like to be a bat? In T. Nagel, Mortal questions. Cambridge, England: Cambridge University Press. Pp. 165–180.

Naka, K. I., and **Rushton, W. A. H.** (1966) S-potentials from colour units in the retina of fish Cyprinidae. Journal of Physiology, 185, 536–555.

Nakayama, K., and **Shimojo, S.** (1990) Da Vinci stereopsis: Depth and subjective occluding contours from unpaired image points. Vision Research, 30, 1811–1825.

Nakayama, K., Shimojo, S., and **Ramachandran, V. S.** (1990) Transparency: Relation to depth, subjective contours, luminance, and neon color spreading. Perception, 19, 497–513.

Nakayama, K., Shimojo, S., and **Silverman, G. H.** (1989) Stereoscopic depth: Its relation to image segmentation, grouping and the recognition of occluded objects. Perception, 18, 55–68.

Nathans, J. (1989) The genes for color vision. Scientific American, 260, 42–49.

Navon, D. (1977) Forest before trees: The precedence of global features in visual perception. Cognitive Psychology, 9, 353–383.

Navon, D., and **Norman, J.** (1983) Does global precedence really depend on visual angle? Journal of Experimental Psychology: Human Perception and Performance, 9, 955–965.

Nawrot, M., and **Blake, R.** (1991) The interplay between stereopsis and structure from motion. Perception & Psychophysics, 49, 230–244.

Negus, V. (1956) The air-conditioning mechanism of the nose. British Medical Journal, 1, 367–371.

Nelson, J. I. (1986) Unsolved problems in the cellular basis of stereopsis. In J. D. Pettigrew, K. J. Sanderson, and W. R. Levick (eds.), Visual neuroscience. Cambridge, England: Cambridge University Press. Pp. 405–420.

Nelson, J. I., Kato, H., and **Bishop, P. O.** (1977) Discrimination of orientation and position disparities by binocularly activated neurons in cat striate cortex. Journal of Neurophysiology, 40, 260–283.

Newall, S. M., Burnham, R. W., and **Clark, J. R.** (1957) Comparison of successive with simultaneous color matching. Journal of the Optical Society of America, 47, 43–56.

Newsome, W. T., Britten, K. H., and **Movshon, J. A.** (1989) Neuronal correlates of a perceptual decision. Nature, 341, 52–54.

Newsome, W. T., and **Paré, E. B.** (1988) A selective impairment of motion perception following lesions of the middle temporal visual area (MT). Journal of Neuroscience, 8, 2201–2211.

Newton, I. (1704/1952) Opticks, or a treatise of the reflections, refractions, inflections & colours of light (4th ed.). New York: Dover.

Niemeyer, W., and **Starlinger, I.** (1981) Do the blind hear better? Investigations on auditory processing in congenital or early acquired blindness: II. Central functions. Audiology, 20, 510–515.

Nilsson, T. H., and **Nelson, T. M.** (1981) Delayed monochromatic hue matches indicate characteristics of visual memory. Journal of Experimental Psychology: Human Perception and Performance, 7, 141–150.

Nisbett, R., and **Wilson, T. D.** (1977) Telling more than we can know: Verbal reports on mental processes. Psychological Review, 84, 231–259.

Nixon, J. C., and **Glorig, A.** (1961) Noise-induced permanent threshold shift at 2000 cps and 4000 cps. Journal of the Acoustical Society of America, 33, 904–908.

Noble, W. (1983) Hearing, hearing impairment, and the audible world: A theoretical essay. Audiology, 22, 325–338.

Norcia, A. M., and **Tyler, C. W.** (1985) Spatial frequency sweep VEP: Visual acuity development during the first year of life. Vision Research, 25, 1399–1403.

Nordby, K. (1990) Vision in a complete achromat: A personal account. In R. Hess, L. Sharpe, and K. Nordby (eds.), Night vision: Basic, clinical and applied aspects. Cambridge: Cambridge University Press. Pp. 290–315.

Norman, J. F., and **Lappin, J. S.** (1992) The detection of surface curvature defined by optical motion. Perception & Psychophysics, 51, 386–396.

Ogawa, H., Yamashita, S., and **Sato, M.** (1974) Variation in gustatory nerve fiber discharge pattern with change in stimulus concentration and quality. Journal of Neurophysiology, 37, 443–457.

Oldfield, S. R., and **Parker, S. P. A.** (1984a) Acuity of sound localization: A topography of auditory space. I. Normal hearing conditions. Perception, 13, 581–600.

Oldfield, S. R., and **Parker, S. P. A.** (1984b) Acuity of sound localization: A topography of auditory space. II. Pinna cues absent. Perception, 13, 601–617.

Oldfield, S. R., and **Parker, S. P. A.** (1986) Acuity of sound localization: A topography of auditory space. III. Monaural hearing conditions. Perception, 15, 67–81.

Olson, H. F. (1967) Music, physics, and engineering (2nd ed.). New York: Dover.

Orban, G. A., Vandenbussche, E., and **Vogels, R.** (1984) Human orientation discrimination tested with long stimuli. Vision Research, 24, 121–128.

O'Shea, R. P. (1991) Thumb's rule tested: Visual angle of thumb's width is about 2 deg. Perception, 20, 415–418.

O'Shea, R. P., Blackburn, S. G., and **Ono, H.** (1993) Aerial perspective, contrast, and depth perception. Paper presented at the Association for Research in Vision and Opthalmology, Sarasota, Fla.

Otto, I., Grandguillaume, P., Boutkhil, L., Burnod, Y., and **Guigon, E.** (1992) Direct and indirect cooperation between temporal and parietal networks for invariant object recognition. Journal of Cognitive Neuroscience, 4, 35–57.

Owen, D. (1980) Camouflage and mimicry. Chicago: University of Chicago Press.

Owen, D. H., and **Machamer, P. K.** (1979) Bias-free improvement in wine discrimination. Perception, 8, 199–209.

Owens, D. A. (1984) The resting state of the eyes. American Scientist, 72, 378–387.

Owsley, C. J., Sekuler, R., and **Siemsen, D.** (1983) Contrast sensitivity throughout adulthood. Vision Research, 23, 689–699.

Packwood, J., and **Gordon, B.** (1975) Stereopsis in normal domestic cat, Siamese cat, and cat raised with alternating monocular occlusion. Journal of Neurophysiology, 38, 1485–1499.

Palmer, S. E., Rosch, E., and **Chase, P.** (1981) Canonical perspective and the perception of objects. In J.

Long and A. Baddeley (eds.), Attention and performance, vol. 9. Hillsdale, N.J.: Erlbaum. Pp. 135–151.

Pangborn, R. M. (1960) Influence of color on the discrimination of sweetness. American Journal of Psychology, 73, 229–238.

Pantle, A., and **Petersik, J. T.** (1979) Factors controlling the competing sensations produced by a bistable stroboscopic motion display. Vision Research, 19, 143–154.

Pantle, A., and **Picciano, L.** (1976) A multistable movement display: Evidence for two separate motion systems in human vision. Science, 193, 500–502.

Parker, D. E. (1980) The vestibular apparatus. Scientific American, 243, 118–135.

Pascual-Leone, A., and **Torres, F.** (1993) Plasticity of the sensorimotor cortex representation of the reading finger in Braille. Brain.

Paterson, C. A. (1979) Crystalline lens. In R. E. Records (ed.), Physiology of the human eye and visual system. New York: Harper & Row. Pp. 232–260.

Pearlman, A. L., Birch, J., and **Meadows, J. C.** (1979) Cerebral color blindness: An acquired defect in hue discrimination. Annals of Neurology, 5, 253–261.

Peli, E., Goldstein, R. B., Young, G. M., Trempe, C. L., and **Buzney, S. M.** (1991) Image enhancement for the visually impaired. Investigative Opthalmology and Visual Science, 32, 2337–2350.

Pelli, D. G., Robson, J. G., and **Wilkins, A. J.** (1988) The design of a new letter chart for measuring contrast sensitivity. Clinical Vision Science, 2, 187–199.

Penfield, W., and **Faulk, M. E.** (1955) The insuyla. Further observation on its function. Brain, 78, 445–470.

Penfield, W., and **Perrot, P.** (1963) The brain's record of auditory and visual experience. Brain, 86, 595–696.

Perky, C. W. (1910) An experimental study of imagination. American Journal of Psychology, 21, 422–452.

Perrett, D. I., Oram, M. W., Harries, M. H., Bevan, R., Hietanen, J. K., Benson, P. J., and **Thomas, S.** (1991) Viewer-centered and object-centered coding of heads in the macaque temporal cortex. Experimental Brain Research, 86, 159–173.

Perrott, D. R., Ambarsoom, H., and **Tucker, J.** (1987) Changes in head position as a measure of auditory localization performance: Auditory psychomotor coordination under monaural and binaural listening conditions. Journal of the Acoustical Society of America, 82, 1637–1645.

Peterhans, E., and **von der Heydt, R.** (1991) Subjective contours—Bridging the gap between psychophysics and physiology. Trends in Neurosciences, 14, 112–119.

Petersen, S. E., Robinson, D. L., and **Morris, J. D.** (1987) Contributions of the pulvinar to visual spatial attention. Neuropsychology, 25, 97–105.

Petersik, J. T. (1978) Possible role of transient and sustained visual mechanisms in the determination of similarity judgments. Perceptual and Motor Skills, 47, 683–698.

Peterson, S. E., Fox, P. T., Posner, M. I., Mintun, M., and Raichle, M. E. (1988) Positron emission tomographic studies of the cortical anatomy of single word processing. Nature, 331, 585–589.

Pfaffmann, C. (1955) Gustatory nerve impulses in rat, cat, and rabbit. Journal of Neurophysiology, 18, 429–440.

Pfaffmann, C., and Bartoshuk, L. M. (1989) Psychophysical mapping of a human case of left unilateral ageusia. Chemical Senses, 14, 738.

Pfaffmann, C., and Bartoshuk, L. M. (1990) Taste loss due to herpes zoster oticus: An update after 19 months. Chemical Senses, 15, 657–658.

Phillips, D. P., and Farmer, M. E. (1990) Acquired word deafness, and the temporal grain of sound representation in the primary auditory cortex. Behavioural Brain Research, 40, 85–94.

Phillips, J. R., Johansson, R. S., and Johnson, K. O. (1992) Responses of human mechanoreceptive afferents to embossed dot arrays scanned across fingerpad skin. Journal of Neuroscience, 12, 827–839.

Pick, A. D. (1979) Listening to melodies: Perceiving events. In A. D. Pick (ed.), Perception and its development: A tribute to Eleanor J. Gibson. Hillsdale, N.J.: Erlbaum. Pp. 145–165.

Pirenne, M. H. (1967) Vision and the eye (2nd ed.). London: Chapman & Hall.

Pirenne, M. H. (1970) Optics, painting, and photography. Cambridge, England: Cambridge University Press.

Pittenger, J. B., and Shaw, R. E. (1975) Aging faces as viscal-elastic events: Implications for a theory of nonrigid shape perception. Journal of Experimental Psychology: Human Perception and Performance, 1, 374–382.

Pittenger, J. B., Shaw, R. E., and Mark, L. S. (1979) Perceptual information for the age level of faces as a higher-order invariant of growth. Journal of Experimental Psychology: Human Perception and Performance, 5, 478–493.

Platt, J. R., and Racine, R. J. (1985) Effect of frequency, timbre, experience, and feedback on musical tuning skills. Perception & Psychophysics, 38, 543–553.

Poggio, G. F., and Fischer, B. (1978) Binocular interaction and depth sensitivity in the striate and prestriate cortex of the behaving monkey. Journal of Neurophysiology, 40, 1392–1405.

Poggio, T. (1984) Vision by man and machine. Scientific American, 250, 106–116.

Poggio, T., Verri, A., and Torre, V. (1991) Green theorems and qualitative properties of the optical flow (Memo No. 1289). M.I.T., Artificial Intelligence Laboratory, Cambridge.

Pokorny, J., Graham, C. H., and Lanson, R. N. (1968) Effect of wavelength on foveal grating acuity. Journal of the Optical Society of America, 58, 1410–1414.

Pollack, I., and Rose, M. (1967) Effect of head movement on the localization of sounds in the equatorial plane. Perception & Psychophysics, 2, 591–596.

Polyak, S. L. (1941) The retina. Chicago: University of Chicago Press.

Pomerantz, J. R. (1981) Perceptual organization in information processing. In M. Kubovy and J. R. Pomerantz (eds.), Perceptual organization. Hillsdale, N.J.: Erlbaum. Pp. 141–180.

Pomerantz, J. R., and Kubovy, M. (1986) Theoretical approaches to perceptual organization. In K. R. Boff, L. Kaufman, and J. P. Thomas (eds.), Handbook of perception and human performance. New York: John Wiley & Sons. Pp. 36.1–34.36.

Pons, T. P., Garraghty, P. E., Friedman, D. P., and Mishkin, M. (1987) Physiological evidence for serial processing in somatosensory cortex. Science, 237, 417–420.

Porter, R. H. (1991) Human reproduction and the mother-infant relationship. In T. V. Getchell, R. L. Doty, L. M. Bartoshuk, and J. B. Snow (eds.), Smell and taste in health and disease. New York: Raven Press. Pp. 429–444.

Posner, M. I. (1992) Attention as a cognitive and neural system. Current Directions in Psychological Science, 1, 11–14.

Potter, M. C. (1966) On perceptual recognition. In J. S. Bruner (ed.), Studies in cognitive growth. New York: John Wiley & Sons. Pp. 103–134.

Prinz, W. (1992) Why don't we perceive our brain states? European Journal of Cognitive Psychology, 4, 1–20.

Prinzmetal, W. (1992) The word-superiority effect does not require a t-scope. Perception & Psychophysics, 51, 473–484.

Pritchard, R. M. (1961) Stabilized images on the retina. Scientific American, 204, 72–78.

Pritchard, R. M., Heron, W., and Hebb, D. O. (1960) Visual perception approached by the method of stabilized images. Canadian Journal of Psychology, 14, 67–77.

Pritchard, T. C. (1991) The primate gustatory system. In T. V. Getchell, R. L. Doty, L. M. Bartoshuk, and J. B. Snow (eds.), Smell and taste in health and disease. New York: Raven Press. Pp. 109–126.

Proust, M. (1928) Swann's way. New York: Random House.

Puccetti, R., and Dykes, R. W. (1978) Sensory cortex and the mind-brain problem. Behaviour and Brain, 1, 337–344.

Pylyshyn, Z. W. (1981) The imagery debate: Analogue media versus tacit knowledge. Psychological Review, 88, 16–45.

Ramachandran, V. S. (1988) Perceiving shape from shading. Scientific American, 259, 76–83.

Ramachandran, V. S. (1992) Blind spots. Scientific American, 266, 86–91.

Ramachandran, V. S., and **Anstis, S. M.** (1986) The perception of apparent motion. Scientific American, 254, 102–109.

Ramachandran, V. S., and **Cavanagh, P.** (1987) Motion capture anisotrophy. Vision Research, 27, 97–106.

Ramirez, I. (1990) Why do sugars taste good? Neuroscience & Biobehavioral Reviews, 14, 125–134.

Randolph, M., and **Semmes, J.** (1974) Behavioral consequences of selective subtotal ablations in the postcentral gyrus of the Macaca mulatta. Brain Research, 70, 55–70.

Ratliff, F. (1965) Mach bands: Quantitative studies on neural networks in the retina. San Francisco: Holden-Day.

Ratliff, F. (1972) Contour and contrast. Scientific American, 226, 90–101.

Ratliff, F. (1976) On the psychophysical basis of universal color names. Proceedings of American Philosophical Society, 120, 311–330.

Ratliff, F. (1984) Why Mach bands are not seen at the edges of a step. Vision Research, 24, 163–165.

Rayner, K. (1978) Eye movements in reading and information processing. Psychological Bulletin, 85, 618–660.

Rayner, K., and **Bertera, J. H.** (1979) Reading without a fovea. Science, 206, 468–469.

Rayner, K., Inhoff, A. W., Morrison, R. E., Slowiaczek, M. L., and **Bertera, J. H.** (1981) Masking of foveal and parafoveal vision during eye fixations in reading. Journal of Experimental Psychology: Human Perception and Performance, 7, 167–179.

Rayner, K., and **Pollatsek, A.** (1987) Eye movements in reading: A tutorial review. In M. Coltheart (ed.), Attention and performance, vol. 12: The psychology of reading. Hove, England: Erlbaum. Pp. 327–362.

Reagan, R. (1990) An American Life. New York: Simon & Schuster.

Reber, A. S. (1992) The cognitive unconscious: An evolutionary perspective. Consciousness and Cognition, 1, 93–133.

Recanzone, G. H., Jenkins, W. M., Hradek, G. T., and **Merzenich, M. M.** (1992) Progressive improvement in discriminative abilities in adult owl monkeys performing a tactile frequency discrimination task. Journal of Neurophysiology, 67, 1015–1030.

Recanzone, G. H., Merzenich, M. M., Jenkins, W. M., Grajski, K. A., and **Dinse, H. R.** (1992) Topographic reorganization of the hand representation in cortical area 3b of owl monkeys trained in a frequency discrimination task. Journal of Neurophysiology, 67, 1031–1056.

Recanzone, G. H., Schreiner, C. E., and **Merzenich, M. M.** (1993) Plasticity in the frequency representation in the primary auditory cortex following discrimination training in adult owl monkeys. Journal of Neuroscience.

Rechtschaffen, A., and **Mednick, S.** (1955) The autokinetic word technique. Journal of Abnormal and Social Psychology, 51, 346.

Records, R. E. (1979a) Eyebrows and eyelids. In R. E. Records (ed.), Physiology of the human eye and visual system. New York: Harper & Row. Pp. 1–24.

Records, R. E. (1979b) Retina: Metabolism and photochemistry. In R. E. Records (ed.), Physiology of the human eye and visual system. New York: Harper & Row. Pp. 296–318.

Rees, J. and **Botwinick, J.** (1971) Detection and decision factors in auditory behavior of the elderly. Journal of Gerontology, 26, 133–136.

Reeves, A. (1982) Letter to the editors. Vision Research, 22, 711.

Regan, D. (1982) Visual information channeling in normal and disordered vision. Psychological Review, 89, 407–444.

Regan, D. (1988) Low contrast letter charts and sinewave grating tests in ophthalmological and neurological disorders. Clinical Vision Science, 2, 235–250.

Regan, D. (1992) Visual judgements and misjudgements in cricket, and the art of flight. Perception, 21, 91–116.

Regan, D., Beverley, K. I., and **Cynader, M.** (1979) The visual perception of motion in depth. Scientific American, 241, 136–151.

Rehn, T. (1978) Perceived odor intensity as a function of airflow through the nose. Sensory Processes, 2, 198–205.

Reichardt, W. (1961) Autocorrelation, a principle for the evaluation of sensory information by the central nervous system. In W. A. Rosenblith (ed.), Sensory communication. New York: John Wiley & Sons. Pp. 303–318.

Reicher, G. M. (1969) Perceptual recognition as a function of meaningfulness of stimulus material. Journal of Experimental Psychology, 81, 275–280.

Reid, T. (1813/1970) An inquiry into the human mind. Chicago: University of Chicago Press.

Rezek, D. L. (1987) Olfactory deficits as a neurologic sign in dementia of the Alzheimer type. Archives of Neurology, 44, 1030–1032.

Richards, W. (1971) The fortification illusions of migraines. Scientific American, 224, 88–98.

Richardson, J. T. E., and **Zucco, G. M.** (1989) Cognition and olfaction: A review. Psychological Bulletin, 105, 352–360.

Rieser, J. J., Ashmead, D. H., Talor, C. R., and **Youngquist, G. A.** (1990) Visual perception and the guidance of locomotion without vision of previously seen targets. Perception, 19, 675–689.

Riggs, L. A., Ratliff, F., Cornsweet, J. C., and **Cornsweet, T. N.** (1953) The disappearance of steadily fixated visual test objects. Journal of the Optical Society of America, 43, 495–501.

Riggs, L. A., Volkmann, F. C., and **Moore, R. K.** (1981) Suppression of the blackout due to blinks. Vision Research, 21, 1075–1079.

Ripoll, H., and **Fleurance, P.** (1988) What does keeping one's eye on the ball mean? Ergonomics, 31, 1647–1654.

Ripps, H. (1982) Night blindness revisited: From man to molecules. Investigative Ophthalmology & Visual Science, 23, 588–609.

Ritter, M. (1984) Size constancy as a function of fixation distance and retinal disparity. In L. Spillmann and B. R. Wooten (eds.), Sensory experience, adaptation, and perception. Hillsdale, N.J.: Erlbaum. Pp. 189–200.

Rizzo, M., Nawrot, M., Blake, R., and **Damasio, A.** (1992) A human visual disorder resembling Area V4 dysfunction in the monkey. Neurology, 42, 1175–1180.

Robson, J. G. (1966) Spatial and temporal contrast-sensitivity functions of the visual system. Journal of the Optical Society of America, 56, 1141–1142.

Rock, I., and **Mitchener, K.** (1992) Further evidence of failure of reversal of ambiguous figures by uninformed subjects. Perception, 21, 39–45.

Rock, I., and **Palmer, S.** (1990) The legacy of Gestalt psychology. Scientific American, 263, 84–90.

Rodin, J., Bartoshuk, L., Peterson, C., and **Schank, D.** (1990) Bulimia and taste: Possible interactions. Journal of Abnormal Psychology, 99, 32–39.

Rogers, B. J., and **Collett, T. S.** (1989) The appearance of surfaces specified by motion parallax and binocular disparity. Quarterly Journal of Experimental Psychology, 41A, 697–717.

Rogers, B. J., and **Graham, M. E.** (1979) Motion parallax as an independent cue for depth perception. Perception, 8, 125–134.

Rogers, B. J., and **Graham, M. E.** (1984) Aftereffects from motion parallax and stereoscopic depth: Similarities and interactions. In L. Spillmann and B. R. Wooten (eds.), Sensory experience, adaptation, and perception. Hillsdale, N.J.: Erlbaum. Pp. 603–619.

Rogowitz, B. (1984) The breakdown of size constancy under stroboscopic illumination. In L. Spillmann and B. R. Wooten (eds.), Sensory experience, adaptation, and perception. Hillsdale, N.J.: Erlbaum. Pp. 201–214.

Roland, P. E. (1976) Focal increase of cerebral blood flow during stereognostic testing in man. Archives of Neurology, 33, 551–558.

Roland, P. E. and **Mortenson, E.** (1987) Somatosensory detection of microgeometry, macrogeometry and kinesthesia in man. Brain Research Reviews, 12, 1–42.

Rolls, B. (1986) Sensory-specific satiety. Nutrition Reviews, 44, 93–101.

Rolls, B., Van Duijvenvoorde, P. M., and **Rolls, E. T.** (1984) Pleasantness changes and food intake in a varied four-course meal. Appetite, 5, 337–348.

Ronchi, V. (1970) The nature of light: An historical survey. Cambridge: Harvard University Press.

Roper, S. D. (1992) The microphysiology of peripheral taste organs. Journal of Neuroscience, 12, 1127–1134.

Rose, J. E., Brugge, J. F., Anderson, D. J., and **Hind, J. E.** (1967) Phase-locked response to low-frequency tones in single auditory nerve fibers of the squirrel monkey. Journal of Neurophysiology, 30, 769–793.

Rosenfeld, A. (1988) Computer vision. Advances in Computers, 27, 265–308.

Rozin, P. (1978) The use of characteristic flavorings in human culinary practice. In C. M. Apt (ed.), Flavor: Its chemical, behavioral, and commercial aspects. Proceedings of the Arthur D. Little Symposium. Boulder, Colo.: Westview Press. Pp. 101–128.

Rozin, P. (1979) Preference and affect in food selection. In J. H. A. Kroeze (ed.), Preference behavior and chemoreception. London: Information Retrieval. Pp. 289–302.

Rozin, P. (1982) "Taste-smell confusions" and the duality of the olfactory sense. Perception & Psychophysics, 31, 397–401.

Rozin, P. (1990) Social and moral aspects of food and eating. In I. Rock (ed.), The legacy of Solomon Asch: Essays in cognition and social psychology. Hillsdale, N.J.: Erlbaum. Pp. 97–110.

Rubert, S. L., Hollender, M. H., and **Mehrhof, E. G.** (1961) Olfactory hallucination. Archives of General Psychiatry, 5, 121–126.

Rubin, M. L., and **Walls, G. L.** (1969) Fundamentals of visual science. Springfield, Ill.: Thomas.

Rucker, C. W. (1971) A history of the ophthalmoscope. Rochester, Minn.: Whiting.

Rueckl, J. G., Cave, K. R., and **Kosslyn, S. M.** (1989) Why are "what" and "where" processed by separate cortical systems? A computational approach. Journal of Cognitive Neuroscience, 1, 171–186.

Runeson, S., and **Frykholm, G.** (1983) Kinematic specifications of dynamics as an informational basis for person-and-action perception: Expectation, gender recognition, and deceptive intention. Journal of Experimental Psychology: General, 112, 585–615.

Rushton, W. A. H. (1965) Visual adaptation. The Ferrier Lecture. Proceedings of the Royal Society of London, Series B, 162, 20–46.

Rushton, W. A. H. (1979) King Charles II and the blind spot. Vision Research, 19, 225.

Russel, M. J. (1976) Human olfactory communication. Nature, 260, 520–522.

Russell, I. J. (1987) The physiology of the organ of Corti. British Medical Bulletin, 43, 802–820.

Russell, J. A., and **Ward, L. M.** (1982) Environmental psychology. Annual Review of Psychology, 33, 651–688.

Rzeszotarski, M. S., Royer, F. L., and **Gilmore, G. C.** (1983) An introduction to two-dimensional fast Fourier transforms and their applications. Behavior Research Methods and Instrumentation, 15, 308–318.

Sacks, O. (1985) The man who mistook his wife for a hat, and other clinical tales. New York: Summit Books.

Safire, W. (1979) Mondegreens: I led the pigeons to the flag. New York Times Magazine, May 27, Pp. 9–10.

Salzman, C. D., Murasugi, C. M., Britten, K. H., and **Newsome, W. T.** (1992) Microstimulation in visual Area MT: Effects on direction discrimination performance. Journal of Neuroscience, 12, 2331–2355.

Sample, P. A., Boynton, R. M., and **Weinreb, R. N.** (1988) Isolating the color vision loss in primary open-angle glaucoma. American Journal of Ophthalmology, 106, 686–691.

Samuel, A. G. (1983) We really is worse than you or them, and so are ma and pa: Reply. Journal of Experimental Psychology: Human Perception and Performance, 9, 321–322.

Samuel, A. G. (1989) Insights from a failure of selective adaptation: Syllable-initial and syllable-final consonants are different. Perception & Psychophysics, 45, 485–493.

Savelsbergh, G. J. P., Whiting, H. T. A., and **Bootsma, R. J.** (1991) Grasping tau. Journal of Experimental Psychology: Human Perception and Performance, 17, 315–322.

Schaal, B. (1988) Olfaction in infants and children: Developmental and functional perspectives. Chemical Senses, 13, 145–190.

Schab, F. R. (1991) Odor memory: Taking stock. Psychological Bulletin, 109, 242–251.

Schacter, D. L. (1989) On the relation between memory and consciousness: Dissociable interactions and conscious experience. In H. L. Roediger III and F. I. M. Craik (eds.), Varieties of memory and consciousness: Essays in honor of Endel Tulving. Hillsdale, N.J.: Erlbaum. Pp. 355–389.

Schall, J. D. (1991) Neural basis of saccadic eye movements in primates. In A. G. Leventhal (ed.), The neural basis of visual function. London: Macmillan. Pp. 388–442.

Scharf, B., and **Buus, S.** (1986) Audition I: Stimulus, physiology, thresholds. In K. R. Boff, L. Kaufman, and J. P. Thomas (eds.), Handbook of perception and human performance. New York: John Wiley & Sons. Pp. 14.1–14.71.

Scharf, B., Quigley, S., Aoki, C., Peachey, N., and

Reeves, A. (1987) Focused auditory attention and frequency selectivity. Perception & Psychophysics, 42, 215–223.

Schechter, P. J., and **Henkin, R. I.** (1974) Abnormalities of taste and smell after head trauma. Journal of Neurology, Neurosurgery, and Psychiatry, 37, 802–810.

Schiff, W. (1965) Perception of impending collision. Psychological Monographs, 79, 1–26.

Schiffman, H. R. (1967) Size estimation of familiar objects under informative and reduced conditions of viewing. American Journal of Psychology, 80, 229–235.

Schiffman, S. S. (1974) Physiochemical correlates of olfactory quality. Science, 185, 112–117.

Schiffman, S. S. (1983) Taste and smell in disease. New England Journal of Medicine, 308, 1275–1279, 1337–1343.

Schiffman, S. S., and **Dackis, C.** (1975) Taste of nutrients: Amino acids, vitamins, and fatty acids. Perception & Psychophysics, 17, 140–146.

Schiffman, S. S., and **Erickson, R. P.** (1980) The issue of primary tastes versus a taste continuum. Neuroscience & Biobehavioral Reviews, 4, 109–117.

Schiffman, S. S., Reynolds, M. L., and **Young, F. L.** (1981) Introduction to multidimensional scaling. New York: Academic Press.

Schiller, P. H., and **Koerner, F.** (1971) Discharge characteristics of single units in superior colliculus of the alert rhesus monkey. Journal of Neurophysiology, 34, 920–936.

Schiller, P. H., and **Logothetis, N. K.** (1990) The color-opponent and broad-band channels in the primate visual system. Trends in Neurosciences, 13, 392–398.

Schiller, P. H., Sandell, J. H., and **Maunsell, J. H. R.** (1986) Functions of the ON and OFF channels of the visual system. Nature, 322, 824–825.

Schlagel, R. H. (1984) A reasonable reply to Hume's scepticism. British Journal of the Philosophy of Science, 35, 359–374.

Schlagger, B. L., and **O'Leary, D. D. M.** (1991) Potential of visual cortex to develop an array of functional units to somatosensory cortex. Science, 252, 1556–1560.

Schneider, G. E. (1969) Two visual systems. Science, 163, 895–902.

Schneider, R. A., and **Wolf, S.** (1955) Olfactory perception thresholds for citral utilizing a new type of olfactorium. Journal of Applied Physiology, 8, 337–342.

Schultz, G., and **Melzack, R.** (1991) The Charles Bonnet syndrome: "Phantom visual images." Perception, 20, 809–826.

Schwartz, B. S., Doty, R. L., Monroe, C., Frye, R., and **Barker, S.** (1989) Olfactory function in chemical workers exposed to acrylate and methacrylate vapors. American Journal of Public Health, 79, 613–618.

Scott, A. B. (1979) Ocular motility. In R. E. Records (ed.), Physiology of the human eye and visual system. New York: Harper & Row. Pp. 577–642.

Scott, T. R., and **Plata-Salaman, C. R.** (1991) Coding of taste quality. In T. V. Getchell, R. L. Doty, L. M. Bartoshuk, and J. B. Snow, Jr. (eds.), Smell and taste in health and disease. New York: Raven Press. Pp. 345–368.

Seagraves, M. A., Goldberg, M. E., Deng, S. Y., Bruce, C. J., Ungerleider, L. G., and **Mishkin, M.** (1987) The role of striate cortex in the guidance of eye movements in the monkey. Journal of Neuroscience, 7, 776–794.

Searle, J. (1987) Minds and brains without programs. In C. Blakemore and S. Greenfield (eds.), Mindwaves. Oxford: Blackwell. Pp. 209–233.

Seashore, C. E. (1938) Psychology of music. New York: McGraw-Hill.

Segal, S. J., and **Fusella, V.** (1970) Influence of imaged pictures and sounds on detection of visual and auditory signals. Journal of Experimental Psychology, 83, 458–464.

Sekuler, A. B., and **Palmer, S. E.** (1992) Perception of partly occluded objects: A microgenetic analysis. Journal of Experimental Psychology: General, 121, 95–111.

Sekuler, R. W. (1965) Spatial and temporal determinants of visual backward masking. Journal of Experimental Psychology, 70, 401–406.

Sekuler, R., and **Ganz, L.** (1963) A new aftereffect of seen movement with a stabilized retinal image. Science, 139, 1146–1148.

Sekuler, R., Owsley, C. J., and **Berenberg, R.** (1986) Contrast sensitivity during provoked visual impairment in multiple sclerosis. Ophthalmic and Physiological Optics, 6, 229–232.

Sergent, J., Ohta, S., and **MacDonald, B.** (1992) Functional neuroanatomy of face and object processing. Brain, 115, 15–36.

Sergent, J., and **Poncet, M.** (1990) From covert to overt recognition of faces in a prosopagnostic patient. Brain, 113, 989–1004.

Sergent, J. A., and **Villemure, J.-G.** (1989) Prosopagnosia in a right hemispherectomized patient. Brain, 112, 975–995.

Seyfarth, R. M., and **Cheney, D. L.** (1984) The natural vocalizations of non-human primates. Trends in Neurosciences, 7, 66–73.

Shankland, R. S. (1972) The development of architectural acoustics. American Scientist, 60, 201–209.

Shannahoff-Khalsa, D. (1986) Breathing for the brain. American Health, 5, 16–18.

Shapley, R., and **Perry, V. H.** (1986) Cat and monkey retinal ganglion cells and their visual functional roles. Trends in Neurosciences, 9, 229–235.

Sharma, S., and **Moskowitz, H.** (1972) Effect of marijuana on the visual autokinetic phenomenon. Perceptual and Motor Skills, 35, 891–894.

Sharpe, D. T. (1974) The psychology of color and design. Chicago: Nelson-Hall.

Sharpe, L. T., and **Nordby, K.** (1990) Total colourblindness: An introduction. In R. F. Hess, L. T. Sharpe, and K. Nordby (eds.), Night vision: Basic, clinical and applied aspects. Cambridge, England: Cambridge University Press. Pp. 253–289.

Shaw, E. A. G. (1974) Transformation of sound pressure level from the free field to the eardrum in the horizontal plane. Journal of the Acoustical Society of America, 56, 1848–1861.

Shaw, R., and **Bransford, J.** (1977) Introduction: Psychological approaches to the problem of knowledge. In R. Shaw and J. Bransford (eds.), Perceiving, acting, and knowing. Hillsdale, N.J.: Erlbaum. Pp. 1–39.

Sheehan, W. (1988) Planets and perception: Telescopic views and interpretations, 1609–1909. Tempe, Ariz: University of Arizona Press.

Shepard, R. N. (1981) Psychophysical complementarity. In M. Kubovy and J. R. Pomerantz (eds.), Perceptual organization. Hillsdale, N.J.: Erlbaum. Pp. 279–341.

Shepard, R. N. and **Cooper, L. A.** (1982) Mental images and their transformations. Cambridge: M.I.T. Press.

Shepherd, G. M. (1988) Neurobiology (2nd ed.). New York: Oxford University Press.

Shepherd, G. M., and **Firestein, S.** (1991) Making scents of olfactory transduction. Current Biology, 1, 204–206.

Sherrick, C. E., and **Cholewiak, R. W.** (1986) Cutaneous sensitivity. In K. Boff, L. Kaufman, and J. Thomas (eds.), Handbook of perception and human performance, vol. 1. New York: Wiley-Interscience. Pp. 12.1–12.58.

Shiffrar, M., and **Freyd, J. J.** (1990) Apparent motion of the human body. Psychological Science, 1, 257–264.

Siegel, J. A., and **Siegel, W.** (1977) Absolute identification of notes and intervals by musicians. Perception & Psychophysics, 21, 143–152.

Siegel, R. K. (1984) Hostage hallucinations: Visual imagery induced by isolation and life-threatening stress. Journal of Nervous and Mental Disease, 172, 264–272.

Siegel, R. M., and **Andersen, R. A.** (1990) The perception of structure from visual motion in monkey and man. Journal of Cognitive Neuroscience, 2, 306–319.

Sillar, K. T., and **Roberts, A.** (1988) A neuronal mechanism for sensory gating during locomotion in a vertebrate. Nature, 331, 262–265.

Simmons, F. B., Epley, J. M., Lummis, R. C., Gutt-

man, N., Frishkopf, L. S., Harmon, L. D., and Zwicker, E. (1965) Auditory nerve: Electrical stimulation in man. Science, 148, 104–106.

Sinnott, J., Beecher, M., Moody, D., and Stebbins, W. (1976) Speech and sound discrimination by monkeys and humans. Journal of the Acoustical Society of America, 60, 687–695.

Skinner, B. F. (1957) Verbal behavior. New York: Appleton-Century-Crofts.

Smith, M., Smith, L. G., and Levinson, B. (1982) The use of smell in differential diagnosis. Lancet, 2, 1452.

Smith-Swintosky, V. L., Plata-Salaman, C. R., and Scott, T. R. (1991) Gustatory neural coding in the monkey cortex: Stimulus quality. Journal of Neurophysiology, 66, 1156–1165.

Snyder, A. W., and Barlow, H. B. (1988) Revealing the artist's touch. Nature, 331, 117–118.

Snyder, S. H., Sklar, P. B., Hwang, P. M., and Pevsner, J. (1989) Molecular mechanisms of olfaction. Trends in Neurosciences, 12, 35–38.

Sorensen, P. (1992) Morphing magic. Computer Graphics World, 15, 36–43.

Southall, J. P. C. (1937/1961) Introduction to physiological optics. New York: Dover.

Sparks, D. L. (1988) Neural cartography: Sensory and motor maps in the superior colliculus. Brain, Behavior and Evolution, 31, 49–56.

Sparks, D. L., and Nelson, J. S. (1987) Sensory and motor maps in the mammalian superior colliculus. Trends in Neurosciences, 10, 312–317.

Sperling, G., Budiansky, J., Spivak, J. G., and Johnson, M. C. (1971) Extremely rapid visual search: The maximum rate of scanning letters for the presence of a numeral. Science, 174, 307–311.

Sperry, R. W. (1980) Mind-brain interaction: Mentalism, yes; dualism, no. Neurosciences, 5, 195–206.

Spillmann, L. (1971) Foveal perceptive fields in the human visual system measured with simultaneous contrast in grids and bars. Pflügers Archiv Gesamte Physiologie, 326, 281–299.

Spitzer, H., Desimone, R., and Moran, J. (1988) Increased attention enhances both behavioral and neuronal performance. Science, 240, 338–340.

Stabell, U., Stabell, B., and Fugelli, A. (1992) Mechanisms of long-term dark adaptation. Scandinavian Journal of Psychology, 33, 12–19.

Starlinger, I., and Niemeyer, W. (1981) Do the blind hear better? Investigations on auditory processing in congenital or early acquired blindness: I. Peripheral functions. Audiology, 20, 503–509.

Steinbach, M. J., and Money, K. E. (1973) Eye movements of the owl. Vision Research, 13, 889–891.

Steinman, R. M. (1976) Role of eye movements in maintaining a phenomenally clear and stable world. In R. A. Monty and J. W. Senders (eds.), Eye movements and psychological processes. Hillsdale, N.J.: Erlbaum. Pp. 121–154.

Steinman, R. M., Cushman, W. B., and Martins, A. J. (1982) The precision of gaze. Human Neurobiology, 1, 97–109.

Steinman, R. M., Kowler, E., and Collewijn, H. (1990) New directions for oculomotor research. Vision Research, 30, 1845–1864.

Steinschneider, M., Arezzo, J., and Vaughn, H. G. (1982) Speech-evoked activity in the auditory radiations and cortex of the awake monkey. Brain Research, 252, 353–365.

Stevens, J. C. (1979) Thermo-tactile interactions: Some influences of temperature on touch. In D. R. Kenshalo (ed.), Sensory function of the skin of humans. New York: Plenum Press.

Stevens, J. C. (1992) Aging and spatial acuity of touch. Journal of Gerontology: Psychological Sciences, 47, 35–40.

Stevens, J. C., and Cain, W. S. (1986) Aging and the perception of nasal irritation. Physiology & Behavior, 37, 323–328.

Stevens, J. K., Emerson, R. C., Gerstein, G. L., Kallos, T., Neufield, G. R., Nichols, C. W., and Rosenquist, A. C. (1976) Paralysis of the awake human: Visual perception. Vision Research, 16, 93–98.

Stevens, K. A. (1981) The information content of texture gradients. Biological Cybernetics, 42, 95–105.

Stevens, K. A. (1983) Evidence relating subjective contours and interpretations involving interposition. Perception, 12, 491–500.

Stevens, K. A., and Brookes, A. (1988) Integrating stereopsis with monocular interpretations of planar surfaces. Vision Research, 28, 371–386.

Stevens, S. S. (1951) Mathematics, measurement, and psychophysics. In S. S. Stevens (ed.), Handbook of experimental psychology. New York: John Wiley & sons. Pp. 1–49.

Stevens, S. S. (1956) The direct estimation of sensory magnitude—Loudness. American Journal of Psychology, 69, 1–25.

Stevens, S. S. (1960) Psychophysics of sensory function. American Scientist, 48, 226–252.

Stevens, S. S. (1975) Psychophysics: An introduction to its perceptual, neural, and social prospects. New York: John Wiley & Sons.

Stevens, S. S., and Guirao, M. (1967) Loudness functions under inhibition. Perception & Psychophysics, 2, 459–465.

Stevens, S. S., and Newman, E. B. (1934) The localization of pure tone. Proceedings of the National Academy of Sciences, 20, 593–596.

Stevens, S. S., and Warshofsky, F. (1965) Sound and hearing. Chicago: Time-Life Books.

Stone, H., and **Pryor, G.** (1967) Some properties of the olfactory system of man. Perception & Psychophysics, 2, 516–518.

Stouffer, J. L., and **Tyler, R. S.** (1990) Characterization of tinnitus by tinnitus patients. Journal of Speech and Hearing Disorders, 55, 439–453.

Stypulkowski, P. H. (1990) Mechanisms of salicylate ototoxicity. Hearing Research, 46, 113–146.

Suga, N. (1990) Biosonar and neural computation in bats. Scientific American, 262, 60–68.

Summerfield, Q. (1975) How a full account of segmental perception depends on prosody and vice versa. In A. Cohen and S. G. Nooteboom (eds.), Structure and process in speech perception. New York: Springer-Verlag. Pp. 51–68.

Summerfield, Q. (1992) Lipreading and audio-visual speech perception. Philosophical Transactions of the Royal Society of London, B, 335, 71–78.

Sur, M., Garraghty, P. E., and **Roe, A. W.** (1988) Experimentally induced visual projects into auditory thalamus and cortex. Science, 242, 1437–1441.

Swets, J. A. (1973) The relative operating characteristic in psychology. Science, 182, 990–1000.

Swets, J. A. (1979) ROC analysis applied to the evaluation of medical imaging techniques. Investigative Radiology, 14, 109–121.

Swets, J. A., Tanner, W. P., Jr., and **Birdsall, T. G.** (1961) Decision processes in perception. Psychological Review, 68, 301–340.

Swift, J. (1726/1890) Gulliver's travels. London: George Routledge and Sons.

Symonds, C., and **MacKenzie, I.** (1957) Bilateral loss of vision from cerebral infarction. Brain, 80, 415–455.

Talamo, B. R., Rudel, R., Kosik, K. S., Lee, V. M.-Y., Adelman, L., and **Kauer, J. S.** (1989) Pathological changes in olfactory neurons in patients with Alzheimer's disease. Nature, 337, 736–739.

Talbot, J. D., Marrett, S., Evans, A. C., Meyer, E., Bushnell, M. C., and **Duncan, G. H.** (1991) Multiple representations of pain in human cerebral cortex. Science, 251, 1355–1358.

Tanaka, K., Fukada, Y., and **Saito, H.** (1989) Underlying mechanisms of the response specificity of expansion/contraction and rotation cells in the dorsal part of the medial superior temporal area of the macaque monkey. Journal of Neurophysiology, 62, 642–656.

Tanaka, K., and **Saito, H.** (1989) Analysis of motion of the visual field by direction, expansion/contraction, and rotation cells clustered in the dorsal part of the medial superior temporal area of the macaque monkey. Journal of Neurophysiology, 62, 626–641.

Tanaka, Y., Kamo, T., Yoshida, M., and **Yamadori, A.** (1991) So-called cortical deafness. Brain, 114, 2385–2401.

Tartter, V. C. (1991) Identifiability of vowels and speakers from whispered syllables. Perception & Psychophysics, 49, 365–372.

Taylor, C. A. (1965) The physics of musical sounds. New York: Elsevier.

Taylor, M. M., and **Williams, E.** (1966) Acoustic trauma in the sports hunter. Laryngoscope, 76, 969–979.

Taylor, W. (1988) Biological effects of the hand-arm vibration syndrome: Historical perspective and current research. Journal of the Acoustical Society of America, 83, 415–422.

Teghtsoonian, R., Teghtsoonian, M., Berglund, B., and **Berglund, U.** (1978) Invariance of odor strength with sniff vigor: An olfactory analogue to size constancy. Journal of Experimental Psychology: Human Perception and Performance, 4, 144–152.

Teller, D. Y. (1979) The forced-choice preferential looking procedure: A psychophysical technique for use with human infants. Infant Behavior and Development, 2, 135–153.

Teller, D. Y. (1989) The domain of visual science. In L. Spillmann and J. S. Werner (eds.), Visual perception: The Neurophysiological Foundations. New York: Academic Press. Pp. 11–21.

Teller, D. Y., and **Movshon, J. A.** (1986) Visual development. Vision Research, 26, 1438–1506.

Terhardt, E., and **Ward, W. D.** (1982) Recognition of musical key: Exploratory study. Journal of the Acoustical Society of America, 72, 26–33.

Teuber, H.-L. Battersby, W. S., and **Bender, M. B.** (1960) Visual field defects after penetrating missile wounds of the brain. Cambridge: Harvard University Press.

Thompson, E., Palacios, A., and **Varcla, F. J.** (1992) Ways of coloring: Comparative color vision as a case study for cognitive science. Behavioral and Brain Sciences, 15, 1–74.

Thompson, P. (1984) The coding of velocity of motion in the human visual system. Vision Research, 24, 41–45.

Thomson, J. A. (1980) How do we use visual information to control locomotion? Trends in Neurosciences, 3, 247–250.

Thornbury, J. M., and **Mistretta, C. M.** (1981) Tactile sensitivity as a function of age. Journal of Gerontology, 36, 34–39.

Thorson, J., Lange, G. D., and **Biederman-Thorson, M.** (1969) Objective measure of the dynamics of a visual movement illusion. Science, 164, 1087–1088.

Thurlow, W. R., and **Runge, P. S.** (1967) Effect of induced head movements on localization of direction of sounds. Journal of the Acoustical Society of America, 42, 480–488.

Till, R. E. (1978) Age-related differences in binocular

backward-masking with visual noise. Journal of Gerontology, 33, 702–710.

Timney, B., and Muir, D. W. (1976) Orientation anisotropy: Incidence and magnitude in Caucasian and Chinese subjects. Science, 193, 699–700.

Titchener, E. B. (1915) A beginner's psychology. New York: Macmillan.

Todd, J. T., and Akerstrom, R. A. (1987) Perception of three-dimensional form from patterns of optical texture. Journal of Experimental Psychology: Human Perception and Performance, 13, 242–255.

Todd, J. T., and Mingolla, E. (1984) Simulations of curved surfaces from patterns of optical texture. Journal of Experimental Psychology: Human Perception and Performance, 10, 734–739.

Todd, J. T., and Norman, J. F. (1991) The visual perception of smoothly curved surfaces from minimal apparent motion sequences. Perception & Psychophysics, 50, 509–523.

Todrank, J., and Bartoshuk, L. M. (1991) A taste illusion: Taste sensation localized by touch. Physiology & Behavior, 50, 1027–1031.

Tonndorf, J. (1987) The analogy between tinnitus and pain: A suggestion for a physiological basis of chronic tinnitus. Hearing Research, 28, 271–275.

Tonndorf, J. (1988) The external ear. In A. F. Jahn and J. Santos-Sacchi (eds.), Physiology of the ear. New York: Raven Press. Pp. 29–39.

Torebjork, H. E., Vallbo, A. B., and Ochoa, J. L. (1987) Intraneural microstimulation in man: Its relation to specificity of tactile sensations. Brain, 110, 1509–1530.

Torrealba, F., Guillery, R. W., Eysel, U., Polley, E. H., and Mason, C. A. (1982) Studies of retinal representations within the cat's optic tract. Journal of Comparative Neurology, 211, 377–396.

Tranel, D., and Damasio, A. R. (1985) Knowledge without awareness: An autonomic index of facial recognition by prosopagnosics. Science, 228, 1453–1454.

Tranel, D., Damasio, A. R., and Damasio, H. (1988) Intact recognition of facial expression, gender, and age in patients with impaired recognition of face identity. Neurology, 38, 690–696.

Treisman, A. (1986) Features and objects in visual processing. Scientific American 255, 114–125.

Treisman, A., and Schmidt, N. (1982) Illusory conjunctions in the perception of objects. Cognitive Psychology, 14, 107–141.

Trotler, Y., Celebrini, S., Stricanne, B., Thorpe, S., and Imbert, M. (1992) Modulation of neural stereoscopic processing in primate Area V1 by the viewing distance. Science, 257, 1279–1281.

Tyler, C. W. (1981) Specific deficits of flicker sensitivity in glaucoma and ocular hypertension. Investigative Ophthalmology & Visual Science, 20, 204–212.

Uchikawa, K., and Boynton, R. M. (1987) Categorical color perception of Japanese observers: Comparison with that of Americans. Vision Research, 27, 1825–1833.

Uhlrich, D. J., Essock, E. A., and Lehmkuhle, S. (1981) Cross-species correspondence of spatial contrast sensitivity functions. Behavioral Brain Research, 2, 291–299.

Ullman, S. (1979) The interpretation of visual motion. Cambridge: M.I.T. Press.

Vallbo, A. B., and Hagbarth, K. E. (1968) Activity from skin mechanoreceptors recorded percutaneously in awake human subject. Experimental Neurology, 21, 270–289.

Vallbo, A. B., and Johansson, R. S. (1984) Properties of cutaneous mechanoreceptors in the human hand related to touch sensation. Human Neurobiology, 3, 3–14.

Van Doren, C. L., Pelli, D. G., and Verrillo, R. T. (1987) A device for measuring tactile spatiotemporal sensitivity. Journal of the Acoustical Society of America, 81, 1906–1916.

Varney, N. R. (1988) The prognostic significance of anosmia in patients with closed-head trauma. Journal of Clinical and Experimental Neuropsychology, 10, 250–254.

Verheijen, F. J. (1963) Apparent relative movement of "unsharp" and "sharp" visual patterns. Nature, 199, 160–161.

Vernon, P. E. (1977) Absolute pitch: A case study. British Journal of Psychology, 68, 485–489.

Verrillo, R. T. (1962) Investigation of some parameters of the cutaneous threshold for vibration. Journal of the Acoustical Society of America, 34, 1768–1773.

Volkmann, F. C., Riggs, L. A., and Moore, R. K. (1980) Eyeblinks and visual suppression. Science, 207, 900–902.

von der Heydt, R., Peterhans, E., and Baumgartner, G. (1984) Illusory contours and cortical neuron responses. Science, 234, 1260–1262.

von Noorden, G. K. (1981) New clinical aspects of stimulus deprivation amblyopia. American Journal of Ophthalmology, 92, 416–421.

Wade, N. J. (1988) On the late invention of the stereoscope. Perception, 16, 785–818.

Wald, G. (1950) Eye and camera. Scientific American, 183, 32–41.

Wales, R., and Fox, R. (1970) Increment detection thresholds during binocular rivalry suppression. Perception & Psychophysics, 8, 90–94.

Walker, J. (1984) How to stop a spinning object by humming and perceive curious blue arcs around a light. Scientific American, 250, 136–144.

Wall, J. T. (1988) Variable organization in cortical maps of the skin as an indication of the lifelong adaptive capacities of circuits in the mammalian brain. Trends in Neurosciences, 12, 549–557.

Wallace, P. (1977) Individual discrimination of humans by odor. Physiology & Behavior, 19, 577–579.

Wallach, H. (1963) The perception of neutral colors. Scientific American, 208, 107–116.

Wallach, H., and Floor, L. (1971) The use of size matching to demonstrate the effectiveness of accommodation and convergence as cues for distance. Perception & Psychophysics, 10, 423–428.

Wallach, H., and O'Connell, D. N. (1953) The kinetic depth effect. Journal of Experimental Psychology, 45, 205–217.

Walls, G. L. (1942) The vertebrate eye and its adaptive radiation. New York: Hafner.

Walls, G. L. (1960) Land! Land! Psychological Bulletin, 57, 29–48.

Wandell, B. A. (1987) Computational methods for color constancy. In Frontiers of visual science. Washington, D.C: National Academy Press.

Ward, W. D. (1966) Temporary threshold shift in males and females. Journal of the Acoustical Society of America, 40, 478–485.

Ward, W. D. (1968) Susceptibility to auditory fatigue. In W. D. Neff (ed.), Contributions to sensory physiology, vol. 3. New York: Academic Press. Pp. 195–225.

Ward, W. D. (1970) Musical perception. In J. V. Tobias (ed.), Foundations of modern auditory theory, vol. 1. New York: Academic Press. Pp. 407–447.

Ward, W. D., and Glorig, A. (1961) A case of firecracker-induced hearing loss. Laryngoscope, 71, 1590–1596.

Warren, R. M. (1970) Perceptual restoration of missing speech sounds. Science, 167, 392–393.

Warren, S., Hämäläinen, H. A., and Gardner, E. P. (1986) Objective classification of motion- and direction-sensitive neurons in primary somatosensory cortex of awake monkeys. Journal of Neurophysiology, 56, 598–632.

Warren, W. H., Jr., Blackwell, A. W., and Morris, M. W. (1989) Age differences in perceiving the direction of self-motion from optical flow. Journal of Gerontology: Psychological Sciences, 44, Pp. 147–153.

Warren, W. H., Jr., Morris, M. W., and Kalish, M. L. (1988) Perception of translational heading from optical flow. Journal of Experimental Psychology: Human Perception and Performance, 14, 646–660.

Warren, W. H., Jr., Young, D. S., and Lee, D. N. (1986) Visual control of step length during running over irregular terrain. Journal of Experimental Psychology: Human Performance and Perception, 12, 259–266.

Wasserman, G. S. (1978) Color vision: An historical perspective. New York: John Wiley & Sons.

Wässle, H., Peichl, L., and Boycott, B. B. (1981) Dendritic territories of cat retinal ganglion cells. Nature, 292, 344–345.

Watson, A. B., and Pelli, D. G. (1983) QUEST: A Bayesian adaptive psychometric method. Perception & Psychophysics, 33, 113–120.

Watt, R. J., and Andrews, D. P. (1981) APE: Adaptive probit estimation of psychometric functions. Current Psychological Reviews, 1, 205–214.

Watts, R. G., and Bahill, A. T. (1990) Keep your eye on the ball: The science and folklore of baseball. New York: W. H. Freeman.

Weale, R. A. (1982) A biography of the eye. London: Lewis.

Weale, R. A. (1986) Retinal senescence. In N. Osborne and J. Chader (eds.), Progress in retinal research, vol. 5. Oxford: Pergamon Press. Pp. 53–73.

Weinstein, S. (1968) Intensive and extensive aspects of tactile sensitivity as a function of body part, sex and laterality. In D. R. Kenshalo (ed.), The skin senses. Springfield, Ill.: Thomas.

Weisenberger, J. M., and Miller, J. D. (1987) The role of tactile aids in providing information about acoustic stimuli. Journal of the Acoustical Society of America, 82, 906–916.

Weisskopf, V. F. (1976) Is physics human? Physics Today, 29, 23–29.

Weisstein, N. (1980) The joy of Fourier analysis. In C. S. Harris (ed.), Visual coding and adaptability. Hillsdale, N.J.: Erlbaum. Pp. 365–380.

Weisstein, N., and Harris, C. S. (1974) Visual detection of line segments: An object-superiority effect. Science, 186, 752–755.

Welch, R. B., and Warren, D. H. (1980) Immediate perceptual response to intersensory discrepancy. Psychological Bulletin, 88, 638–667.

Wells, G. L., Lindsay, R. C. L., and Ferguson, T. J. (1979) Accuracy, confidence, and juror perceptions in eyewitness identification. Journal of Applied Psychology, 64, 440–448.

Wenger, M. A., Jones, F. N., and Jones, M. H. (1956) Physiological psychology. New York: Holt, Rinehart, & Winston.

Werker, J. F., and Tees, R. C. (1992) The organization and reorganization of human speech perception. Annual Review of Neuroscience, 15, 377–402.

Werner, G., and Whitsel, B. L. (1973) Functional organization of the somatosensory cortex. In A. Iggo (ed.), Handbook of sensory physiology, vol. 2: Somatosensory system. New York: Springer-Verlag.

Werner, J. S., Cicerone, C. M., Kliegl, R., and DellaRosa, D. (1984) Spectral efficiency of blackness induction. Journal of the Optical Society of America A, 1, 981–986.

Werntz, D. A., Bickford, R. G., and Shannahoff-

Khalsa, D. (1987) Selective hemispheric stimulation by unilateral forced nostril breathing. Human Neurobiology, 6, 165–171.

Wertheimer, M. (1912/1961) Experimental studies on the seeing of motion. T. Shipley (trans. and ed.), Classics in psychology. New York: Philosophical Library. Pp. 1032–1088.

Wertheimer, M. (1923/1958) Principles of perceptual organization. In D. C. Beardslee and M. Wertheimer (eds.), Readings in perception. Princeton, N.J.: Van Nostrand. Pp. 115–135.

Wertheimer, M. (1957) Perception and the Rorschach. Journal of Projective Techniques, 21, 209–216.

Wertheimer, M. (1961) Psychomotor coordination of auditory and visual space at birth. Science, 134, 1692–1693.

Westfall, R. S. (1980) Never at rest: A biography of Isaac Newton. Cambridge, England: Cambridge University Press.

Wever, E. G. (1978) The reptile ear. Princeton, N.J.: Princeton University Press.

Wever, E. G., and **Bray, C. W.** (1937) The perception of low tones and the resonance-volley theory. Journal of Psychology, 3, 101–114.

Wheatstone, C. (1838/1964) Some remarkable phenomena of binocular vision. In W. N. Dember (ed.), Visual perception: The nineteenth century. New York: John Wiley & Sons. Pp. 114–129.

Wheeler, D. D. (1970) Processes in word recognition. Cognitive Psychology, 1, 59–85.

White, H. E., and **Levatin, P.** (1962) "Floaters" in the eye. Scientific American, 206, 119–127.

Wiesel, T. N., and **Hubel, D. H.** (1960) Receptive fields of ganglion cells in the cat's retina. Journal of Physiology, 153, 583–594.

Wiesel, T. N., and **Hubel, D. H.** (1966) Spatial and chromatic interactions in the lateral geniculate body of the rhesus monkey. Journal of Neurophysiology, 29, 1115–1156.

Wiesenfelder, H., and **Blake, R.** (1991) Apparent motion can survive binocular rivalry suppression. Vision Research, 31, 1589–1600.

Wightman, F., and **Kistler, D. J.** (1980) A new "look" at auditory space perception. In G. van den Brink and F. A. Bilsen (eds.), Psychophysical, physiological and behavioral studies in hearing. Delft: Delft University Press. Pp. 441–448.

Wightman, F. L., and **Kistler, D. J.** (1989a) Headphones simulation of free-field listening: I. Stimulus synthesis. Journal of the Acoustical Society of America, 85, 858–867.

Wightman, F. L., and **Kistler, D. J.** (1989b) Headphones simulation of free-field listening: II. Psychophysical validation. Journal of the Acoustical Society of America, 85, 868–878.

Wightman, F. L., Kistler, D., and **Arruda, M.** (1989) The hierarchy of sound localization cues revealed by experiments in a simulated free-field. Association for Research in Otolaryngology, 12, 65.

Wilkins, P. A., and **Acton, W. I.** (1982) Noise and accidents: A review. Annals of Occupational Hygiene, 25, 249–260.

Williams, D. R. (1988) Topography of the foveal cone mosaic in the living human eye. Vision Research, 28, 433–454.

Williams, D. R. (1991) Progress in vision research. Optics and Photonics News, 2, 8–9.

Williams, D. R., MacLeod, D. I. A., and **Hayhoe, M. M.** (1981) Punctate sensitivity of the blue-sensitive mechanism. Vision Research, 21, 1357–1375.

Williams, D., Phillips, G., and **Sekuler, R.** (1986) Hysteresis in the perception of motion direction as evidence for neural cooperativity. Nature, 324, 253–255.

Wilson, B. S., Finley, C. C., Lawson, D. T., Wolford, R. D., Eddington, D. K., and **Rabinowitz, W. M.** (1991) Better speech recognition with cochlear implants. Nature, 352, 236–238.

Wilson, H. R., Ferrera, V. P., and **Yo, C.** (1992) A psychophysically motivated model of two-dimensional motion perception. Visual Neuroscience, 9, 79–98.

Wilson, H. R., Mets, M. B., Nagy, S. E., and **Kressel, A. B.** (1988) Albino spatial vision as an instance of arrested visual development. Vision Research, 28, 979–990.

Wilson, J. P., and **Sutton, G. J.** (1981) Acoustic correlates of tonal tinnitus. In Tinnitus, CIBA Foundation Symposium, vol. 85. London: Pitman. Pp. 82–100.

Winderickz, J., Lindsey, D. T., Sanocki, E., Teller, D. Y., Motulsky, A. G., and **Deeb, S. S.** (1992) Polymorphism in red photopigment underlies variation in colour matching. Nature, 356, 431–433.

Winter, R. (1976) The smell book: Scents, sex, and society. Philadelphia: Lippincott.

Wise, L. Z., and **Irvine, D. R. F.** (1985) Topographic organization of interaural intensity difference sensitivity in deep layers of cat superior colliculus: Implications for auditory spacial representation. Journal of Neurophysiology, 54, 185–211.

Wist, E. R. (1976) Dark adaptation and the Hermann grid illusion. Perception & Psychophysics, 20, 10–12.

Wolfe, J. M. (1984) Global factors in the Hermann gird illusion. Perception, 13, 33–40.

Wollberg, Z., and **Newman, J. D.** (1972) Auditory cortex of squirrel monkey: Response patterns of single cells to species-specific vocalizations. Science, 175, 212–214.

Wood, J. B., and **Harkins, S. W.** (1987) Effects of age, stimulus selection, and retrieval environment on odor identification. Journal of Gerontology, 42, 584–588.

Woodworth, R. S. (1938) Experimental psychology. New York: Holt.

Woodworth, R. S., and **Schlosberg, H.** (1954) Experimental psychology (2nd ed.). New York: Holt.

Wright, E. (1992) The original of E. G. Boring's "young girl/mother-in-law" drawing and its relation to the pattern of a joke. Perception, 21, 273–275.

Wright, R. H. (1966) Why is an odour? Nature, 209, 551–554.

Wurtz, R. H., and **Goldberg, M. E.** (1972) Activity of superior colliculus in behaving monkey. Journal of Physiology, 35, 587–596.

Wurtz, R. H., Goldberg, M. E., and **Robinson, D. L.** (1982) Brain mechanisms of visual attention. Scientific American, 244, 124–135.

Wysocki, C. J., and **Beauchamp, G.** (1984) Ability to smell androstenone is genetically determined. Proceedings of the National Academy of Science, 81, 4899–4902.

Wysocki, C. J., Pierce, J. D., and **Gilbert, A. N.** (1991) Geographic, cross-cultural, and individual variation in human olfaction. In T. V. Getchell, R. L., Doty, L. M. Bartoshuk, and J. B. Snow, Jr. (eds.), Smell and taste in health and disease. New York: Raven Press. Pp. 287–314.

Yellott, J. I., Jr. (1982) Spectral analysis of spatial sampling by photoreceptors: Topological disorder prevents aliasing. Vision Research, 22, 1205–1210.

Yonas, A. (1984) Reaching as a measure of infant spatial perception. In G. Gottlieb and N. A. Krasnegor (eds.), Measurement of audition and vision in the first year of postnatal life: A methodological review. Norwood, N.J.: Ablex.

Yost, W. A. (1991) Auditory image perception and analysis: The basis for hearing. Hearing Research, 56, 8–18.

Yost, W. A., and **Nielsen, D. W.** (1985) Fundamentals of hearing (2nd ed.). New York: Holt, Rinehart & Winston.

Young, F. A. (1981) Primate myopia. American Journal of Optometry and Physiological Optics, 58, 560–566.

Young, P. T. (1928) Auditory localization with acoustical transposition of the ears. Journal of Experimental Psychology, 11, 399–429.

Young, T. (1801/1948) Observations on vision. In W. Dennis (ed.), Reading in the history of psychology. New York: Appleton-Century-Crofts. Pp. 96–101.

Yuille, A. L., and **Grzywacz, N. M.** (1988) A computational theory for the perception of coherent visual motion. Nature, 333, 71–74.

Yuodelis, C., and **Hendrickson, A.** (1986) A qualitative analysis of the human fovea during development. Vision Research, 26, 847–855.

Zacks, J. (1970) Temporal summation phenomena at threshold: Their relation to visual mechanisms. Science, 170, 197–199.

Zeki, S., Watson, J. D. G., Lueck, C. J., Friston, K. J., Kennard, C., and **Frackowiak, R. S. J.** (1991) A direct demonstration of functional specialization in human visual cortex. Journal of Neuroscience, 11, 641–649.

Zellner, D. A., Bartoli, A. M., and **Eckard, R.** (1991) Influence of color on odor identification and likeing ratings. American Journal of Psychology, 104, 547–561.

Zellner, D. A., and **Kautz, M. A.** (1990) Color affects perceived odor intensity. Journal of Experimental Psychology: Human Perception and Performance, 16, 391–397.

Zelman, S. (1973) Correlation of smoking history with hearing loss. Journal of the American Medical Association, 223, 920.

Zihl, J., von Cramon, D., and **Mai, N.** (1983) Selective disturbance of movement vision after bilateral brain damage. Brain, 106, 313–340.

Zihl, J., von Cramon, D., Mai, N., and **Schmid, C.** (1991) Disturbance of movement vision after bilateral posterior brain damage, further evidence and follow up observations. Brain, 114, 2235–2252.

Zimbardo, P. G., Andersen, S. M., and **Kabat, L. G.** (1981) Induced hearing deficit generates experimental paranoia. Science, 212, 1529–1531.

Zisman, F., and **Adams, A. J.** (1982) Spectral sensitivity of cone mechanisms in juvenile diabetes. In G. Verriest (ed.), Colour vision deficiencies, VI. Proceedings of the Sixth Symposium of the International Research Group of Colour Vision Deficiencies. The Hague: W. Junk. Pp. 127–131.

Zollinger, H. (1988) Categorical color-perception: Influence of cultural factors on the differentiation of primary and derived basic color terms in color naming by Japanese children. Vision Research, 28, 1379–1382.

Zrenner, E. (1983) Neurophysiological aspects of color vision in primates. Berlin: Springer-Verlag.

Zurek, P. M. (1981) Spontaneous narrowband acoustic signals emitted by human ears. Journal of the Acoustical Society of America, 69, 514–523.

Zwicker, E. (1964) Negative afterimage in hearing. Journal of the Acoustical Society of America, 36, 2413–2415.

Zwicker, E., and **Scharf, B.** (1965) A model of loudness summation. Psychological Review, 72, 3–26.

Credits and Acknowledgments

Chapter 1

Page 2: Mountcastle, V. B., from "The view from within: Pathways to the study of perception." Johns Hopkins Medical Journal, 1975, 136, 109–131. Used by permission.

Page 4: Courtesy Glyn Cloyd.

Page 5: Sperry, R. W., from "Mind-brain interaction: Mentalism, yes; dualism, no." Neurosciences, 1980, 5, 195–206. Used by permission.

Page 6: Searle, J., from "Minds and brains without programs." In C. Blakemore and S. Greenfield (eds.), Mindwaves, 1987. Oxford: Blackwell. Pp. 209–233. Used by permission.

Page 14: Figure 1.3. Courtesy George Gerster/Comstock.

Page 22: Figure 1.7. Courtesy George Bellerose/Stock, Boston.

Chapter 2

Page 39: Figure 2.7. Courtesy Glyn Cloyd.

Page 48: Figure 2.17. Courtesy Glyn Cloyd.

Page 53: Figure 2.22. Courtesy Glyn Cloyd.

Chapter 3

Page 70: From the poem "Age four" from *Sojourner microcosms: New and selected poems, 1959–1977* by Anselm Hollo © 1977. Published by Blue Wind Press.

Page 90: Figure 3.20. Anstis, S. M., from "A chart demonstrating variations in acuity with retinal position." Vision Research, 1974, 14, 589–592. Used with permission.

Page 93: Anstis, S. M., from "A chart demonstrating variations in acuity with retinal position." Vision Research, 1974, 14, 589–592. Used with permission.

Chapter 4

Page 127: Figure 4.14. Hubel, D. H., Wiesel, T. N., and Stryker, M. P., from "Anatomical demonstration of orientation columns in macaque monkey." Journal of Comparative Neurology, 1978, 177, 361–380. Used with permission.

Page 129: Figure 4.15. Fellemen, D. J., and Van Essen, D. C., from "Distributed hierarchical processing in the primate cerebral cortex." Cerebral Cortex, 1991, 1, 1–17. Used by permission.

Page 132: Marr, D., from "Early processing of visual information." Philosophical Transactions of the Royal Society, Series B, 1976, 275, 483–524. Used by permission.

Page 137: Todd, J. T., and Mingolla, E., from "Simulations of curved surfaces from patterns of optical texture." Journal of Experimental Psychology: Human Perception and Performance, 1984, 10, 734–739 © 1983, American Psychological Association. Used by permission.

Page 138: Todd, J. T., and Mingolla, E., from "Simulations of curved surfaces from patterns of optical texture." Journal of Experimental Psychology: Human Perception and Performance, 1984, 10, 734–739 © 1983, American Psychological Association. Used by permission.

Chapter 5

Page 144: Figure 5.1. Courtesy Leonard Lee Rue IV/Photo Researchers.

Page 147: Figure 5.5. Courtesy Robert Sekuler.

Page 148: Figure 5.6, Julesz, B., from "A brief outline of the texton theory of human vision." Trends in Neurosciences, 1984, 7, 41–45. Used with permission.

Page 150: Figure 5.8. Courtesy Judth Canty/Stock, Boston.

Page 162: Figure 5.19. Courtesy Karin Boothroyd.

Page 163: Figure 5.21. Courtesy Gregory Philips.

Page 164: Figure 5.23, Courtesy Richard M. Held.

Page 165: Figure 5.25. Used by permission Children's Television Workshops; computer image processing courtesy Gregory Philips.

Page 170: Figure 5.30. Courtesy Richard Kirkham.

Page 170: Figure 5.31. Courtesy Gregory Philips.

Page 171: Figure 5.32. Courtesy Gregory Philips.

Chapter 6

Page 186: Weisskopf, V. F., from "Is physics human?" Physics Today, 1976, 29, 23–29. Used by permission.

Chapter 7

Page 236: Figure 7.15. Courtesy Baron Wolman/Woodfin Camp & Associates.

Page 239: Figure 7.19. Courtesy Frank Siteman/Stock, Boston.

Page 241: Figure 7.21. Courtesy Dennis Markley.

Chapter 8

Page 260: Figure 8.8, Warren, W. H., Jr., Blackwell, A. W., and Morris, M. W., from "Age differences in perceiving the direction of self-motion from optical flow." Journal of Gerontology: Psychological Sciences, 1988, 44, Pp. 147–153. Used with permission.

Page 284: Anstis, S. M., from "Apparent movement." In R. Held, H. W. Leibowitz, and H. L. Teuber (eds.), Handbook of sensory physiology, 1978, vol. 8. Berlin: Springer-Verlag. Pp. 655–673. Used with permission.

Chapter 9

Page 308: Figure 9.14. Courtesy of David Lim.

Page 321: Figure 9.22. Courtesy of Evan Relkin.

Page 321: Figure 9.23. Courtesy of Evan Relkin.

Chapter 10

Page 337: Figure 10. Heffner, R. S., and Heffner, H. E., from "Hearing in mammals: The least weasel." Journal of Mammology, 1985, 66, 745–755. Used with permission.

Page 365: Figure 10.18. Courtesy of Kathy Bendo (top, left and right photos); courtesy of Lyndon Baines Johnson Library (bottom photo), used with permission.

Chapter 11

Page 402: Figure 11.10. Lederman, S. J., from "Skin and touch." *The Encyclopedia of Human Biology,* © 1991, Academic Press. Reprinted with permission.

Chapter 12

Page 422: Figure 12.7. Levitan, I. B., and Kaczmarek, L. K., from *The neuron. Cell and molecular biology,* 1991, Oxford Press. Adapted with permission.

Page 429: Figure 12.11. Cain, W. S., from "Odor identification by males and females: Predictions versus performance." Chemical Senses, 1982, 7, 129–142.

Page 429: Figure 12.15. Courtesy of Inglis Miller.

Chapter 13

Page 457: Benton, A. L., from "The neuropsychology of facial recognition." American Psychologist, 1980, 35, 176–186, © 1980, American Psychological Association. Reprinted by permission.

Page 464: Figure 13.3. Courtesy Glyn Cloyd.

Page 470: Figure 13.6. Biederman, I., Glass, A. L., and Stacey, E. W., Jr., from "Searching for objects in real-world scenes." Journal of Experimental Psychology. 1973, 97, 22–27. Used with permission.

Page 471: Figure 13.7. Palmer, S. E., Rosch, E., and Chase, P., from "Canonical perspective and the perception of objects." In J. Long and A. Baddeley (eds.), Attention and performance, 1981, vol. 9. Hillsdale, N. J.: Erlbaum. Pp. 135–151. Used with permission.

Page 471: Figure 13.8. Palmer, S. E., Rosch, E., and Chase, P., from "Canonical perspective and the perception of objects," In J. Long and A. Baddeley (eds.), Attention and performance, 1981, vol. 9. Hillsdale, N.J.: Erlbaum. Pp. 135–151. Used with permission.

Page 472: Figure 13.9. Biederman, I., from "Higher-level vision." In D. N. Osherson, S. Kosslyn, and J. Hollerbach (eds.), An invitation to cognitive science: visual cognition and action. Cambridge: M.I.T. Press, Pp. 41–72. Adapted with permission.

Page 479: Figure 13.15. Prinzmetal, W., "The word-superiority effect does not require a t-scope." Perception & Psychophysics, 1992, 51, 473–484. Adapted with permission.

Page 485: Figure 13.18. Courtesy of Lewis Harvey.

Name Index

Subject Index